NEUROSCIENCE RESEARCH PROGRESS

WORKING MEMORY: CAPACITY, DEVELOPMENTS AND IMPROVEMENT TECHNIQUES

NEUROSCIENCE RESEARCH PROGRESS

Additional books in this series can be found on Nova's website
under the Series tab.

Additional E-books in this series can be found on Nova's website
under the E-book tab.

PSYCHOLOGY OF EMOTIONS, MOTIVATIONS AND ACTIONS

Additional books in this series can be found on Nova's website
under the Series tab.

Additional E-books in this series can be found on Nova's website
under the E-book tab.

NEUROSCIENCE RESEARCH PROGRESS

WORKING MEMORY: CAPACITY, DEVELOPMENTS AND IMPROVEMENT TECHNIQUES

EDEN S. LEVIN
EDITOR

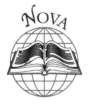

Nova Science Publishers, Inc.
New York

Copyright © 2011 by Nova Science Publishers, Inc.

All rights reserved. No part of this book may be reproduced, stored in a retrieval system or transmitted in any form or by any means: electronic, electrostatic, magnetic, tape, mechanical photocopying, recording or otherwise without the written permission of the Publisher.

For permission to use material from this book please contact us:
Telephone 631-231-7269; Fax 631-231-8175
Web Site: http://www.novapublishers.com

NOTICE TO THE READER

The Publisher has taken reasonable care in the preparation of this book, but makes no expressed or implied warranty of any kind and assumes no responsibility for any errors or omissions. No liability is assumed for incidental or consequential damages in connection with or arising out of information contained in this book. The Publisher shall not be liable for any special, consequential, or exemplary damages resulting, in whole or in part, from the readers' use of, or reliance upon, this material. Any parts of this book based on government reports are so indicated and copyright is claimed for those parts to the extent applicable to compilations of such works.

Independent verification should be sought for any data, advice or recommendations contained in this book. In addition, no responsibility is assumed by the publisher for any injury and/or damage to persons or property arising from any methods, products, instructions, ideas or otherwise contained in this publication.

This publication is designed to provide accurate and authoritative information with regard to the subject matter covered herein. It is sold with the clear understanding that the Publisher is not engaged in rendering legal or any other professional services. If legal or any other expert assistance is required, the services of a competent person should be sought. FROM A DECLARATION OF PARTICIPANTS JOINTLY ADOPTED BY A COMMITTEE OF THE AMERICAN BAR ASSOCIATION AND A COMMITTEE OF PUBLISHERS.

Additional color graphics may be available in the e-book version of this book.

LIBRARY OF CONGRESS CATALOGING-IN-PUBLICATION DATA

Working memory : capacity, developments, and improvement techniques / editor, Eden S. Levin.
 p. cm.
 Includes index.
 ISBN 978-1-61761-980-9 (hardcover)
 1. Short-term memory. I. Levin, Eden S. II. Title.

BF378.S54W67 2010
153.1'3--dc22
              2010036164

Published by Nova Science Publishers, Inc. † New York

CONTENTS

Preface		vii
Chapter 1	Working Memory and the Autistic Mind R. Hansen, L. Deling, E. Olufs, R. Pytlik, and F. R. Ferraro	1
Chapter 2	Measurement of Working Memory Karlee D. Fellner and John R. Reddon	33
Chapter 3	Effects of Visuo-Spatial Working Memory on Wayfinding Ability Laura Piccardi and Raffaella Nori	81
Chapter 4	Working Memory and Prefrontal Cortex and Their Relation with the Brain Reward System and Drug Addiction Ester Miyuki Nakamura-Palacios	109
Chapter 5	Working Memory in the Service of Verbal Episodic Encoding: A Cognitive Neuropsychological Perspective Matthew J. Wright, Peter Bachman and Ellen Woo	141
Chapter 6	Working Memory in Preterm and Full-Term Infants Jing Sun and Nicholas Buys	175
Chapter 7	The Assessment and Training of Working Memory for Prevention and Early Intervention in Case of Reading, Writing and Arithmetical Difficulties in Children Antonella D'Amico	201
Chapter 8	Working Memory in Sentence Comprehension and Production Matthew J. Traxler, David Caplan, Debra L. Long and Gloria S. Waters	225
Chapter 9	Working Memory Components and Virtual Reorientation: A Dual-Task Study Alessandro O. Caffò, Luciana Picucci, Manuela N. Di Masi and Andrea Bosco	249

Chapter 10	Using fMRI to Examine the Brain – Bases of Working Memory *Michael A. Motes, Ehsan Shokri Kojori, Neena K. Rao,* *Ilana J. Bennett and Bart Rypma*	**267**
Chapter 11	Aging and Short-Term Memory for Face Identity of Emotional Faces *Sandra J. E. Langeslag and Jan W. van Strien*	**287**
Chapter 12	Varying Background Colours Reveals that Enhanced Short-Term Memory for Angry Faces Is a Valence and Not an Arousal Effect *Sandra J. E. Langeslag, Margaret C. Jackson, Jan W. van Strien* *and David E. J. Linden*	**301**
Chapter 13	Working Memory Deficits in Schizophrenia: Neurobiological Correlates and Treatment *Haiyun Xu, Hong-Ju Yang and Gregory M. Rose*	**313**
Chapter 14	Tobacco, Nicotine and Cotinine: For Memory, Neurological, and Psychiatric Disorders *V. Echeverria, P. Rajeev and R. Zeitlin*	**349**
Chapter 15	Working Memory and Functional Outcome in Patients with Major Depressive Disorder *Yasuhiro Kaneda*	**373**
Chapter 16	Control of Working memory Contents During Task-Switching *James A. Grange*	**381**
Chapter 17	Development of Neural Mechanisms of Working Memory *V. Vuontela and S. Carlson*	**417**
Index		**441**

PREFACE

Working memory is the executive and attentional aspect of cognition which operates on the data held in short-term memory (which may be thought of as the RAM for working memory's CPU processes) and which is involved in the interim integration, processing, disposal, and retrieval of information. Working memory tasks include the active monitoring or manipulation of information or behaviors. This book presents current research from across the globe in the study of working memory capacity, developments and improvement techniques. Some of the topics discussed herein include working memory and the autistic mind; the effects of visuo-spatial working memory and the ability to move successfully through the environment; as well as working memory and the prefrontal cortex.

Chapter 1 - The current chapter will focus on working memory abilities and development, primarily examining individuals with autism ages 5 to 20 years. With Baddeley and Hitch's model as a starting point, the authors will explore the research surrounding how working memory typically develops, deviations found in the autistic population compared to typical working memory performance and development, and the role such differences may play when considering possible intervention strategies to use with individuals with autism spectrum disorders. Recent findings in the working memory literature will be examined, including task effects that facilitate and inhibit performance, experimental design factors that may play a role in the contradictory results within the area of working memory in individuals with autism spectrum disorders, and neurological factors that may contribute to cognitive differences.

In general, working memory capacity increases with age in the typically developing population, with specific increases seen in short-term memory capabilities, verbal span abilities, visual span abilities, and complex working memory processes. Specialized working memory components and strategies also develop with age. There is currently little evidence of a general working memory deficit in individuals with autism; however, research suggests that certain domains of working memory may show impairments or delayed development in individuals with autism. Verbal span abilities appear to be largely intact within the ASD population with deficits on tasks that rely on spontaneous rehearsal strategies that prove helpful as the task complexity increases. The visuospatial sketchpad of children and adolescents with autism seems grossly intact with some deficits demonstrated in oculomotor and spatial tasks requiring more mature development. Within the central executive, studies have shown individuals with autism to have intact performance on simple inhibition tasks. However, they often show impaired performance on measures of planning and complex inhibition tasks. On tasks that involve the episodic buffer component, children and adolescents with autism tend to encode specific features of events rather than global features, making memory strategies less efficient. Some of these deficits have been attributed to neurobiological differences found in individuals with autism, including an increased total brain volume, overreliance of the right hemisphere, reduced activation of the dorsolateral prefrontal cortex, atypical activity in the cingulate cortex, and underconnectivity in several circuitry systems. Although little research has specifically been conducted on working memory interventions for individuals with autism, understanding specific working memory strengths and weaknesses can help guide approaches to improving working memory functioning. Within other populations, working memory training has been effective in targeting specific working memory factors that are possibly implicated in autism as well, including metamemory skills, overt rehearsal strategies, and elaboration. Additional research is needed on the capacity and development of working memory in children with autism as current findings are often inconsistent.

Chapter 2 - Working memory is the mechanism involved in the temporary manipulation and storage of information. It contributes to a number of cognitive functions, including learning, retrieving long-term memory, inhibiting irrelevant information, and working with novel problems. Working memory has limited capacity, and thus has significant implications for individual differences in learning and cognitive functioning.

Measurement of working memory is used to assess intellectual and cognitive ability, including individual cognitive development and declines and deficits in performance related to aging, dementia, neurological disorders, medical conditions, genetic disorders, developmental disabilities, learning disabilities, and psychiatric conditions. Working memory tasks include simple span (visuospatial and phonological short-term memory) and complex span tasks (visuospatial, phonological, and executive working memory). Commonly used memory assessment scales include the Wechsler Memory Scale, Wide Range Assessment of Memory and Learning, Swanson Cognitive Processing Test, Working Memory Test Battery for Children, and Automated Working Memory Assessment. Cognitive scales which contain an assessment of working memory include the Wechsler intelligence scales, Cognitive Assessment System, Stanford Binet Intelligence Scale, Woodcock-Johnson, Differential Ability Scales, Kaufman Assessment Battery for Children, Universal Nonverbal Intelligence Test, and NEPSY Developmental Neuropsychological Assessment.

Despite the number of measures designed to assess working memory, there is controversy over the consistency and overall adequacy of its measurement. This is largely because it is challenging to measure working memory directly, as it is influenced by factors such as processing speed, knowledge, executive functioning, long-term memory, and attention. In addition, tasks provide only a small sample of overall working memory. Also problematic is that working memory itself is a complex construct that is not fully understood by the scientific community. Controversy aside, the assessment of working memory is essential in the measurement of cognitive functioning in order to identify individual strengths and weaknesses and to inform individual remediation/treatment.

Chapter 3 – The present review analyse the relationship between visuo-spatial working memory (VSWM) in wayfinding, which is the ability to move successfully through the environment. As the results of research on individual differences in wayfinding are mixed, various explanation have to be considered. In this chapter, the authors will analyze these findings in light of the different component of VSWM proposed by Logie (1995, 2003) and a more recent model by Cornoldi and Vecchi (2003).

The authors will also investigate the development of VSWM and how its changes in older adults, causing a decrease in wayfinding ability. For example, evidence from studies of route learning and memory for object location indicates an aging-related decrement in piloting, particularly in unfamiliar surroundings. On the one hand, the decline in landmark-based navigation could be the result of diminished path integration skill, particularly if path integration typically provides a supplemental informational for piloting. On the other hand, the more basic path integration process may retain its operational integrity beyond the time that association-based piloting begins to reflect a general age-related decline in learning rate. In this chapter, the authors considered these different explanations in relation to theories about VSWM. Finally, the authors consider the results of studies on brain-damagedpatients demonstrating the importance of the ventromedial prefrontal cortex, which is necessary to maintain active the goal destination in VSWM for use in navigation.

Chapter 4 – Cellular and molecular mechanisms involved in learning and memory processes are very similar or the same as those involved in the drug-induced reorganization of neural circuitry that occurs during addiction. Using a classic working memory task in animal learning, the radial maze, the authors have demonstrated that different drugs of abuse (for instance, ethanol, Δ9-tetrahydrocanabinol and nicotine) administered into the medial prefrontal cortex (mPFC) affect the performance of a delayed-task, suggesting that these drugs somehow change the spatial working memory processing. These effects may involve dopaminergic and/or glutamatergic mediation in the mPFC because they were prevented by SCH 23390, clozapine or memantine. The mPFC in rodents, which is functionally related to the dorsolateral prefrontal cortex (DLPFC) in primates and human beings, is part of the brain reward circuitry and highly involved in the processing of working memory. Working memory manipulates items in short-term memory to plan, organize, and process information required to generate future thoughts or actions. Its integrity is required in the processing of important cognitive functions such as learning, goal-directed behavior, decision-making, understanding and reasoning, all function that are substantially affected in drug addiction and dependence. In a randomized double-blind placebo-controlled clinical trial the authors showed that gabapentin, an anticonvulsant drug, reduced alcohol consumption and craving, and also improved frontal cognitive performance involving working memory processing. In a recent study considering different types of alcoholics according to Lesch's typology the authors found that frontal dysfunction was more seen to a greater extent in Type IV alcoholics, even in those that showed preserved mental function measured by mini-mental status examination. Considering this pitiful evidence, the authors started to search for any treatment that would possibly decrease this frontal cortical dysfunction, especially the processing of working memory. The authors found interesting data showing that transcranial direct current stimulation (tDCS) over the left DLPFC improved the working memory and reduced alcohol craving. Thus, the authors are currently investigating the effects of tDCS over the left DLPFC in the P3 waveform registered by Event Related Potential (ERP) in alcoholics. So far, in a sample of alcoholics, they have found that tDCS results in a change the P3 waveform in frontal and central region that may be related to changes in brain activity. Completion of this study and adding future investigations that combine pharmacological and non-pharmacological strategies may unravel this intriguing relationship between working memory in the prefrontal cortex and drug addiction, and hopefully establish new therapeutic possibilities.

Chapter 5 – While dissociations between working memory and episodic memory have been shown, both of these processes appear to partially overlap at the behavioral and neuroanontomical levels. Episodic encoding and working memory both appear to depend on the integrity and integration of processes carried out within the lateral prefrontal cortex and both appear to be related to effective verbal learning. The neuroanatomic substrate of semantic memory also appears to overlap with these processes in the prefrontal cortex. In the current chapter, the authors review interactions between verbal working memory, semantic memory, and episodic memory in individuals suffering from closed head injury, human immunodeficiency virus/acquired immunodeficiency syndrome, Alzheimer's disease, and Schizophrenia in an attempt to elucidate the cognitive neuropsychology of verbal memory encoding. The authors' review suggests that working memory enhances encoding, but not retention, of verbal episodic memories across these memory-disordered populations.

Chapter 6 – *Introduction:* This study investigated working memory in preterm and full-term infants at 8 months after expected date of delivery. Working memory is defined as "the ability to maintain an appropriate problem solving set for the attainment of a future goal" [1, p. 201]. An important characteristic of working memory is that it is prospective, that is, its purpose is to attain a goal, and it not only enables information to be held in mind but also to be manipulated. Working memory emerges in infancy and continues to develop throughout childhood. Working memory is believed to underlie some learning problems in children at school age. Although numerous studies have reported that the overall development of preterm infants is comparable to that of full-term infants at the same corrected age, it is unclear to what extent the development of specific cognitive abilities is affected by prematurity and/or other factors such as medical complications. As preterm infants have a high rate of learning difficulties, it is possible that factors associated with prematurity specifically affect the development of some regions of the brain associated with the regulation of working memory.

Methods: The current study aimed to examine the effects of maturation and length of exposure to extrauterine environmental stimuli on the development of working memory, by comparing the development of preterm infants with that of full-term infants at both the same corrected age and the same chronological age. A case-control study design was used for the study. Thirty-seven preterm infants without identified disabilities and 74 full-term and gender matched healthy full-term infants participated in the study. The preterm infants were all less than 32 weeks gestation and less than 1500 grams birthweight. All infants were assessed on working memory tasks at 8 months after the expected date of delivery (when preterm infants were actually 10-11 months chronological age).

Results: The findings of the study showed that preterm infants performed significantly more poorly than full-term infants at 8 months after the expected date of delivery on measures of working memory. The results suggest that the effects of maturation are greater than the effects of exposure to extrauterine environmental stimuli on the development of working memory. Furthermore, the preterm infants were divided into two subgroups on the basis of (a) low or high medical risk factors, (b) birthweight of < 1000 g versus 1000-1500 g, and (c) gestation age of < 28 weeks versus 28-32 weeks, in order to assess the effects of these variables on the performance of working memory. Medical risk, lower birthweight and lower gestation age were all found to adversely affect performance on working memory.

Discussions and Conclusions: It is argued that medical risk, lower birthweight and lower gestation factors may influence the development of specific areas of the brain which govern working memory, and given that the prefrontal regions are particularly immature they may be especially vulnerable to damage or disruption. The present study provides further insights into the emergence of working memory in infants and the feasibility of evaluating these abilities in infants who are at risk for further learning difficulties and attention deficits.

Chapter 7 – The first part of the chapter reviews the recent literature regarding the involvement of working memory functions in scholastic learning and its role as an underlying factor of reading, writing and arithmetical difficulties. In the second part of the chapter the authors find an experience of assessment and training of working memory for the prevention of reading, writing and mathematical learning difficulties. On the basis of this study, an Italian working memory test battery and a training programme have been developed, including a series of activities involving both verbal and visual-spatial working memory with different degrees of central executive demand.

Chapter 8 – Sentence comprehension and production both involve temporary activation, storage, and manipulation of partially structured representations. Comprehenders sometimes buffer individual words and phrases as they register and process new input and relate new to previously presented input. Speakers must activate conceptual representations, search for corresponding lexicalized concepts, place them in the appropriate order, and apply the proper inflections before they can begin articulation. All of this activity requires some ability retain information in an active state and manipulate this information. Considerable research on both healthy and neurologically impaired individuals has focused on describing the working memory system or systems that support this temporary activation and manipulation of information. This paper provides an overview of the theoretical and methodological issues that characterize research in this area, with a particular emphasis on sentence processing. The authors will make a number of suggestions for improving the methods used to research working memory in sentence comprehension and production.

Chapter 9 – In the history of cognitive psychology, one of the most studied, analyzed, cited, revised and criticized theoretical model was the Baddeley & Hitch's (1974) Working Memory Model. A binding attribute of working memory is its limited capacity, as evidenced by the studies on span measures. The methodology most often used to investigate such limited capacity is dual-task paradigm. In the present experiment a dual task procedure was employed to evaluate the requirements of working memory resources in a virtual spatial memory task, a dual task procedure was employed to shed light on the hypothesis that spatial language would be an essential for the integration of geometric and non-geometric (feature) information. Nowadays, contrasting results do not permit to accomplish with this hypothesis and integration of different classes of information remains at level of open debate. The present experiment was aimed at providing new evidence for the aforementioned topic employing the virtual version of the reorientation task and two well-known concurrent tasks: articulatory suppression for verbal and spatial tapping tasks for visuo-spatial working memory components, respectively. These tasks were already employed in navigation-based experiments. If visuo-spatial working memory is substantially involved in reorientation, then it might expect that spatial tapping would impair the encoding relationships among target, landmark and geometric characteristics of the environment largely than articulatory suppression. On the other hand, a large decrease in performance following articulatory suppression will lead to conclude that the language hypothesis might be correct. Sixty participants were randomly assigned to one of three different dual task experimental conditions: Articulatory Suppression Task, Spatial Tapping Task and No Concurrent Task. The articulatory suppression task involved a sequence of monosyllabic syllables when pronounced by Italian speakers i. e. Ba/Be/Bi/Bo/Bu/Da/De/Di/Do/Du. The spatial tapping task involved the participant in tapping repeatedly on wooden keys of a custom-made keypad.

Data showed a main effect of the dual task interference, with a significant decrease in performance as effect of visuo-spatial as well as verbal dual task. Moreover, the difference between the two dual tasks was also significant demonstrating that visuo-spatial interference worsened the performance significantly more than verbal one. These results seem to shed new light on current debate, since they lead to conclude that reorientation task engages critically visuo-spatial, and with a minor extent, verbal component of working memory.

Chapter 10 – Considerable knowledge has been gained about the brain bases of working memory through research with functional magnetic resonance imaging (fMRI). However, using fMRI to explore the component processes that support working memory is difficult due to the timing of component processes and the lag of the hemodynamic response underlying the blood oxygen level dependent (BOLD) response in fMRI. Resolving controversies regarding the role of various brain regions in encoding, maintaining, retrieving, searching, and comparing information held in working memory requires isolating BOLD signal changes in response to the engagement of each of these component processes. A variety of fMRI experimental design and analysis techniques have been used for this purpose. These have included regression analyses with models based on canonical or subject-derived hemodynamic response functions, varying the duration of component process intervals, using component process intervals that exceed the ideal time needed for the hemodynamic response to return to baseline, regression modeling of parts of component process intervals, and including partial-trials in which only a subset of the component processes are engaged. The present chapter provides an overview of the technical challenges in using fMRI to examine the brain bases of working memory component processes, briefly reviews study designs and analysis methods that have been used to explore the brain bases of working memory, and offers suggestions for future research directions.

Chapter 11 – Age differences have been observed in emotional modulation of long-term memory (LTM) but have not yet been investigated in short-term memory (STM) in a comparable manner. In this study, age differences in the effect of stimulus emotionality on STM for stimulus content were examined. Younger (18-29 years) and older (61-77 years) adults completed a STM task with angry, happy, and neutral faces. Memory for face identity was increased for angry and neutral compared to happy faces. The response bias was most conservative for angry, and most liberal for happy faces. No age differences were observed in this emotional modulation of STM. It is argued that this is not due to lack of statistical power or to participant characteristics, but rather to the constraint nature of the task (probe-guided retrieval and short retention interval). The current findings do not suggest that emotional modulation of STM changes across the lifespan.

Chapter 12 – There is debate on whether the effect of stimulus emotionality on memory is a valence or an arousal effect. In a previous study, short-term memory (STM) was enhanced for angry compared to happy and neutral faces, and music-induced contextual arousal did not modulate this effect. The absence of such a contextual arousal effect could, however, have been due to the cross-modal nature of the study, as the contextual arousal was induced auditorily while the to-be-remembered stimuli were presented visually. In this study, we investigated the influence of visually-induced contextual arousal on the same STM task to determine whether the angry face benefit in STM is a valence or an arousal effect. Contextual arousal was successfully manipulated by presenting the background colours red, pink, and light pink. STM discrimination was enhanced for angry faces, and was not modulated by contextual arousal. High contextual arousal elicited by the red or pink backgrounds was accompanied by a more liberal response bias, regardless of facial expression. Because of this dissociation and because the effects of facial expression and background colour did not interact, it is concluded that the angry face benefit in STM is a valence and not an arousal effect. It is suggested that these stimulus valence and contextual arousal effects have different underlying mechanisms.

Chapter 13 – Working memory is a cognitive process dedicated to the transitory maintenance and online manipulation of information. Patients with schizophrenia, a heterogeneous brain disease, show several types of working memory deficits, including in visuospatial working memory, phonological working memory, and executive functioning. These deficits may underlie other schizophrenia symptoms and predict patient outcomes. Furthermore, there is increasing evidence suggesting that working memory deficits may provide a behavioral marker of genetic liability for schizophrenia. While the dominant role of the prefrontal dysfunction in working memory deficits of patients with schizophrenia has been appreciated, there is increasing evidence suggesting the existence of disturbed functional connectivity within brain networks subserving domain-specific components of working memory in schizophrenia. This functional deficit may result from dysfunctional neurotransmitter systems, of which the dopaminergic system has been best characterized, and/or white matter abnormalities which have been shown to be a consistent pathological finding in brains of schizophrenia patients. Working memory deficits in schizophrenia can be somewhat relieved by antipsychotics and various cognitive rehabilitation approaches. Atypical, but not typical, antipsychotics have shown some promise for relieving working memory deficits in patients with schizophrenia. Cognitive rehabilitation, an alternative to pharmacological treatment of cognitive deficits in patients with schizophrenia, also shows promise, but further work needs to be done to optimize this approach. Developing effective treatments for working memory impairments in schizophrenia patients remains an important therapeutic goal.

Chapter 14 – Epidemiological studies have associated tobacco consumption with a lower incidence of Alzheimer's disease (AD) and Parkinson's disease (PD). The neuroprotective effect of tobacco has been mainly attributed to the stimulation by nicotine of the $\alpha 7$ nicotinic acetylcholine receptors (nAChRs), which are implicated in neuronal survival, attention, and memory. A reduction in cholinergic function including lower levels of the expression of nAChRs in the hippocampus correlates with memory impairment in AD and schizophrenia. Although nicotine improves memory, sensory gating, and attention, its toxicity and undesired effects such as negative cardiovascular effects have terminated its therapeutic applications. Interestingly, its main metabolite cotinine shows similar neuroprotective and mnemonic properties but has a ten-fold longer half-life than nicotine and a good safety profile in humans. In neurodegenerative conditions including AD and PD, the accumulation of aggregated forms of the β-amyloid peptide correlates with cognitive impairment. Cotinine has been shown to reduce Aβ aggregation in vitro. Additionally, since cotinine is a weak agonist of the nAChRs, the authors postulate that cotinine improves neuronal survival and memory at least in part by acting as a positive modulator of the $\alpha 7$ nAChRs. The potentiation of $\alpha 7$ nAChRs by cotinine can be beneficial in a broad range of neurological disorders such as schizophrenia, AD, attention-deficit hyperactivity disorder, and PD in which the modulation of these receptors can ameliorate working memory and attention. Based on actual evidence and these ideas, the relevance and potential therapeutic use of cotinine in several neurological disorders are discussed in this chapter.

Chapter 15 – *Objective:* Patients with major depressive disorder (MDD) have been reported to perform less well in neurocognitive tests than normal control subjects. The author tested the hypotheses that a specific type of cognitive function, namely verbal working memory (WM), in patients with MDD is predictive of the functional outcome.

Study 1: In this naturalistic cross-sectional study, the subjects consisted of 54 clinic adult out-patients. The assessments were performed using the 7-item Hamilton Rating Scale for Depression (HAM-D7) for the severity of depression, and the Digit Sequencing Task (DST) for evaluation of verbal WM. Functional outcome was rated on a scale of 0 (non-impaired) to 3 (severely impaired). The author found that, in the patients with current episode of MDD, functional outcome was significantly correlated with HAM-D7 scores, but not with DST scores. Meanwhile, in a sample of full remitted or partial remitted (mildly depressed) patients, functional outcome was significantly correlated with both DST and HAM-D7 scores. Moreover, in a sample of full remitted or partial remitted (mildly depressed) patients, the DST scores significantly contributed to the prediction of the functional outcome, but the HAM-D7scores did not.

Study 2: In this naturalistic longitudinal study, the subjects consisted of 24 adult outpatients. Significant decrease of the HAM-D7 scores was observed during the 12-week study period, whereas the DST scores showed no significant increase. At baseline, the functional outcome was significantly correlated with the scores on HAM-D7, but, at 12 weeks, it was significantly correlated with both HAM-D7 and DST scores. According to a multiple regression analysis, the DST scores at baseline significantly contributed to prediction of the functional outcome at 12 weeks.

Conclusion: These studies suggest the existence of a correlation between a deficit of verbal WM and the functional outcome after treatment in patients with MDD. Enhancement of verbal WM function may be useful to achieve normalization of functioning as an important component of remission in addition to symptomatic remission.

Chapter 16 - Every day life requires frequent switches between tasks in order to achieve goaldirected behaviour. For example, driving presents us with a complicated environment wherein many sub-tasks—speed monitoring, steering, recollection of directions from memory etc.—must be switched between in order to arrive safely at our destination. However, as working memory is limited in capacity, the question arises as to how a new task is implemented in working memory in the face of conflicting activation from the now-irrelevant task. The mechanisms that allow such fluid switching are measured by utilising the socalled task-switching paradigm. Within this paradigm, participants switch between two or three simple cognitive tasks (e.g. odd/even; higher/lower than 5 judgements on number stimuli). Recent research from the task-switching paradigm has suggested that task performance is afforded by activation of task-relevant representations in working memory. Such an established representation guides behaviour by directing attention to task-relevant stimuli and actions whilst filtering out task-irrelevant information. The present chapter provides a critical review of behavioural results in the taskswitching paradigm, outlining the controversies that have surrounded this popular paradigm in recent years. This chapter also reviews the concept of inhibitory mechanisms in task-switching, serving to suppress the activation levels of the previously relevant task. Inhibition is inferred by slower reaction times returning to a recently executed task after one intervening trial (an ABA sequence) compared to returning to a task not recently executed (a CBA sequence, where A, B, & C are arbitrary labels for tasks). This reaction time cost is thus an important phenomenon for exploring the dynamics of inhibitory processes of working memory contents during task-switching.

Chapter 17 - Working memory (WM), the ability to hold and manipulate information online, improves during childhood as shown by an increase in WM capacity and a positive correlation between age and measures of WM performance. Intact function of WM is essential in many forms of complex cognition such as learning, reasoning, problem solving and language comprehension. WM function has a strong impact on academic achievement and is related to adaptive functioning at school. Children with deficits in WM have learning difficulties that are often accompanied by behavioural problems.

The neural processes subserving WM performance and brain structures supporting this system continue to develop throughout childhood till adolescence and early adulthood. The prefrontal cortex (PFC), that is one of the last brain regions to mature, has a central role in the function of WM. WM network involves also distributed areas in parietal, temporal and striatal regions. It has been suggested that neuroanatomical brain development occurs in parallel with behavioural and cognitive maturation during childhood and adolescence. In this chapter, the authors focus on the neural mechanisms that support the function of WM, their developmental trajectories and relation of their development to the maturation of cognitive abilities. The authors will also discuss the development of the brain's "default-mode" network that is active in the absence of cognitive task performance, i.e. during a resting state and shows attenuation of activation (deactivation) when the brain becomes engaged in attention requiring cognitive task performance. Deactivation mechanisms are important in the performance of WM tasks: inability to deactivate is associated with impaired task performance and is evident in patients with certain neuropsychological disorders.

In: Working Memory: Capacity, Developments and...
Editor: Eden S. Levin

ISBN: 978-1-61761-980-9
© 2011 Nova Science Publishers, Inc.-

Chapter 1

WORKING MEMORY AND THE AUTISTIC MIND

*R. Hansen, L. Deling, E. Olufs,
R. Pytlik, and F. R. Ferraro*[*]
University of North Dakota, Grand Forks, North Dakota, USA

ABSTRACT

The current chapter will focus on working memory abilities and development, primarily examining individuals with autism ages 5 to 20 years. With Baddeley and Hitch's model as a starting point, we will explore the research surrounding how working memory typically develops, deviations found in the autistic population compared to typical working memory performance and development, and the role such differences may play when considering possible intervention strategies to use with individuals with autism spectrum disorders. Recent findings in the working memory literature will be examined, including task effects that facilitate and inhibit performance, experimental design factors that may play a role in the contradictory results within the area of working memory in individuals with autism spectrum disorders, and neurological factors that may contribute to cognitive differences.

In general, working memory capacity increases with age in the typically developing population, with specific increases seen in short-term memory capabilities, verbal span abilities, visual span abilities, and complex working memory processes. Specialized working memory components and strategies also develop with age. There is currently little evidence of a general working memory deficit in individuals with autism; however, research suggests that certain domains of working memory may show impairments or delayed development in individuals with autism. Verbal span abilities appear to be largely intact within the ASD population with deficits on tasks that rely on spontaneous rehearsal strategies that prove helpful as the task complexity increases. The visuospatial sketchpad of children and adolescents with autism seems grossly intact with some deficits demonstrated in oculomotor and spatial tasks requiring more mature development.

---

[*] Corresponding author: Chester Fritz Distinguished Professor, Director, General/Experimental Ph.D. Program, Fellow, National Academy of Neuropsychology, Dept. Psychology - University of North Dakota, Corwin-Larimore Rm. 215, 319 Harvard Street Stop 8380, Grand Forks, ND 58202-8380, 701-777-2414 (O), 701-777-3454 (FAX), and F. R. Ferraro, f_ferraro@und.nodak.edu

Within the central executive, studies have shown individuals with autism to have intact performance on simple inhibition tasks. However, they often show impaired performance on measures of planning and complex inhibition tasks. On tasks that involve the episodic buffer component, children and adolescents with autism tend to encode specific features of events rather than global features, making memory strategies less efficient. Some of these deficits have been attributed to neurobiological differences found in individuals with autism, including an increased total brain volume, overreliance of the right hemisphere, reduced activation of the dorsolateral prefrontal cortex, atypical activity in the cingulate cortex, and underconnectivity in several circuitry systems. Although little research has specifically been conducted on working memory interventions for individuals with autism, understanding specific working memory strengths and weaknesses can help guide approaches to improving working memory functioning. Within other populations, working memory training has been effective in targeting specific working memory factors that are possibly implicated in autism as well, including metamemory skills, overt rehearsal strategies, and elaboration. Additional research is needed on the capacity and development of working memory in children with autism as current findings are often inconsistent.

Keywords: working memory, autism spectrum disorder, development

WORKING MEMORY AND THE AUTISTIC MIND

What is Working Memory?

Working memory is an active multicomponent system that allows an individual to retain information in order to process, respond, and translate material into long-term memory (Alloway, Rajendran, & Archibald, 2009). Baddeley and Hitch's 1974 model of working memory has provided a foundation on which much current research has been built (for review, see Repovs & Baddeley, 2006). The model remains relevant today with subsequent modifications incorporating newer findings into a revised model. Baddeley and Hitch originally proposed three integral components to working memory: the phonological loop, visuospatial sketchpad, and the central executive (Baddeley & Hitch, 1974; Baddeley, 1994). Baddeley (2000) then updated the model to include the episodic buffer to explain cognitive findings not accounted for by the other aforementioned components

The *phonological loop* is comprised of two parts—a phonological store and articulatory rehearsal process. The phonological store allows auditory or phonological input to be retained for a few seconds before being subject to decay (Baddeley, Thomson, & Buchanan, 1975). The articulatory rehearsal process involves vocally or subvocally reviewing the input from the phonological store, allowing the material to remain longer in the phonological store for encoding into short-term memory. Consequently, the capacity of the phonological loop is limited by the amount of content that can be voiced in real time within the approximate two-seconds time frame allowed by the phonological store, yet material can be stored indefinitely if such memory strategies are continued.

The *visuospatial sketchpad* refers to the amount of cognitive "space" available to attend to and retain information that is either visual or spatial (Baddeley & Hitch, 1994; Logie, 1995). These visual and spatial stores are considered to be mutually exclusive but still use the same visuospatial sketchpad to manipulate information into memory. Logie (1995) expanded the Baddeley & Hitch model by proposing that the visuospatial sketchpad dissociates into two subsystems: 1) a *visual cache* available to store stable information about shape, color and appearance and 2) an *inner scribe* retaining dynamic information about movement sequences, action pathways and locations of objects. Studies attempting to quantify the specific unit capacity of the visuospatial sketchpad report contradictory and inconclusive findings (for review, see Davis & Holmes, 2005). Some evidence has been found suggesting that short-term visual memory is restricted to three to five objects regardless of the number of individual features and independent of spatial location (Cowan, 2001; Luck & Vogel, 1997). However, others (e.g., Wilken & Ma, 2004) have found support for more flexible, visual short-term memory with varying capacity dependent on the number of attended features, the quality and integration of the internal representation, and the possibility of interference or aid in different modalities (i.e., phonological input, semantic cues, etc.). This adaptable visuospatial memory model may explain why memory performance declines as more features are required to be retained and why using strategies such as manipulating information into an integrated, representative object can increase the number of recalled items (Alvarez & Cavanagh, 2004; Treisman & Zhang, 2006).

Coordinating the flow of information between the phonological and visuospatial storage components, the *central executive* component of the working memory model acts as the "control center" for not only temporary storage and long-term retrieval but also the manipulation of material needed in more complex cognitive tasks, such as learning, reasoning, and comprehending (Alloway, et al., 2009). Baddeley (1993) equated the central executive's role to conscious awareness since it deals less with storage and retrieval and more with coordinating how resources are allocated to cognitive tasks. Accordingly, the central executive manages the attentional processes of working memory - sustaining, selecting, and shifting – allowing for subsequent encoding and retrieval of both current and past memories (Baddeley & Hitch, 1994; Repovs & Baddeley, 2006). The central executive is assumed to have a limited capacity to store information in addition to a limited pool of resources to draw upon; however, central executive functioning seems more influenced by attention capabilities. Thus, individual differences in overall working memory capacity seem to be less about the specific number of items that can be stored and more about the ability to control attention in maintaining material, retrieving information quickly and suppressing distractors (Engle, 2002; Kane & Engle, 2000).

Baddeley's 2000 addition to the model, the *episodic buffer*, serves as the "translator" of multi-dimensional information to a representation that can be more easily understood and retained. This is achieved by integrating separate bits of information from the different components of the working memory system and long-term memory into unitary scenes, or episodes, which can be more efficiently accessed and understood. Additionally, the episodic buffer facilitates the contemplation of potential outcomes and future planning as it can combine complex information from multiple sources in order to create and manipulate novel representations (Repovs & Baddeley, 2006). As the newest and consequently least understood component of working memory, the exact role of the episodic buffer in working memory capacity is still unclear. However, the episodic buffer appears to be important in manipulating and integrating different codes of received and stored information while influencing processing speed and overall working memory efficiency (Baddeley & Hitch, 2000). A number of empirical findings showing individual differences in working memory that were not explained by the original tripartite working memory model have been recently attributed to the episodic buffer, such as evidence of chunking (Wolters & Raffone, 2008), redintegration (Campoy & Baddeley, 2008; Hulme, Maughan, & Brown, 1991) and strategies utilizing combined verbal and visual encoding (Chincotta, Underwood, Ghani, Papadopoulou, & Wresinski, 1999; Logie & Pearson, 2000).

These four components of the working memory model —phonological loop, visuospatial sketchpad, central executive, and episodic buffer—operate independently while interacting together to function as working memory. Working memory is a vital contributor to effective cognitive functioning as it involves the fluid ability to store, manipulate and encode information for later retrieval and use in executing complex cognitive tasks. Thus, underdevelopment and impairments within the working memory system can hinder not only the successful mastery of specific academic and vocational skills for children, but also the global development of appropriate life skills needed for everyday living. Applying Baddeley and Hitch's working memory model in the field of cognitive development has been valuable when investigating special populations and the extent to which working memory deficits may underlie developmental disorders. Working memory research continues to prove useful in adding insight into the possible etiological factors and mechanisms of such developmental disorders including those within the autism spectrum.

How Does Working Memory Develop?

Baddeley and Hitch's model has been well explored within the adult population with converging behavioral, neuropsychological and neuroimaging evidence supporting the model (for review, see Collette & Van der Linden, 2002). However, there are still many inconsistencies in the literature about whether Baddeley and Hitch's domain-specific, working memory model is applicable to developing children (e.g., Chuah & Maybery, 1999; Bayliss, Jarrold, Baddeley, Gunn, & Leigh, 2005). While cognitive developmental psychologists agree that overall working memory performance increases as normally developing children age into adulthood, the debate continues as to whether this increase in performance is due to an increase in working memory capacity, the emergence of different working memory subcomponents, improvement in working memory efficiency or a combination of these and other factors contributing to working memory functioning. As research continues to investigate the development of working memory, findings will not only increase understanding about the features of working memory in typically developing children, but can help clarify the impact working memory may have on the cognitive functioning of children with autism spectrum disorders (ASD).

Working Memory Capacity

A considerable number of findings over the past two decades concur that age has a strong relationship with increases in short-term memory capabilities (e.g., Gathercole, Pickering, Ambridge, & Wearing, 2004; Isaacs & Vargha-Khadem, 1989; Visu-Petra, Cheie & Benga, 2008). For example, different methodologies used to measure phonological short-term memory, including digit span, word recall and non-word repetition tasks, have consistently demonstrated a steep, linear relationship between age and performance up to age eight years, with gradual improvements and eventual tapering in performance increases by early adolescence (Gathercole & Baddeley, 1998; Gathercole & Pickering, 2000). The ability to recall verbal material increases with span size from two to three memory items at age four years to the typical adult levels of six or seven items by twelve years of age (Hulme, Muir, Thomson, & Lawrence, 1984; Gathercole, 1999). Assessment of visuospatial memory development has indicated a similar relationship between age and memory capacity; visual span has been found to steadily increase from three to four items for five-year-olds and then plateaus after age eleven to fourteen items for adolescents and young adults (Miles & Morgan, 1996; Wilson, Scott, & Power, 1987). However, visual span findings may be confounded by the tendency for older participants to employ verbal recoding strategies to maintain visual representations (Gathercole, Adams & Hitch, 1994). Complex working memory processes mediated by the executive control component show a slightly different developmental pattern with improvements extending into adulthood. For example, studies using listening span tasks have shown a positive relationship between development and span size with consistent improvements in listening span capacity occurring up through age sixteen (Gathercole & Pickering, 1999). Executive functioning measures such as backward digit span and day/night Stroop tasks have also indicated a prolonged course of developmental improvements in capacity (Isaacs & Vargha-Khadem, 1989).

Emergence of Working Memory Components

In addition to working memory capacity increasing with advancing age, evidence for the emergence of different working memory components throughout the course of development has also been demonstrated. The phonological store of Baddeley and Hitch's model has been found to typically emerge by approximately three years of age (Ford & Silber, 1994; Gathercole & Adams, 1993). However, spontaneous rehearsal strategies used to maintain the otherwise decaying store of phonological codes have been found to arrive later in development, not appearing until about age 7 years of age (Flavell, Friedrichs, & Hoyt, 1970; Gathercole & Hitch, 1993). In adulthood, the phonological loop and the visuospatial sketchpad are interactive, but independent, components (Hitch, 1990). There is some evidence that for younger children, the phonological loop and the visuospatial sketchpad are not distinct entities until approximately seven years of age (Alloway, Gathercole, & Pickering, 2006). This dissociation may develop with maturation as the tendency to recode nonverbal information into verbal input strengthens reliance on the phonological loop (Brandimonte, Hitch & Bishop, 1992; Kemps, 2000). Research has also indicated different developmental patterns for the separate visual and spatial components within the visuospatial memory system (i.e., *visual cache* and *inner scribe*). Several studies of children aged five to fourteen (Cowan et al., 2003; Logie & Pearson, 1997; Mammarella, Pazzaglia & Cornoldi, 2008) found that performance improvements on visual memory measures developed more rapidly than performance on tasks assessing spatial memory, suggesting that visual memory develops faster in children than spatial memory. Furthermore, use of cognitive strategies mediated by the episodic buffer, such as chunking and redintegration, also emerge at different developmental stages. Chunking capabilities have been found to arrive after the age of seven years (Gilchrist, Cowan, & Naveh-Benjamin, 2009), while evidence of employing redintegration strategies have been found in children younger than age four.

Increased Efficiency in Working Memory through Maturation of Skills and Speed

As development brings increases in working memory capacity and the emergence of more specialized memory components and strategies, working memory processes expectedly become more efficient with increasing age. Baddeley, Gathercole and Papagno (1998) noted that between the emergence of the phonological store and the arrival of spontaneous verbal strategies, verbal short-term memory capacity continues to increase with age. This memory span increase can be explained by an increase in not only articulation speed (Hulme & Tordoff, 1989), but also in rehearsal speed (Gathercole et al, 2004). That is, not only does a child learning to talk faster allow for faster recall of information, this increase in speed also allows improved retrieval from the short-term memory store before the material is subject to decay. Once spontaneous rehearsal strategies begin to be employed, a child's increased rate of speaking presumably reflects an increased rate of inner speech used in subvocal rehearsal strategies as well, allowing for more material from the phonological store to be continuously recycled and retained. Consequently, verbal memory becomes more proficient and memory spans expand until articulation rates reach adult levels of speed (around age eleven or twelve years); thus, no further gains in verbal memory efficiency are found (Gathercole, 2008).

Increased efficiency in the visuospatial memory system can also be assumed to occur with the maturation of general vision circuitry since visual attention allows for material to be encoded, retained and recalled. Several dimensions of vision improve with development including general acuity, the extent of scanning, the rate at which a figure is examined and the temporal and spatial consistency of viewing objects (DeMarie & Ferron, 2003). Indeed, research has demonstrated both smooth and saccadic eye movements can interfere with visuospatial working memory (Hale, Myerson, Rhee, Weiss, & Abrams, 1996; Lawrence, Myerson, Oonk, & Abrams, 2001). More specifically, voluntary eye movements produced greater disruptions to spatial memory span than impairments that can be accounted for by other non-visual attention shifts and interferences (Pearson & Sahraie, 2003). Thus, as a child gains better oculomotor control and faster viewing processes, visuospatial memory can improve as well. Additionally, visuospatial working memory may become more efficient with increasing age as a child shifts from employing early visuospatial strategies to adding mature inner speech and rehearsal strategies that consequently enhance visuospatial short-term memory (Holmes & Adams, 2006.)

Coinciding with frontal lobe development, increases in working memory capacity may also reflect the development of executive control. Most notably, working memory improves with the ability to maintain attention and focus on relevant material, particularly when other events may compete for attention and take away from the cognitive resources available for other working memory processes (Swanson, 1999). These results can be expected considering the corresponding neuroanatomical evidence for the prefrontal lobe's role in executive functioning and this brain region's longer course of development with full development not occurring until into the mid twenties (O'Reilly, Braver & Cohen, 1999).

Integrative processes mediated by the episodic buffer increase the speed, efficiency and thus capacity of the entire working memory system. For example, learning to use the cognitive strategy of chunking has been a proposed factor for age-related increases in working memory efficiency (Cowan et al., 2003; Baddeley, 2003). Some argue that the development of memory span seen in childhood is due to an increase in the *size* of each chunk used to maintain verbal information with the *number* of chunks one is able retain being invariant across ages (Ottem, Lian, & Karlsen, 2007). Others propose that the number of chunks increases with age - two to three chunks are used in young children with chunk capacity peaking at about four chunks in young adults (Gilchrist et al., 2009). Redintegration strategies using long-term knowledge to facilitate memory recall also become more effective as crystallized knowledge accumulates throughout maturation, providing more abundant resources for memorial strategies. The maturation of cognitive skills and the synergistic effect of employing multiple memory domains and strategies add speed and efficiency that are reflected in the age-related increases of working memory abilities.

Development of the working memory system throughout childhood undoubtedly has an integral role in eventual adulthood cognitive functioning. Specifically, the phonological loop has been found essential in the acquisition of language, syntax and long-term learning of the phonological forms of new words (Alloway, Gathercole, Adams, & Willis, 2005). Visuospatial short-term memory may play a key role in the learning of spatial objects, such as faces, and has also been found to support the acquisition of arithmetic skills (Holmes & Adams, 2006; McKenzie, Bull, & Gray, 2003). The functioning of a child's central executive has been consistently associated with a variety of higher level abilities, including reading comprehension, advanced mathematical capabilities, planning and reasoning development (Bull, Johnston, & Roy, 1999; Swanson & Beebe-Frankenberger, 2004). Considering the important and pervasive role working memory has in the typical development of a child, impairment in such processes could certainly contribute to developmental disorders such as autism. Investigating the nature of working memory strengths and weaknesses prevalent in such developmental disorders can give better insight into the disorders themselves, and can aid in implementing appropriate support and interventions based on a specific working memory profile. Furthermore, investigating the complete working memory system employed by individuals with ASD can help determine if generalized working memory impairments or even specific core deficits within the working memory system underlie behavioral, cognitive and social deficits seen in ASD individuals or if other factors inherent to ASD are contributing to poor performance on tasks involving working memory processes.

Is Working Memory Impaired in Children with Autism Spectrum Disorders?

Currently, there is no clear consensus on whether or not individuals with autism spectrum disorders (ASD) have a working memory deficit. Research on the memory profile of ASD children is relatively sparse. Not only must researchers work around limitations posed by the practicalities of assessing a disabled *and* pediatric population, but the wide range of general abilities and functioning within the autism spectrum can also be problematic for studying this special population. Some researchers have found typical performance in working memory tasks, including verbal and visuospatial domains (Bennetto, Pennington &, Rogers, 1996; Ozonoff & Strayer, 2001). Others have reported working memory difficulties confined to only the verbal domain (Alloway, et al., 2009), visuospatial domain (Williams, Goldstein, Carpenter & Minshew, 2005) or the executive control processes of planning, problem-solving and other complex operations (Ozonoff & Jensen, 1999; Verté, Geurts, Roeyers, Oosterlaan, & Sergeant, 2005). Further findings have indicated working memory impairments when autistic participants were compared to controls matched by chronological age but not when compared to IQ-matched controls (Belleville, Rouleau, & Caza, 1998; Russell, Jarrold, & Henry, 1996). Often times, studies reaching opposing conclusions differ in the choice of comparison groups, the developmental level of the participants, the targeted age range of the study, the experimental tasks given, and the matching measures utilized to compare participants (Russo, Flanagan, Iarocci, Berringer, Zelazo, & Burack, 2007). These experimental design factors make generalizations difficult; thus, establishing conclusions about working memory profiles within autism spectrum disorders will likely require more time to collect multiple sources of convergent findings. Though not an exhaustive review, the authors will use the framework of the Baddeley and Hitch's working memory model to help integrate the differing findings for working memory capabilities specific to children and adolescent ASD populations.

Phonological Loop

Considering that qualitative impairments in verbal abilities are diagnostic criteria for autism spectrum disorders (DSM-IV; APA, 1994), it could be argued that such verbal difficulties would weaken verbal working memory capabilities in ASD individuals. However, findings are varied with poor performance found in some but not all measures used to assess functioning of verbal short-term memory. Results appear more congruent when results are separated by the phonological loop's subcomponents for capacity and maintenance (i.e., the phonological store and the articulatory rehearsal strategies) and when considering the complexity of the experimental tasks.

When measuring simple verbal span capacity, several studies indicate similar levels of performance by the ASD group relative to both IQ- and age-matched controls. Joseph and colleagues (Joseph, Steele, Meyer, & Tager-Flusberg, 2005) found no significant differences between autism and control groups of school-aged children, with a typical verbal span size of about 5 words that correlated with age and language level in both groups. These findings are consistent with other studies showing typical ranges of phonological store capacity for ASD children and adolescents (Minshew & Goldstein, 2001; Russell et al., 1996; Williams, Goldstein, Carpenter & Minshew, 2005).

In contrast, ASD individuals have been shown to struggle with remembering the temporal order of information (for review, see Bennetto et al., 1996) – a process aided by rehearsal strategies (Bjorklund, 1990). Use of rehearsal strategies have been demonstrated in individuals with autism (Bebko & Ricciuti, 2000; Smith, Gardiner, & Bowler, 2007; Russell et al., 1996). However, Bebko and Ricciuti (2000) found children with ASD use rehearsal strategies at a lower rate and required more prompting to use such strategies than similarly aged peers with typical development. They also found that though recall levels for the HFA group fell within typical ranges for short-term memory capacity in same-aged children, their performance was more similar with children several years younger. Furthermore, 36% of the HFA sample ($n = 11$) was found to be non-rehearsers despite being beyond the age (CA and VMA $M = 9.6$ years) at which spontaneous rehearsal strategies emerge. These and other's findings (Joseph, Steele, et al., 2005) provide evidence for at least a delay in the emergence of spontaneous rehearsal in the development of the ASD working memory system.

ASD performance on verbal working memory tasks also seems to vary depending on the complexity of the tasks employed by different studies. For example, in a study conducted by Alloway and colleagues (2009), children with Asperger's Syndrome were found to be proficient in a Listening Recall subtest requiring a true/false verification of the sentence and recall of the final word of each sentence. However, in a similar but more involved listening recall measure, Williams and colleagues (2006b) found significant impairments for the HFA group on tasks requiring the child to repeat progressively longer, meaningful sentences. These findings and others (Gabig, 2008; Miniscalco, Hagberg, Kadesjö, Westerlund, & Gillberg, 2007) support the idea that with increasing task complexity, working memory deficits become more apparent in individuals with autism.

Overall, ASD verbal memory span capacities were found to be largely intact despite language deficits inherent to disorders within the autism spectrum. However, working memory performance may be dampened by a delayed emergence of spontaneous rehearsal strategies and an inability to recruit adequate executive resources to match increasing task demands. Further research is needed to investigate if communication difficulties experienced by ASD children lead to specific verbal working memory deficits (e.g., employing rehearsal strategies) or if executive deficits underlie more generalized working memory impairment that could contribute to language problems.

Visuospatial Sketchpad

In addition to cognitive tasks that theoretically enlist the phonological loop of Baddeley and Hitch's working memory model, measures have been devised to assess functioning of the visuospatial sketchpad. Using a variety of such visuospatial working memory tests, studies have demonstrated both typical and atypical performance for ASD individuals. For example, children with autism showed impaired performance on the CANTAB Spatial Working Memory computerized test across multiple studies (Goldberg et al., 2005; Happé, Booth, Charlton, Hughes, 2006; Landa & Goldberg, 2005; Sinzig, Morsch, Bruning, Schmidt, & Lehmkuhl, 2008; Steele, Minshew, Luna, & Sweeney, 2007). Russell and colleagues found that performance of relatively low-ability ASD participants was inferior on visuospatial working memory tasks when matched by chronological age to typically developing controls; however, performance levels were similar and in some cases superior when ASD participants were matched by mental age (Russell et al., 1996: Russell, 1997). Furthermore, Ozonoff and Strayer (2001) failed to find any visuospatial working memory deficits in HFA children and adolescents on a running memory task for the type of shape previously presented and a spatial-memory span task for the location of a shape presented on the previous trial. ASD preschoolers were also shown to perform at typical levels on visuospatial measures including object retrieval, memory for stationary /scrambled boxes and spatial reversal tasks (Griffith, Pennington, Wehner & Rogers, 1999). More recently, others have found no differences between children with typical development and autism spectrum disorders in memory capacity or decay rates for visual information (McMorris, Hancock, & Bebko, 2010).

Inconsistent results may be explained by the different methodologies used to assess visuospatial working memory and the specific visuospatial subcomponents that mediate the tasks' processes. In typical development, visuospatial memory relies on both the visual cache for static, feature-based information and the inner scribe for information on movement and placement. When assessing visual working memory, performance declines with an increase in the number of objects and features to be remembered (Alvarez & Cavanagh, 2004). This is pertinent for interpreting findings with ASD subjects in that research has well established that individuals with autism have a specific perceptual-cognitive style for relying on a more bottom-up, piece-by-piece, feature-based approach to processing visual stimuli rather than the top-down, global, integrated perceptual processes used in individuals with typical development (for review, see Brosnan, Scott, Fox, & Pye, 2004). Furthermore, typically developing children younger than seven years seem to lack the ability to selectively attend to visual information that was identified by the experiment as important to remember. Instead, young children attempted to remember every piece of information that they were presented (Siegler et al., 2006). Considering this general immaturity in selectively attending to visual information combined with ASD children's tendency to perceive an overload of detailed features, performance on visuospatial memory tasks with increasing capacity demands on the visual cache should expectedly be compromised, particularly in younger or more developmentally delayed ASD children. Indeed, several studies do provide evidence for increasing impairment that parallels not only mental age but the complexity of the visual working memory task (Landa & Goldberg, 2005; Williams, Goldstein, & Minshew, 2006).

In addition to integrating visual information into less-detailed, representative objects, verbally recoding visual representations has also been shown to be effective in bolstering typical visuospatial working memory (Miles & Morgan, 1996). This verbal recoding strategy has been detected in typically developing children by the age of seven years. However, individuals with ASD have been shown to rely more on visual representations than verbal representations (Sahyoun, Belliveau, Soulières, Schwartz, & Mody, 2010). When comparing performance between the verbal and non-verbal versions of different visuospatial working memory tasks, children with autism demonstrated poorer performance under verbal conditions than did typical control subjects matched for verbal ability (Joseph, Steele et al., 2005). Findings imply that children with autism prefer using visual strategies in both verbal and non-verbal visospatial working memory tasks, whereas typically developing children rely more on verbal strategies (Joseph, McGrath, & Tager-Flusberg, 2005; Poirier & Martin, 2008; Russell, Jarrold, & Hood, 1999). This less effective reliance on visual over verbal processing may contribute to impairments found in the ASD visuospatial working memory system.

Finally, general findings that eye movements and oculomotor control may impact functioning of the inner scribe and hence weaken spatial working memory are particularly pertinent to understanding spatial memory processing in the autistic population. A growing number of studies repeatedly indicate pervasive, multi-modal visual symptoms in ASD individuals, including differences in eye movement patterns and control (for review, see Coulter, 2009). Using the Oculomotor Delayed Response Task, Luna and colleagues (2007) demonstrated decreased accuracy in initial primary saccades and final resting eye position across HFA groups ages 8 to 33 years. Further, the difference in accuracy between memory and the visually guided saccades was more pronounced for the autistic group. Despite continued impairment, the autistic group did show developmental improvements in eye movements from childhood to adolescence. However, the control group (matched for CA, IQ and gender) showed mature oculomotor control around 19 years of age, while the autism group did not reach maturity until 25 years of age. These results not only support other evidence of oculomotor abnormalities in autism (Takarae, Minshew, Luna, & Sweeney, 2004), but demonstrate the negative impact vision symptoms may have on visual working memory capacity (Luna, Doll, Hegedus, Minshew, & Sweeney, 2007).

Overall, inconsistent results have been reported for tasks that require visuospatial working memory. Contradictions among the findings may be due to studies' varying levels of task complexity, differing verbal and intellectual abilities of ASD participants and the specific modality (e.g., static features, spatial location, etc) assessed within the visuospatial memory system. Factors inherent to autism spectrum disorders, such as bottom-up processing, visual-over-verbal encoding and atypical oculomotor control, may be related to the visuospatial working memory strengths and weaknesses exhibited by ASD individuals.

Central Executive

As the central executive coordinates the other subcomponents of the working memory system, it is involved in a myriad of complex, integrative processes that together reflect general working memory capabilities. There are a wide variety of measures and modalities that have been used to investigate the capacity and capabilities of the central executive and related executive functioning processes. However, due to its multi-modal role, it is difficult to delineate if complex working memory capacity is a reflection of the central executive itself or if performance is being affected by a specific domain within the working memory system. Consequently, conclusions about the role of working memory in autism spectrum disorders have been debated, and studies often include a variety of executive functioning processes that may or may not be specifically attributed to Baddeley and Hitch's central executive component of working memory (for review, see Hill, 2004). Experimental techniques that reliably identify highly specific processes contributing to complex working memory are limited even within the typical developing population of children; therefore, only a brief overview of findings correlated with the central executive processes of synchronization, inhibition and attention will be presented.

Initial suggestions of working memory impairment in autism arose from poor performance relative to typically developing peers on the Tower of Hanoi and Tower of London tasks – a finding that has been widely replicated across different age groups and levels of impairment in ASD individuals (e.g., Benetto, Pennington, & Rogers, 1996; Goldberg et al., 2005; Ozonoff & Jensen, 1999). In fact, group differences on these Tower tasks are currently more robust than any other executive measure used to study autism and has been found to be the single best predictor of group membership out of a broad neuropsychological battery (Ozonoff, Pennington, & Rogers, 1991). As classic measures of planning, Tower tasks require simultaneous synchronization of maintaining and manipulating verbal (rules for the task and inner speech to guide moves) and visual (mental and real images of disks) material. Thus, performance on planning tasks can be considered related to the "control center" processes of the central executive. Autism studies using Tower tasks and other measures of planning support impairment in complex working memory processes. However, other factors that may contribute to poor Tower performance, such as inhibition deficits, language difficulties, and developmental delays, have been recognized (Goldberg et al., 2005; Tager-Flusberg & Joseph, 2005; Verté et al., 2005).

Performance on inhibition tasks shows quite variable performance by children with ASD and adolescents. More specifically, on the Stroop Color and Word Test, children with high-functioning autism showed intact abilities when compared to a group with Attention Deficit/Hyperactivity Disorder (ADHD), a sibling control group, and a normal control group (Goldberg et al., 2005 (card version); Christ, Holt, White, & Green, 2007 (computerized and card versions)). However, while participants with ASD showed no difference on response time (computerized version) when compared to a typically functioning control group, they correctly inhibited significantly fewer incongruent items and tended to be slower (Robinson, Goddard, Dritschel, Wisley, & Howlin, 2009). This may be due to the fact that the authors gave a computerized, single trial version of the Stroop that may have been more sensitive to inhibition difficulties than the standard card version (Robinson et al., 2009). Using the Go/No Go Task, intact inhibition was found in individuals with ASD when compared to a typically functioning, language impaired, and ADHD group (Noterdaeme, Amorosa, Mildenberger, Sitter, & Minow, 2001; Raymaekers, Antrop, van der Meere, Wiersema, & Roeyers, 2007). However, when ASD children/adolescents have comorbid symptoms of ADHD, they perform significantly less well than healthy controls (Sinzig et al., 2008). On the similarly simple Day-Night task, children with autism again showed an intact ability when compared to a typically functioning control group. The authors suggested that because the Day-Night task requires a verbal response, subvocal rehearsal was disrupted. Consequently, performances were comparable between both groups since any advantage that typically functioning children may have had from verbal self-reminding would be absent (Joseph, McGrath et al., 2005). In contrast, autistic children and adolescents demonstrated impairment in tasks that combine both inhibition and complex working memory processes (e.g., NEPSY Knock-Tap, Change Task, The Circle Drawing Task, TEA-Ch Walk Don't Walk, etc.) as these tasks require inhibiting a prepotent response while maintaining a conflicting response rule (Bishop & Norbury, 2005; Geurts et al., 2004; Vérte et al., 2005). Overall, it seems that purer measures of inhibition, such as the Stroop Color and Word Test, Go/No Go and Day/Night tasks, indicate intact inhibition while measures that require additional abilities show performance impairment in the autistic population.

In tandem with inhibitory abilities to ignore distractions, attentional abilities to maintain focus on relevant material are related to the functioning of the central executive in coordinating cognitive resources available for other working memory processes (Swanson, 1999). Research on autism and attention has found varied and inconsistent results (for review, see Ames & Fletcher-Watson, 2010). A significant confound to attention research within autism spectrum disorders is the comorbidity of ASD and ADHD. A review estimated almost half of children with autism spectrum disorders also suffer from ADHD symptoms of inattention, impulsivity and hyperactivity (Goldstein & Schwebach, 2004). Not all autism studies control for ADHD comorbidity, and thus the sole impact of attentional deficits on working memory is difficult to assess (Yoshida & Uchiyama, 2004).

Sinzig and colleagues (2008) addressed the confounds of comorbid ADHD symptoms in ASD working memory performance. Overall, they replicated previous findings of robust deficits in inhibition and complex working memory tasks for children with ADHD, and supported findings of impairment in children with ASD in planning and cognitive flexibility. Interestingly, children with dual-diagnoses of ADHD and ASD experienced more difficulties with inhibitory tasks and test duration but not with working memory tasks. Goldberg and colleagues (2005) also studied children with HFA, ADHD and typical development and found no group differences on response inhibition, planning, or set-shifting tasks. Geurts et al. (2004) demonstrated typical performance by children with HFA in tasks assessing interference control and complex working memory, but found significantly greater impairment than the ADHD group in planning and flexibility tasks. Such heterogeneous findings make interpretations of the role of attention on executive control functioning inconclusive.

In sum, impairments in executive control processes of planning and complex tasks of inhibition have been found in ASD children. Attention deficits, if present, also have a negative impact on some executive control functioning. However, the overlap of ADHD and ASD symptoms on working memory should be considered when researching and interpreting conclusions about impairments.

Episodic Buffer

As the newest addition to the model, research on the role of the episodic buffer in ASD working memory profiles is limited. However, some findings have demonstrated impairment in integrative strategies theoretically managed by the episodic buffer. For example, autistic individuals have been found to benefit less from the semantic relationships in recalling word lists compared to matched controls (Bowler, Gardiner, Grice, & Saavalainen, 2000; Minshew & Goldstein, 2001). This finding may reflect an inability to use long-term knowledge to facilitate short-term memory - a process used in redintegration and chunking strategies. ASD individuals may fail to encode the relational and global features of sets of stimuli due to their focus on individual items, thus making their memory processes less efficient. Findings inferring an organizational deficit in aiding recall are also consistent with the bias for local over global processing in autism (Hill & Frith, 2003; Rimland & Fein, 1988).

To address the initial question "Is working memory impaired in children with autism spectrum disorders?" the response must consider at least four factors: the type of comparison group, the developmental level of the participants, the experimental tasks given, and the matching measures used to compare participants. Since there is currently little consistent evidence of a general working memory deficit in individuals with autism, focusing on the specific working memory components that may be impaired or at least delayed could provide a more accurate profile of working memory in ASD that includes both the strengths and weaknesses found within the working memory system. Furthermore, when considering that overall working memory performance increases with typical development into adulthood, it could be argued that working memory deficits found in children with autism spectrum disorders are due to delayed or arrested development of different emerging working memory subcomponents and general working memory efficiency. Verbal span abilities of ASD children appear to be largely intact with impairment occurring when tasks rely on spontaneous rehearsal strategies used by older children with typical development. The visuospatial sketchpad of children and adolescents with autism also seems grossly intact with some deficits demonstrated in oculomotor and spatial tasks that require more mature development of the oculomotor circuitry and visuospatial sketchpad. As for the central executive, studies have shown individuals with autism to have intact performance on simple inhibition tasks. However, they often show impaired performance on the more developed processes needed in planning and complex inhibition tasks. When considering the role of the episodic buffer in ASD working memory systems, children and adolescents with autism tend to encode specific features of events rather than global features, similar to the memory strategies used by younger children. Consequently, strategies employed by the episodic buffer are less efficient and unable to improve working memory capabilities, particularly as tasks become more complex.

To date, research has been limited and findings have been too inconsistent to make generalized conclusions about working memory functioning in children with ASD. Stronger operational definitions for constructs, such as working memory and executive functioning, along with consistent use of tasks to assess specific working memory domains may help resolve some of the conflicting results found for both typically and atypically developing children. Investigating the neurological basis of working memory processes in autism can also provide converging data to support neuropsychological and behavioral findings. Considering the vast individual and group differences within the ASD population, a multidimensional approach is needed to understand the role working memory may contribute generally to disorders within the spectrum and individually to the cognitive strengths and weakness of children with ASD.

What Neurological Factors Could Be Contributing to Possible Working Memory Deficits in Autism?

Neurological studies offer a promising area of research in parsing out cognitive processing differences between children with typical development from those with autism spectrum disorders. Several brain structures have been implicated in autism, including the cerebral cortex, basal ganglia, amygdala, hippocampus, brain stem, corpus callosum and cerebellum (for review, see Brambilla et al, 2003). Neurochemical studies are also investigating the role serotonin, dopamine, acetylcholine, oxytocin and other neurotransmitters play in contributing to autistic behavioral symptoms and abnormal brain development (Lam, Aman & Arnold, 2006; Minshew & Williams, 2007). Several findings of cerebral activity differences have also been noted, including hypoactivation for processing facial stimuli, reduced activation of the bilateral brain regions and overreliance on temporal and occipital regions (for review, see O'Hearn, Asato, Ordaz, & Luna, 2008). These and other neurological differences found in individuals with autism may account for potential working memory deficits reported in this population. However, interpretative caution is warranted considering the inconsistencies in findings, co-morbid factors and disagreement over assigning specific neurobiological functioning to different brain regions. With brain imaging techniques continually improving and allowing for more current and in-depth findings with each new study, only a brief overview of neurological findings that may be pertain to constructs included in the Baddeley and Hitch working memory model is presented.

Individuals with autism spectrum disorders have been found to recruit a reduced number of brain regions assigned to the verbal aspects of working memory. Neuroimaging studies have also reported individuals with autism to over-rely on the right hemisphere brain regions when processing verbal and visual tasks. These differences could be specifically contributing to the performance differences found in cognitive tasks involving the phonological loop of working memory. In fact, Koshino and colleagues (2005) found that though HFA participants had similar performance in a n-back working memory letter task to age and IQ matched controls, the fMRI results suggested that HFA participants relied more on visual processes including right lateralized activation in the prefrontal and parietal regions and more activation in the posterior regions including inferior temporal and occipital regions. In contrast, the control-group participants demonstrated activation in circuitry used for verbal rather than visual codes (left lateralized activation of the parietal and posterior regions). These results may help explain inconsistencies found in the literature (e.g., Williams, Happé, & Jarrold, 2008) with evidences of comparable performance in simpler tasks used to assess verbal working memory – visual processes may be sufficient for simpler tasks but not for more complex verbal working memory processes (O'Hearn, Asato, Ordaz, & Luna, 2008).

Cortical abnormalities have also been found in ASD individuals that include decreased activity in the dorsolateral prefrontal cortex and posterior cingulate regions during oculomotor working memory tasks (Luna et al., 2002). This reduced activation may account for the difficulties seen in ASD individuals when attempting to maintain spatial location information in working memory tasks, particularly in processes that require functional integration of the prefrontal cortex with other distributed circuitry. Furthermore, higher levels of activation were found in the frontal eye fields and parietal lobule than in controls and lower levels of activation were shown in the dorsolateral prefrontal cortex, supplementary motor areas, and cingulate cortex (Hubl, et al., 2003). These findings indicate that while autistic individuals do access the basic brain circuitry for oculomotor function, they seem to rely more on these basic regions to perform higher order visuospatial tasks. Furthermore, fMRI studies have corroborated behavioral evidence of ASD individuals to use a local rather than global approach for visual information processing that may account for differences in working memory strategies (Ring et al., 1999). Consequently, more complex visuospatial working memory skills may be compromised.

Neurophysiological research suggests that the prefrontal cortex plays an important role in several cognitive processes mediated by working memory's central executive, including response inhibition and attention (Casey, Giedd, & Thomas, 2000). Age-related changes in the prefrontal cortex have been found in typical development, with the dorsolateral prefrontal cortex being one of the last brain regions to anatomically mature and activation of the superior frontal and parietal cortices increasing between the ages of nine and eighteen years (Klingberg, Forssberg, & Westerberg, 2002). Normal pruning phases help develop early synaptic density and prevent overgrowth of the prefrontal cortex while strengthening the remaining synaptic connections. Interestingly, the onset of brain overgrowth in children with ASD coincides with the onset of autistic symptoms, implicating its role in the pathological process of functional and structural brain abnormalities (Hardan, Minshew, Harenski, & Keshavan, 2001). In addition to a general increase in total brain volume attributed to deficient pruning processes, a prominent and consistent neurobiological abnormality found in individuals with autism is an enlarged parieto-temperal lobe (Brieber, et al., 2007; Hardan, Muddasani, Vemulapalli, Keshavan, & Minshew, 2006). Without proper pruning of these critical areas, cerebral activation tends to be diffuse and undifferentiated in individuals with autism and may have a direct impact on working memory functioning.

Further differences in connectivity and pattern activation have been found in persons with autism. Just and colleagues (2004) found atypical timing, connectivity synchronization and overall activation patterns in autistic individuals while performing sentence comprehension tasks. Reduced cortical connectivity such as that found by Just and colleagues could provide an explanation for reduced performance on working memory tasks that require a larger cognitive load with integration from several domains. This could help explain differences found in the research when considering the tasks used to investigate autistics' use of the specific components of working memory. Though structural abnormalities and activation differences have been reported, the literature also includes findings for intact circuitry in individuals with autism that supports working memory, including the insula, intraparietal sulcus, basal ganglia, thalamus, supramarginal gyrus, frontal eye fields, supplementary eye fields, presupplementary motor area, precuneus, and cerebellum (for review, see Toal et al., 2010). Such findings provide converging evidence that the neural systems in autism seem intact but may not be fully developed to incorporate distributed circuitry for higher order processes (Just, Cherkassky, Keller, & Minshew, 2004). Inherently, impairment in the circuitry that mediates complex processes can account for poor working memory performance, particularly in tasks employing multiple domains and requiring more cognitive resources.

Could Working Memory Interventions be Useful in Treating Autism?

Consistent with the inconclusive research about whether or not individuals with ASD have working memory deficits, research exploring possible working memory interventions for individuals with ASD is scarce. Strategies and interventions that have been explored as means of improving working memory involve teaching specific memory strategies, specific training programs, and classroom-based interventions. While currently little to no research has been conducted on improving working memory in individuals diagnosed with ASD, there is literature on working memory interventions for other populations, and these interventions may be beneficial to children with autism as well.

There is evidence that working memory capacities can be increased through specific interventions. It appears that working memory has less to do with general intelligence and more to do with the memory strategies used. Researchers have found that superior memory ability is not the result of higher intellectual function or differences in brain structures but the result of the use of spatial memory strategies that engage the hippocampus, an area of the brain critical for memory (Maguire, Valentine, Wilding, & Kapur, 2003). Therefore, the use of working memory strategies should help facilitate superior memory ability. If these memory strategies can be taught to individuals, regardless of intelligence or natural ability, it could improve their memory capacities and therefore increase their performance in tasks that tax working memory.

It is important to implement working memory interventions with children with working memory deficits, as adequate working memory is necessary for the academic success of children. Working memory is vital for supporting children's classroom learning, as children must be able to engage in dual tasks that require storing certain information while simultaneously mentally manipulating other information. Children with working memory deficits have difficulty with learning activities that require dual tasks, such as those common in classroom activities (Gathercole & Alloway, 2008). Children with reduced working memory capacity are at a distinct disadvantage in learning the information presented in the classroom, and this can impede their academic progress in the long run and place them below their peers in the ability to learn new information, even though the child may have equivalent intelligence. The working memory research suggests that the deficits that occur in children with ASD are commonly present when the children are given tasks that require more complex working memory skills (Gabig, 2008; Miniscalco et al., 2007; Williams et al., 2006). Classroom learning consists primarily of complex memory tasks, such as the dual tasks described previously. Children with ASD have additional difficulties that lead to trouble with school learning, and a low working memory capacity can further hinder their ability to attend to several tasks in the classroom.

Schools, teachers, parents, or anyone working with a child with a working memory deficit should take an active role in helping children with low working memory capacities increase their memory skills in order to help them attend to the classroom and daily living activities. One of the major differences between young children and older children is the automatic and appropriate use of optimal learning strategies. However, schools up to this point have not specifically taught students effective strategic learning skills, hindering students' capacity to become independent learners (Raforth, 2006). In fact, training working memory strategies could be particularly useful to teach young children, as they do not seem to automatically use optimal memory strategies, even if the strategies are in their repertoire (St. Clair-Thompson, Stevens, Hunt, & Bolder, 2010).

Theories behind Improving Working Memory

There are several theories on how one can best improve an individual's working memory capacity. Working memory naturally develops and improves as children get older. Developmental improvements in complex attention are driven by increases in processing speed and storage capacity, two factors that increase with age (Bayliss, et al., 2005). These increases in working memory and processing speed are two factors that lead to developmental increases in inductive reasoning (Kail, 2007). As these processes increase working memory capacity naturally during human development, it may be that increasing children's capacity or processing speed with training would improve the working memory of children with developmental disabilities, such as children with ASD. However, few studies have looked at interventions that work to improve processing speed and storage capacity in children. Instead, interventions tend to focus on strategy training.

DeMarie and Ferron (2003) found evidence for a three-factor model of how memory improves with age and development. Each of these three factors could therefore be targeted by interventions to improve working memory by providing children with these strategies before they would have developed them on their own. The three factors that have been examined are: metamemory, strategy, and capacity skills. The metamemory factor was not supported in younger children, but was in older children and adults.

Metamemory refers to a child's understanding of their own memory process. This onset of metamemory maturity helps explain the increase in memory strategy use and subsequent memory improvement in older children (Raforth, 2006). Strategic memory is the second factor that leads to increases in working memory ability with age (DeMarie & Ferron, 2003). Younger children tend to use optimal memory strategies less frequently and less effective strategies more often than older children, suggesting that while younger children know about the optimal strategy to use, they are less accurate in their use of it. The use of optimal strategies increases with age (Friedrich, 1974). As children age, strategic memory behavior emerges and becomes more effective and organized, resulting in increased knowledge, metamemory, and capacity.

The third factor associated with working memory improvement is memory capacity (DeMarie & Ferron, 2003). Memory capacity refers to how many items a person can hold in working memory. The traditional position posited by Miller (1956) is that short-term memory holds approximately seven plus or minus two units of information. Therefore, people have limitations on the amount of information that can be stored in working memory, making it difficult to increase capacity through interventions. Working memory capacity increases with human development. This is evidenced by the fact that when younger and older children use identical memory strategies, older children remember more information than younger children (Friedrich, 1974).

Strategy Interventions

The majority of working memory interventions focus on the training of specific working memory strategies to individuals. One type of strategic memory intervention that has been researched is phonological short-term memory interventions. Across a wide range of studies, it has been found that children younger than eight years of age encode visually presented information using only their visuo-spatial working memory system. However, after the age of eight, children developmentally begin to use a more phonological approach to encode and remember the same visual information. In the majority of cases, it seems that the encoding of visual stimuli into phonological codes is partially what leads to improved visuo-spatial information in children. This dual encoding of visual and phonological coding of visually presented information serves two purposes. First, it allows for a more stable way of maintaining information and provides children with a choice of representational forms that they can focus their attention on, depending on what the task itself requires (Pickering, 2001). Hitch et al. (1988) found that young children who verbally labeled objects that were presented visually recalled the objects better than children who did not provide a name of the object, supplying further evidence that the process of coding information phonologically as well as visually leads to improvements in recall.

A common type of memory strategy is overt rehearsal. In this rehearsal strategy, the individual will repeat what they have heard, read, or written. This is what is occurring when students re-read their notes over and over again (Raforth, 2006). Another type of strategic memory intervention is verbal working memory interventions. One of the most common strategies for verbal working memory interventions is the elaboration strategy. In this strategy, individuals create connections with the material in a way that adds meaning to the material. At first, the elaboration strategies children use are ineffective because they are not memorable enough for the child. Instead, the performance of older children and adults is better because they have learned to create connections that have specific meaning to them (Raforth, 2006). Children with ASD could be taught to use elaboration strategies more effectively by teaching them to create connections with special meaning to the material to be learned.

Another type of working memory strategy is the use of mneumonic devices. One type of mneumonic device is a spatial imagery strategy referred to as the Method of Loci. As stated previously in this chapter, individuals with superior working memory capacity tend to use spatial learning strategies (Maguire et al., 2002). In a study comparing the effects of two different mneumonic strategies, the Loci Mneumonic and strategic training, participants demonstrated improved working memory capabilities with both methods (Cavallini, Pagnin, & Vecchi, 2003). The Loci Mneumonic technique requires participants to first generate a series of known locations, and then add to the scene the object or name that is to be remembered. The strategic training was based on the fact that different types of material are best remembered using different working memory strategies, and so it teaches the participants to choose the best strategy for the material being presented. A second study trained adults to use an imagery-based strategy in which they were to create an image for each word presented while trying to make connections between the images. The results further suggest that strategic training interventions may have improve working memory capabilities younger and older adults alike (Carretti, Borella, & De Beni, 2007).

Chaining, an imagery-based memory strategy, has been shown to have the potential to increase the working memory capacity of adults. In a study by McNamara and Scott (2001), participants were trained to use a particular chaining strategy called of story formation. Story formation is a strategy in which an individual creates a story using the words presented in a list to create associations between the words. After the training, improvements were made in the participants' working memory abilities. In addition, these results were not found when a control group was allowed to practice the words the same amount of time but were not instructed on how to use a particular strategy. This suggests that the training of specific memory strategies has the ability to improve working memory capacity beyond that resulting from practice alone. Overall, these combined results suggest that teaching children how to use imagery strategies to remember information could lead to an increase in working memory capacity. This type of intervention may also be effective for children with ASD. Children with ASD may have difficulties with story or narrative memory tasks (Gabig, 2008; Miniscalco et al., 2007, & Williams et al., 2006). Therefore, teaching children with ASD to use story formation or elaboration strategies may improve this deficit in working memory by increasing working memory abilities in children with ASD that may generalize to other activities children engage in, such as life skills and classroom learning.

Lastly, strategy interventions have been examined that focus on teaching attention strategies with the goal of maintaining an individual's attention on the task at hand. Cicerone (2002) examined an intervention for attentional deficits that can occur after a mild traumatic brain injury. The intervention focused on the conscious and deliberate use of strategies to allocate one's attentional resources and manage the rate of information during task performance. The results suggested that the primary reason for the increase in working memory and a reduction in attentional dysfunction of individuals completing the training was based on working memory performance increases that occurred because of the intervention. All together, it appears that strategy training is an effective way to increase people's working memory capacity. If this type of training is useful for a variety of different people, it is possible that these strategies would also be useful for children with ASD. It could increase the child's complex working memory ability and teach children how to use the memory strategies they have appropriately.

Memory Capacity

Memory capacity also can make a difference in determining the usefulness of a working memory intervention, and there is some evidence that working memory capacity will not limit the improvements an individual can make with working memory interventions. Turley-Ames and Whitfield (2003) found that individuals with smaller memory span capabilities are able to improve their working memory performance through different training activities. Low memory span individuals benefitted more from rehearsal strategic training than imagery or semantic training. High memory span individuals, on the other hand, did not benefit from any of the training activities, possibly because they were already skilled at applying a specific, effective memory strategy to task performance. Overall, this suggests that even when individuals have low memory span they can still be helped with strategic training, especially rehearsal training. If children with autism have low working memory capacity, certain interventions should still be beneficial to them and will increase their working memory ability.

Working Memory Training Programs

Specific training programs have also been proposed as effective interventions for increasing working memory capabilities. Training programs intended to treat attention and memory deficits have been shown to result in significant improvements in tests of learning and memory in children with acquired brain injuries (Sjo, Spellerberg, Weidner, & Kihlgren, 2010) and adults aged 65 and older (Smith et al., 2009). Memory training programs have also been used successfully with typically developing students in a classroom setting. St. Clair-Thompson et al. (2010) used a memory training program called Memory Boosters with children ages five to eight. The children were first tested on measures of the phonological loop, visuospatial sketchpad, and central executive components of working memory. Memory Booster starts with a story and then provides instructions to the child about the memory strategy of rehearsal. As the children progress through the training program, they are taught additional memory strategies to use on the program tasks. Throughout the entire computer training program, children receive verbal encouragement, feedback from the computer, and rewards in the form of watching cartoons. Results showed that the training program led to significant improvements in the tasks assessing the phonological loop and central executive components of working memory, and in the particular, the improvements in listening recall were quite large. In addition, the improvements in working memory generalized beyond the tasks trained by the program. This study demonstrated that memory improvements can occur through training in strategy interventions instead of direct practice of memory tasks alone. The training program also led to an overall improvement in classroom tasks, suggesting that these strategies may help children improve their academic participation.

There is additional evidence that training programs are effective at increasing performance on working memory tasks. Klingberg, Forssberg, and Westerberg (2002) used an intense, adaptive training program for working memory tasks. For all the working memory tasks the computer ran the individual through, the difficulty of the task was adjusted by changing the number of stimuli that were to be remembered. Overall, daily training significantly improved performance on visuo-spatial working memory tasks and nonverbal complex reasoning tasks that were not specifically taught by the computer program. These results were the same for both individuals with ADHD and control individuals. Overall, the results showed that the amount of information an individual can hold in their working memory system can be increased through intense, adaptive computerized training. Most importantly, the training effect also generalized to other tasks requiring working memory, suggesting that the results could also generalize to everyday situations. An individual with ASD would possibly be able to use the skills they learned with the training program and use it in other areas of their daily activities in ways that may foster more independence.

These computerized training programs may be the most useful intervention for children with ASD because they do not appear to demonstrate as many working memory deficits when the task is computerized (Ozonoff & Strayer, 2001; Alloway et al., 2009; Silk, 2006). Therefore, by teaching children working memory strategies on the computer, they may benefit from increased working memory skills that will generalize to other tasks in their lives while maintaining their interest and attention.

Classroom Working Memory Interventions

Up to this point the interventions discussed have focused on the isolated training of individuals through strategy training or training programs to improve their working memory capabilities. There has also recently been a movement to implement working memory interventions through the schools and classrooms of children with working memory difficulties. In general, there are two approaches to classroom-based interventions. The first is through direct strategy instruction by teachers in the classroom. The idea behind direct strategy interventions is that schools are best able to directly teach children independent learning skills. Raforth (2006) suggested that schools can develop a list of strategic learning objectives, identify memory strategies that can be gained by students to accomplish these objectives, specific instructional strategies and activities that can be used to teach the learning strategies, and ways to provide feedback on the learning strategies to students. In addition, Raforth stresses the importance of schools adopting and embedding the strategic learning objectives across the curriculum. This will allow students with reduced working memory capabilities to gain the skills necessary to help them succeed with their peers in a regular classroom.

The second type of intervention suggested is to reduce the working memory load of students in the classroom, instead of attempting to increase the children's working memory capacity. In this intervention, teachers control the classroom environment in a way that prevents working memory overload. Gathercole and Alloway (2008), along with Elliot, Riddick, and Adams, developed an educational intervention that focuses on promoting an understanding of working memory and its practical consequences for classroom learning. The intervention is primarily focused on working with the teachers to highlight several areas where teachers can reduce the working memory load of their students. The intervention first encourages teachers to be aware of and recognize the warning signs of working memory failures in students. The second area the intervention provides guidance in is how to structure learning activities in a way that maintains the intended learning goals but still reduces working memory load. . Third, the intervention provides information to the teachers on how to reduce the memory load of activities to an amount that is reasonable for children by reducing the overall amount of material that students have to remember, reducing the unfamiliarity of new information while increasing its meaningfulness, simplifying verbal instructions, and encouraging the use of memory aids. Lastly, the intervention focuses on informing teachers of ways to develop the student's own strategies for overcoming the working memory failures they may have, therefore promoting long-term learning. This intervention has the potential to help children with ASD, as they would be able to remain in the classroom with their peers while the working memory requirements for the classroom are reduced, allowing children with ASD to benefit more from the lessons of the classroom and interactions with peers.

What Can We Conclude about Working Memory and the Autistic Mind?

The current Baddeley and Hitch model of working memory seems to be a suitable framework for researching working memory in the ASD population. Overall findings indicate both intact and impaired working memory capabilities for children with autism, dependent on the particular working memory domain being investigated, the task used to assess the component, and the level of development or general abilities of the ASD participants. A better consensus on operationally defining working memory performance and more task- to-task comparisons of results may better explain inconsistencies in the literature. Continued research in neurological factors involved in the working memory system may help reveal organic etiologies of specific working memory differences and similarities found between typically developing children and children with autism spectrum disorders.

In sum, the literature suggests ASD children to have discrete areas of delayed development or impairments compared to the typical working memory system, such as the visuospatial domains that involve oculomotor networks and some aspects of the central executive such as planning and complex tasks of inhibition. Working memory performance may also be compromised by a delayed emergence or low bias for relying on verbal and integrative memorial strategies compared to control groups. Individuals with autism may only show working memory deficits when tasks involve heavy working memory demands versus those tasks that involve a low cognitive load. Furthermore, comorbid attention deficits, if present, have also been found to negatively impact some areas of working memory functioning in ASD children. Converging data from neuroanatomical and functional imaging studies support findings of domain-specific working memory impairments including atypical brain structures (e.g., prefrontal cortex, hippocampus, corpus callosum, etc.) and cerebral activity (e.g., reduced bilateral activation, overreliance on temporal and occipital regions, underconnectivity, etc.). Since overall working memory performance increases with normal development into adulthood, it could be argued that working memory deficits within ASD children are due to delayed or arrested development of different emerging working memory subcomponents and general working memory efficiency. Thus, interventions that target specific domains in working memory capacity rather than general working memory abilities may prove useful in working with ASD children.

Due to its profound effect on daily functioning, working memory should be considered an important area for both research and therapeutic interventions with autistic children as it has been found to be a predictor of not only success in the academic arena, but in life skills as well. Considering the vast individual and group differences within the ASD population, a multidimensional approach is needed to understand the role working memory may contribute generally to disorders within the spectrum and uniquely to the cognitive strengths and weakness of individual children with ASD.

REFERENCES

[1] Abell, F., Krams, M., Ashburner, J., Passingham, R., Friston, K., Frackowiak, R., Happé, F., Frith, C. & Frith, U. (1999). The neuroanatomy of autism: A voxel-based whole brain analysis of structural scans. *NeuroReport: For Rapid Communication of Neuroscience Research, 10(8)*, 1647-1651. doi:10.1097/00001756-199906030-00005.

[2] Alloway, T. P., Gathercole, S. E., Adams, A. & Willis, C. (2005). Working memory abilities in children with special educational needs. *Educational and Child Psychology, 22(4)*, 56-67.

[3] Alloway, T. P., Rajendran, G. & Archibald, L. M. D. (2009). Working memory in children with developmental disorders. *Journal of Learning Disabilities, 42(4)*, 372-382.

[4] Alvarez, G. A. & Cavanagh, P. (2004). Research article the capacity of visual short-term memory is set both by visual information load and by number of objects. *Psychological Science, 15(2)*, 106-111. doi:10.1111/j.0963-7214.2004.01502006.x

[5] Ames, C. & Fletcher-Watson, S. (2010). A review of methods in the study of attention in autism. *Developmental Review, 30(1)*, 52-73. doi:10.1016/j.dr.2009.12.003

[6] Baddeley, A. (2003). Working memory: Looking back and looking forward. *Nature Reviews Neuroscience, 4(10)*, 829-839. doi:10.1038/nrn1201

[7] Baddeley, A. D., Thomson, N. & Buchanan, M. (1975). Word length and structure of short-term memory. *Journal of Verbal Learning and Verbal Behavior*, 575-589.

[8] Baddeley, A. D. & Hitch, G. J. (1974). Working memory. In G. H. Bower (Ed.), *The psychology of learning and motivation Vol. 8* (pp. 47–89). New York: Academic Press.

[9] Baddeley, A. D. & Hitch, G. J. (1994). Developments in the concept of working memory. *Neuropsychology, 8(4)*, 485-493. doi:10.1037/0894-4105.8.4.485

[10] Baddeley, A. D. & Hitch, G. J. (2000). Development of working memory: Should the pascual-leone and the baddeley and hitch models be. *Journal of Experimental Child Psychology, 77(2)*, 128.

[11] Baddeley, A., Gathercole, S. & Papagno, C. (1998). *The phonological loop as a language learning device*. US: American Psychological Association. doi:10.1037/0033-295X.105.1.158

[12] Bayliss, D. M., Jarrold, C., Gunn, D. M., Baddeley, A. D. & Leigh, E. (2005). Mapping the developmental constraints on working memory span performance. *Developmental Psychology, 41(4)*, 579-597.

[13] Bebko, J. M. & Ricciuti, C. (2000). Executive functioning and memory strategy use in children with autism: The influence of task constraints on spontaneous rehearsal. *Autism: The International Journal of Research & Practice, 4(3)*, 299.

[14] Belleville, S., Rouleau, N. & Caza, N. (1998). Effect of normal aging on the manipulation of information in working memory. *Memory & Cognition, 26(3)*, 572-583.

[15] Bennetto, L., Pennington, B. F. & Rogers, S. J. (1996). *Intact and impaired memory functions in autism*. United Kingdom: Blackwell Publishing. doi:10.2307/1131734

[16] Bishop, D. V. M. & Norbury, C. F. (2005). Executive functions in children with communication impairments, in relation to autistic symptomatology 2: Response inhibition. *Autism, 9(1)*, 29-43. doi:10.1177/1362361305049028

[17] Bjorklund, D. F. (1990). In Bjorklund D. F. (Ed.), *Children's strategies: Contemporary views of cognitive development*. Hillsdale, NJ England: Lawrence Erlbaum Associates, Inc.

[18] Bowler, D. M., Gardiner, J. M., Grice, S. & Saavalainen, P. (2000). Memory illusions: False recall and recognition in adults with Asperger's syndrome. *Journal of Abnormal Psychology, 109(4)*, 663-672. doi:10.1037/0021-843X.109.4.663

[19] Brambilla, P., Hardan, A., di Nemi, S. U., Perez, J., Soares, J. C. & Barale, F. (2003). Brain anatomy and development in autism: Review of structural MRI studies. *Brain Research Bulletin, 61(6)*, 557. doi:10.1016/j.brainresbull.2003.06.001

[20] Brandimonte, M. A., Hitch, G. J. & Bishop, D. V. (1992). *Influence of short-term memory codes on visual image processing: Evidence from image transformation tasks*. US: American Psychological Association. doi:10.1037/0278-7393.18.1.157

[21] Brieber, S., Neufang, S., Bruning, N., Kamp-Becker, I., Remschmidt, H., Herpertz-Dahlmann, B., et al. (2007). Structural brain abnormalities in adolescents with autism spectrum disorder and patients with attention deficit/hyperactivity disorder. *Journal of Child Psychology & Psychiatry, 48(12)*, 1251-1258. doi:10.1111/j.1469-7610.2007.01799.x.

[22] Brosnan, M. J., Scott, F. J., Fox, S. & Pye, J. (2004). Gestalt processing in autism: Failure to process perceptual relationships and the implications for contextual understanding. *Journal of Child Psychology & Psychiatry, 45(3)*, 459-469. doi:10.1111/j.1469-7610.2004.00237.x

[23] Bull, R., Johnston, R. S. & Roy, J. A. (1999). Exploring the roles of the visual-spatial sketch pad and central executive in children's arithmetical skills: Views from cognition and developmental neuropsychology. *Developmental Neuropsychology, 15(3)*, 421-442. doi:10.1080/87565649909540759

[24] Campoy, G. & Baddeley, A. (2008). Phonological and semantic strategies in immediate serial recall. *Memory, 16(4)*, 329-340. doi:10.1080/09658210701867302

[25] Carretti, B., Borella, E. & De Beni, R. (2007). Does strategic memory training improve the working memory performance of younger and older adults? *Experimental Psychology, 54(4)*, 311-320. doi:10.1027/1618-3169.54.4.311

[26] Casey, B. J., Giedd, J. N. & Thomas, K. M. (2000). Structural and functional brain development and its relation to cognitive development. *Biological Psychology, 54*(1-3), 241-257. doi:10.1016/S0301-0511(00)00058-2.

[27] Cavallini, E., Pagnin, A. & Vecchi, T. (2003). The rehabilitation of memory in old age: Effects of mnemonics and metacognition in strategic training. *Clinical Gerontologist, 26(1)*, 125-141.

[28] Chincotta, D., Underwood, G., Ghani, K. A., Papadopoulou, E. & Wresinski, M. (1999). *Memory span for arabic numerals and digit words: Evidence for a limited-capacity, visuo-spatial storage system*. United Kingdom: Taylor & Francis. doi:10.1080/027249899391098

[29] Christ, S. E., Holt, D. D., White, D. A. & Green, L. (2007). Inhibitory control in children with autism spectrum disorder. *Journal of Autism and Developmental Disorders, 37(6)*, 1155-1165. doi:10.1007/s10803-006-0259-y

[30] Chuah, Y. M. L. & Maybery, M. T. (1999). *Verbal and spatial short-term memory: Common sources of developmental change?* Journal of Experimental Child Psychology.

[31] Collette, F. & Van der Linden, M. (2002). Brain imaging of the central executive component of working memory. *Neuroscience & Biobehavioral Reviews, 26(2)*, 105.

[32] Cowan, N. (2001). The magical number 4 in short-term memory: A reconsideration of mental storage capacity. *Behavioral & Brain Sciences, 24(1)*, 87.

[33] Cowan, N., Towse, J. N., Hamilton, Z., Saults, J. S., Elliott, E. M., Lacey, J. F., Moreno, M. V. & Hitch, G. J. (2003). Children's working-memory processes: A response-timing analysis. *Journal of Experimental Psychology: General, 132(1)*, 113-132. doi:10.1037/0096-3445.132.1.113

[34] Davis, G. & Holmes, A. (2005). The capacity of visual short-term memory is not a fixed number of objects. *Memory & Cognition, 33(2)*, 185-195.

[35] DeMarie, D. & Ferron, J. (2003). Capacity, strategies, and metamemory: Tests of a three-factor model of memory development. *Journal of Experimental Child Psychology, 84(3)*, 167. doi:10.1016/S0022-0965(03)00004-3

[36] Engle, R. W. (2002). Working memory capacity as executive attention. *Current Directions in Psychological Science, 11(1)*, 19-23. doi:10.1111/1467-8721.00160

[37] Flavell, J. H., Friedrichs, A. G. & Hoyt, J. D. (1970). *Developmental changes in memorization processes*. Netherlands: Elsevier Science. doi:10.1016/0010-0285(70)90019-8

[38] Ford, S. & Silber, K. P. (1994). *Working memory in children: A developmental approach to the phonological coding of pictorial material*. United Kingdom: British Psychological Society.

[39] Friedrich, D. (1974). Developmental analysis of memory capacity and information-encoding strategy. *Developmental Psychology, 10(4)*, 559-563. doi:10.1037/h0036590

[40] Gabig, C. S. (2008). Verbal working memory and story retelling in school-age children with autism. *Language, Speech, & Hearing Services in Schools, 39(4)*, 498-511. doi:10.1044/0161-1461(2008/07-0023)

[41] Gathercole, S. E. (1999). Cognitive approaches to the development of short-term memory. *Trends in Cognitive Sciences, 3(11)*, 410-419. doi:10.1016/S1364-6613(99)01388-1
[42] Gathercole, S. E. (2008). Working memory in the classroom. *The Psychologist, 21(5)*, 382-385.
[43] Gathercole, S. & Adams, A. (1993). Phonological working memory in very young children. *Developmental Psychology, 29(4)*, 770.
[44] Gathercole, S. E., Adams, A. & Hitch, G. J. (1994). *Do young children rehearse? An individual-differences analysis.* US: Psychonomic Society.
[45] Gathercole, S. E. & Alloway, T. P. (2008). Working memory and classroom learning. In C. A. Fiorello (Ed.), *Applied cognitive research in K–3 classrooms.* (pp. 17-40). New York, NY US: Routledge/Taylor & Francis Group.
[46] Gathercole, S. E. & Hitch, G. J. (1993). In Morris P. E. (Ed.), *Developmental changes in short-term memory: A revised working memory perspective.* Hillsdale, NJ England: Lawrence Erlbaum Associates, Inc.
[47] Gathercole, S. E. & Pickering, S. J. (1999). Estimating the capacity of phonological short-term memory. *International Journal of Psychology, 34*(5-6), 378-382. doi:10.1080/002075999399729
[48] Gathercole, S. E., Pickering, S. J., Ambridge, B. & Wearing, H. (2004). The structure of working memory from 4 to 15 years of age. *Developmental Psychology, 40(2)*, 177-190. doi:10.1037/0012-1649.40.2.177
[49] Geurts, H. M., Verté, S., Oosterlaan, J., Roeyers, H. & Sergeant, J. A. (2004). How specific are executive functioning deficits in attention deficit hyperactivity disorder and autism? *Journal of Child Psychology & Psychiatry, 45(4)*, 836-854. doi:10.1111/j.1469-7610.2004.00276.x
[50] Gilchrist, A. L., Cowan, N. & Naveh-Benjamin, M. (2009). Investigating the childhood development of working memory using sentences: New evidence for the growth of chunk capacity. *Journal of Experimental Child Psychology, 104(2)*, 252-265. doi:10.1016/j.jecp.2009.05.006
[51] Goldberg, M. C., Mostofsky, S. H., Cutting, L. E., Mahone, E. M., Astor, B. C., Denckla, M. B. & Landa, R. J. (2005). Subtle executive impairment in children with autism and children with ADHD. *Journal of Autism and Developmental Disorders, 35(3)*, 279-293. doi:10.1007/s10803-005-3291-4
[52] Goldstein, S. & Schwebach, A. J. (2004). The comorbidity of pervasive developmental disorder and attention deficit hyperactivity disorder: Results of a retrospective chart review. *Journal of Autism & Developmental Disorders, 34(3)*, 329-339.
[53] Griffith, E. M., Pennington, B. F., Wehner, E. A. & Rogers, S. J. (1999). Executive functions in young children with autism. *Child Development, 70(4)*, 817-32.
[54] Hale, S., Myerson, J., Rhee, S. H., Weiss, C. S. & Abrams, R. A. (1996). Selective interference with the maintenance of location information in working memory. *Neuropsychology, 10(2)*, 228-240. doi:10.1037/0894-4105.10.2.228
[55] Happé, F., Booth, R., Charlton, R. & Hughes, C. (2006). Executive function deficits in autism spectrum disorders and attention-deficit/hyperactivity disorder: Examining profiles across domains and ages. *Brain & Cognition, 61(1)*, 25-39. doi:10.1016/j.bandc.2006.03.004

[56] Hardan, A., Minshew, N., Harenski, K. & Keshavan, M. (2001). Posterior Fossa Magnetic Resonance Imaging in Autism. *Journal of the American Academy of Child & Adolescent Psychiatry, 40(6)*, 666.

[57] Hardan, A., Muddasani, S., Vemulapalli, M., Keshavan, M. & Minshew, N. (2006). An MRI Study of Increased Cortical Thickness in Autism. *American Journal of Psychiatry, 163(7)*, 1290-1292.

[58] Hill, E. L. (2004). Executive dysfunction in autism. *Trends in Cognitive Sciences, 8(1)*, 26. doi:10.1016/j.tics.2003.11.003

[59] Hill, E. L. & Frith, U. (2003). Understanding autism: Insights from mind and brain. In E. Hill (Ed.), *Autism: Mind and brain.* (pp. 1-19). New York, NY US: Oxford University Press.

[60] Hitch, G. J. (1990). Developmental fractionation of working memory. In T. Shallice (Ed.), *Neuropsychological impairments of short-term memory.* (pp. 221-246). New York, NY US: Cambridge University Press.

[61] Holmes, J. & Adams, J. W. (2006). Working memory and children's mathematical skills: Implications for mathematical development and mathematics curricula. *Educational Psychology, 26(3)*, 339-366. doi:10.1080/01443410500341056

[62] Hubl, D., Bölte, S., Feineis-Matthews, S., Lanfermann, H., Federspiel, A., Strik, W., Poustka, F. & Dierks, T. (2003). Functional imbalance of visual pathways indicates alternative face processing strategies in autism. *Neurology, 61(9)*, 1232-1237.

[63] Hulme, C., Maughan, S. & Brown, G. D. (1991). *Memory for familiar and unfamiliar words: Evidence for a long-term memory contribution to short-term memory span.* Netherlands: Elsevier Science. doi:10.1016/0749-596X(91)90032-F

[64] Hulme, C., Thomson, N., Muir, C. & Lawrence, A. (1984). Speech rate and the development of short-term memory span. *Journal of Experimental Child Psychology, 38(2)*, 241-253. doi:10.1016/0022-0965(84)90124-3

[65] Hulme, C. & Tordoff, V. (1989). Working memory development: The effects of speech rate, word length, and acoustic similarity on serial recall. *Journal of Experimental Child Psychology, 47(1)*, 72-87. doi:10.1016/0022-0965(89)90063-5

[66] Isaacs, E. B. & Vargha-Khadem, F. (1989). *Differential course of development of spatial and verbal memory span: A normative study.* United Kingdom: British Psychological Society.

[67] Joseph, R. M., McGrath, L. M. & Tager-Flusberg, H. (2005). Executive dysfunction and its relation to language ability in verbal school-age children with autism. *Developmental Neuropsychology, 27(3)*, 361-378. doi:10.1207/s15326942dn2703_4

[68] Joseph, R. M., Steele, S. D., Meyer, E. & Tager-Flusberg, H. (2005). Self-ordered pointing in children with autism: Failure to use verbal mediation in the service of working memory? *Neuropsychologia, 43(10)*, 1400-1411. doi:10.1016/j.neuropsychologia.2005.01.010

[69] Just, M. A., Cherkassky, V. L., Keller, T. A. & Minshew, N. J. (2004). Cortical activation and synchronization during sentence comprehension in high-functioning autism: Evidence of underconnectivity. *Brain: A Journal of Neurology, 127(8)*, 1811-1821. doi:10.1093/brain/awh199

[70] Kail, R. V. (2007). Longitudinal evidence that increases in processing speed and working memory enhance children's reasoning. *Psychological Science, 18(4)*, 312-313. doi:10.1111/j.1467-9280.2007.01895.x

[71] Kane, M. J. & Engle, R. W. (2000). Working-memory capacity, proactive interference, and divided attention: Limits on long-term memory retrieval. *Journal of Experimental Psychology: Learning, Memory, and Cognition, 26(2)*, 336-358. doi:10.1037/0278-7393.26.2.336

[72] Kemps, E. (2000). Structural complexity in visuo-spatial working memory. *Current Psychology Letters: Behaviour, Brain & Cognition, 3*, 59-70.

[73] Klingberg, T., Forssberg, H. & Westerberg, H. (2002). Increased Brain Activity in Frontal and Parietal Cortex Underlies the Development of Visuospatial Working Memory Capacity during Childhood. *Journal of Cognitive Neuroscience, 14(1)*, 1-10. doi:10.1162/089892902317205276.

[74] Koshino, H., Carpenter, P., Minshew, N., Cherkassky, V., Keller, T. & Just, M. (2005). Functional connectivity in an fMRI working memory task in high-functioning autism. *NeuroImage, 24(3)*, 810-821. doi:10.1016/j.neuroimage.2004.09.028.

[75] Lam, K. S. L., Aman, M. G. & Arnold, L. E. (2006). Neurochemical correlates of autistic disorder: A review of the literature. *Research in Developmental Disabilities, 27(3)*, 254-289. doi:10.1016/j.ridd.2005.03.003

[76] Landa, R. J. & Goldberg, M. C. (2005). Language, social, and executive functions in high functioning autism: A continuum of performance. *Journal of Autism and Developmental Disorders, 35(5)*, 557-573. doi:10.1007/s10803-005-0001-1

[77] Lawrence, B. M., Myerson, J., Oonk, H. M. & Abrams, R. A. (2001). The effects of eye and limb movements on working memory. *Memory, 9(4-6)*, 433-444. doi:10.1080/09658210143000047

[78] Logie, R. H. (1995). *Visuo-spatial working memory*. Hove, England: Lawrence Erlbaum Associates Ltd.

[79] Logie, R. H. & Pearson, D. G. (1997). The inner eye and the inner scribe of visuo-spatial working memory: Evidence from developmental fractionation. *European Journal of Cognitive Psychology, 9(3)*, 241-257. doi:10.1080/095414497382806

[80] Luck, S. J. & Vogel, E. K. (1997). The capacity of visual working memory for features and conjunctions. *Nature, 390*(6657), 279.

[81] Luna, B., Minshew, N. J., Garver, K. E., Lazar, N. A., Thulborn, K. R., Eddy, W. F. & Sweeney, J. A. (2002). Neocortical system abnormalities in autism: An fMRI study of spatial working memory. *Neurology, 59(6)*, 834-840.

[82] Luna, B., Doll, S. K., Hegedus, S. J., Minshew, N. J. & Sweeney, J. A. (2007). Maturation of executive function in autism. *Biological Psychiatry, 61(4)*, 474-481. doi:10.1016/j.biopsych.2006.02.030

[83] Maguire, E. A., Valentine, E. R., Wilding, J. M. & Kapur, N. (2003). Routes to remembering: The brains behind superior memory. *Nature Neuroscience, 6(1)*, 90.

[84] Mammarella, I. C., Pazzaglia, F. & Cornoldi, C. (2008). Evidence for different components in children's visuospatial working memory. *British Journal of Developmental Psychology, 26(3)*, 337-355. doi:10.1348/026151007X236061

[85] McKenzie, B., Bull, R. & Gray, C. (2003). The effects of phonological and visual-spatial interference on children's arithmetical performance. *Educational and Child Psychology, 20(3)*, 93-108.

[86] McMorris, C.A., Hancock, L.H. & Bebko, J.M. (2010). *Iconic memory: Examining the visual information processing abilities of children with Autism Spectrum Disorders.*

Poster presented at the 2010 International Meeting for Autism Research, Philadelphia, May 2010

[87] Miles, C. & Morgan, M. J. (1996). Developmental and individual differences in visual memory span. *Current Psychology, 15(1)*, 53.

[88] Miniscalco, C., Hagberg, B., Kadesjö, B., Westerlund, M. & Gillberg, C. (2007). Narrative skills, cognitive profiles and neuropsychiatric disorders in 7-8-year-old children with late developing language. *International Journal of Language & Communication Disorders, 42(6)*, 665-681. doi:10.1080/13682820601084428

[89] Minshew, N. J. & Goldstein, G. (2001). *The pattern of intact and impaired memory functions in autism* Wiley-Blackwell.

[90] Minshew, N. J. & Williams, D. L. (2007). The new neurobiology of autism: Cortex, connectivity, and neuronal organization. *Archives of Neurology, 64(7)*, 945-950. doi:10.1001/archneur.64.7.945

[91] Noterdaeme, M., Amorosa, H., Mildenberger, K., Sitter, S. & Minow, F. (2001). Evaluation of attention problems in children with autism and children with a specific language disorder. *European Child & Adolescent Psychiatry, 10(1)*, 58-66. doi:10.1007/s007870170048

[92] O'Hearn, K., Asato, M., Ordaz, S. & Luna, B. (2008). Neurodevelopment and executive function in autism. *Development and Psychopathology, 20(4)*, 1103-1132. doi:10.1017/S0954579408000527

[93] O'Reilly, R. C., Braver, T. S. & Cohen, J. D. (1999). A biologically based computational model of working memory. In P. Shah (Ed.), *Models of working memory: Mechanisms of active maintenance and executive control.* (pp. 375-411). New York, NY US: Cambridge University Press.

[94] Ottem, E., Lian, A. & Karlsen, P. (2007). Reasons for the growth of traditional memory span across age. *European Journal of Cognitive Psychology, 19(2)*, 233-270. doi:10.1080/09541440600684653.

[95] Ozonoff, S. & Jensen, J. (1999). Specific executive function profiles in three neurodevelopmental disorders. *Journal of Autism and Developmental Disorders, 29(2)*, 171-177. doi:10.1023/A:1023052913110

[96] Ozonoff, S., Pennington, B. F. & Rogers, S. J. (1991). *Executive function deficits in high-functioning autistic individuals: Relationship to theory of mind.* United Kingdom: Blackwell Publishing. doi:10.1111/j.1469-7610.1991.tb00351.x

[97] Ozonoff, S. & Strayer, D. L. (2001). Further evidence of intact working memory in autism. *Journal of Autism and Developmental Disorders, 31(3)*, 257-263. doi:10.1023/A:1010794902139

[98] Pearson, D. G. & Logie, R. H. (2000). In Nualláin S. Ó. (Ed.), *Working memory and mental synthesis: A dual-task approach.* Amsterdam Netherlands: John Benjamins Publishing Company.

[99] Pearson, D. G. & Sahraie, A. (2003). Oculomotor control and the maintenance of spatially and temporally distributed events in visuo-spatial working memory. *Quarterly Journal of Experimental Psychology: Section A, 56(7)*, 1089.

[100] Pickering, S. J. (2001). The development of visuo-spatial working memory. *Memory, 9*(4-6), 423-432. doi:10.1080/09658210143000182

[101] Poirier, M. & Martin, J. S. (2008). In Bowler D. (Ed.), *Working memory and immediate memory in autism spectrum disorders*. New York, NY US: Cambridge University Press.

[102] Raforth, M.A. (2006). Strategic learning. In G.G. Bear & K.M. Minke (Eds.), *Children's needs III: Development, prevention, and intervention* (pp. 473-483). Bethesda, MD: National Association of School Psychologists.

[103] Raymaekers, R., Antrop, I., van, d. M., Wiersema, J. R. & Roeyers, H. (2007). HFA and ADHD: A direct comparison on state regulation and response inhibition. *Journal of Clinical and Experimental Neuropsychology, 29(4)*, 418-427. doi:10.1080/13803390600737990

[104] RepovŠ, G. & Baddeley, A. (2006). The multi-component model of working memory: Explorations in experimental cognitive psychology. *Neuroscience, 139(1)*, 5-21. doi:10.1016/j.neuroscience.2005.12.061

[105] Rimland, B. & Fein, D. (1988). Special talents of autistic savants. In D. Fein (Ed.), *The exceptional brain: Neuropsychology of talent and special abilities.* (pp. 474-492). New York, NY US: Guilford Press.

[106] Ring, H., Baron-Cohen, S., Wheelwright, S., Williams, S., Brammer, M., Andrew, C., et al. (1999). Cerebral correlates of preserved cognitive skills in autism: A functional MRI study of Embedded Figures Task performance. *Brain: A Journal of Neurology, 122(7)*, 1305-1315. doi:10.1093/brain/122.7.1305.

[107] Robinson, S., Goddard, L., Dritschel, B., Wisley, M. & Howlin, P. (2009). Executive functions in children with autism spectrum disorders. *Brain and Cognition, 71(3)*, 362-368. doi:10.1016/j.bandc.2009.06.007

[108] Russell, J., Jarrold, C. & Henry, L. (1996). Working memory in children with autism and with moderate learning difficulties. *Journal of Child Psychology and Psychiatry, 37(6)*, 673-686. doi:10.1111/j.1469-7610.1996.tb01459.x

[109] Russell, J., Jarrold, C. & Hood, B. (1999). Two intact executive capacities in children with autism: Implications for the core executive dysfunctions in the disorder. *Journal of Autism and Developmental Disorders, 29(2)*, 103-112. doi:10.1023/A:1023084425406

[110] Russo, N., Flanagan, T., Iarocci, G., Berringer, D., Zelazo, P. D. & Burack, J. A. (2007). *Deconstructing executive deficits among persons with autism: Implications for cognitive neuroscience* doi:10.1016/j.bandc.2006.04.007

[111] Sahyoun, C. P., Belliveau, J. W., Soulières, I., Schwartz, S. & Mody, M. (2010). Neuroimaging of the functional and structural networks underlying visuospatial vs. linguistic reasoning in high-functioning autism. *Neuropsychologia, 48(1)*, 86-95. doi:10.1016/j.neuropsychologia.2009.08.013

[112] Silk, T. J. (2006). Visuospatial processing and the function of prefrontal-parietal networks in autism spectrum disorders: A functional MRI study. *The American Journal of Psychiatry, 163(8)*, 1440-1443.

[113] Sinzig, J., Morsch, D., Bruning, N., Schmidt, M. H. & Lehmkuhl, G. (2008). Inhibition, flexibility, working memory and planning in autism spectrum disorders with and without comorbid ADHD-symptoms. *Child and Adolescent Psychiatry and Mental Health, 2* doi:10.1186/1753-2000-2-4

[114] Sjö, N. M., Spellerberg, S., Weidner, S. & Kihlgren, M. (2010). Training of attention and memory deficits in children with acquired brain injury. *Acta Paediatrica, 99(2)*, 230-236. doi:10.1111/j.1651-2227.2009.01587.x

[115] Smith, B. J., Gardiner, J. M. & Bowler, D. M. (2007). Deficits in free recall persist in Asperger's syndrome despite training in the use of list-appropriate learning strategies. *Journal of Autism & Developmental Disorders, 37(3)*, 445-454. doi:10.1007/s10803-006-0180-4

[116] Smith, G. E., Housen, P., Yaffe, K., Ruff, R., Kennison, R. F., Mahncke, H. W. & Zelinski, E. M. (2009). A cognitive training program based on principles of brain plasticity: Results from the improvement in memory with plasticity-based adaptive cognitive training (IMPACT) study. *Journal of the American Geriatrics Society, 57(4)*, 594-603. doi:10.1111/j.1532-5415.2008.02167.x

[117] St Clair-Thompson, H., Stevens, R., Hunt, A. & Bolder, E. (2010). Improving children's working memory and classroom performance. *Educational Psychology, 30(2)*, 203-219. doi:10.1080/01443410903509259

[118] Steele, S. D., Minshew, N. J., Luna, B. & Sweeney, J. (2007). Spatial working memory deficits in autism. *Journal of Autism & Developmental Disorders, 37(4)*, 605-612. doi:10.1007/s10803-006-0202-2

[119] Swanson, H. L. (1999). What develops in working memory? A life span perspective. *Developmental Psychology, 35(4)*, 986-1000. doi:10.1037/0012-1649.35.4.986

[120] Swanson, H. L. & Beebe-Frankenberger, M. (2004). The relationship between working memory and mathematical problem solving in children at risk and not at risk for serious math difficulties. *Journal of Educational Psychology, 96(3)*, 471-491. doi:10.1037/0022-0663.96.3.471

[121] Tager-Flusberg, H. & Joseph, R. M. (2005). Theory of mind, language, and executive functions in autism: A longitudinal perspective. In B. Sodian (Ed.), *Young children's cognitive development: Interrelationships among executive functioning, working memory, verbal ability, and theory of mind.* (pp. 239-257). Mahwah, NJ US: Lawrence Erlbaum Associates Publishers.

[122] Takarae, Y., Minshew, N. J., Luna, B. & Sweeney, J. A. (2004). Oculomotor abnormalities parallel cerebellar histopathology in autism. *Journal of Neurology, Neurosurgery & Psychiatry, 75(9)*, 1359-1361. doi:10.1136/jnnp.2003.022491

[123] Toal, F., Daly, E. M., Page, L., Deeley, Q., Hallahan, B., Bloemen, O., Cutter, W. J., Brammer, M. J., Curran, S., Robertson, D., Murphy, C., Murphy, K. C. & Murphy, D. G. M. (2010). Clinical and anatomical heterogeneity in autistic spectrum disorder: A structural MRI study. *Psychological Medicine, 40(7)*, 1171-1181. doi:10.1017/S0033291709991541

[124] Treisman, Anne, and Zhang Weiwei. 2006. "Location and binding in visual working memory." *Memory & Cognition* 34, no. 8: 1704-1719.

[125] Verté, S., Geurts, H. M., Roeyers, H., Oosterlaan, J. & Sergeant, J. A. (2005). Executive functioning in children with autism and tourette syndrome. *Development and Psychopathology, 17(2)*, 415-445. doi:10.1017/S0954579405050200

[126] Visu-Petra, L., Cheie, L. & Benga, O. (2008). Short-term memory performance and metamemory judgments in preschool and early school-age children: A quantitative and qualitative analysis. *Cogniţie Creier Comportament, 12(1)*, 71-101.

[127] Wilken, P. & Ma, W. J. (2004). A detection theory account of change detection. *Journal of Vision, 4(12)*, 1120-1135. doi:10.1167/4.12.11

[128] Williams, D. L., Goldstein, G., Carpenter, P. A. & Minshew, N. J. (2005). Verbal and spatial working memory in autism. *Journal of Autism & Developmental Disorders, 35(6)*, 747-756. doi:10.1007/s10803-005-0021-x.

[129] Williams, D. L., Goldstein, G. & Minshew, N. J. (2006). The profile of memory function in children with autism. *Neuropsychology, 20(1)*, 21-29. doi:10.1037/0894-4105.20.1.21.

[130] Williams, D., Happé, F. & Jarrold, C. (2008). Intact inner speech use in autism spectrum disorder: evidence from a short-term memory task. *Journal of Child Psychology & Psychiatry, 49(1)*, 51-58. doi:10.1111/j.1469-7610.2007.01836.x.

[131] Wilson, J. L., Scott, J. H. & Power, K. G. (1987). Developmental differences in the span of visual memory for pattern. *British Journal of Developmental Psychology, 5(3)*, 249-255.

[132] Wolters, G. & Raffone, A. (2008). Coherence and recurrency: Maintenance, control and integration in working memory. *Cognitive Processing, 9(1)*, 1-17. doi:10.1007/s10339-007-0185-8.

[133] Yoshida, Y. & Uchiyama, T. (2004). The clinical necessity for assessing attention Deficit/Hyperactivity disorder (AD/HD) symptoms in children with high-functioning pervasive developmental disorder (PDD). *European Child & Adolescent Psychiatry, 13(5)*, 307-314. doi:10.1007/s00787-004-0391-1.

Chapter 2

MEASUREMENT OF WORKING MEMORY

Karlee D. Fellner[1] and John R. Reddon[2]
[1]University of British Columbia, Vancouver, British Columbia, Canada
[2]Alberta Hospital Edmonton, Edmonton, Alberta, Canada

ABSTRACT

Working memory is the mechanism involved in the temporary manipulation and storage of information. It contributes to a number of cognitive functions, including learning, retrieving long-term memory, inhibiting irrelevant information, and working with novel problems. Working memory has limited capacity, and thus has significant implications for individual differences in learning and cognitive functioning.

Measurement of working memory is used to assess intellectual and cognitive ability, including individual cognitive development and declines and deficits in performance related to aging, dementia, neurological disorders, medical conditions, genetic disorders, developmental disabilities, learning disabilities, and psychiatric conditions. Working memory tasks include simple span (visuospatial and phonological short-term memory) and complex span tasks (visuospatial, phonological, and executive working memory). Commonly used memory assessment scales include the Wechsler Memory Scale, Wide Range Assessment of Memory and Learning, Swanson Cognitive Processing Test, Working Memory Test Battery for Children, and Automated Working Memory Assessment. Cognitive scales which contain an assessment of working memory include the Wechsler intelligence scales, Cognitive Assessment System, Stanford Binet Intelligence Scale, Woodcock-Johnson, Differential Ability Scales, Kaufman Assessment Battery for Children, Universal Nonverbal Intelligence Test, and NEPSY Developmental Neuropsychological Assessment.

Despite the number of measures designed to assess working memory, there is controversy over the consistency and overall adequacy of its measurement. This is largely because it is challenging to measure working memory directly, as it is influenced by factors such as processing speed, knowledge, executive functioning, long-term memory, and attention. In addition, tasks provide only a small sample of overall working memory. Also problematic is that working memory itself is a complex construct that is not fully understood by the scientific community. Controversy aside, the assessment of working memory is essential in the measurement of cognitive functioning in order to identify individual strengths and weaknesses and to inform individual remediation/treatment.

INTRODUCTION

Working memory is conceptualized as the mechanism responsible for the temporary storage and manipulation of information in the service of complex cognition (Baddeley, 1983, 2003, 2007; Dehn, 2008; Repovs & Baddeley, 2006; Richardson et al., 1996). Although this construct has been defined in various ways, researchers generally agree that working memory is divided into visuospatial and verbal storage components, and involves executive and attentional processes, encoding, strategic processes, and long-term memory retrieval (Baddeley & Jarrold, 2007; Dehn, 2008). One of the most prominent models of working memory is the multicomponent model originally proposed by Baddeley and Hitch (1974). This model is frequently cited in working memory research, as numerous studies and assessment tools are based on it (Alloway, Gathercole, Kirkwood, & Elliot, 2008; Baddeley, 2002; Conway et al., 2005; Repovs & Baddeley, 2006; Richardson et al., 1996; Turner & Engle, 1989). Given that many tasks designed to measure working memory are based on Baddeley and Hitch's (1974) multicomponent model, it is important to have an understanding of the issues in order to understand working memory measures (Alloway et al., 2008; Cocchini, Logie, Sala, MacPherson, & Baddeley, 2002; Repovs & Baddeley, 2006).

The current multicomponent model consists of four components: the central executive, phonological loop, visuospatial sketchpad, and episodic buffer (Baddeley, 2002, 2007; Baddeley & Jarrold, 2007; Repovs & Baddeley, 2006). The central executive is a limited capacity attentional control system that connects the contents of working memory to long-term memory, and divides, focuses, and switches attention (Baddeley, 2007; Baddeley & Jarrold, 2007; Repovs & Baddeley, 2006). It is one of the least understood components of working memory, yet given its crucial role in guiding working memory function, it is one of the most important (Baddeley, 2002; Baddeley & Jarrold, 2007; Repovs & Baddeley, 2006).

The phonological loop and visuospatial sketchpad are subsidiary storage systems that are controlled by the central executive (Baddeley, 2007; Repovs & Baddeley, 2006). The phonological loop temporarily stores speech-based and acoustic information (Baddeley, 2007; Baddeley & Larsen, 2007a, 2007b; Repovs & Baddeley, 2006). This information is referred to as a memory trace, and is lost quickly unless it is maintained through subvocal rehearsal (Baddeley, 2007; Baddeley & Larsen, 2007a, 2007b; Repovs & Baddeley, 2006). This system is thought to have evolved in order to facilitate language acquisition (Baddeley, Gathercole, & Papagno, 1998; Baddeley & Jarrold, 2007; Baddeley & Larsen, 2007a, 2007b; Coolidge & Wynn, 2005). The other storage system, visuospatial sketchpad, is involved in the storage and maintenance of spatial and visual information (Baddeley, 2007; Baddeley & Jarrold, 2007; Bruyer & Scailquin, 1998). This system consists of separate visual and spatial subcomponents that use independent rehearsal mechanisms (Baddeley & Jarrold, 2007; Bruyer & Scailquin, 1998; Coolidge & Wynn, 2005; Repovs & Baddeley, 2006; Zimmer, Speiser, & Seidler, 2003). Visual working memory is primarily associated with visual perception and imagery, while spatial working memory is related to attention and physical action (Bruyer & Scailquin, 1998; Repovs & Baddeley, 2006).

Baddeley later proposed the addition of a fourth component, the episodic buffer, as a consciously accessible, limited capacity storage system that integrates information from the other three components and long-term memory (Baddeley, 2000, 2007; Baddeley & Jarrold, 2007; Repovs & Baddeley, 2006). Integration and maintenance of information in the episodic buffer is dependent on the central executive (Baddeley, 2000; Repovs & Baddeley, 2006). The episodic buffer is a relatively new concept, and thus is not yet fully understood (Baddeley, 2007; Repovs & Baddeley, 2006).

Working memory serves an integral function as an interface between planned behavior, sensory perception, short-term memory, and long-term memory (Dehn, 2008; Repovs & Baddeley, 2006). It is essential to a number of complex cognitive functions, including learning, problem-solving, reading comprehension, long-term memory retrieval, inhibiting irrelevant information, and abstract reasoning (Baddeley, 1992; Dehn, 2008; Shelton, Elliot, Hill, Calamia, & Gouvier, 2009). Important variations in working memory have also been found to be associated with neurological, medical, and genetic disorders as well as developmental disabilities, learning disabilities, and psychiatric disorders (see "Working Memory Assessment in Clinical Applications" section). Thus, working memory plays a significant role across fields of psychology (Shelton et al., 2009). The implications of limitations in working memory underscore the need for valid, reliable measures of this construct in both applied and research settings (Baddeley, 2007; Conway, Jarrold, Kane, Miyake, & Towse, 2008; Dehn, 2008; Shelton et al., 2009). Unfortunately, the division among fields in psychology has resulted in divergent methods of measurement between disciplines, and at times, a substantial discrepancy between tools used in research and practice (Conway et al., 2008; Shelton et al., 2009). This disconnect is problematic, and has led to some controversy over methods used to assess working memory in practical settings.

MEASUREMENT OF WORKING MEMORY

Historical Development

Measurement of cognitive ability was first emphasized by Sir Francis Galton in the 19th century in his book "Inquiries into Human Faculty and its Development" (Galton, 1883). Soon after, Ebbinghaus (1885/1913) published the first psychological report regarding measurement of immediate memory. In this document, he reported his own recall span of nonsense syllables and the number of repetitions required to accurately recall progressively longer lists. Ebbinghaus' book piqued interest in variation in immediate memory, and the first empirical paper on memory span was published by Jacobs (1887) two years later. Jacobs measured "span of prehension" (Jacobs, 1887, p. 79) through using digits, letters, and nonsense syllables to test the number of items that people could recall. Jacobs (1887) also emphasized the importance of this span in cognitive ability. Subsequently, reports that memory span was impaired among institutionalized individuals were published (e.g., Galton, 1887), and simple span tasks became integrated into the first intelligence tests (Binet & Simon, 1905; Burt, 1909; Cattell & Galton, 1890).

These first measures primarily emphasized immediate storage of small amounts of information, and resemble the simple span tasks that continue to be used in the assessment of short-term memory today (Baddeley, 2007; Conway et al., 2005; Kane et al., 2004). It is important to distinguish between working memory and short-term memory in discussing working memory measurement. In contrast to these original measures of short-term memory, measures of working memory involve the manipulation of information held in short-term storage (Alloway et al., 2008; Baddeley, 2007; Conway et al., 2005; Conway, Kane, & Engle, 2003; Kane et al., 2004; Shelton et al., 2009; Towse, Hitch, & Hutton, 2000). Short-term memory and working memory differ in several ways. Working memory holds information from various cognitive processes and relies on long-term memory, while short-term memory only holds information from the perceptual environment and can operate independently from long-term memory (Baddeley, 2007; Dehn, 2008). As well, short-term memory passively stores domain-specific (that is, verbal and visual) information. On the other hand, working memory involves active information processing and is less domain-specific in its integration of general executive processes (Alloway et al., 2008; Baddeley, 2007; Bayliss, Jarrold, Baddeley, & Gunn, 2005; Conway et al., 2003; Dehn, 2008; Kane et al., 2004; Towse et al., 2000). This distinction is important in working memory measurement, as short-term and working memory tasks measure different constructs and show distinct relationships with various applications and cognitive constructs (Alloway et al., 2008; Baddeley, 2007; Bayliss, Jarrold, Baddeley, & Gunn, 2005; Carretti, Borella, Cornoldi, & De Beni, 2009; Daneman & Merikle, 1996; Kane et al., 2004; Leather & Henry, 1994; Luo, Chen, Zen, & Murray, 2010; Oakhill & Kyle, 2000; Shelton et al., 2009; Towse et al., 2000).

The first mention of the need to investigate the processing role of immediate memory was by Miller, Galanter, and Pribram (1960), and the first model to integrate processing into a theory of working memory was Baddeley and Hitch's multicomponent model (1974). Along with the emerging emphasis on processing came the need for measures of working memory that assessed more than simple storage capacity. Daneman and Carpenter (1980) published the first working memory span task that measured both storage and processing. This served as a model for the development of a number of complex span tasks – tasks that involve the simultaneous presentation of to-be-recalled information and a secondary processing task such as verifying equations or comprehending sentences (Conway et al., 2005). Some of the original tasks that were developed include reading span (Daneman & Carpenter, 1980), counting span (Case, Kurland, & Goldberg, 1982), and operation span (Turner & Engle, 1989). Aside from standardized assessment batteries, complex tasks are among the most commonly used cognitive measurement tools in applied settings (Conway et al., 2005). They have also been used extensively in research regarding individual differences, and have contributed to elaboration and further understanding of working memory theory.

Task Measures of Working Memory

Simple span tasks.

Despite the emphasis on processing in working memory and the distinction between short-term and working memory, simple span tasks that measure short-term memory continue to be used in working memory measurement. In particular, they are included in standardized batteries that are used primarily in applied settings. This is not completely unwarranted, given that short-term memory is a component of working memory (Baddeley, 2007). Simple span tasks are used to measure both visuospatial and phonological short-term memory, and are briefly described below.

Visuospatial short-term memory.

The primary tasks used to assess visuospatial short-term memory include block-tapping span and visual digit-span (Dehn, 2008). Block-tapping span, also known as the Corsi block task (Milner, 1971; Towse & Houston-Price, 2001; Vandierendonck, Kemps, Fastame, & Szmalec, 2004), involves an arrangement of nine randomly placed blocks. The examiner taps increasing numbers of blocks in a predetermined sequence at the rate of one per second, and the examinee is asked to replicate the tapping sequence. This task requires simple recall of visual information, drawing on the visuospatial short-term memory store (Milner, 1971; Vandierendonck et al., 2004).

In the visual digit span task, the examinee is shown printed digits and asked to recall them in sequential order. The digits are typically presented individually at a rate of one per second to reduce opportunities to use memory strategies like chunking (Dehn, 2008). Variations of these visuospatial tasks may be used as well, with the basic underlying principle being the short-term storage of visual or spatial stimuli.

Phonological short-term memory.

A number of simple span tasks are used to measure phonological short-term memory, including forward digit span, word span, pseudoword span, and letter span. Forward digit span is the most frequently used measure of short-term memory span in psychology and education (Alloway et al., 2008; Dehn, 2008). It was first used by Jacobs (1887), and has been incorporated in intelligence scales ever since (Dehn, 2008). Forward digit span typically involves the presentation of digits at a rate at one per second, though the procedure may be varied depending on the purpose of the assessment (Alloway et al., 2008; Dehn, 2008; Shelton et al., 2009).

Word span involves recall of a series of words that are typically presented at a rate of one per second (Dehn, 2008; Gathercole, Willis, Emslie, & Baddeley, 1991). Words are usually one or two syllables long, and should be unrelated so long-term memory and working memory interfere with recall as little as possible. Pseudoword span is similar to word span, but uses nonsense words in place of actual words (Gathercole et al., 1991). This provides a purer measure of phonological short-term memory, as the examinee cannot rely on strategies that use long-term memory. As with word span, pseudowords should have only one or two syllables and should not rhyme (Dehn, 2008).

Letter span is equivalent to digit span, but uses letters rather than numbers. It is particularly useful with examinees who have delayed or deficient math skills, as this has been shown to impact digit span, which leads to underestimates of phonological short-term memory capacity (Dehn, 2008).

Complex span tasks.

Complex tasks require the simultaneous storage and processing of information, and are thought to give a more accurate measure of working memory as it is applied in daily life

(Baddely, 2007; Conway et al., 2003; Dehn, 2008; Kane et al., 2004; Towse et al., 2000). Accordingly, complex span measures have shown much higher correlations than simple span measures with real-world applications such as complex cognition and academic performance (Ackerman, Beier, & Boyle, 2005; Alloway et al., 2008; Baddeley, 2007; Bayliss, Jarrold, Baddeley, & Gunn, 2005; Colom, Abad, Quiroga, Shih, & Flores-Mendoza, 2008; Conway, Cowan, Bunting, Therriault, & Minkoff, 2002; Conway et al., 2003, 2005; Dehn, 2008; Kane et al., 2004; Shelton et al., 2009; Towse et al., 2000). Thus, individual results on complex span tasks offer useful information regarding executive working memory and its implications for daily functioning (Baddeley, 2007; Conway et al., 2003; Daneman & Merikle, 1996; Dehn, 2008; Kane et al., 2004; Towse et al., 2000). Complex span tasks can measure visuospatial working memory, phonological working memory, and executive working memory. These tasks tap both domain-general and domain-specific working memory. In other words, both visuospatial and phonological tasks also involve executive working memory, and therefore are not pure measures of either storage system (Baddeley, 2007; Bayliss, Jarrold, Gunn, & Baddeley, 2003; Conway et al., 2003; Coolidge & Wynn, 2005; Dehn, 2008).

Visuospatial working memory.
Visuospatial working memory tasks measure the function of the visuospatial sketchpad of the multicomponent model of working memory (Baddeley, 2007; Baddeley & Hitch, 1974; Repovs & Baddeley, 2006). This is typically measured through counting span and backward block-tapping span (Dehn, 2008), though a number of additional measures have been developed. Counting span was originally developed by Case and colleagues (1982) as a measure of visual working memory capacity. The original task had participants count the number of green dots in a display of mixed green and yellow dots, and following the presentation of a series of dot displays, recall count totals in serial order (Case et al., 1982). A number of modified versions of counting span have been investigated, for example, using random target shapes instead of dots (Engle, Tuholski, Laughlin, & Conway, 1999). This task involves digit recall while counting and discriminating among objects in a display.

Backward block-tapping span is a modification of the Corsi block task that involves reverse recall of a sequence of block-tapping. While forward block-tapping measures short-term memory, backward block-tapping measures working memory given the processing required to transform (i.e., invert) the serial order of responses (Dehn, 2008; Vandierendonck et al., 2004). Other variations of the Corsi task have also been studied, including a version that combines block-tapping with digit span by incorporating digits in the blocks (Towse & Houston-Price, 2001). Another task that measures visuospatial working memory is the matrix task, which involves the examiner reading aloud sentences that describe spatial locations of letters on a grid. The examinee then writes the letters in the appropriate positions on the grid (Brooks, 1967; Salway & Logie, 1995). This requires the simultaneous processing and storage of spatial information.

Phonological working memory. Phonological working memory tasks measure the capacity of the phonological loop of Baddeley and Hitch's (1974) model (Baddeley, 2007; Baddeley & Larsen, 2007a, 2007b; Repovs & Baddeley, 2006). A number of complex span tasks measure phonological working memory, including reading span, operation span, and listening span.

Reading span was the first task developed to measure both storage and processing in working memory (Daneman & Carpenter, 1980). As such, it has served as a prototype for the subsequent development of a variety of measures of phonological and executive working memory (Dehn, 2008). The original reading span task required the examinee to read a number of sentences aloud and recall the last word from each in serial order (Daneman & Carpenter, 1980). In the same study, Daneman and Carpenter added a true-false component to ensure that participants attended to the sentences, preventing strategy use. Several modifications have since been made to this task, including versions that require participants to verify the grammatical accuracy of the sentence (Turner & Engle, 1989), and versions that require this in addition to recall of an unrelated word or individual letter rather than a word in the sentence (Conway et al., 2005; Engle et al., 1999; Kane et al., 2004). Reading span remains one of the most widely used measures of working memory in cognitive research.

Operation span was developed by Turner and Engle (1989) to investigate whether the correlation between reading comprehension and complex span was dependent on the nature of the secondary task. They modified reading span by replacing the sentences with mathematical equations, which participants had to verify as correct or incorrect. Turner and Engle then had the examinee read aloud a target word for serial recall following the operations. They found that operation span predicted reading comprehension ability despite the fact reading was not involved in the secondary task. This study demonstrated the existence of a common mechanism of working memory among complex span tasks.

In listening span, the examiner reads a number of sentences to the examinee and asks him or her to recall the last word in each sentence (Siegel & Ryan, 1989; Swanson & Howell, 2001). As with the complex span tasks already mentioned, this may be modified in a variety of ways to present additional challenge. For example, the individual may be asked a verification question about the sentence (Stothard & Hulme, 1992), or a cloze procedure may be used in which the examinee later recalls the words he or she used to complete the sentence (Siegel & Ryan, 1989).

Although they are not technically complex span tasks because there is no secondary processing task, there are two additional measures for assessing phonological working memory: memory for sentences and memory for stories. Memory for sentences involves recall of complete sentences (Jeffries, Ralph, & Baddeley, 2004), while memory for stories involves the retelling of short stories. These measures are thought to tap pure phonological working memory because the central executive is not involved. They also measure more than short-term memory because they involve meaning-based encoding and activation of long-term semantic memory (Dehn, 2008; Jeffries et al., 2004). Overall, measures of verbal working memory have been heavily researched and are widely used in both research and applied settings.

Executive working memory.
Tasks that measure executive working memory tap the central executive component of Baddeley and Hitch's (1974) model. Most of these measures tap both the central executive and the domain-specific skill used in the task (Coolidge & Wynn, 2005; Repovs & Baddeley, 2006). The central executive is primarily measured using alternative working memory tests, such as dual-processing tasks (Dehn, 2008; Repovs & Baddeley, 2006; Savage, Lavers, & Pillay, 2007); however, there are a few complex span tasks that tap this component (Dehn, 2008). For example, both backward word span and backward digit span are used to measure executive working memory. They are administered in the same way as forward word span and digit span, but the examinee is asked to recall the stimuli in reverse order, requiring

additional processing (Alloway et al., 2008). Computation span is another complex span task that is used (de Jong, 1998). In this test, the examinee orally reads simple math problems and states the answer aloud, following which the examiner reads out a digit. After a series of calculations, the individual is asked to recall the presented digits in order. Another recently developed task is reasoning span, which involves remembering the one-word solutions to a sequence of anaphora reasoning problems (Garcia-Madruga, Gutierrez, Carriedo, Luzon, & Vila, 2007). Despite the general popularity of complex span tasks in working memory measurement, some of the more common tasks used to measure the central executive use an alternative format.

Alternative measures.

In addition to complex span tasks, alternative tasks have been developed to measure working memory, particularly the central executive. Research on these measures is increasing as separate functions of this complex component continue to be identified and studied (Baddeley, 2007; Barch et al., 2009). Such tasks include trail-making, Stroop, *n*-back, random generation, star counting, and verbal-spatial association. Trail-making tasks require the examinee to quickly connect letters and numbers on a page in alphabetical and numerical order (Dehn, 2008). This assesses the ability to switch between retrieval and operations (Dehn, 2008). The Stroop task measures attention and the ability to inhibit irrelevant information or automatic responses. The basic form of the task involves reading a list of color words printed in discrepant colors (Dehn, 2008).

The *n*-back task requires the examinee to continuously report whether each item in a list matches the item that appeared *n* items ago (Conway et al., 2005; Dehn, 2008; Kirschner, 1958). This task has been used widely in the literature, however, there is controversy as to whether the *n*-back is a valid measure of working memory, particularly given that it does not measure the same construct as complex span tasks (Conway et al., 2005; Dehn, 2008; Kane, Conway, Miura, & Colfiesh, 2007; Miller, Price, Okun, Montijo, & Bowers, 2009; Shelton et al., 2009).

Random generation is a relatively simple task requiring examinees to randomly generate letters, numbers, or categorical words without repetitions (Dehn, 2008; Salway & Logie, 1995). Star counting measures inhibition in executive working memory. The examinee counts rows of stars that have addition and subtraction signs inserted at various points to indicate whether subsequent stars should be added or subtracted from the count total (Das-Smaal, de Jong, & Koopmans, 1993; de Jong & Das-Smaal, 1990). The second part of the task requires the examinee to reverse the meaning of the signs, incorporating further inhibition (Das-Smaal et al., 1993; de Jong, 1998; de Jong & Das-Smaal, 1990; Dehn, 2008; Savage et al., 2007).

Verbal-spatial association, or the verbal-to-spatial mapping task, requires the examinee to remember the spatial location of words presented on a computer screen (Cowan, Saults, & Morey, 2006). It is thought to be the first task to assess Baddeley's episodic buffer (Baddeley, 2000; Cowan et al., 2006). A new measure was recently designed to tap both visuospatial working memory and the episodic buffer (Price, 2009). The computerized object and abstract designs test (COAD) presents a dot grid containing various linear designs that are presented sequentially on a computer screen. Following presentation of the lines, the examinee must draw the figure on a sheet of paper (Price, 2009). This requires conscious processing, accessing long-term memory, visuospatial working memory, and binding of these functions in the episodic buffer (Price, 2009).

Additional tests such as running memory span and keep track tasks have also been developed, but have little research confirming their validity (Conway et al., 2005). At this point, the most popular, well-researched instruments used in the measurement of working memory are complex span tasks (Conway et al., 2005). Complex tasks, as well as a number of other tasks, are also frequently incorporated in memory and cognitive assessment batteries.

Memory Scales

In applied settings and clinical research, working memory is often assessed using memory scales. There are some scales designed to measure working memory specifically, while others measure broad memory capacities. Unfortunately, broad scales tend to disregard modern theories of working memory, including measures of working memory under a concentration or attention subscale (Dehn, 2008). The few tests that focus exclusively on working memory are fairly recent and undeveloped, however, unlike general memory tests they are often based on working memory theory, and are thus more adequate for clinical use (Dehn, 2008).

Wechsler Memory Scale – fourth edition (WMS-IV).

The WMS-IV (Wechsler, 2009) is a comprehensive memory assessment tool designed for individuals aged 16 to 90 years old. Index scores provide an indication of Auditory Memory, Visual Memory, Visual Working Memory, Immediate Memory, and Delayed Memory. The Visual Working Memory Index consists of two subtests: spatial addition and symbol span. While the previous version of the WMS (WMS-III; Wechsler, 1997b) measured both visual and auditory working memory, the WMS-IV was modified to measure only visual working memory in order to eliminate the construct overlap between the Wechsler Adult Intelligence Scale – third edition (WAIS-III; Wechsler, 1997a) and WMS-III (Pearson Assessments, 2009; Pearson Education, 2008). With these changes, the Wechsler Adult Intelligence Scale – fourth edition (WAIS-IV; Wechsler, 2008) and WMS-IV working memory indices are complementary, as the WAIS-IV Working Memory Index is intended to measure phonological working memory (Pearson Assessments, 2009).

Spatial addition replaced the Corsi block span task that was in the WMS-III (Pearson Education, 2008). In this subtest, the examinee is shown a grid with blue dots, red dots, or both for five seconds, following which he or she is shown a second grid with additional dots. The examinee is asked to add the spatial locations of the blue dots and cancel out blue dots that spatially overlap, and indicate the locations of the remaining blue dots with blue and white cards (Pearson Education, 2008). The results of this subtest correlate with the arithmetic subtest of the Working Memory Index on the WAIS-IV, and because of the high correlation, the publisher recommends that the WMS Visual Working Memory Index be used only when there is a specific hypothesis about visuospatial working memory, or a reason to believe that the WAIS-IV working memory index was not a valid measure of working memory (Pearson Assessments, 2009).

Symbol span is a visuospatial equivalent to digit span. The examinee views a page of symbols for five seconds, following which he or she must choose the correct symbols from a page in serial order. Symbol span involves only a forward recall condition (Pearson

Education, 2008), and thus may more accurately represent a measure of visuospatial short-term memory.

Wide Range Assessment of Memory and Learning – second edition (WRAML-2).
The WRAML-2 (Adams & Sheslow, 2003) is designed for individuals aged 5 to 90 years old, and consists of a Visual Memory Index, Verbal Memory Index, Attention/Concentration Index, and a Working Memory Index. Phonological working memory is measured with story memory and sentence memory tasks, while visuospatial working memory is measured using a picture memory task (Adams & Sheslow, 2003). Executive working memory is measured using the verbal working memory and symbolic working memory subtests. The verbal working memory task requires the examinee to separate animal words from non-animal words and arrange them by size before repeating the words in order. The symbolic working memory task requires the examinee to listen to a list of letters and numbers and subsequently indicate by pointing on a card the correct sequence of letters followed by numbers (Adams & Sheslow, 2003). The WRAML-2 has demonstrated validity, however, it uses simple span tasks to measure attention and concentration and there is no separate measure of working memory (Dehn, 2008).

Test of Memory and Learning – second edition (TOMAL-2).
The TOMAL-2 (Reynolds & Voress, 2007) is a comprehensive assessment battery designed for individuals aged 5 to 59 years old. Core indexes include Verbal Memory, Nonverbal Memory, and Composite Memory, while supplementary indexes include Verbal Delayed Recall, Learning, Attention and Concentration, Sequential Memory, Free Recall, and Associate Recall (Reynolds & Voress, 2007). The authors do not acknowledge working memory as a distinct construct, but instead place working memory subtests under measures of attention and concentration and sequential recall. Memory for stories is found under the Verbal Memory factor. The other two working memory tasks are under Attention and Concentration, and include digits backward and letters backward (Reynolds & Voress, 2007). The TOMAL-2 also includes several tests of short-term memory, including facial memory, abstract visual memory, memory for location, digits and letters forward, and manual imitation (Reynolds & Voress, 2007). Given that this test does not directly assess working memory, results must be used with caution when making inferences about working memory.

Swanson Cognitive Processing Test (S-CPT).
The S-CPT (Swanson, 1995) measures in-depth working memory in individuals aged 4.5 to 78.6 years. All of the tasks require simultaneous storage and processing of information, tapping executive working memory (Dehn, 2008). Many of the tasks in the S-CPT are derivations of Daneman and Carpenter's (1980) sentence span measure. Swanson (1995) also attempts to measure the influence of strategy knowledge and use through presenting the examinee with possible strategies for remembering information on certain tasks. In addition, the S-CPT measures a range of memory processes including retrieval, visuospatial, phonological, episodic, and semantic (Dehn, 2008; Swanson, 1995). Subtests include rhyming words, visual matrix, auditory digital sequence, mapping and directions, story retelling,

picture sequence, phrase sequence, spatial organization, semantic association, semantic categorization, and nonverbal sequencing (Swanson, 1995).

A primary advantage of the S-CPT is that the composite score is probably the best comprehensive measure of working memory available (Dehn, 2008). Importantly, this test is based on published research on valid measures of working memory. Accordingly, the S-CPT is correlated with learning and higher level memory processes (Swanson, 1995). Despite the benefits, concerns have been raised about the S-CPT regarding allowing extensive strategy use (St. Clair-Thompson, 2007), inadequacy of the standardization sample, complex administration and scoring rules, and having only two composite scores (Callahan, 1998).

Working Memory Test Battery for Children (WMTB-C).

The WMTB-C (Pickering & Gathercole, 2001) is a battery based directly on Baddeley and Hitch's (1974) multicomponent model of working memory. It is designed for children aged 5 to 15 years old and measures the visuospatial sketchpad, phonological loop, and central executive by producing three corresponding composites. Central executive subtests consist of complex span procedures, including backward digit recall, listening span, and counting recall. However, the tasks used to measure phonological and visuospatial working memory are simple span measures of short-term memory. Subtests that measure phonological storage include digit recall, word list recall, non-word list recall, and word list matching. Subtests that measure visuospatial storage include the Corsi blocks task and mazes memory (Pickering & Gathercole, 2001). Aside from its use of simple span tasks, the WMTB-C is a reliable and valid measure of short-term and working memory, and it has an advantage over many other batteries in its strong theoretical basis (Dehn, 2008).

Children's Memory Scale (CMS).

The CMS (Cohen, 1997) is a general memory scale designed to assess memory in children aged 5 to 16 who have neurodevelopmental or neurological disorders. This test does not explicitly measure working memory, but rather, assesses memory functioning in three domains: Visual/Nonverbal, Auditory/Verbal, and Attention/Concentration (Cohen, 1997). The Attention/Concentration index contains subtests that measure both short-term and working memory. Phonological working memory is measured by a memory for stories subtest (stories), executive working memory is measured using forward and backward digit span (numbers), and a sequences subtest that requires the examinee to recall a forward version of a well-known sequence (e.g., alphabet) followed by a backward version that has had interspersed items (Cohen, 1997). The CMS is valuable in the assessment of long-term storage and learning (Napolitano, 2001; Stein, 2001), though it is not as helpful for working memory assessment because it contains few working memory subtests and does not include an index (Dehn, 2008).

Automated Working Memory Assessment (AWMA).

The AWMA (Alloway, 2007a) is a computerized test of working memory designed to identify working memory problems in individuals aged 4 to 22 years old. The battery is based on Baddeley's (2000) four component model of working memory, however, because measures of visuospatial and phonological working memory involve executive working memory, specific tasks are aimed to measure only visuospatial and phonological working memory (Alloway et al., 2008). Importantly, the AWMA distinguishes between the measurement of short-term memory and the measurement of working memory (Alloway, 2007a), producing composites for Verbal Short-Term Memory (digit recall, word recall, nonword recall), Verbal Working Memory (listening recall, counting recall, backwards digit), Visuospatial Short-Term Memory (dot matrix, mazes memory, block recall), and Visuospatial Working Memory (odd-one-out, Mr. X, spatial span). The AWMA is a useful instrument for assessing short-term and working memory, and demonstrates a particularly important step in working memory assessment in its differentiation of working memory from short-term memory (Alloway et al., 2008; Baddeley, 2007; Dehn, 2008).

Rating Scales.
Recent research is showing promise in the use of parent and teacher rating scales for identification of children with working memory difficulties, as correlations between these measures and measures of working memory function have been demonstrated (Alloway, Gathercole, Holmes, et al., 2009; Alloway, Gathercole, Kirkwood, & Elliot, 2009; Mahone, Martin, Kates, Hay, & Horska, 2009). Although ratings of working memory involve indirect measurement they do have the potential to help identify individuals that would benefit from a more thorough assessment.

Cognitive Scales

Measures of short-term memory have been included in cognitive assessment batteries since their development in the early 20th century. Complex working memory tasks have also been incorporated, and with increasing awareness of the integral role of working memory in learning and cognitive functioning, measures of short-term and working memory are incorporated in nearly all tests of cognitive abilities (Dehn, 2008).

The Wechsler Scales.
Both the Wechsler Adult Intelligence Scale – fourth edition (WAIS-IV; Wechsler, 2008) and Wechsler Intelligence Scale for Children – fourth edition (WISC-IV; Wechsler, 2003) include short-term and working memory subtests. Both batteries include the same subtests on the Working Memory Index: digit span, letter-number sequencing, and arithmetic. The arithmetic subtest is actually a supplemental subtest that is not routinely administered in that it is intended for substitution when either digit span or letter-number sequencing cannot be administered. However, given that there are only two working memory subtests included on the composite working memory index, arithmetic is often administered for edification. Letter-number sequencing has been shown to be the most valid measure of the working memory construct in the Wechsler scales (Shelton et al., 2009). It involves recalling a verbally presented list of mixed letters and numbers in numerical followed by alphabetical order, drawing on both storage and processing. There are a few issues with the other measures, digit span and arithmetic. Digit span includes both digit span forward and backward, and thus confounds short-term and working memory. Fortunately, scaled scores are provided for both forward and backward tasks so they may be compared. Potentially more problematic is the use of the arithmetic subtest, as it is not an established measure of working memory. Here, the

individual listens to orally presented math problems and is asked to solve them mentally within a time limit. Although this process requires working memory, it is also highly dependent on mathematical ability, and thus may not be a valid measure (Dehn, 2008; Keith, Fine, Taub, Reynolds, & Kranzler, 2006; Shelton et al., 2009). There has been much controversy over the validity of this subtest, yet revisions of the Wechsler scales have continued to use it in the Working Memory Index. Thus, the Wechsler scales should be supplemented with other tests when detailed assessment of working memory is needed (Dehn, 2008; Shelton et al., 2009). Overall, scores on the Working Memory Index generally correlate with lab scores on working memory tasks (Shelton et al., 2009).

Alternatively, the Wechsler Intelligence Scale for Children – fourth edition, Integrated (WISC-IV Integrated; Wechsler et al., 2004) includes in-depth assessment of short-term and working memory through adding 16 supplemental processing subtests to the original WISC-IV battery (Wechsler, 2003). This allows measurement of phonological, visuospatial, and broad short-term and working memory. Subtests categorized as "registration" tasks measure short-term memory, and subtests categorized as "mental manipulation" tasks measure working memory. In addition to the subtests on the original WISC-IV, the WISC-IV Integrated includes visual digit span, spatial span (Corsi block task) with forward and backward conditions, letter span rhyming and non-rhyming, letter-number sequencing process approach, and arithmetic process approach. The modified letter-number sequencing task includes embedded words that may provide long-term retrieval cues if the examinee picks up on them. The modified arithmetic task involves completion of the original arithmetic task, readministration of items scored zero in part one, and finally, administration of a written arithmetic subtest for items that were scored zero in part two (Wechsler et al., 2004). The WISC-IV Integrated thus provides a more thorough assessment of working memory than the WISC-IV.

Stanford-Binet Intelligence Scales – fifth edition (SB5).

Like the Wechsler intelligence scales, the SB5 (Roid, 2003) is a general measure of intelligence. In addition to the Full Scale IQ, the SB5 produces a Verbal IQ and Nonverbal IQ, and verbal and nonverbal scores for each index. It measures five factors: Fluid Reasoning, Knowledge, Quantitative Processing, Visual-Spatial Processing, and Working Memory. The Working Memory index in the current version of the test replaced the Short-Term Memory index in the fourth edition (Johnson, 2005). Working memory subtests include memory for sentences and Daneman and Carpenter's (1980) listening span task (last word). Nonverbal working memory is measured using a variation of the Corsi block span that involves forward and backward span and requires the examinee to mentally sort block taps on blocks of different colored strips (Roid, 2003). Overall, the SB5 provides a relatively good measure of visuospatial and phonological working memory, particularly as digit tasks are excluded which reduces confounds due to arithmetic ability. However, as with the Wechsler scales, the SB5 must be supplemented with other subtests if a comprehensive assessment of working memory is needed (Dehn, 2008).

Cognitive Assessment System (CAS).

The CAS (Naglieri & Das, 1997) measures cognitive processes based on the Planning, Attention, Simultaneous, and Successive (PASS) theory (Naglieri, 2005; Naglieri & Das, 2005). Though working memory is not explicitly identified as part of the CAS, it is measured within the simultaneous and successive processing scales, and through a Stroop task (expressive attention) included in the Attention index and a trail-making task (planned connections) included in the Planning index. The Simultaneous Processing index includes figure memory, a visuospatial short-term memory task that requires the examinee to draw a geometric shape he or she was shown five seconds prior (Naglieri & Das, 1997). The Successive Processing index includes a word span task (word series) measuring phonological short-term memory, a memory for sentences task (sentence repetition) measuring phonological working memory through repetition of nonsense sentences, and a task called sentence questions that measures verbal and executive working memory through asking questions about the nonsense statements in the sentence repetition task (Naglieri, 2005). Although the CAS does not claim to measure working memory, it measures this construct directly, particularly given that interference and long-term semantic memory are excluded from the tasks (Dehn, 2008).

Woodcock-Johnson III (WJ III).

The WJ III consists of two batteries, the WJ III Test of Cognitive Abilities (WJ III COG; Woodcock, McGrew, & Mather, 2001a) and the WJ III Tests of Achievement (WJ III ACH; Woodcock, McGrew, & Mather, 2001b). The WJ III COG includes subtests to measure general intelligence and a range of cognitive abilities. This battery encourages examiners to select subtests based on factors they are looking to measure (Schrank, 2005). The Working Memory composite includes a backward digit span task (numbers reversed) and an auditory working memory subtest. This subtest measures phonological and executive working memory through the sorting and serial recall of interspersed digits and words (Woodcock et al., 2001a). The Working Memory composite may be combined with the Memory Span composite to provide a measure of the broader cognitive ability cluster Short-Term Memory. The Memory Span index includes memory for words and memory for sentences as measures of phonological short-term memory. The Short-Term Memory cluster is confounded by its inclusion of the Working Memory composite, and thus is not a measure of pure short-term memory. The Working Memory composite score may be used to represent executive working memory (Dehn, 2008), and may be supplemented with the memory for stories task (story recall) included on the WJ III ACH (Woodcock et al., 2001b). Overall, the WJ III provides adequate tests of some components of working memory, but is by no means a thorough measure.

Differential Ability Scales – second edition (DAS II).

The DAS II (Elliot, 2006) is a measure of cognitive abilities that includes three primary composites, Spatial Ability, Verbal Ability, and Nonverbal Reasoning Ability, and three optional clusters, School Readiness, Processing Speed, and Working Memory. Working Memory is measured with digits backward (recall of digits backward) and a subtest called recall of sequential order. In this subtest, the examinee is read a list of body parts and instructed to recall them from highest to lowest location on the body. As difficulty increases, other object names are interspersed with the list of body parts (Elliot, 2006). Phonological short-term memory is measured using digit span (recall of digits forward), and visuospatial short-term memory is measured using recall of designs and recognition of pictures (Elliot, 2006). The DAS II also assesses processing speed, visual processing, and phonological processing, which are closely related to working memory. This makes profile analysis especially useful. Another advantage is that the Working Memory cluster is not confounded by measures of short-term memory (Dehn, 2008).

Kaufman Assessment Battery for Children – second edition (KABC-II).

The KABC-II (Kaufman & Kaufman, 2004) measures cognitive abilities on five scales: Learning, Memory, Simultaneous processing, Planning, and Knowledge. The KABC-II is grounded in two theories of intelligence, Luria's neuropsychological model (Luria, 1980) and the Cattell-Horn-Carroll theory (Carroll, 1993; Horn & Blankson, 2005; McGrew, 2005). The test may therefore be interpreted according to either model (Kaufman, Kaufman, Kaufman-Singer, & Kaufman, 2005). The Memory scale includes a subtest called word order that measures executive working memory. For this subtest, the examinee touches a series of silhouettes of common objects in the order the examiner names them. On higher level items, interference is introduced through having the examinee complete a color naming task between the stimulus and response (Kaufman et al., 2005). The other two subtests on the Memory scale are measures of short-term memory, and include a forward digit span task (number recall) and hand movements. The hand movements task involves the examinee repeating hand movements in the same order as presented by the examiner (Kaufman et al., 2005). Although the KABC-II is a useful measure overall, the measurement of short-term and working memory is limited given the small number of subtests (Dehn, 2008).

Universal Nonverbal Intelligence Test (UNIT).

The UNIT (Bracken & McCallum, 1998) is a purely nonverbal assessment of intelligence. It was designed to accurately assess intelligence in linguistic minorities, children with hearing difficulties, and children with expressive or receptive language disabilities (McCallum & Bracken, 2005). The UNIT consists of three memory subtests and three reasoning subtests that make up four composites: Symbolic Memory, Nonsymbolic Memory, Symbolic Reasoning, and Nonsymbolic Reasoning. Symbolic Memory includes the symbolic memory and object memory subtests. In symbolic memory, the examinee is shown a sequence of universal symbols which he or she must recreate with response cards. In object memory, the examinee is shown a visual array of familiar objects for five seconds. After the array is removed, the examinee must place chips on the original objects as they appear in a second array that includes foils. Nonsymbolic memory consists of the spatial memory subtest which involves recreating a pattern of colored dots on a grid (Bracken & McCallum, 1998). The UNIT is limited in its measurement of working memory processes, however, it provides in-depth assessment of short-term visuospatial retention, and is useful with examinees that require a purely nonverbal battery (Dehn, 2008).

NEPSY II: A developmental neuropsychological assessment.

The NEPSY II (Korkman, Kirk, & Kemp, 2007) is a neuropsychological assessment tool that measures six domains: Attention and Executive Functioning, Language, Memory and Learning, Sensorimotor Functioning, Social Perception, and Visuospatial Processing. Within the Memory and Learning domain, visuospatial short-term memory is measured using memory for faces and memory for designs. In this same domain, verbal working memory is measured using a memory for stories task (narrative memory), a memory for sentences task (sentence repetition), and word list interference, which involves word recall following interference, and thus also measures executive working memory. Within the Language domain, phonological short-term memory is measured using repetition of nonsense words, which is basic pseudoword span (Korkman et al., 2007). The primary advantage of using the NEPSY II in working memory assessment is that it offers detailed assessment of executive functioning and language within the same battery, allowing for analysis of factors that may influence working memory performance (Dehn, 2008).

WORKING MEMORY MEASUREMENT AND INTELLIGENCE

A critical role of working memory assessment has been its contribution to the study of intelligence (Baddeley, 2003, 2007). Simple span tasks have been included in intelligence batteries since their development. Thus, associations between working memory and intelligence have been heavily studied over the years. Although issues in working memory measurement have complicated research at times, working memory generally demonstrates a high correlation with general intelligence, or Spearman's g (Ackerman et al., 2005; Baddeley, 2007; Colom et al. 2008; Colom, Flores-Mendoza, Quiroga, & Privado, 2005; Colom, Flores-Mendoza, & Rebollo, 2003; Colom, Rebollo, Palacios, Juan-Espinosa, & Kyllonen, 2004; Conway et al., 2002, 2003, 2005; Coolidge & Wynn, 2005; Embretson, 1995; Kane et al., 2004; Kaufman, DeYoung, Gray, Brown, & Mackintosh, 2009; Mackintosh & Bennett, 2003; Martinez & Colom, 2009; Oberauer, Sub, Wilhelm, & Wittmann, 2008; Salthouse & Pink, 2008; Sub, Oberauer, Wittman, Wilhelm, & Schulze, 2002; Troche & Rammsayer, 2009; Unsworth, Brewer, & Spillers, 2009).

In a review of the research on intelligence and working memory, Conway et al. (2003) found that working memory capacity accounts for one-third to one-half of the variance in general intelligence. Importantly, the tasks used to measure working memory have been shown to impact this relationship (Ackerman et al., 2005; Colom et al., 2008; Conway et al., 2003; Kane et al., 2004; Oberauer et al., 2008). Complex tasks that measure both storage and processing generally demonstrate stronger relationships than simple span tasks, which primarily measure short-term memory (Ackerman et al., 2005; Alloway et al., 2008; Bayliss, Jarrold, Baddeley, & Gunn, 2005; Colom et al., 2003; Conway et al., 2002, 2003, 2005; Kane et al., 2004; Shelton et al., 2009; Towse et al., 2000). Regardless, strong correlations between working memory and intelligence have been consistently demonstrated in the literature (Ackerman et al., 2005; Colom et. al., 2003, 2004, 2005, 2008; Conway et al., 2002, 2003, 2005; Embretson, 1995; Kane et al., 2004; Kaufman et al., 2009; Mackintosh & Bennett, 2003; Martinez & Colom, 2009; Oberauer et al., 2008; Salthouse & Pink, 2008; Sub et al., 2002; Troche & Rammsayer, 2009; Unsworth et al., 2009). This relationship has also been observed in children (Miller & Vernon, 1996; Tillman, Nyberg, & Bohlin, 2008) and adolescents (Fry & Hale, 1996). Some studies have found substantially high correlations, claiming that working memory is almost perfectly predicted by general intelligence (92% explained variance; Colom et al., 2004). Although it is clearly one of the primary cognitive processes underlying intelligence, many researchers have cautioned against this assumption (Ackerman et al., 2005; Conway et al., 2003; Embretson, 1995; Kane et al., 2004; Kaufman et al., 2009; Necka, 1992).

The precise nature of the relationship between working memory and intelligence remains ambiguous. For instance, some studies have reported that a domain-general function measured in both visuospatial and phonological tasks is associated with intelligence (Colom et al., 2003; Kane et al., 2004). Some studies have reported that working memory capacity is most highly correlated with IQ (Conway et al., 2002; Necka, 1992; Polczyk & Necka, 1997), while others have found alternative functions of working memory to be more related. Colom and colleagues (2008) concluded that short-term storage accounts for most of the relationship between working memory and intelligence. Another study found that, in regard to visuospatial working memory, it was encoding strategy rather than capacity that was behind the relationship (Cusack, Lehmann, Veldsman, & Mitchell, 2009). Salthouse and Pink (2008) also obtained results indicating that capacity is not likely the aspect of working memory most associated with intelligence, theorizing that greater intelligence is associated with greater ability to adapt to new working memory tasks and perform them effectively. Unsworth and Engle (2005) found that attentional control in working memory measures may be what links them to intelligence. Oberauer and colleagues (2008) found that measuring relational integration in working memory predicted intelligence at least as well as tasks measuring simultaneous storage and processing. One study reported that secondary memory processes accounted for all the variance in intelligence that was predicted by working memory, denouncing the unique role of working memory in the prediction of intelligence (Mogle, Lovett, Stawski, & Sliwinski, 2008). However, when this study was investigated by another research team, these conclusions were found to be false, as both working memory and secondary memory were uniquely associated with intelligence (Unsworth et al., 2009). Some of these inconsistencies in results may be related to issues in working memory measurement, or alternatively, could be associated with findings that high intelligence individuals show much greater domain specificity in working memory (Kane et al., 2004), which may produce varied outcomes depending on the sample.

There has also been some research investigating the relationship between working memory and different components of intelligence. For example, Haavisto and Lehto (2004) examined correlations between measures of working memory and fluid and crystallized intelligence. They found that phonological working memory was associated with crystallized intelligence, while visuospatial working memory was associated with fluid intelligence (Haavisto & Lehto, 2004). Martinez and Colom (2009) demonstrated that working memory predicted fluid intelligence, but not crystallized or spatial intelligence when the variance due to fluid intelligence was removed. This remains consistent with existing literature on the relationship between working memory and general intelligence, as fluid intelligence is often considered representative of Spearman's *g* (Horn & Blankson, 2005; Martinez & Colom, 2009). Sub and colleagues (2002) also reported findings that specific working memory resources are associated with specific domains within general intelligence. Overall, it is clear that working memory and *g* are related to one another. Only further research with more defined theories and measures will clarify the specific nature of this relationship.

WORKING MEMORY MEASUREMENT AND AGING

Measurement of working memory has also been prominent in research on aging and cognitive decline in later life. The literature has consistently shown that aging is associated with declines in working memory function (e.g., Bailey, Dunlosky, & Hertzog, 2009; Bopp & Verhaeghen, 2009; Borella, Carretti, & De Beni, 2008; Brebion, Smith & Ehrlich, 1997; Briggs, Raz, & Marks, 1999; Caggiano, Jiang, & Parasuraman, 2006; Campbell & Charness, 1990; Chen & Li, 2007; De Beni, Borella, & Carretti, 2007; Dobbs & Rule, 1989; Gazzaley, Sheridan, Cooney, & D'Esposito, 2007; Hartley, Speer, Jonides, Reuter-Lorenz, & Smith, 2001; Hartman, Bolton, & Fehnel, 2001; Hartman, Dumas, & Nielsen, 2001; Haut, Chen, & Edwards, 1999; Hedden & Park, 2001; Hertzog, Dixon, Hultsch, & MacDonald, 2003; Mutter, Haggbloom, Plumlee, & Schirmer, 2006; Piolino et al., 2010; Pratt, Boyes, Robins, & Manchester, 1989; Ros, Latorre, & Serrano, 2010; Salthouse, Babcock, & Shaw, 1991; Vaughn, Basak, Hartman, & Verhaeghen, 2008; Verhaeghen & Hoyer, 2007; Voelcker-Rehage, Stronge, & Alberts, 2006). Deficits have also been shown in specific components of working memory. Many studies have demonstrated impairment of visuospatial working memory in later life (Baddeley, Cocchini, Sala, Logie, & Spinnler, 1999; Cornoldi, Bassani, Berto, & Mammarella, 2007; Mammarella, Fairfield, De Beni, & Cornoldi, 2009; Mikels, Larkin, Reuter-Lorenz, & Carstensen, 2005; Rowe, Hasher, & Turcotte, 2008). Chen, Hale, and Myerson (2003) found that specifically, older adults exhibit significant deficits in spatial working memory, but not visual object working memory. Aside from visuospatial working memory, Hartman and Warren (2005) found that older adults demonstrated significant impairments in temporal working memory due to decreases in associative ability and particular difficulty with order information.

Along this line of research, investigators have also examined specific functions of working memory that are impaired and may thus underlie the deficits in working memory observed in later life. Some researchers have demonstrated working memory deficits due to decreased capacity (Babcock & Salthouse, 1990; Foos, 1989; Kumar, Rakitin, Nambisan, Habeck, & Stern, 2008). Some studies have emphasized particular impairment under high loads (Gazzaley et al., 2007; Kliegel & Jager, 2006; Mitchell, Johnson, Raye, Mather, & D'Esposito, 2000; Van der Linden, Bredart, & Beerten, 1994), which has been shown to be associated with deficiencies in binding (Mitchell et al., 2000; Piolino et al., 2010). Several researchers have found that deficits in working memory are largely associated with impairments in inhibition of irrelevant material (Cornoldi et al., 2007; Hedden & Park, 2001; Kliegel & Jager, 2006; Mammarella et al., 2009; Van Gerven, Van Boxtel, Meijer, Willems, & Jolles, 2007) and interference (Rowe et al., 2008; Rowe, Hasher, & Turcotte, 2009; Schmiedek, Li, & Lindenberger, 2009). Some studies have shown that active maintenance is the primary source of working memory dysfunction (Baddeley et al., 1999; Caggiano et al., 2006), while some have demonstrated that updating in the central executive is particularly associated with deficits (Chen & Li, 2007; Hartman, Bolton, et al., 2001; Hartman, Dumas, et al., 2001; Van der Linden et al., 1994). Some researchers have also demonstrated that deficits in focus switching are associated with observed declines in working memory (Vaughan et al., 2008; Verhaeghen & Hoyer, 2007). Voelcker-Rehage and colleagues (2006) also demonstrated that cognitive-motor deficits are associated with declines in performance under dual-task conditions. Finally, a number of studies have shown that decreases in working memory scores are associated with age-related decreases in processing speed (Babcock & Salthouse, 1990; Bailey et al., 2009; Chaytor & Schmitter-Edgecombe, 2004; Fisk & Warr, 1996; Hartley et al., 2001; Kumar et al., 2008; Salthouse, 1992).

Given the relationship between working memory and intelligence, it is not surprising that researchers have found that declines in working memory are associated with age-related cognitive declines (Borella et al., 2008; Chen & Li, 2007; Nettelbeck & Burns, 2010; Salthouse, 1991). Working memory has also been shown to be associated with declines in perceptual-motor skill (Kennedy, Partridge, & Raz, 2008) and slowing of information processing (Briggs et al., 1999). Age-related declines in working memory have also been shown to contribute to decreases in matrix reasoning performance (Salthouse, 1993), decreases in discrimination learning, particularly for non-occurrence conditions (Mutter et al., 2006), and difficulty with delayed execution of actions (Kliegel & Jager, 2006). Working memory impairment has also been shown to correlate with decreases in episodic memory (Hertzog et al., 2003) and autobiographical memory (Piolino et al., 2010; Ros et al., 2010). Specifically, Ros and colleagues (2010) observed a decrease in specific autobiographical memories and an increase in general memories. Declines in working memory have also been demonstrated to decrease reading comprehension (Brebion et al., 1997; De Beni et al., 2007) and accuracy of story retelling (Pratt et al., 1989). Thus, age-related declines in working memory have important implications for changes in everyday behaviors and abilities.

Fortunately some research has found that extensive working memory practice may be helpful in increasing some working memory functions (Li et al., 2008). In addition, despite general declines in working memory with age, some abilities are preserved, such as working memory for emotional material (Mikels et al., 2005), inhibition of domain-general interference (Rose, Myerson, Sommers, & Hale, 2009), reliance on familiar information in working memory performance (Schmeidek et al., 2009), structural and operational working memory capacity (Salthouse et al., 1991), and content-with-context binding in working memory (Bopp & Verhaeghen, 2009). Thus, the decline in working memory is not necessarily global.

Finally, along with research on aging, much research has been done on working memory and dementia. In individuals with Alzheimer's Disease (AD), working memory deficits have been shown to be associated with loss of financial capacity (Earnst et al., 2001). Research has consistently found declines in working memory associated with both AD and its precursor, mild cognitive impairment (MCI; Baddeley et al., 1999; Baddeley, Bressi, Sala, Logie, & Spinnler, 1991; Baddeley, Logie, Bressi, Sala, & Spinnler, 1986; Belleville, Chertkow & Gauthier, 2007; Belleville, Rouleau, Van der Linden, & Collette, 2003; Earnst et al., 2001; Haut et al., 1998; Huntley & Howard, 2010; Price et al., 2010; Small, Andersen, & Kempler, 1997). MCI is associated with impairments in semantic coding due to strategic functioning of the episodic buffer (Price et al., 2010), attentional control that continues to decline with the development of AD (Belleville et al., 2007), and visuospatial and executive working memory (Huntley & Howard, 2010). Huntley and Howard (2010) found that there were no significant phonological working memory impairments in mild AD, rather, these deficits developed later in the progression of the disease. Individuals with AD have also demonstrated severe impairments in alphabetic recall (Belleville et al., 2003), dual-task performance (Baddeley et al., 1991), central executive working memory (Baddeley et al., 1986; Baddeley et al., 1999), and semantic processing of written passages (Haut et al., 1998). Given that AD is a chronic degenerative brain disease that is largely diagnosed based on memory impairment (Fellner &

Reddon, 2010), the consistent demonstration of severe working memory deficit in this population is not surprising.

WORKING MEMORY MEASUREMENT IN CLINICAL APPLICATIONS

Measurement of working memory is invaluable in applied settings, as research has shown working memory function to be related to a number of neurological disorders, medical conditions, genetic disorders, developmental delays and disabilities, learning disabilities, and psychiatric diagnoses. This research has had significant implications in the identification and treatment of many of these conditions. Although there remain inconsistencies in the literature in regard to particular conditions, the work that has been done remains valuable, and many questions are open for future research. An important reminder here is of the need for further research on the assessment of working memory in an effort toward refinement of the construct and standardization of theoretically-based measures that can be used reliably across research and practice. This would create greater consistency in research results, and contribute to advances in remediation.

In what follows next, some of clinical correlates of working memory that have been found in the research literature are reviewed.

Neurological Disorders

Several neurological disorders impact the functioning of working memory. Research with children with cerebral palsy has demonstrated deficits in executive functioning, visuospatial working memory, and phonological working memory (Jenks et al., 2007; Jenks, de Moor, & van Lieshout, 2009; Peeters, Verhoeven, & de Moor, 2009). Such studies have found that the deficits in executive functioning and visuospatial working memory are strongly related to arithmetic difficulties these children experience (Jenks et al., 2007, 2009), and deficits in phonological working memory capacity are thought to result from auditory perception and speech impairments in these children (Peeters et al., 2009). General deficiencies in working memory have also been found in children with hydrocephalus (Boyer, Yeates, & Enrile, 2006). Working memory deficits have also been identified in some individuals with multiple sclerosis, particularly when high demands are placed on the central executive component (D'Esposito et al., 1996; Lengenfelder et al., 2006).

Impairments in working memory have also been observed in individuals with Parkinson's disease (Bublak, Muller, Gron, Reuter, & von Gramon, 2002; Gilbert, Belleville, Bherer, & Chouinard, 2005; Hochstadt, Nakano, Lieberman, & Friedman, 2006; Kensinger, Shearer, Locascio, Growdon, & Corkin, 2003; Possin, Filoteo, Song, & Salmon, 2008; Siegert, Weatherall, Taylor, & Abernethy, 2008; West, Ergis, Winocur, & Saint-Cyr, 1998), though there has been some debate as to the nature of the impairment (Siegert et al., 2008). Some studies have identified impairment in the central executive in manipulation of information, with no significant deficit in short-term storage (Bublak et al., 2002; Gilbert et al., 2005; Kensinger et al., 2003; West et al., 1998). However, a meta-analysis conducted by Siegert and colleagues (2008) revealed significant impairment on verbal working memory, and importantly, on both short-term and working memory in visuospatial tasks. The greater deficit in visuospatial memory suggests that working memory impairment may not be solely in the central executive in Parkinson's disease (Siegert et al., 2008). Though there may be debate between researchers regarding specific memory impairments associated with neurological disorders, it is generally agreed upon that many neurological disorders involve some dysfunction of working memory.

Medical Conditions

In addition to neurological disorders, a number of other medical conditions have been shown to impact working memory function. Vicari, Caravale, Carlesimo, Casadei, and Allemand (2004) demonstrated that low birth weight, preterm infants who did not have cognitive disorders had significant impairment in visuospatial working memory at ages three and four years old. In a study investigating working memory in eight to nine year olds who had been exposed to cocaine prenatally, Mayes, Snyder, Langlois, and Hunter (2007) found that these children had a relative deficit in visuospatial working memory compared to controls. Nulsen, Fox, and Hammond (2010) in a meta-analysis found that cumulative use of ecstacy was associated with increasing impairment in verbal (22 studies) and visuospatial (9 studies) measures of working memory. Measures of short-term memory were also impacted but not related to lifetime usage (30 verbal studies and 12 visuospatial studies). A review of the literature studying working memory in individuals with Fetal Alcohol Spectrum Disorder (FASD) found that prenatal exposure to alcohol is associated with deficits in working memory, particularly in the central executive (Rasmussen, 2005).

Working memory has also been shown to be a significant predictor of cognitive complaints in individuals with HIV, and may result from a decline in working memory as a result of HIV infection (Bassel, Rourke, Halman, & Smith, 2002). Long term deficits in working memory have also been observed as a result of cranial radiation therapy for leukemia in childhood, and are thought to be associated with the observed declines in measures of intelligence (Schatz, Kramer, Ablin, & Matthay, 2000). Finally, research has found working memory deficits associated with traumatic brain injury (TBI; Levin et al., 2004; Mandalis, Kinsella, Ong, & Anderson, 2007; Newsome et al., 2008; Vallat-Azouvi, Weber, Legrand, & Azouvi, 2007). Levin and colleagues (2004) found that within three months of injury, all the children in their study showed improved working memory function. However, between one and two years post-injury, children with severe TBI showed a decline in working memory while children with milder TBI showed continued improvement in working memory as a result of development and recovery (Levin et al., 2004). Mandalis and colleagues (2007) found that children with TBI had deficits in the central executive and phonological loop, and that these deficits were related to difficulties with new learning due to poor encoding. Similarly, working memory impairment has been found in adults with TBI, particularly in central executive tasks requiring controlled processing (Vallat-Azouvi et al., 2007).

Genetic Disorders

Some genetic disorders have also been found to have associated deficits in working memory. Lanfranchi, Cornoldi, Drigo, and Vianello (2009) found that children with Fragile X syndrome have impaired central executive functioning, as evidenced by significant differences from controls on working memory tasks requiring medium and high levels of control. In a study on children with early-treated phenylketonuria (PKU), results indicated that older children with PKU had significantly poorer working memory scores than controls on both visuospatial and phonological tasks (White, Nortz, Mandernach, Huntington, & Steiner, 2002). In addition, a number of studies have found that individuals with Down syndrome have deficits in the central executive and phonological working memory, though visuospatial working memory tends to be appropriate for their mental age (Baddeley & Jarrold, 2007; Gathercole & Alloway, 2006; Jarrold, Baddeley, & Hewes, 1999; Lanfranchi, Carretti, Spano, & Cornoldi, 2009; Lanfranchi, Jerman, & Vianello, 2009; Numminen, Service, Ahonen, & Ruoppila, 2001). One study found a deficit in simultaneous visuospatial working memory tasks, but not in sequential visuospatial working memory tasks, which may indicate appropriate visuospatial abilities with impairment in central executive functioning (Lanfranchi, Caretti, et al., 2009). The opposite profile has been observed in individuals with Williams syndrome, who tend to display substantial impairment of visuospatial working memory (Gathercole & Alloway, 2006; Jarrold et al., 1999).

Intellectual and Developmental Disabilities

Not surprisingly, a number of studies have found that deficits in working memory are associated with cognitive and developmental disabilities. Working memory impairments have been found repeatedly in individuals with intellectual disabilities (Carretti, Belacchi, & Cornoldi, 2010; Henry & Winfield, 2010; Maehler & Shuchardt, 2009; Numminen et al., 2000; Numminen, Lehto, & Ruoppila, 2001; Numminen, Service, & Ruoppila, 2002; Schuchardt, Gebhardt, & Maehler, 2010; Van der Molen, Van Luit, Jongmans, & Van der Molen, 2007). Studies differentiating between the components of working memory have found that individuals with intellectual disability have deficits in the visuospatial sketchpad and central executive that match the ability of mental age-matched controls (Numminen et al., 2000; Schuchardt et al., 2010; Van der Molen et al., 2007). However, even when compared to controls with equivalent mental age, individuals with intellectual disability display a severe deficit in phonological working memory. Thus, it is possible that these persons demonstrate a developmental lag in visuospatial and executive working memory, but have structurally different phonological working memory (Schuchardt et al., 2010; Van der Molen et al., 2007). Numminen, Lehto, et al. (2001) also showed that adults with intellectual disability compared to controls matched for fluid intelligence (children between the ages of three and six) demonstrated phonological and visuospatial working memory deficits, but performed equally as well or better than controls on tasks based on knowledge, skills, or familiar semantic information. Thus, it appears that individuals with intellectual disability draw on long-term memory for the performance of working memory tasks when possible (Numminen, Service, et al., 2001). Research on academic performance in individuals with intellectual disability has shown that phonological working memory is associated with reading and writing skills, while executive working memory is related to number skills (Henry & Winfield, 2010; Numminen et al., 2000). Finally, literature examining executive working memory in more detail has found that individuals with intellectual disability have particular impairment in updating and inhibition (Carretti et al., 2010; Numminen, Lehto, et al., 2001).

In addition to intellectual disability, a number of other developmental disabilities have shown correlations with working memory function. There have been inconsistent findings regarding the relationship between Autism Spectrum Disorders (ASD) and working memory (Gokcen, Bora, Erermis, Kesikci, & Aydin, 2009). Russell, Jarrold, and Henry (1996) found deficits in the executive working memory of children with autism when compared to normal controls, while Torii, Shimoyama, and Sugita (2010) found children with autism had no deficits in working memory function itself, but rather only in use of semantic strategy. This impairment in semantic strategy is consistent with the social deficits observed in autism (Torii et al., 2010). Alloway, Rajendran, and Archibald (2009) found that children with Asperger syndrome had deficits in verbal short-term memory, and another study investigating parents of children with ASD demonstrated deficits in verbal working memory (Gokcen et al., 2009). Taken together, these findings emphasize the importance of task selection in the measurement of working memory, as it is possible that difficulties with interpretation of meaning in individuals with ASD is associated with the deficits in verbal working memory that have been observed (Gokcen et al., 2009; Torii et al., 2010).

Results from studies on individuals with specific language impairment (SLI) have been very consistent, indicating a domain-specific impairment in phonological short-term and working memory (Alloway, Rajendran, et al., 2009; Alloway & Archibald, 2008; Gathercole & Alloway, 2006; Montgomery, 1995, 2000; Norrelgen, Lacerda, & Forssberg, 2002). Children with SLI demonstrate a particularly severe deficit in the pseudoword repetition task, which is identified as a phenotypic marker of SLI (Gathercole & Alloway, 2006). Working memory impairments have also been demonstrated in individuals with developmental coordination disorder (DCD). Children with DCD have deficits in both verbal and visuospatial short-term and working memory (Alloway, 2007b; Alloway, Rajendran, et al., 2009; Alloway & Archibald, 2008; Alloway & Temple, 2007), with particularly marked impairment in visuospatial working memory (Alloway, 2007b; Alloway, Rajendran, et al., 2009). Working memory deficits in individuals with SLI and DCD are likely related to many of the associated symptoms, as well as difficulties in learning and academic achievement.

Substantial research has been done on the correlations between working memory and attention deficit hyperactivity disorder (ADHD). Findings have been inconsistent with this population. Some studies have reported general working memory deficits in individuals with ADHD (Alloway, Gathercole, Holmes, et al., 2009; Buzy, Medoff, & Schweitzer, 2009; Karatekin & Asarnow, 1998; Martinussen, Hayden, Hogg-Johnson, & Tannock, 2005; McInnes, Humphries, Hogg-Johnson, & Tannock, 2003; Rapport et al., 2008; Stevens, Quittner, Zuckerman, & Moore, 2002), some have emphasized deficits in visuospatial working memory (Barnett et al., 2001; Marchetta, Hurks, Krabbendam, & Jolles, 2008; McInnes et al., 2003; Westerberg, Hirvikoski, Forssberg, & Klingberg, 2004), and others have emphasized demands on executive working memory (Kofler, Rapport, Bolden, Sarver, & Raiker, 2010). Other researchers have found that individuals with ADHD do not exhibit deficits in working memory (de Freitas Messina, Tiedemann, de Andrade, & Primi, 2006; Jonsdottir, Bouma, Sergeant, & Scherder, 2005; Palladino, 2006; Siegel & Ryan, 1989), while still others have reported normal working memory functioning in general accompanied by deficits in inhibitory executive processes (Brocki, Nyberg, Thorell, & Bohlin, 2007; Cornoldi et al., 2001; Karatekin, 2004; Kerns, McInerney & Wilde, 2001; Ross, Harris, Olincy, & Radant, 2000; Sonuga-Barke, Dalen, Daley, & Remington, 2002). Research has even reported that impaired inhibitory processes are not involved either (Engelhardt, Nigg, Carr, & Ferreira, 2008). Given the conflicting results in the literature, there is not enough evidence to conclude that impaired working memory is a characteristic of ADHD (Gathercole & Alloway, 2006). A number of confounding factors are possible, such as the tasks used to measure working memory or the possibility that working memory results are confounded by hyperactive behavior (Alloway, Gathercole, Holmes, et al., 2009; Gathercole & Alloway, 2006).

Despite inconsistencies in some of the research on correlates between working memory and intellectual and developmental disabilities, there are many disabilities that show strong links with working memory impairment, which is very useful in informing diagnosis and interventions. Hopefully, as models and measures of working memory continue to be refined, we will obtain increasingly specific and helpful results from applied clinical research.

Learning Disabilities

Another field that has seen much research on correlates with working memory is the study of learning disabilities (LD). Unfortunately, there have also been mixed results in working memory research in this field. Some studies on individuals with general LD have reported a general working memory deficiency in this population (Gathercole, Alloway, Willis, & Adams, 2006; Maehler & Schuchardt, 2009; Swanson, 1993b, 2000, 2003; Swanson & Sachse-Lee, 2001b), while others have found deficits in short-term but not working memory (Bayliss, Jarrold, Baddeley, & Leigh, 2005). Research on individuals with mathematical learning disabilities has also produced mixed results perhaps because because the relationships between math ability and working memory are complicated by such factors age, skill level, and type of skill (Raghubar, Barnes, & Hecht, 2010). Some studies have reported primarily general working memory deficits (Geary, Hoard, Byrd-Craven, & DeSoto, 2004; Keeler & Swanson, 2001; Mabbot & Bisanz, 2008; Passolunghi & Siegel, 2001; Wilson & Swanson, 2001), while some have reported only counting deficits, but no working memory impairments (Hitch & McAuley, 1991). Generally, however, most of the literature examining math disabilities reports deficits in visuospatial working memory and some aspect of the central executive, typically pertaining to inhibition or high-load storage and processing of information (Andersson & Lyxell, 2007; McLean & Hitch, 1999; Passolunghi & Cornoldi, 2008; Passolunghi & Siegel, 2004; Schuchardt, Maehler, & Hasselhorn, 2008; van der Sluis, van der Leij, & de Jong, 2005).

A substantial amount of research has also been done on individuals with reading disabilities, and has also reported mixed findings (Savage et al., 2007). As with general LD, some studies have found a relatively general working memory deficit in individuals with reading disabilities (de Jong, 1998; Ram-Tsur, Faust, & Zivotofsky, 2008; Smith-Spark & Fisk, 2007; Swanson, 1993a; Swanson, & Ashbaker, 2000; Swanson, Ashbaker, & Lee, 1996; Swanson & Berninger, 1995; Swanson, Howard, & Saez, 2006; Swanson & Sachse-Lee, 2001a; Torii et al., 2010), while others have found that only phonological working memory is impaired (Barbosa, Miranda, Santos, & Bueno, 2009; Kibby & Cohen, 2008; Schuchardt et al., 2008; Steinbrink & Klatte, 2007), and yet others have reported only deficits in phonological storage (Kibby, Marks, Morgan, & Long, 2004; Robertson & Joanisse, 2010) or no deficit in working memory at all (van der Sluis et al., 2005). Some researchers have found a phonological working memory deficit in addition to some impairments in executive working memory (Berninger et al., 2006; Jeffries & Everatt, 2004). Alternatively, some studies have found that deficits in the central executive are primarily associated with reading difficulties (Swanson, 1999; Swanson, Cochran, & Ewers, 1989; Swanson & Jerman, 2007). Central executive deficits have also been found to be implicated in specific difficulties in reading comprehension (Swanson et al., 2006; Swanson & Berninger, 1995), as well as verbal working memory (Nation, Adams, Bowyer-Crane, & Snowling, 1999). A meta-analysis conducted by Swanson, Zheng, and Jerman (2009) found that children with reading disabilities have deficits in components of the phonological loop and central executive. Specifically, they found that the primary issue in the phonological loop was access to speech codes, and difficulty in the executive system was involved in the simultaneous monitoring of storage and processing of information (Swanson et al., 2009). Savage and colleagues (2007) reported similar results in their review of the literature. They found that despite the mixed evidence in the literature, generally speaking there is a phonological processing deficit in individuals with dyslexia, while impairments associated with reading comprehension remain less clear considering there are a number of potential issues that may contribute to comprehension difficulties (Savage et al., 2007).

There are several potential methodological issues that have likely contributed to the inconsistencies in the LD literature. For instance, it is essential that researchers distinguish between types of reading and mathematical difficulties, as different mechanisms may be associated with different subtypes (Savage et al., 2007). Again, an issue of primary importance is the difference in working memory measures between researchers. The use of valid, standardized measures that are consistent among researchers would contribute to more coherent results regarding areas of strength and weakness in working memory (Savage et al., 2007).

Psychiatric Conditions

Deficits in working memory have also been shown to be associated with a variety of psychological concerns and psychiatric diagnoses. Working memory deficits have been shown to be associated with Dysthymia and depression (Arnett et al., 1999; Deldin, Deveney, Kim, Casas, & Best, 2001; Franklin et al., 2010; Joormann & Gotlib, 2008; Nebes et al., 2000). In looking at children with Dysthymia, Franklin and colleagues (2010) found that the children demonstrated deficits in visuospatial working memory, particularly the executive component. Nebes and colleagues (2000) found that depressed elderly people showed impaired working memory performance compared to non-depressed controls, and Arnett and colleagues (1999) found that depressed multiple sclerosis patients demonstrated particular impairment in the central executive. Other studies have shown that differences in working memory in depressed individuals are related to increased processing of negative information, and particular difficulty removing irrelevant negative information from working memory

(Deldin et al., 2001; Joorman & Gotlib, 2008). In addition to correlates with depression, research has found that bipolar disorder is associated with deficits in visuospatial working memory (Allen et al., 2010) and some aspects of executive working memory (Allen et al., 2010; Larson, Shear, Krikorian, Welge, & Strakowski, 2005). Bora and colleagues (2008) have also found phonological and executive working memory deficits in first degree relatives of individuals with bipolar disorder, indicating a possible marker of genetic vulnerability to the disorder.

Research has also shown associations between visual working memory and phobias (Reinecke, Rinck, & Becker, 2006). Correlations have also been shown between working memory and trauma, as well as eye movement desensitization and reprocessing therapy for trauma (Gunter & Bodner, 2008; Lilley, Andrade, Turpin, Sabin-Farrell, & Holmes, 2009). Dobbs, Dobbs, and Kiss (2001) found that cognitive deficits associated with chronic fatigue syndrome (CFS) were partially related to control processes of the central executive, while Deluca and colleagues (2004) found no differences between individuals with CFS and healthy controls on measures of working memory, rather they only demonstrated deficits in processing speed. General impairments in working memory have also been found in individuals with borderline personality disorder (Stevens, Burkhardt, Hautzinger, Schwarz, & Unckel, 2004), and verbal working memory impairments have been found in those with schizotypal personality disorder (McClure et al., 2007). Visuospatial and central executive working memory deficits have also been found in individuals with schizotypy (Matheson & Langdon, 2008; Park, Holzman, & Lenzenweger, 1995; Tallent & Gooding, 1999), and thus may be a marker for risk of developing schizophrenia (Wood et al., 2003).

Schizophrenia is the most heavily researched psychiatric diagnosis in working memory studies. Research with people diagnosed with schizophrenia has generally been consistent, showing a pervasive deficit in working memory associated with the disorder (Barch, Csernansky, Conturo, & Snyder, 2002; Brown et al., 2007; Chey, Lee, Kim, Kwon, & Shin, 2002; Forbes, Carrick, McIntosh, & Lawrie, 2009; Granholm, Morris, Sarkin, Asarnow, & Jeste, 1997; Karatekin & Asarnow, 1998; Lee & Park, 2005; Ross et al., 2000; Stone, Gabrieli, Stebbins, & Sullivan, 1998; Stratta, Prosperini, Daneluzzo, Bustini, & Rossi, 2001; Sullivan, Shear, Zipursky, Sagar, & Pfefferbaum, 1997; Zanello, Curtis, Ba, & Merlo, 2009). This is typically attributed to the prefrontal lobe dysfunction characteristic of schizophrenia (Chey et al., 2002; Forbes et al., 2009; Lee & Park, 2005; Stone et al., 1998; Zanello et al., 2009). Many studies have investigated specific components of working memory as well, finding deficits in the central executive (Oram, Geffen, Geffen, Kavanagh, & McGrath, 2005; Pantelis et al., 2004), visuospatial sketchpad (Burglen et al., 2004; Cocchi et al., 2007; Coleman et al., 2002; Fuller et al., 2009; Gold, Wilk, McMahon, Buchanan, & Luck, 2003; Pantelis et al., 2004; Piskulic, Olver, Norman, & Maruff, 2007; Snyder et al., 2008), and phonological loop (Fleming, Goldberg, Gold, & Weinberger, 1995). Literature has also reported findings on specific deficiencies within working memory, such as slowed consolidation (Fuller, Luck, McMahon, & Gold, 2005) and binding (Burglen et al., 2004; Salame, Burglen, & Danion, 2006). Cameron and colleagues (2002) also reported on the specific details of working memory subcomponents involved in negative, positive and disorganized symptoms of schizophrenia. Detailed meta-analyses have verified these consistencies in the literature as well (Forbes et al., 2009; Lee & Park, 2005). Thus, assessment of working memory is extremely valuable in clinical populations.

CONCLUSION: ISSUES IN THE MEASUREMENT OF WORKING MEMORY

Despite the number of tasks, scales, and measures designed to assess working memory, there remains a great deal of controversy and debate regarding measurement. One basic issue is that the construct of working memory itself continues to be somewhat ambiguous and undefined. Working memory is a purely theoretical concept, and there are a number of different models and hypotheses regarding its structure and functions. Therefore, it is not fully clear what measures of working memory are actually measuring (Baddeley, 2007; Bayliss, Jarrold, Baddeley, & Gunn, 2005; Conway et al., 2003, 2005; McCabe, 2008; Savage et al., 2007; Towse et al., 2000; Towse & Hitch, 1995). In addition, there are no specific tasks that are pure measures of the particular working memory components they claim to measure (Conway et al., 2005), and thus tasks often measure more than one process or ability. For instance, a complex task may involve the central executive and verbal ability, and if an individual has a specific verbal deficit, the measure will underestimate his or her working memory function. In this situation, the individual's working memory score may not correlate with his or her general cognitive abilities (Baddeley, 2007; Conway et al., 2005).

Given the wide range of tasks that measure working memory, it is unclear how these tasks relate to one another or to specific functions of working memory (Conway et al., 2003; Savage et al., 2007; Shelton et al., 2009; Towse et al., 2000; Towse & Hitch, 1995; Unsworth & Engle, 2007). For example, the degree to which storage and processing are involved in complex span tasks, and which aspects of each of these functions are involved in any given task, is unclear (Conway et al., 2005; Savage et al., 2007; Towse & Hitch, 1995; Unsworth & Engle, 2007). In addition, despite overall research findings that simple and complex span tasks measure different constructs, some studies have reported that they actually measure the same cognitive processes (Unsworth & Engle, 2007). The ecological validity of working memory measures has also been questioned when related to everyday processing, as the processing required in tasks is not the same as required in daily life (Savage et al., 2007). As well, despite the fact that complex span tasks do not rely heavily on prior knowledge (Baddeley, 2007), many tasks incorporate *some* knowledge, and individuals who have prior knowledge of the material show better performance (Tirre & Pena, 1992).

Another primary issue is that there are no agreed upon measures that are used consistently across research studies (Baddeley, 2007; Conway et al., 2005; Savage et al., 2007; Shelton et al., 2009; Unsworth & Engle, 2007). A variety of simple span, complex span, and alternative tasks are all referred to as working memory tasks, yet they may measure different constructs (Conway et al., 2005; Shelton et al., 2009). Furthermore, even when similar tasks are used in different studies, administration, scoring, and interpretation are often inconsistent (Conway et al., 2005; Towse & Hitch, 1995; Unsworth & Engle, 2007). For a review of working memory span tasks that outlines recommendations for consistent administration and scoring, see Conway and colleagues (2005). Unsworth and Engle (2007) demonstrated that different methods of scoring significantly impact correlations with cognitive abilities and clinical diagnoses. Thus, many areas of working memory research have discrepancies in their findings (Savage et al., 2007; Unsworth & Engle, 2007).

Because working memory measurement is used in applied settings and diverse fields of psychological research, there is often a substantial discrepancy between tools used in research and practice (Conway et al., 2008; Shelton et al., 2009). The relationship between validated tasks used in cognitive research and psychometric batteries used in clinical settings has not been fully tested, and confounds such as those mentioned about the Wechsler scales remain in practical settings (Shelton et al., 2009). This has important diagnostic implications, as many laboratory tests of working memory have been shown to be associated with a variety of conditions, while some of the tasks used in clinical settings have not (Shelton et al., 2009). Thus there is a pressing need for standardization and consistency in the use of valid working memory measures.

Despite the challenges with working memory assessment, it has been invaluable across various fields in psychology. A distinct advantage of working memory measures is that they are less culturally influenced than other cognitive measures, as they do not rely heavily on prior knowledge (Baddeley, 2007). This makes them useful in assessment with diverse populations, and also likely contributes to their high correlation with fluid intelligence, and accordingly, general intelligence (Baddeley, 2007). Still, a substantial amount of research on working memory measurement is needed in order to develop valid measures that may be used consistently across research and practice (Conway et al., 2003, 2005; Savage et al., 2007; Shelton et al., 2009).

ACKNOWLEDGMENTS

We thank Dr. David M. Gill for his review of the manuscript.

REFERENCES

Ackerman, P. L., Beier, M. E., & Boyle, M. O. (2005). Working memory and intelligence: The same or different constructs? *Psychological Bulletin, 131*, 30-60.

Adams, W., & Sheslow, D. (2003). *Wide Range Assessment of Memory and Learning – second edition.* Lutz, FL: Psychological Assessment Resources.

Allen, D. N., Randall, C., Bello, D., Armstrong, C., Frantom, L., Cross, C., & Kinney, J. (2010). Are working memory deficits in bipolar disorder markers for psychosis? *Neuropsychology, 24*, 244-254.

Alloway, T. P. (2007a). *Automated Working Memory Assessment (AWMA).* London: Harcourt Assessment.

Alloway, T. P. (2007b). Working memory, reading, and mathematical skills in children with developmental coordination disorder. *Journal of Experimental Child Psychology, 96*, 20-36.

Alloway, T. P., & Archibald, L. (2008). Working memory and learning in children with developmental coordination disorder and specific language impairment. *Journal of Learning Disabilities, 41*, 251-262.

Alloway, T. P., Gathercole, S. E., Holmes, J., Place, M., Elliot, J. G., & Hilton, K. (2009). The diagnostic utility of behavioral checklists in identifying children with ADHD and children with working memory deficits. *Child Psychiatry and Human Development, 40*, 353-366.

Alloway, T. P., Gathercole, S. E., Kirkwood, H., & Elliot, J. (2008). Evaluation of the validity of the Automated Working Memory Assessment. *Educational Psychology, 28*, 725-734.

Alloway, T. P., Gathercole, S. E., Kirkwood, H., & Elliot, J. (2009). The working memory rating scale: A classroom-based behavioral assessment of working memory. *Learning and Individual Differences, 19*, 242-245.

Alloway, T. P., Rajendran, G., & Archibald, L. (2009). Working memory in children with developmental disorders. *Journal of Learning Disabilities, 42*, 372-382.

Alloway, T. P., & Temple, K. J. (2007). A comparison of working memory skills and learning in children with developmental coordination disorder and moderate learning difficulties. *Applied Cognitive Psychology, 21*, 473-487.

Andersson, U., & Lyxell, B. (2007). Working memory deficit in children with mathematic difficulties: A general or specific deficit? *Journal of Experimental Child Psychology, 96*, 197-228.

Arnett, P. A., Higginson, C. I., Voss, W. D., Bender, W. I., Wurst, J. M., & Tippin, J. M. (1999). Depression in multiple sclerosis: Relationship to working memory capacity. *Neuropsychology, 13*, 546-556.

Babcock, R. L., & Salthouse, T. A. (1990). Effects of increased processing demands on age differences in working memory. *Psychology and Aging, 3*, 421-428.

Baddeley, A. (1992). Working memory: The interface between memory and cognition. *Journal of Cognitive Neuroscience, 4*, 281-288.

Baddeley, A. (2003). Working memory: Looking back and looking forward. *Neuroscience, 4*, 829-839.

Baddeley, A. (2007). *Working memory, thought, and action.* New York: Oxford.

Baddeley, A., Cocchini, G., Sala, S. D., Logie, R. H., & Spinnler, H. (1999). Working memory and vigilance: Evidence from normal aging and Alzheimer's disease. *Brain and Cognition, 41*, 87-108.

Baddeley, A., & Jarrold, C. (2007). Working memory and Down syndrome. *Journal of Intellectual Disability Research, 51*, 925-931.

Baddeley, A., Logie, R., Bressi, S., Sala, S. D., & Spinnler, H. (1986). Dementia and working memory. *The Quarterly Journal of Experimental Psychology, 38*, 603-618.

Baddeley, A. D. (1983). Working memory. *Philosophical Transactions of the Royal Society of London (B), 302*, 311-324.

Baddeley, A. D. (2000). The episodic buffer: A new component of working memory? *Trends in Cognitive Sciences, 4*, 417-423.

Baddeley, A. D. (2002). Is working memory still working? *European Psychologist, 7*, 85-97.

Baddeley, A. D., Bressi, S., Sala, S. D., Logie, R., & Spinnler, H. (1991). The decline of working memory in Alzheimer's disease. *Brain, 114*, 2521-2542.

Baddeley, A. D., Gathercole, S. E., & Papagno, C. (1998). The phonological loop as a language learning device. *Psychological Review, 105*, 158-173.

Baddeley, A. D., & Hitch, G. (1974). Working memory. In G. A. Bower (Ed.), *Recent advances in learning and motivation* (Vol. 8, pp. 47-90). New York: Academic Press.

Baddeley, A. D., & Larsen, J. D. (2007a). The phonological loop: Some answers and some questions. *The Quarterly Journal of Experimental Psychology, 60*, 512-518.

Baddeley, A. D., & Larsen, J. D. (2007b). The phonological loop unmasked? A comment on the evidence for a "perceptual-gestural" alternative. *The Quarterly Journal of Experimental Psychology, 60*, 497-504.

Bailey, H., Dunlosky, J., & Hertzog, C. (2009). Does differential strategy use account for age-related deficits in working-memory performance. *Psychology and Aging, 24*, 82-92.

Barbosa, T., Miranda, M. C., Santos, R. F., & Bueno, O. F. A. (2009). Phonological working memory, phonological awareness and language in literacy difficulties in Brazilian children. *Reading and Writing, 22*, 201-218.

Barch, D. M., Berman, M. G., Engle, R., Jones, J. H., Jonides, J., MacDonald III, A., ... Nee, D. E. (2009). CNTRICS final task selection: Working memory. *Schizophrenia Bulletin, 35*, 136-152.

Barch, D. M., Csernansky, J. G., Conturo, T., & Snyder, A. Z. (2002). Working and long-term memory deficits in schizophrenia: Is there a common prefrontal mechanism? *Journal of Abnormal Psychology, 111*, 478-494.

Barnett, R., Maruff, P., Vance, A., Luk, E. S. L., Costin, J., Wood, C., & Pantels, C. (2001). Abnormal executive function in attention deficit hyperactivity disorder: The effect of stimulant medication and age on spatial working memory. *Psychological Medicine, 31*, 1107-1115.

Bassel, C., Rourke, S. B., Halman, M. H., & Smith, M. L. (2002). Working memory performance predicts subjective cognitive complains in HIV infection. *Neuropsychology, 16*, 400-410.

Bayliss, D. M., Jarrold, C., Baddeley, A. D., & Gunn, D. M. (2005). The relationship between short-term memory and working memory: Complex span made simple? *Memory, 13*, 414-421.

Bayliss, D. M., Jarrold, C., Baddeley, A. D., & Leigh, E. (2005). Differential constraints on the working memory and reading abilities of individuals with learning difficulties and typically developing children. *Journal of Experimental Child Psychology, 92*, 76-99.

Bayliss, D. M., Jarrold, C., Gunn, D. M., & Baddeley, A. D. (2003). The complexities of complex span: Explaining individual differences in working memory in children and adults. *Journal of Experimental Psychology, 132*, 71-92.

Belleville, S., Chertkow, H., & Gauthier, S. (2007). Working memory and control of attention in persons with Alzheimer's disease and mild cognitive impairment. *Neuropsychology, 21*, 458-469.

Belleville, S., Rouleau, N., Van der Linden, M., & Collette, F. (2003). Effect of manipulation and irrelevant noise on working memory capacity of patients with Alzheimer's dementia. *Neuropsychology, 17*, 69-81.

Berninger, V. W., Abbott, R. D., Thomson, J., Wagner, R., Swanson, H. L., Wijsman, E. M., & Raskind, W. (2006). Modeling phonological core deficits within a working memory architecture in children and adults with developmental dyslexia. *Scientific Studies of Reading, 10*, 165-198.

Binet, A., & Simon, T. (1905). Méthodes nouvells pour le diagnostic du niveau intellectual des anormaux. *L'Année Psychologique, 11*, 191-244.

Bopp, K. L., & Verhaeghen, P. (2009). Working memory and aging: Separating the effects of content and context. *Psychology and Aging, 24*, 968-980.

Bora, E., Vahip, S., Akdeniz, F., Ilerisoy, H., Aldemir, E., & Alkan, M. (2008). Execuitve and verbal working memory dysfunction in first-degree relatives of patients with bipolar disorder. *Psychiatry Research, 161*, 318-324.

Borella, E., Carretti, B., & De Beni, R. (2008). Working memory and inhibition across the adult life-span. *Acta Psychologica, 128*, 33-44.

Boyer, K. M., Yeates, K. O., & Enrile, B. G. (2006). Working memory and information processing speed in children with myelomeningocele and shunted hydrocephalus: Analysis of the Children's Paced Auditory Serial Addition Test. *Journal of the International Neuropsychological Society, 12*, 305-313.

Bracken, B. A., & McCallum, R. S. (1998). *The Universal Nonverbal Intelligence Test*. Itasca, IL: Riverside.

Brebion, G., Smith, M. J., & Ehrlich, M. F. (1997). Working memory and aging: Deficit or strategy differences? *Aging, Neuropsychology, and Cognition, 4*, 58-73.

Briggs, S. D., Raz, N., & Marks, W. (1999). Age-related deficits in generation and manipulation of mental images: I. The role of sensorimotor speed and working memory. *Psychology and Aging, 14*, 427-435.

Brocki, K. C., Nyberg, L., Thorell, L. B., & Bohlin, G. (2007). Early concurrent and longitudinal symptoms of ADHD and ODD: Relations to different types of inhibitory control and working memory. *Journal of Child Psychology and Psychiatry, 48*, 1033-1041.

Brooks, L. R. (1967). The suppression of visualization by reading. *Quarterly Journal of Experimental Psychology, 19*, 289-299.

Brown, G. G., Lohr, J., Notestine, R., Turner, T., Gamst, A., & Eyler, L. T. (2007). Performance of schizophrenia and bipolar patients on verbal and figural working memory tasks. *Journal of Abnormal Psychology, 116*, 741-753.

Bruyer, R., & Scailquin, J. C. (1998). The visuospatial sketchpad for mental images: Testing the multicomponent model of working memory. *Acta Psychologia, 98*, 17-36.

Bublak, P., Muller, U., Gron, G., Reuter, M., & von Cramon, D. Y. (2002). Manipulation of working memory information is impaired in Parkinson's disease and related to working memory capacity. *Neuropsychology, 16*, 577-590.

Burglen, F., Marczewski, P., Mitchell, K. J., van der Linden, M., Johnson, M. K., Danion, J. M., & Salame, P. (2004). Impaired performance in a working memory binding task in patients with schizophrenia. *Psychiatry Research, 125*, 247-255.

Burt, C. (1909). Experimental tests of general intelligence. *British Journal of Psychology, 3*, 94-177.

Buzy, W. M., Medoff, D. R., & Schweitzer, J. B. (2009). Intra-individual variability among children with ADHD on a working memory task: An ex-Gaussian approach. *Child Neuropsychology, 15*, 441-459.

Caggiano, D. M., Jiang, Y., & Parasuraman, R. (2006). Aging and repetition priming for targets and distracters in a working memory task. *Aging, Neuropsychology, and Cognition, 13*, 552-573.

Callahan, C. M. (1998). Review of the Swanson-Cognitive Processing Test. In J. C. Impara & B. S. Plake (Eds.), *The thirteenth mental measurements yearbook*. Lincoln, NE: Buros Institute of Mental Measurements. Retrieved from Mental Measurements Yearbook database.

Cameron, A. M., Oram, J., Geffren, G. M., Kavanagh, D. J., McGrath, J. J., & Geffen, L. B. (2002). Working memory correlates of three symptom clusters in schizophrenia. *Psychiatry Research, 110*, 49-61.

Campbell, J. I. D., & Charness, N. (1990). Age-related declines in working-memory skills: Evidence from a complex calculation task. *Developmental Psychology, 26*, 879-888.

Carretti, B., Belacchi, C., & Cornoldi, C. (2010). Difficulties in working memory updating in individuals with intellectual disability. *Journal of Intellectual Disability Research, 54*, 337-345.

Carretti, B., Borella, E., Cornoldi, C., & De Beni, R. (2009). Role of working memory in explaining the performance of individuals with specific reading comprehension difficulties: A meta-analysis. *Learning and Individual Differences, 19*, 246-251.

Carroll, J. B. (1993). *Human cognitive abilities: A survey of factor-analytic studies.* New York: Cambridge University Press.

Case, R., Kurland, M. D., & Goldberg, J. (1982). Operational efficiency and the growth of short-term memory span. *Journal of Experimental Child Psychology, 33*, 386-404.

Cattell, J. M., & Galton, F. (1890). Mental tests and measurements. *Mind, 15*, 373-381.

Chaytor, N., & Schmitter-Edgecombe, M. (2004). Working memory and aging: A cross-sectional and longitudinal analysis using a self-ordered pointing task. *Journal of the International Neuropsychological Society, 10*, 489-503.

Chen, J., Hale, S., & Myerson, J. (2003). Effects of domain, retention interval, and information load on young and older adults' visuospatial working memory. *Aging, Neuropsychology, and Cognition, 10*, 122-123.

Chen, J., & Li, D. (2007). The roles of working memory updating and processing speed in mediating age-related differences in fluid intelligence. *Aging, Neuropsychology, and Cognition, 14*, 631-646.

Chey, J., Lee, J., Kim, Y., Kwon, S., & Shin, Y. (2002). Spatial working memory span, delayed response and executive function in schizophrenia. *Psychiatry Research, 110*, 259-271.

Cocchi, L., Schenk, R., Volken, H., Bovet, P., Parnas, J., & Vianin, P. (2007). Visuo-spatial processing in a dynamic and static working memory paradigm in schizophrenia. *Psychiatry Research, 152*, 129-142.

Cocchini, G., Logie, R. H., Sala, S. D., MacPherson, S. E., & Baddeley, A. D. (2002). Concurrent performance of two memory tasks: Evidence for domain-specific working memory systems. *Memory & Cognition, 30*, 1086-1095.

Cohen, M. J. (1997). *Children's Memory Scale.* San Antonio, TX: Psychological Corporation.

Coleman, M. J., Cook, S., Matthysse, S., Barnard, J., Lo, Y., Levy, D. L., & Holzman, P. S. (2002). Spatial and object working memory impairments in schizophrenia patients: A Bayesian item-response theory analysis. *Journal of Abnormal Psychology, 111*, 425-435.

Colom, R., Abad, F. J., Quiroga, M. A., Shih, P. C., & Flores-Mendoza, C. (2008). Working memory and intelligence are highly related constructs, but why? *Intelligence, 36*, 584-606.

Colom, R., Flores-Mendoza, C., Quiroga, M. A., & Privado, J. (2005). Working memory and general intelligence: The role of short-term storage. *Personality and Individual Differences, 39*, 1005-1014.

Colom, R., Flores-Mendoza, C., & Rebollo, I. (2003). Working memory and intelligence. *Personality and Individual Differences, 34*, 33-39.

Colom, R., Rebollo, I., Palacios, A., Juan-Espinosa, M., & Kyllonen, P. C. (2004). Working memory is (almost) perfectly predicted by g. *Intelligence, 32*, 277-296.

Conway, A. R. A., Cowan, N., Bunting, M. F., Therriault, D. J., & Minkoff, S. R. B. (2002). A latent variable analysis of working memory capacity, short-term memory capacity, processing speed, and general fluid intelligence. *Intelligence, 30*, 163-183.

Conway, A. R. A., Jarrold, C., Kane, M. J., Miyake, A., & Towse, J. N. (2008). *Variation in working memory.* New York: Oxford.

Conway, A. R. A., Kane, M. J., Bunting, M. F., Hambrich, D. Z., Wilhelm, O., & Randall, W. E. (2005). Working memory span tasks: A methodological review and user's guide. *Psychonomic Bulletin & Review, 12,* 769-786.

Conway, A. R. A., Kane, M. J., & Engle, R. W. (2003). Working memory capacity and its relation to general intelligence. *TRENDS in Cognitive Sciences, 7,* 547-552.

Coolidge, F. L., & Wynn, T. (2005). Working memory, its executive functions, and the emergence of modern thinking. *Cambridge Archeological Journal, 15,* 5-26.

Cornoldi, C., Bassani, C., Berto, R., & Mammarella, N. (2007). Aging and the intrusion superiority effect in visuo-spatial working memory. *Aging, Neuropsychology, and Cognition, 14,* 1-21.

Cornoldi, C., Marzocchi, G. M., Belotti, M., Caroli, M. G., De Mao, T., & Braga, C. (2001). Working memory interference control deficit in children referred by teachers for ADHD symptoms. *Child Neuropsychology, 7,* 230-240.

Cowan, N., Saults, J. S., & Morey, C. C. (2006). Development of working memory for verbal-spatial associations. *Journal of Memory and Language, 55,* 274-289.

Cusack, R., Lehmann, M., Veldsman, M., & Mitchell, D. J. (2009). Encoding strategy and not visual working memory capacity correlates with intelligence. *Psychonomic Bulletin & Review, 16,* 641-647.

D'Esposito, M., Onishi, K., Thompson, H., Robinson, K., Armstrong, C., & Grossman, M. (1996). Working memory impairments in Multiple Sclerosis: Evidence from a dual-task paradigm. *Neuropsychology, 10,* 51-56.

Daneman, M., & Carpenter, P. A. (1980). Individual differences in working memory and reading. *Journal of Verbal Learning and Verbal Behavior, 19,* 450-466.

Daneman, M., & Merikle, P. M. (1996). Working memory and language comprehension: A meta-analysis. *Psychonomic Bulletin & Review, 3,* 422-433.

Das-Smaal, E. A., de Jong, P. F., & Koopmans, J. R. (1993). Working memory, attentional regulation and the Star Counting Test. *Personality and Individual Differences, 14,* 815-824.

de Beni, R., Borella, E., & Carretti, B. (2007). Reading comprehension in aging: The role of working memory and metacomprehension. *Aging, Neuropsychology, and Cognition, 14,* 189-212.

de Freitas Messina, L., Tiedemann, K. B., de Andrade, E. R., & Primi, R. (2006). Assessment of working memory in children with attention-deficit/hyperactivity disorder. *Journal of Attention Disorders, 10,* 28-35.

de Jong, P. F. (1998). Working memory deficits of reading disabled children. *Journal of Experimental Child Psychology, 70,* 75-96.

de Jong, P. F., & Das-Smaal, E. A. (1990). The Star Counting Test: An attention test for children. *Personality and Individual Differences, 11,* 597-604.

Dehn, M. J. (2008). *Working memory and academic learning: Assessment and intervention.* Wiley: Hoboken, NJ.

Deldin, P. J., Deveney, C. M., Kim, A. S., Casas, B. R., & Best, J. L. (2001). A slow wave investigation of working memory biases in mood disorders. *Journal of Abnormal Psychology, 110,* 267-281.

Deluca, J., Christodoulou, C., Diamond, B. J., Rosenstein, E. D., Kramer, N., & Natelson, B. H. (2004). Working memory deficits in chronic fatigue syndrome: Differentiating between speed and accuracy of information processing. *Journal of the International Neuropsychological Society, 10*, 101-109.

Dobbs, A. R., & Rule, B. G. (1989). Adult age differences in working memory. *Psychology and Aging, 4*, 500-503.

Dobbs, B. M., Dobbs, A. R., & Kiss, I. (2001). Working memory deficits associated with chronic fatigue syndrome. *Journal of the International Neuropsychological Society, 7*, 285-293.

Earnst, K. S., Wadley, V. G., Aldridge, T. M., Steenwyk, A. B., Hammond, A. E., Harrell, L. E., & Marson, D. C. (2001). Loss of financial capacity in Alzheimer's disease: The role of working memory. *Aging, Neuropsychology, and Cognition, 8*, 109-119.

Ebbinghaus, H. (1885/1913). *Memory: A contribution to experimental psychology*. New York: Teachers College.

Elliot, C. D. (2006). *Differential Ability Scales – second edition*. San Antonio, TX: Psychological Corporation.

Embretson, S. E. (1995). The role of working memory capacity and general control processes in intelligence. *Intelligence, 20*, 169-189.

Engle, R. W., Tuholski, S. W., Laughlin, J. E., & Conway, A. R. A. (1999). Working memory, short-term memory and general fluid intelligence: A latent variable approach. *Journal of Experimental Psychology, 128*, 309-331.

Engelhardt, P. E., Nigg, J. T., Carr, L. A., & Ferreira, F. (2008). Cognitive inhibition and working memory in attention-deficit/hyperactivity disorder. *Journal of Abnormal Psychology, 117*, 591-605.

Fellner, K. D., & Reddon, J. R. (2010). Organic disorders. In J. Thomas & H. Hersen (Eds.), *Handbook of Clinical Psychology Competencies* (pp. 1009-1037). New York: Springer.

Fisk, J. E., & Warr, P. (1996). Age and working memory: The role of perceptual speed, the central executive, and the phonological loop. *Psychology and Aging, 11*, 316-323.

Fleming, K., Goldberg, T. E., Gold, J. M., & Weinberger, D. R. (1995). Verbal working memory dysfunction in schizophrenia: Use of a Brown-Peterson paradigm. *Psychiatry Research, 56*, 155-161.

Foos, P. W. (1989). Adult age differences in working memory. *Psychology and Aging, 4*, 269-275.

Forbes, N. F., Carrick, L. A., McIntosh, A. M., & Lawrie, S. M. (2009). Working memory in schizophrenia: A meta-analysis. *Psychological Medicine, 39*, 889-905.

Franklin, T., Lee, A., Hall, N., Hetrick, S., Ong, J., Haslam, N., ... Karsz, F. (2010). The association of visuospatial working memory with dysthymic disorder in pre-pubertal children. *Psychological Medicine, 40*, 253-261.

Fry, A. F., & Hale, S. (1996). Processing speed, working memory, and fluid intelligence: Evidence for a developmental cascade. *Psychological Science, 7*, 237-241.

Fuller, R. L., Luck, S. J., Braun, E. L., Robinson, B. M., McMahon, R. P., & Gold, J. M. (2009). Impaired visual working memory consolidation in schizophrenia. *Neuropsychology, 23*, 71-80.

Fuller, R. L., Luck, S. J., McMahon, R. P., & Gold, J. M. (2005). Working memory consolidation is abnormally slow in schizophrenia. *Journal of Abnormal Psychology, 114*, 279-290.

Galton, F. (1883). *Inquiries into human faculty and its development*. London: Macmillan.

Galton, F. (1887). Supplementary notes on "prehension" in idiots. *Mind, 12*(45), 79-82.

Garcia-Madruga, J. A., Gutierrez, F., Carriedo, N., Luzon, J. M., & Vila, J. O. (2007). Mental models in propositional reasoning and working memory's central executive. *Thinking & Reasoning, 13*, 370-393.

Gathercole, S. E., & Alloway, T. P. (2006). Practitioner review: Short-term and working memory impairments in neurodevelopmental disorders: Diagnosis and remedial support. *Journal of Child Psychology and Psychiatry, 47*, 4-15.

Gathercole, S. E., Alloway, T. P., Willis, C., Adams, A. M. (2006). Working memory in children with reading disabilities. *Journal of Experimental Child Psychology, 93*, 265-281.

Gathercole, S. E., Willis, C., Emslie, H., & Baddeley, A. D. (1991). The influences of number of syllables and wordlikeness on children's repetition of nonwords. *Applied Pscyholinguistics, 12*, 349-367.

Gazzaley, A., Sheridan, M. A., Cooney, J. W., & D'Esposito, M. (2007). Age-related deficits in component processes of working memory. *Neuropsychology, 21*, 532-539.

Geary, D. C., Hoard, M. K., Byrd-Craven, J., & DeSoto, M. C. (2004). Strategy choices in simple and complex addition: Contributions of working memory and counting knowledge for children with mathematical disability. *Journal of Experimental Child Psychology, 88*, 121-151.

Gilbert, B., Belleville, S., Bherer, L., & Chouinard, S. (2005). Study of verbal working memory in patients with Parkinson's disease. *Neuropsychology, 19*, 106-114.

Gokcen, S., Bora, E., Erermis, S., Kesikci, H., & Aydin, C. (2009). Theory of mind and verbal working memory deficits in parents of autistic children. *Psychiatry Research, 166*, 46-53.

Gold, J. M., Wilk, C. M., McMahon, R. P., Buchanan, R. W., & Luck, S. J. (2003). Working memory for visual features and conjunctions in schizophrenia. *Journal of Abnormal Psychology, 112*, 61-71.

Granholm, E., Morris, S. K., Sarkin, A. J., Asarnow, R. F., & Jeste, D. V. (1997). Pupillary responses index overload of working memory resources in schizophrenia. *Journal of Abnormal Psychology, 106*, 458-467.

Gunter, R. W., & Bodner, G. E. (2008). How eye movements affect unpleasant memories: Support for a working-memory account. *Behaviour Research and Therapy, 46*, 913-931.

Haavisto, M. J., & Lehto, J. E. (2004). Fluid/spatial and crystallized intelligence in relation to domain-specific working memory: A latent-variable approach. *Learning and Individual Differences, 15*, 1-21.

Hartley, A. A., Speer, N. K., Jonides, J., Reuter-Lorenz, P. A., & Smith, E. E. (2001). Is the dissociability of working memory systems for name identity, visual-object identity, and spatial location maintained in old age? *Neuropsychology, 15*, 3-17.

Hartman, M., Bolton, E., & Fehnel, S. E. (2001). Accounting for age differences in the Wisconsin Card Sorting Test: Decreased working memory, not inflexibility. *Psychology and Aging, 16*, 385-399.

Hartman, M., Dumas, J., & Nielsen, C. (2001). Age differences in updating working memory: Evidence from the delayed-matching-to-sample test. *Aging, Neuropsychology, and Cognition, 8*, 14-35.

Hartman, M., & Warren, L. H. (2005). Explaining age differences in temporal working memory. *Psychology and Aging, 20*, 645-656.

Haut, M. W., Chen, S., & Edwards, S. (1999). Working memory, semantics, and normal aging. *Aging, Neuropsychology, and Cognition, 6*, 179-186.

Haut, M. W., Roberts, V. J., Goldstein, F. C., Martin, R. C., Keefover, R. W., & Rankin, E. D. (1998). *Aging, Neuropsychology, and Cognition, 5*, 63-72.

Hedden, T., & Park, D. (2001). Aging and interference in verbal working memory. *Neuropsychology and Aging, 16*, 666-681.

Henry, L., & Winfield, J. (2010). Working memory and educational achievement in children with intellectual disabilities. *Journal of Intellectual Disability Research, 54*, 354-365.

Hertzog, C., Dixon, R. A., Hultsch, D. F., & MacDonald, S. W. S. (2003). Latent change models of adult cognition: Are changes in processing speed and working memory associated with changes in episodic memory? *Psychology and Aging, 18*, 755-769.

Hitch, G., J., & McAuley, E. (1991). Working memory in children with specific arithmetical learning difficulties. *British Journal of Psychology, 82*, 375-386.

Hochstadt, J., Nakano, H., Lieberman, P., & Friedman, J. (2006). The roles of sequencing and verbal working memory in sentence comprehension deficits in Parkinson's disease. *Brain and Language, 97*, 243-257.

Horn, J. L., & Blankson, N. (2005). Foundations for better understanding of cognitive abilities. In D. P. Flanagan & P. L. Harrison (Eds.), *Contemporary intellectual assessment: Theories, tests, and issues* (2nd ed.; pp. 41-68). New York: Guilford Press.

Huntley, J. D., & Howard, R. J. (2010). Working memory in early Alzheimer's disease: A neuropsychological review. *International Journal of Geriatric Psychiatry, 25*, 121-132.

Jacobs, J. (1887). Experiments on "prehension." *Mind, 12*(45), 75-79.

Jarrold, C., Baddeley, A. D., & Hewes, A. K. (1999). Genetically dissociated components of working memory: Evidence from Down's and Williams syndrome. *Neuropsychologia, 37*, 637-651.

Jeffries, E., Ralph, M. A. L., & Baddeley, A. D. (2004). Automatic and controlled processing in sentence recall: The role of long-term and working memory. *Journal of Memory and Language, 51*, 623-643.

Jeffries, S., & Everatt, J. (2004). Working memory: Its role in dyslexia and other specific learning disabilities. *Dyslexia, 10*, 196-214.

Jenks, K. M., de Moor, J., & van Lieshout, E. C. D. M. (2009). Arithmetic difficulties in children with cerebral palsy are related to executive function and working memory. *Journal of Child Psychology and Psychiatry, 50*, 824-833.

Jenks, K. M., de Moor, J., van Lieshout, E. C. D. M., Maathuis, K. G. B., Keus, I., & Gorter, J. W. (2007). The effect of cerebral palsy on arithmetic accuracy is mediated by working memory, intelligence, early numeracy, and instruction time. *Developmental Neuropsychology, 32*, 861-879.

Johnson, J. A. (2005). Review of the Stanford-Binet Intelligence Scales, fifth edition. In R. Spies & B. Plake (Eds.), *The sixteenth mental measurements yearbook*. Lincoln, NE: Buros Institute of Mental Measurements. Retrieved from Mental Measurements Yearbook database.

Jonsdottir, S., Bouma, A., Sergeant, J. A., & Scherder, E. J. A. (2005). The impact of specific language impairment on working memory in children with ADHD combined subtype. *Archives of Clinical Neuropsychology, 20*, 443-456.

Joormann, J., & Gotlib, I. H. (2008). Updating the contents of working memory in depression: Interference from irrelevant negative material. *Journal of Abnormal Psychology, 117*, 182-192.

Kane, M. J., Conway, A. R. A., Miura, T. K., & Colfiesh, G. J. H. (2007). Working memory, attention control, and the n-back task: A question of construct validity. *Journal of Experimental Psychology: Learning, Memory, & Cognition, 33*, 615-622.

Kane, M. J., Hambrick, D. Z., Tuholski, S. W., Wilhelm, O., Payne, T. W., & Engle, R. W. (2004). The generality of working memory capacity: A latent-variable approach to verbal and visuo-spatial memory span and reasoning. *Journal of Experimental Psychology, 133*, 189-217.

Karatekin, C. (2004). A test of the integrity of the components of Baddeley's model of working memory in attention-deficit/hyperactivity disorder (ADHD). *Journal of Child Psychology and Psychiatry, 45*, 912-926.

Karatekin, C., & Asarnow, R. F. (1998). Working memory in childhood-onset schizophrenia and attention-deficit/hyperactivity disorder. *Psychiatry Research, 80*, 165-176.

Kaufman, A. S., & Kaufman, N. L. (2004). *Manual for the Kaufman Assessment Battery for Children – second edition (KABC-II)*. Circle Pines, MN: American Guidance Service.

Kaufman, J. S., Kaufman, A. S., Kaufman-Singer, J., & Kaufman, N. L. (2005). The Kaufman Assessment Battery for Children – second edition and the Kaufman Adolescent and Adult Intelligence Test. In D. P. Flanagan & P. L. Harrison (Eds.), *Contemporary intellectual assessment: Theories, tests, and issues* (2nd ed.; pp. 344-370). New York: Guilford Press.

Kaufman, S. B., DeYoung, C. G., Gray, J. R., Brown, J., & Mackintosh, N. (2009). Associative learning predicts intelligence above and beyond working memory and processing speed. *Intelligence, 37*, 374-382.

Keeler, M. L., & Swanson, H. L. (2001). Does strategy knowledge influence working memory in children with mathematical disabilities? *Journal of Learning Disabilities, 34*, 418-434.

Keith, T. Z., Fine, J. G., Taub, G. E., Reynolds, M. R., & Kranzler, J. H. (2006). Higher order, multisample confirmatory factor analysis of the Wechsler Intelligence Scale for Children – fourth edition: What does it measure? *School Psychology Review, 35*, 108-127.

Kennedy, K. M., Partridge, T., & Raz, N. (2008). Age-related differences in acquisition of perceptual-motor skills: Working memory as a mediator. *Aging, Neuropsychology, and Cognition, 15*, 165-183.

Kensinger, E. A., Shearer, D. K., Locascio, J. J., Growdon, J. H., & Corkin, S. (2003). Working memory in mild Alzheimer's disease and early Parkinson's disease. *Neuropsychology, 17*, 230-239.

Kerns, K. A., McInerney, R. J., & Wilde, N. J. (2001). Time reproduction, working memory, and behavioral inhibition in children with ADHD. *Child Neuropsychology, 7*, 21-31.

Kibby, M. Y., & Cohen, M. J. (2008). Memory functioning in children with reading disabilities and/or attention deficit/hyperactivity disorder: A clinical investigation of their working memory and long-term memory functioning. *Child Neuropsychology, 14*, 525-546.

Kibby, M. Y., Marks, W., Morgan, S., & Long, C. J. (2004). Specific impairment in developmental reading disabilities: A working memory approach. *Journal of Learning Disabilities, 37*, 349-363.

Kirschner, W. K. (1958). Age differences in short-term retention of rapidly changing information. *Journal of Experimental Psychology, 33*, 352-358.

Kliegel, M., & Jager, T. (2006). Delayed-executive prospective memory performance: The effects of age and working memory. *Developmental Neuropsychology, 30*, 819-843.

Kofler, M. J., Rapport, M. D., Bolden, J., Sarver, D. E., & Raiker, J. S. (2010). ADHD and working memory: The impact of central executive deficits and exceeding storage/rehearsal capacity on observed inattentive behaviour. *Journal of Abnormal Child Psychology, 38*, 149-161.

Korkman, M., Kirk, U., & Kemp, S. (2007). *NEPSY-II: A developmental neuropsychological assessment.* San Antonio, TX: The Psychological Corporation.

Kumar, A., Rakitin, B. C., Nambisan, R., Habeck, C., & Stern, Y. (2008). The response-signal method reveals age-related changes in object working memory. *Psychology and Aging, 23*, 315-329.

Lanfranchi, S., Carretti, B., Spano, G., & Cornoldi, C. (2009). A specific deficit in visuospatial simultaneous working memory in Down syndrome. *Journal of Intellectual Disability Research, 53*, 474-483.

Lanfranchi, S., Cornoldi, C., Drigo, S., & Vianello, R. (2009). Working memory in individuals with Fragile X syndrome. *Child Neuropsychology, 15*, 105-119.

Lanfranchi, S., Jerman, O., & Vianello, R. (2009). Working memory and cognitive skills in individuals with Down syndrome. *Child Neuropsychology, 15*, 397-416.

Larson, E. R., Shear, P. K., Krikorian, R., Welge, J., & Strakowski, S. M. (2005). Working memory and inhibitory control among manic and euthymic patients with bipolar disorder. *Journal of the International Neuropsychological Society, 11*, 163-172.

Leather, C. V., & Henry, L. A. (1994). Working memory span and phonological awareness tasks as predictors of early reading ability. *Journal of Experimental Child Psychology, 58*, 88-111.

Lee, J., & Park, S. (2005). Working memory impairments in schizophrenia: A meta-analysis. *Journal of Abnormal Psychology, 114*, 599-611.

Lengenfelder, J., Bryant, D., Diamond, B. J., Kalmar, J. H., Moore, N. B., & DeLuca, J. (2006). Processing speed interacts with working memory efficiency in multiple sclerosis. *Archives of Clinical Neuropsychology, 21*, 229-238.

Levin, H. S., Hanten, G., Zhang, L., Swank, P. R., Ewing-Cobbs, L., Dennis, M., ... Barnes, M. A. (2004). Changes in working memory after traumatic brain injury in children. *Neuropsychology, 18*, 240-247.

Li, S. C., Schmiedek, F., Huxhold, O., Rocke, C., Smith, J., & Lindenberger, U. (2008). Working memory plasticity in old age: Practice gain, transfer, and maintenance. *Psychology and Aging, 23*, 731-742.

Lilley, S. A., Andrade, J., Turpin, G., Sabin-Farrell, R., & Holmes, E. A. (2009). Visuospatial working memory interference with recollections of trauma. *British Journal of Clinical Psychology, 48*, 309-321.

Luo, D., Chen, G., Zen, F., & Murray, B. (2010). Modeling working memory tasks on the item level. *Intelligence, 38*, 66-82.

Luria, A. R. (1980) *Higher cortical functions in man.* New York: Basic Books.

Mabbot, D. J., & Bisanz, J. (2008). Computational skills, working memory, and conceptual knowledge in older children with mathematics learning disabilities. *Journal of Learning Disabilities, 41*, 15-28.

Mackintosh, N. J., & Bennett, E. S. (2003). The fractionation of working memory maps onto different components of intelligence. *Intelligence, 31*, 519-531.

Maehler, C., & Schuchardt, K. (2009). Working memory functioning in children with learning disabilities: Does intelligence make a difference? *Journal of Intellectual Disability Research, 53*, 3-10.

Mahone, E. M., Martin, R., Kates, W. R., Hay, T., & Horska, A. (2009). Neuroimaging correlates of parent ratings of working memory in typically developing children. *Journal of the International Neuropsychological Society, 15*, 31-41.

Mammarella, N., Fairfield, B., De Beni, R., & Cornoldi, C. (2009). Aging and intrusion errors in an active visuo-spatial working memory task. *Aging Clinical an Experimental Research, 21*, 282-291.

Mandalis, A., Kinsella, G., Ong, B., & Anderson, V. (2007). Working memory and new learning following pediatric traumatic brain injury. *Developmental Neuropsychology, 32*, 683-701.

Marchetta, N. D. J., Hurks, P. P. M., Krabbendam, L., & Jolles, J. (2008). Interference control, working memory, concept shifting, and verbal fluency in adults with attention-deficit/hyperactivity disorder (ADHD). *Neuropsychology, 22*, 74-84.

Martinez, K., & Colom, R. (2009). Working memory capacity and processing efficiency predict fluid but not crystallized and spatial intelligence: Evidence supporting the neural noise hypothesis. *Personality and Individual Differences, 46*, 281-286.

Martinussen, R., Hayden, J., Hogg-Johnson, S., & Tannock, R. (2005). A meta-analysis of working memory impairments in children with attention-deficit/hyperactivity disorder. *Journal of the American Academy of Child and Adolescent Psychiatry, 44*, 377-384.

Matheson, S., & Langdon, R. (2008). Schizotypal traits impact upon executive working memory and aspects of IQ. *Psychiatry Research, 159*, 207-214.

Mayes, L., Snyder, P. J., Langlois, E., & Hunter, N. (2007). Visuospatial working memory in school-aged children exposed in utero to cocaine. *Child Neuropsychology, 13*, 205-218.

McCabe, D. P. (2008). The role of covert retrieval in working memory span tasks: Evidence from delayed recall tests. *Journal of Memory and Language, 58*, 480-494.

McCallum, R. S., & Bracken, B. A. (2005). The Universal Nonverbal Intelligence Test: A multidimensional measure of intelligence. In D. P. Flanagan & P. L. Harrison (Eds.), *Contemporary intellectual assessment: Theories, tests, and issues* (2nd ed.; pp. 425-440). New York: Guilford Press.

McClure, M. M., Romero, M. J., Bowie, C. R., Reichenberg, A., Harvey, P. D., & Siever, L. J. (2007). Visual-spatial learning and memory in schizotypal personality disorder: Continued evidence for the importance of working memory in the schizophrenia spectrum. *Archives of Clinical Neuropsychology, 22*, 109-116.

McGrew, K. S. (2005). The Cattell-Horn-Carroll theory of cognitive abilities: Past, present, and future. In D. P. Flanagan & P. L. Harrison (Eds.), *Contemporary intellectual assessment: Theories, tests, and issues* (2nd ed.; pp. 136-181). New York: Guilford Press.

McInnes, A., Humphries, T., Hogg-Johnson, S., & Tannock, R. (2003). Listening comprehension and working memory are impaired in attention-deficit hyperactivity disorder irrespective of language development. *Journal of Abnormal Child Psychology, 31*, 427-443.

McLean, J. F., & Hitch, G. J. (1999). Working memory impairments in children with specific arithmetic learning difficulties. *Journal of Experimental Child Psychology, 74*, 240-260.

Mikels, J. A., Larkin, G. R., Reuter-Lorenz, P. A., & Carstensen, L. L. (2005). Divergent trajectories in the aging mind: Changes in working memory for affective versus visual information with age. *Psychology and Aging, 20*, 542-553.

Miller, G., Galanter, E., & Pribram, K. (1960) *Plans and the structure of behaviour.* New York: Holt, Rinehart and Winston.

Miller, K. M., Price, C. C., Okun, M. S., Montijo, H., & Bowers, D. (2009). Is the n-back task a valid neuropsychological measure for assessing working memory? *Archives of Clinical Neuropsychology, 24*, 711-717.

Miller, L. T., & Vernon, P. A. (1996). Intelligence, reaction time, and working memory in 4- to 6-year-old children. *Intelligence, 22*, 155-190.

Milner, B. (1971) Interhemispheric differences in the localization of psychological processes in man. *British Medical Bulletin, 27*, 272-277.

Mitchell, K. J., Johnson, M. K., Raye, C. L., Mather, M., & D'Esposito, M. (2000). Aging and reflective processes of working memory: Binding and test load deficits. *Psychology and Aging, 15*, 527-541.

Mogle, J. A., Lovett, B. J., Stawski, R. S., & Sliwinski, M. J. (2008). What's so special about working memory? *Psychological Science, 19*, 1071-1077.

Montgomery, J. W. (1995). Examination of phonological working memory in specifically language-impaired children. *Applied Psycholinguistics, 16*, 355-378.

Montgomery, J. W. (2000). Relation of working memory to off-line and real-time sentence processing in children with specific language impairment. *Applied Psycholinguistics, 21*, 117-148.

Mutter, S. A., Haggbloom, S. J., Plumlee, L. F., & Schirmer, A. R. (2006). Aging, working memory, and discrimination learning. *The Quarterly Journal of Experimental Psychology, 59*, 1556-1566.

Naglieri, J. A. (2005). The Cognitive Assessment System. In D. P. Flanagan & P. L. Harrison (Eds.), *Contemporary intellectual assessment: Theories, tests, and issues* (2nd ed.; pp. 441-460). New York: Guilford Press.

Naglieri, J. A., & Das, J. P. (1997). *Cognitive Assessment System.* Itasca, IL: Riverside.

Naglieri, J. A., & Das, J. P. (2005). Planning, Attention, Simultaneous, Successive (PASS) theory. In D. P. Flanagan & P. L. Harrison (Eds.), *Contemporary intellectual assessment: Theories, tests, and issues* (2nd ed.; pp. 120-135). New York: Guilford Press.

Napolitano, S. A. (2001). Review of the Children's Memory Scale. In B. S. Plake & J. C. Impara (Eds.), *The fourteenth mental measurements yearbook.* Lincoln, NE: Buros Institute of Mental Measurements. Retrieved from Mental Measurements Yearbook database.

Nation, K., Adams, J. W., Bowyer-Crane, C. A., & Snowling, M. J. (1999). Working memory deficits in poor comprehenders reflect underlying language impairments. *Journal of Experimental Child Psychology, 73*, 139-158.

Nebes, R. D., Butters, M. A., Mulsant, B. H., Pollock, B. G., Zmuda, M. D., Houck, P. R., & Reynold, C. F., III. (2000). Decreased working memory and processing speed mediate cognitive impairment in geriatric depression. *Psychological Medicine, 30*, 679-691.

Necka, E. (1992). Cognitive analysis of intelligence: The significance of working memory processes. *Personality and Individual Differences, 13*, 1031-1046.

Nettelbeck, T., & Burns, N. R. (2010). Processing speed, working memory and reasoning ability from childhood to old age. *Personality and Individual Differences, 48*, 379-384.

Newsome, M. R., Steinberg, J. L., Scheibel, R. S., Troyanskaya, M., Chu, Z., Hanten, G., ... Lu, H. (2008). Effects of traumatic brain injury on working memory-related brain activation in adolescents. *Neuropsychology, 22,* 419-425.

Norrelgen, F., Lacerda, F., & Forssberg, H. (2002). Temporal resolution of auditory perception and verbal working memory in 15 children with language impairment. *Journal of Learning Disabilities, 35*, 540-546.

Nulsen, C. E., Fox, A. M., & Hammond, G. R. (2010). Differential effects of ecstacy on short-term and working memory: A meta-analysis. *Neuropsychology Review, 20,* 21-32.

Numminen, H., Lehto, J. E., & Ruoppila, I. (2001). Tower of Hanoi and working memory in adult persons with intellectual disability. *Research in Developmental Disabilities, 22*, 373-387.

Numminen, H., Service, E., Ahonen, T., Korhonen, T., Tolvanen, A., Patja, K., & Ruoppila, I. (2000). Working memory structure and intellectual disability. *Journal of Intellectual Disability Research, 44*, 579-590.

Numminen, H., Service, E., Ahonen, T., & Ruoppila, I. (2001). Working memory and everday cognition in adults with Down's syndrome. *Journal of Intellectual Disability Research, 45*, 157-168.

Numminen, H., Service, E., & Ruoppila, I. (2002). Working memory, intelligence and knowledge base in adult persons with intellectual disability. *Research in Developmental Disabilities, 23*, 105-118.

Oakhill, J., & Kyle, F. (2000). The relation between phonological awareness and working memory. *Journal of Experimental Child Psychology, 75*, 152-164.

Oberauer, K., Sub, H. M., Wilhelm, O., & Wittmann, W. W. (2008). Which working memory functions predict intelligence? *Intelligence, 36*, 641-652.

Oram, J. Geffen, G. M., Geffen, L. B., Kavanagh, D. J., & McGrath, J. J. (2005). Exxecutive control of working memory in schizophrenia. *Psychiatry Research, 135*, 81-90.

Palladino, P. (2006). The role of interference control in working memory: A study with children at risk of ADHD. *The Quarterly Journal of Experimental Psychology, 59*, 2047-2055.

Pantelis, C., Harvey, C. A., Plant, G., Fossey, E., Maruff, P., Stuart, G. W., ... Brewer, W. J. (2004). Relationship of behavioural and symptomatic syndromes in schizophrenia to spatial working memory and attentional set-shifting ability. *Psychological Medicine, 34*, 693-703.

Park, S., Holzman, P. S., & Lenzenweger, M. F. (1995). Individual differences in spatial working memory in relation to schizotypy. *Journal of Abnormal Psychology, 104*, 355-363.

Passolunghi, M. C., & Cornoldi, C. (2008). Working memory failures in children with arithmetical difficulties. *Child Neuropsychology, 14*, 387-400.

Passolunghi, M. C., & Siegel, L. S. (2001). Short-term memory, working memory, and inhibitory control in children with difficulties in arithmetic problem solving. *Journal of Experimental Child Psychology, 80*, 44-57.

Passolunghi, M. C., & Siegel, L. S. (2004). Working memory and access to numerical information in children with disability in mathematics. *Journal of Experimental Child Psychology, 88*, 348-367.

Pearson Assessments. (2009). *WMS-III to WMS-IV: Rationale for change.* San Antonio: Pearson Education.

Pearson Education. (2008). *Wechsler Memory Scale – fourth edition: Clinical features of the new edition.* San Antonio: Author.

Peeters, M., Verhoeven, L., & de Moor, J. (2009). Predictors of verbal working memory in children with cerebral palsy. *Research in Developmental Disabilities, 30*, 1502-1511.

Pickering, S. J., & Gathercole, S. E. (2001). *Working Memory Test Battery for Children (WMTB-C).* London: Harcourt Assessment.

Piolino, P., Coste, C., Martinelli, P., Mace, A. L., Quinette, P., Guillery-Girard, B., & Bellevile, S. (2010). Reduced specificity of autobiographical memory and aging: Do the executive and feature binding functions of working memory have a role? *Neuropsychologia, 48*, 429-440.

Piskulic, D., Olver, J. S., Norman, T. R., & Maruff, P. (2007). Behavioural studies of spatial working memory dysfunction in schizophrenia: A quantitative literature review. *Psychiatry Research, 150*, 111-121.

Polczyk, R., & Necka, E. (1997). Capacity and retention capability of working memory modify the strength of the RT/IQ correlation: A short note. *Personality and Individual Differences, 23*, 1089-1091.

Possin, K. L., Filoteo, J. V., Song, D. D., & Salmon, D. P. (2008). Spatial and object working memory deficits in Parkinson's disease are due to impairment in different underlying processes. *Neuropsychology, 22*, 585-595.

Pratt, M. W., Boyes, C., Robins, S., & Manchester, J. (1989). Telling tales: Aging, working memory, and the narrative cohesion of story retellings. *Developmental Psychology, 25*, 628-635.

Price, J. P. (2009). The computerized object and abstract designs test (COAD): A pilot study of a new test of visual working memory. *British Journal of Clinical Psychology, 48*, 109-123.

Price, S. E., Kinsella, G. J., Ong, B., Mullaly, E., Phillips, M., Pangnadasa-Fox, L., … Perre, D. (2010). Learning and memory in amnestic mild cognitive impairment: Contribution of working memory. *Journal of the International Neuropsychological Society, 16*, 342-351.

Raghubar, K. P., Barnes, M. A., & Hecht, S. A. (2010). Working memory and mathematics: A review of developmental, individual difference, and cognitive approaches. *Learning and Individual Differences, 20*, 110-122.

Ram-Tsur, R., Faust, M., & Zivotofsky, A. Z. (2008). Poor performance on serial visual tasks in persons with reading disabilities. *Journal of Learning Disabilities, 41*, 437-450.

Rapport, M. D., Alderson, R. M., Kofler, M. J., Sarver, D. E., Bolden, J., & Sims, V. (2008). Working memory deficits in boys with attention-deficit/hyperactivity disorder (ADHD): The contribution of central executive and subsystem processes. *Journal of Abnormal Child Psychology, 36*, 825-837.

Rasmussen, C. (2005). Executive functioning and working memory in Fetal Alcohol Spectrum Disorder. *Alcoholism: Clinical and Experimental Research, 29*, 1359-1367.

Reinecke, A., Rinck, M., & Becker, E. S. (2006) Spiders crawl easily through the bottleneck: Visual working memory for negative stimuli. *Emotion, 6,* 438-449.

Repovs, G., & Baddeley, A. (2006). The multi-component model of working memory: Explorations in experimental cognitive psychology. *Neuroscience, 139*, 5-21.

Reynolds, C. R., & Voress, J. K. (2007). *Test of Memory and Learning – second edition*. Austin, TX: PRO-ED.

Richardson, J. T. E., Engle, R. W., Hasher, L., Logie, R. H., Stoltzfus, E. R., & Zacks, R. T. (1996). *Working memory and human cognition*. New York: Oxford.

Robertson, E. K., & Joanisse, M. F. (2010). Spoken sentence comprehension in children with dyslexia and language impairment: The roles of syntax and working memory. *Applied Psycholinguistics, 31*, 141-165.

Roid, G. H. (2003). *Stanford-Binet Intelligence Scales – fifth edition*. Itasca, IL: Riverside Publishing.

Ros, L., Latorre, J. M., & Serrano, J. P. (2010). Working memory capacity and overgeneral autobiographical memory in young and older adults. *Aging, Neuropsychology, and Cognition, 17*, 89-107.

Rose, N. S., Myerson, J., Sommers, M. S., & Hale, S. (2009). Are there age differences in the executive component of working memory? Evidence from domain-general interference effects. *Aging, Neuropsychology, and Cognition, 16*, 633-653.

Ross, R. G., Harris, J. G., Olincy, A., & Radant, A. (2000). Eye movement task measures inhibition and spatial working memory in adults with schizophrenia, ADHD, and a normal comparison group. *Psychiatry Research, 95*, 35-42.

Rowe, G., Hasher, L., & Turcotte, J. (2008). Age differences in visuospatial working memory. *Psychology and Aging, 23*, 79-84.

Rowe, G., Hasher, L., & Turcotte, J. (2009). Age and synchrony effects in visuospatial working memory. *The Quarterly Journal of Experimental Psychology, 62*, 1873-1880.

Russell, J., Jarrold, C., & Henry, L. (1996). Working memory in children with autism and with moderate learning difficulties. *Journal of Child Psychology and Psychiatry, 37*, 673-686.

Salame, P., Burglen, F., & Danion, J. M. (2006). Differential disruptions of working memory components in schizophrenia in an object-location binding task using the suppression paradigm. *Journal of the International Neuropsychological Society, 12*, 510-518.

Salthouse, T. A. (1991). Mediation of adult age differences in cognition by reductions in working memory and speed of processing. *Psychological Science, 2*, 179-183.

Salthouse, T. A., (1992). Influence of processing speed on adult age differences in working memory. *Acta Psychologica, 79*, 155-170.

Salthouse, T. A. (1993). Influence of working memory on adult age differences in matrix reasoning. *British Journal of Psychology, 84*, 171-199.

Salthouse, T. A., Babcock, R. L., & Shaw, R. J. (1991). Effects of adult age on structural and operational capacities in working memory. *Psychology and Aging, 6*, 118-127.

Salthouse, T. A., & Pink, J. E. (2008). Why is working memory related to fluid intelligence? *Psychonomic Bulletin & Review, 15*, 364-371.

Salway, A. F. S., & Logie, R. H. (1995). Visuospatial working memory, movement control and executive demands. *British Journal of Psychology, 86*, 253-269.

Savage, R., Lavers, N., & Pillay, V. (2007). Working memory and reading difficulties: What we know and what we don't know about the relationship. *Educational Psychological Review, 19*, 185-221.

Schatz, J., Kramer, J. H., Ablin, A., & Matthay, K. K. (2000). Processing speed, working memory, and IQ: A developmental model of cognitive deficits following cranial radiation therapy. *Neuropsychology, 14*, 189-200.

Schmiedek, F., Li, S. C., & Lindenberger, U. (2009). Interference and facilitation in spatial working memory: Age-associated differences in lure effects in the n-back paradigm. *Psychology and Aging, 24*, 203-210.

Schrank, F. A. (2005). Woodcock-Johnson III Tests of Cognitive Abilities. In D. P. Flanagan & P. L. Harrison (Eds.), *Contemporary intellectual assessment: Theories, tests, and issues* (pp. 371-401). New York: Guilford Press.

Schuchardt, K., Gebhardt, M., & Maehler, C. (2010). Working memory functions in children with different degrees of intellectual disability. *Journal of Intellectual Disability Research, 54*, 346-353.

Schuchardt, K., Maehler, C., & Hasselhorn, M. (2008). Working memory deficits in children with specific learning disorders. *Journal of Learning Disabilities, 41*, 514-523.

Shelton, J. T., Elliot, E. M., Hill, B. D., Calamia, M. R., & Gouvier, W. D. (2009). A comparison of laboratory and clinical working memory tests and their prediction of fluid intelligence. *Intelligence, 37*, 283-293.

Siegel, L. S., & Ryan, E. B. (1989). The development of working memory in normally achieving and subtypes of learning disabilities. *Child Development, 60*, 973-980.

Siegert, R. J., Weatherall, M., Taylor, K. D., & Abernethy, D. A. (2008). A meta-analysis of performance of simple span and more complex working memory tasks in Parkinson's disease. *Neuropsychology, 22*, 450-461.

Small, J. A., Andersen, E. S., & Kempler, D. (1997). Effects of working memory capacity on understanding rate-altered speech. *Aging, Neuropsychology, and Cognition, 4*, 126-139.

Smith-Spark, J. H., & Fisk, J. E. (2007). Working memory functioning in developmental dyslexia. *Memory, 15*, 34-56.

Snyder, P. J., Jackson, C. E., Piskulic, D., Olver, J., Norman, T., & Maruff, P. (2008). Spatial working memory and problem solving in schizophrenia: The effect of symptom stabilization with atypical antipsychotic medication. *Psychiatry Research, 160*, 316-326.

Sonuga-Barke, E. J. S., Dalen, L., Daley, D., & Remington, B. (2002). Are planning, working memory, and inhibition associated with individual differences in preschool ADHD symptoms? *Developmental Neuropsychology, 21*, 255-272.

St. Clair-Thompson, H. L. (2007). The influence of strategies upon relationships between working memory and cognitive skills. *Memory, 15*, 353-365.

Stein, M. B. (2001). Review of the Children's Memory Scale. In B. S. Plake & J. C. Impara (Eds.), *The fourteenth mental measurements yearbook*. Lincoln, NE: Buros Institute of Mental Measurements. Retrieved from Mental Measurements Yearbook database.

Steinbrink, C., & Klatte, M. (2007). Phonological working memory in German children with poor reading and spelling abilities. *Dyslexia, 14*, 271-290.

Stevens, A., Burkhardt, M., Hautzinger, M., Schwarz, J., & Unckel, C. (2004). Borderline personality disorder: Impaired visual perception and working memory. *Psychiatry Research, 125*, 257-267.

Stevens, J., Quittner, A. L., Zuckerman, J. B., & Moore, S. (2002). Behavioral inhibition, self-regulation of motivation, and working memory in children with attention deficit hyperactivity disorder. *Developmental Neuropsychology, 21*, 117-139.

Stone, M., Gabrieli, J. D. E., Stebbins, G. T., & Sullivan, E. V. (1998). Working and strategic memory deficits in schizophrenia. *Neuropsychology, 12*, 278-288.

Stothard, S. E., & Hulme, C. (1992). Reading comprehension difficulties in children: The role of language comprehension and working memory skills. *Reading and Writing, 4*, 245-256.

Stratta, P., Prosperini, P., Daneluzzo, E., Bustini, M., & Rossi, A. (2001). Educational level and age influence spatial working memory and Wisconsin Card Sorting Test performance differently: A controlled study in schizophrenic patients. *Psychiatry Research, 102*, 39-48.

Sub, H. M., Oberauer, K., Wittmann, W. W., Wilhelm, O., & Schulze, R. (2002). Working-memory capacity explains reasoning ability – and a little bit more. *Intelligence, 30*, 261-288.

Sullivan, E. V., Shear, P. K., Zipursky, R. B., Sagar, H. J., & Pfefferbaum, A. (1997). Patterns of content, contextual, and working memory impairments in schizophrenia and nonamnesic alcoholism. *Neuropsychology, 11*, 195-206.

Swanson, H. L. (1993a). Individual differences in working memory: A model testing and subgroup analysis of learning-disabled and skilled readers. *Intelligence, 17*, 285-332.

Swanson, H. L. (1993b). Working memory in learning disability subgroups. *Journal of Experimental Child Psychology, 56*, 87-114.

Swanson, H. L. (1995). *Swanson Cognitive Processing Test (S-CPT): A dynamic assessment measure.* Austin, TX: PRO-ED.

Swanson, H. L. (1999). Reading comprehension and working memory in learning-disabled readers: Is the phonological loop more important than the executive system? *Journal of Experimental Child Psychology, 72*, 1-31.

Swanson, H. L. (2000). Are working memory deficits in readers with learning disabilities hard to change? *Journal of Learning Disabilities, 33*, 551-566.

Swanson, H. L. (2003). Age-related differences in learning disabled and skilled readers' working memory. *Journal of Experimental Child Psychology, 85*, 1-31.

Swanson, H. L., & Ashbaker, M. H. (2000). Working memory, short-term memory, speech rate, word recognition and reading comprehension in learning disabled readers: Does the executive system have a role? *Intelligence, 28*, 1-30.

Swanson, H. L., Ashbaker, M. H., & Lee, C. (1996). Learning-disabled readers' working memory as a function of processing demands. *Journal of Experimental Child Psychology, 61*, 242-275.

Swanson, H. L., & Berninger, V. (1995). The role of working memory in skilled and less skilled readers' comprehension. *Intelligence, 21*, 83-108.

Swanson, H. L., Cochran, K. F., & Ewers, C. A. (1989). Working memory in skilled and less skilled readers. *Journal of Abnormal Child Psychology, 17*, 145-156.

Swanson, H. L., Howard, C. B., & Saez, L. (2006). Do different components of working memory underlie different subgroups of reading disabilities? *Journal of Learning Disabilities, 39*, 252-269.

Swanson, H. L., & Howell, M. (2001). Working memory, short-term memory, and speech rate as predictors of children's reading performance at different ages. *Journal of Educational Psychology, 93*, 720-734.

Swanson, H. L., & Jerman, O. (2007). The influence of working memory on reading growth in subgroups of children with reading disabilities. *Journal of Experimental Child Psychology, 96*, 249-283.

Swanson, H. L., & Sachse-Lee, C. (2001a). A subgroup analysis of working memory in children with reading disabilities: Domain-general or domain-specific deficiency? *Journal of Learning Disabilities, 34*, 249-263.

Swanson, H. L., & Sachse-Lee, C. (2001b). Mathematical problem solving and working memory in children with learning disabilities: Both executive and phonological processes are important. *Journal of Experimental Child Psychology, 79*, 294-321.

Swanson, H. L., Zheng, X., & Jerman, O. (2009). Working memory, short-term memory, and reading disabilities. *Journal of Learning Disabilities, 42*, 260-287.

Tallent, K. A., & Gooding, D. C. (1999). Working memory and Wisconsin Card Sorting Test performance in schizotypic individuals: A replication and extension. *Psychiatry Research, 89*, 161-170.

Tillman, C. M., Nyberg, L., & Bohlin, G. (2008). Working memory components and intelligence in children. *Intelligence, 36*, 394-402.

Tirre, W. C., & Pena, C. M. (1992). Investigation of functional working memory in the reading span test. *Journal of Educational Psychology, 84*, 462-472.

Torii, M., Shimoyama, I., & Sugita, K. (2010). Phonemic and semantic working memory in information processing in children with high function pervasive developmental disorders. *International Medical Journal, 17*, 35-39.

Towse, J. N., & Hitch, G. J. (1995). Is there a relationship between task demand and storage space in tests of working memory capacity? *The Quarterly Journal of Experimental Psychology, 48A*, 108-124.

Towse, J. N., Hitch, G. J., & Hutton, U. (2000). On the interpretation of working memory span in adults. *Memory & Cognition, 28*, 341-348.

Towse, J. N., & Houston-Price, C. M. T. (2001). Combining representations in working memory: A brief report. *British Journal of Developmental Psychology, 19*, 319-324.

Troche, S. J., & Rammsayer, T. H. (2009). The influence of temporal resolution power and working memory capacity on psychometric intelligence. *Intelligence, 37*, 479-486.

Turner, M. L., & Engle, R. W. (1989). Is working memory capacity task dependent? *Journal of Memory & Language, 28*, 127-154.

Unsworth, N., Brewer, G. A., & Spillers, G. J. (2009). There's more to the working memory capacity-fluid intelligence relationship than just secondary memory. *Psychonomic Bulletin & Review, 16*, 931-937.

Unsworth, N., & Engle, R. W. (2005). Working memory capacity and fluid abilities: Examining the correlation between operation span and raven. *Intelligence, 33*, 67-81.

Unsworth, N., & Engle, R. W. (2007). On the division of short-term and working memory: An examination of simple and complex span and their relation to higher order abilities. *Psychological Bulletin, 33*, 1038-1066.

Vallat-Azouvi, C., Weber, T., Legrand, L., & Azouvi, P. (2007). Working memory after severe traumatic brain injury. *Journal of the International Neuropsychological Society, 13*, 770-780.

Van der Linden, M., Bredart, S., & Beerten, A. (1994). Age-related differences in updating working memory. *British Journal of Psychology, 85,* 145-152.

Van der Molen, M. J., Van Luit, J. E. H., Jongmans, M. J., & Van der Molen, M. W. (2007). Verbal working memory in children with mild intellectual disabilities. *Journal of Intellectual Disability Research, 51*, 162-169.

van der Sluis, S., van der Leij, A., & de Jong, P. (2005). Working memory in Dutch children with reading- and arithmetic-related LD. *Journal of Learning Disabilities, 38*, 207-221.

Van Gerven, P. W. M., Van Boxtel, M. P. J., Meijer, W. A., Willems, D., & Jolles, J. (2007). On the relative role of inhibition in age-related working memory decline. *Aging, Neuropsychology, and Cognition, 14*, 95-107.

Vandierendonck, A., Kemps, E., Fastame, M. C., & Szmalec, A. (2004). Working memory components of the Corsi blocks task. *British Journal of Psychology, 95*, 57-79.

Vaughan, L., Basak, C., Hartman, M., & Verhaeghen, P. (2008). Aging and working memory inside and outside the focus of attention: Dissociations of availability and accessibility. *Aging, Neuropsychology, and Cognition, 15*, 703-724.

Verhaeghen, P., & Hoyer, W. J. (2007). Aging, focus switching, and task switching in a continuous calculation task: Evidence toward a new working memory control process.

Vicari, S., Caravale, B., Carlesimo, G. A., Casadei, A. M., & Allemand, F. (2004). Spatial working memory deficits in children at ages 3-4 who were low birth weight, preterm infants. *Neuropsychology, 18*, 673-678.

Voelcker-Rehage, C., Stronge, A. J., & Alberts, J. L. (2006). Age-related differences in working memory and force control under dual-task conditions. *Aging, Neuropsychology, and Cognition, 13*, 366-384.

Wechsler, D. (1997a). *Wechsler Adult Intelligence Scale – third edition*. San Antonio, TX: The Psychological Corporation.

Wechsler, D. (1997b). *Wechsler Memory Scale – third edition*. San Antonio, TX: The Psychological Corporation.

Wechsler, D. (2003). *Wechsler Intelligence Scale for Children-fourth edition*. San Antonio, TX: Psychological Corporation.

Wechsler, D. (2008). *Wechsler Adult Intelligence Scale – fourth edition*. San Antonio, TX: The Psychological Corporation.

Wechsler, D. (2009). *Wechsler Memory Scale – fourth edition*. San Antonio, TX: The Psychological Corporation.

Wechsler, D., Kaplan, E., Fein, D., Kramer, J., Morris, R., Delis, F., & Maerlender, A. (2004). *Wechsler Intelligence Scale for Children – fourth edition – Integrated*. San Antonio, TX: The Psychological Corporation.

West, R., Ergis, A., Winocur, G., & Saint-Cyr, J. (1998). The contribution of impaired working memory monitoring to performance of the self-ordered pointing task in normal aging and Parkinson's disease. *Neuropsychology, 12*, 546-554.

Westerberg, H., Hirvikoski, T., Forssberg, H., & Klingberg, T. (2004). Visuo-spatial working memory span: A sensitive measure of cognitive deficits in children with ADHD. *Child Neuropsychology, 10*, 155-161.

White, D. A., Nortz, M. J., Mandernach, T., Huntington, K., & Steiner, R. D. (2002). Age-related working memory impairments in children with prefrontal dysfunction associated with phenylketonuria. *Journal of the International Neuropsychological Society, 8*, 1-11.

Wilson, K. M., & Swanson, H. L. (2001). Are mathematics disabilities due to a domain-general or a domain-specific working memory deficit? *Journal of Learning Disabilities, 34*, 237-248.

Wood, S. J., Pantelis, C., Proffitt, T., Phillips, L. J., Stuart, G. W., Buchanan, J. A., ... Mahony, K. (2003). Spatial working memory ability is a marker of risk-for-psychosis. *Psychological Medicine, 33*, 1239-1247.

Woodcock, R. W., McGrew, K. S., & Mather, N. (2001a). *Woodcock-Johnson III Tests of Cognitive Abilities*. Itasca, IL: Riverside.

Woodcock, R. W., McGrew, K. S., & Mather, N. (2001b). *Woodcock-Johnson III Tests of Achievement*. Itasca, IL: Riverside.

Zanello, A., Curtis, L., Ba, M. B., & Merlo, M. C. G. (2009). Working memory impairments in first-episode psychosis and chronic schizophrenia. *Psychiatry Research, 165*, 10-18.

Zimmer, H. D., Speiser, H. R., & Seidler, B. (2003). Spatio-temporal working-memory and short-term object-location tasks use different memory mechanisms. *Acta Psychologica, 114*, 41-65.

In: Working Memory: Capacity, Developments and…
Editor: Eden S. Levin

ISBN: 978-1-61761-980-9
© 2011 Nova Science Publishers, Inc.-

Chapter 3

EFFECTS OF VISUO-SPATIAL WORKING MEMORY ON WAYFINDING ABILITY

Laura Piccardi[1,2] *and Raffaella Nori*[3]

[1]Department of Health Sciences, University of L'Aquila, Italy
[2]Research Centre of Neuropsychology, IRCCS Foundation, Saint Lucia, Rome, Italy
[3]Department of Psychology, University of Bologna, Italy

ABSTRACT

The present review analyse the relationship between visuo-spatial working memory (VSWM) in wayfinding, which is the ability to move successfully through the environment. As the results of research on individual differences in wayfinding are mixed, various explanation have to be considered. In this chapter, we will analyze these findings in light of the different component of VSWM proposed by Logie (1995, 2003) and a more recent model by Cornoldi and Vecchi (2003).

We will also investigate the development of VSWM and how its changes in older adults, causing a decrease in wayfinding ability. For example, evidence from studies of route learning and memory for object location indicates an aging-related decrement in piloting, particularly in unfamiliar surroundings. On the one hand, the decline in landmark-based navigation could be the result of diminished path integration skill, particularly if path integration typically provides a supplemental informational for piloting. On the other hand, the more basic path integration process may retain its operational integrity beyond the time that association-based piloting begins to reflect a general age-related decline in learning rate. In this chapter, we considered these different explanations in relation to theories about VSWM. Finally, we consider the results of studies on brain-damagedpatients demonstrating the importance of the ventromedial prefrontal cortex, which is necessary to maintain active the goal destination in VSWM for use in navigation.

Keywords: human orientation, topographical memory, landmark-based navigation, working memory, remembering space

Much research in cognitive psychology (e.g., Tversky, 2000) and environmental psychology (e.g., Golledge, 1999) have been devoted to study navigational learning, particularly what happens during route learning and which cognitive abilities are involved. The working-memory system most likely has a role in navigational tasks (Garden, Cornoldi, & Logie, 2002).

The term *working memory* (WM), proposed by Miller, Galanter, and Pribram (1960), emphasizes the functional role of short-term memory (STM) as part of an integrated system for holding and manipulating information during the performance of complex cognitive tasks (Baddeley & Hitch, 1974). The same term has been used with reference to animal learning to refer to situations in which animals need to retain information across several trials during the same day (e.g., Olton, Walker, & Gage, 1978). The mechanisms involved in typical human WM task are certainly different from those used in animal studies. To clarify this issue, Baddeley and Hitch (1974) proposed that the concept of a single, unitary STM should be replaced by a multicomponent system composed of two slave systems: one, the phonological loop, stores acoustic and verbal information, and the other, the visuo-spatial sketchpad, is its visual equivalent (see figure 1). It is assumed that the overall system is controlled by a limited-capacity attentional system, called the central executive. This tripartite structure was modified and revised in subsequent WM theories. In fact, Baddeley (2000) added a fourth component to the model, the episodic buffer, which is a third storage system that links information among working memory systems and long-term memory.

Regardless of the model, WM plays an important role in everyday tasks. Although the role played by the articulatory loop has been extensively studied in these tasks, the structure of visuo-spatial sketchpad was little explored until the end of the 1980s (e.g., Logie, 1986, 1989). New findings have lead to reformulations of Baddeley and Hitch's (1974) original model and to the new theoretical perspective on visuo-spatial working memory (VSWM).

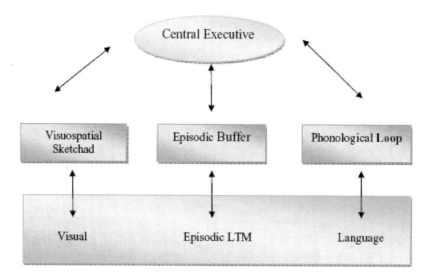

Figure 1. A schematic figure of Baddeley's Working memory model in which the episodic buffer provides an interface between the sub-systems of working memory and long-term memory (source, Baddeley, 2003).

THEORETICAL MODELS OF VISUO-SPATIAL WORKING MEMORY

As the characteristics of VSWM have only been studied recently, the relationships among the different theoretical models are not completely clear. Research over the past few decades has sought to identify the different components involved in VSWM and to clarify their relationship with other memory components. For this purpose, researchers have adopted a wide range of experimental procedures. For example, cognitive neuropsychologists have used functional magnetic resonance imaging (fMRI) and positron emission tomography (PET) to explore the biological/neurological aspects of VSWM (e.g. Levine, Warach & Farah, 1985; Riddoch, Humphreys, Blott, & Hardy, 2003), and cognitive psychologists have used behavioural experiments to clarify this issue (e.g., Pazzaglia & Cornoldi, 1999; Coluccia & Martello, 2004).

In this chapter, we will not provide a complete review of the models presented in the literature but we will discuss only the best models for interpreting experimental results on what happens when we acquire and recall spatial information. Therefore, we will discuss Logie's (1995, 2003) multicomponent model and Cornoldi and Vecchi's (2000, 2003; Cornoldi, 1995) continuum model.

Multicomponent Model

Logie (1995, 2003) assumed that VSWM is divided into two major components: one for processing visual information (*Visual Cache*) and one for processing spatial information (*Inner Scribe*).

The visual cache provides a temporary store for visual information (i.e., colour and shape), and the inner scribe handles information about movement sequences and provides a mechanism through which visual information can be rehearsed in WM. Specifically, information held in the visual cache is subject to decay unless it is maintained. The active inner scribe is responsible for rehearsing the contents of the visual cache and for planning and executing movements. The dissociation between visual and spatial components is supported by reports of studies conducted in both brain-damaged and healthy individuals (e.g., Farah, Hammond, Levine, & Calvo, 1988; Wilson, Baddley, & Young, 1999; Logie & Marchetti 1991; Della Sala, Gray, Baddeley, Allamano, & Wilson, 1999; Quinn & McConnell, 1996; Hamilton, Coates, & Heffernan, 2003; Tresch, Sinnamon, & Seamon, 1993). Some developmental data also support a distinction between a visual and a spatial component (e.g., Logie & Pearson, 1997; Hamilton, Coates, & Heffernan, 2003). Pickering, Gathercole, Hall and Lloyd (2001) reported similar results in a developmental study in which different spatial and visual tasks were adopted. The experimental method used in these studies is called "developmental fractionation" (Hitch, 1990). This term indicates that the cognitive systems responsible for the two tasks seem to develop at different rates and with little overlap in a given age group of children. Recent researches have also demonstrated the possibility of fragmenting the spatial component of VSWM even more. Indeed, Pazzaglia and Cornoldi (1999) showed that the manipulation of the sequential/simultaneous presentation to-be-memorized VSWM stimuli is an important variable, suggesting a differentiation between sequential and simultaneous processes in the inner scribe. Spatial sequential processing requires the recall of a serial position presented in a sequential format, whereas spatial simultaneous processing requires recalling a position presented simultaneously. Therefore, it seems that the visual cache holds visual information such as form, colour, texture, and static layout of objects, and the inner scribe holds both sequential and simultaneous spatial information.

Continuum Model

The model proposed by Cornoldi and Vecchi (2000, 2003; Cornoldi, 1995) is based on two main assumptions: a) the nature of information to be processed, b) the amount of active information processing required. The model is represented as a conical structure; it is organized along a horizontal dimension, which reflects differences in the content of memory (verbal, visuo-spatial), and a vertical dimension, which reflects differences in active and passive processing. Specifically, temporary storage of information requiring a low level of control is located on the lower end of the vertical line, and high-level active tasks (i.e., transformation tasks) occupy the highest positions along the continuum because they require more cognitive resources. In this framework, a visual or spatial sequential/simultaneous task might be passive (i.e., when it requires the simple recall of previously acquired information) or active (i.e., when the task requires integration and manipulation of information to produce an output substantially different from the original input). Note that active processing functions are more sensitive to deterioration and to individual differences than passive ones (e.g., Salthouse & Mitchell, 1989; Vecchi, 1998). The distinction between passive storage and active processing within the VSWM has been posited in many theoretical accounts (e.g., Carpenter & Just, 1989; Cornoldi & Vecchi, 2000; Helstrup, 1989) and has been confirmed in research on imagery in the blind people, in gender differences, and in lifespan development (e.g., Bayliss, Jarrold, Gunn, & Baddeley, 2003; Cavallini, Fastame, Palladino, Rossi, Vecchi, 2003, 2004; Richardson, 1994; Vecchi, 2001). Moreover, a variety of neuropsychological studies on specific learning disabilities support the distinction between passive and active processes in both visual and spatial WM (e.g., Cornoldi, Rigoni, Venneri, & Vecchi, 2000; Rourke, 1989).

ASSESSMENT OF VISUO-SPATIAL WORKING MEMORY

In the literature, few standardized VSWM tests include all components of the visuo-spatial working memory models, and there is no agreement on the format of these tests (Vecchi, Phillips, & Cornoldi, 2001). A number of tasks have been proposed as measures of VSWM. Following we will describe the most used in literature.

1. *The Corsi Block Test* (CBT; Corsi, 1972, Milner, 1971). The apparatus consists of nine cubes placed irregularly on a wooden board. The cubes are numbered on the examiner's side and are tapped by the examiner in sequences of increasing length. Participants are usually required to recall the cubes in the right order. The test was revised recently and contains some variations. For example, a computerised version

contains implications about the process (i.e., the role of vertical dimension, the absence of the continuity element, specifically, the hand movement, between one position and the next) (Cornoldi & Vecchi, 2003). In the "backward" version of the test, participants have to indicate the different positions starting from the last and going back to the first. Several studies have pointed out that the backward version is not a pure measure of VSWM (e.g., Mammarella & Cornoldi, 2005; Vecchi & Richardson, 2001; Vandierendonck, Kemps, Fastame, & Szmalec, 2004; Vandierendonck & Szmalec, 2005). This task is used to measure spatial memory span and, in particular, the sequential component of the inner scribe VSWM subsystem (e.g., Della Sala et al., 1999). It is assumed that the task involves passive processing because it only requires remembering the correct sequence of cubes (Mammarella, Pazzaglia, & Cornoldi, 2006). The test has been used with all age ranges from preschoolers to octogenarians. With the CBT, it is possible to assess deficits in immediate nonverbal memory (De Renzi, Faglioni, & Previdi, 1977; De Renzi & Nichelli, 1975; Morris et al., 1988), developmental changes and gender differences in spatial skills (Capitani, Laiacona, & Ciceri, 1991; Isaacs & Vargha-Khadem, 1989; Orsini et al., 1986), and to clarify theoretical conceptions of visuospatial memory (Jones, Farrand, Stuart, & Morris, 1995). The clinical populations assessed with CBT include learning-disabled children, Korsakoff's patients, demented individuals (e.g., with Alzheimer's and Huntington's disease), and other neurological disorders (for an extensive review of methodological and theoretical considerations see Berch et al., 1998).

2. *The Walking Corsi Test* (WalCT; Piccardi et al., 2008). This is a large version of the CBT (scale 10:1); it is used to evaluate route-memory ability by measuring a pathway span. It was built in an empty room (5m x 6m) in which the walls were completely covered with curtains to hide all external landmarks (i.e., doors, heaters, etc.). Nine black squares (30 cm x 30 cm) were placed on a 2.50 m x 3.00 m light-grey carpet. The scaled position and the relative spatial layout of the squares were the same as in *Corsi Block Test*. In the WalCT, the experimental conditions, administration, and scoring procedures are identical to those of the CBT; the WalCT, however, is particularly sensitive to navigational deficits. Indeed, patients with topographical disorientation failed selectively in WalCT but not on CBT (Piccardi et al., 2010; Piccardi et al., submitted).

3. *The Visual Pattern Test* (VPT; Della Sala, Gray, Baddeley, & Wilson, 1997). In the VRPT, a single matrix is presented in which the 50% of the boxes are outlined in black. The participants' task is to indicate on the response grid which is the same as the test sheet, the positions that were marked during the presentation phase. This test is used to measure the visual but not the spatial component of visuo-spatial working memory. Indeed, many results obtained with the VPT indicate that it does not measure the same type of ability measured by the Corsi Block Test. In fact, Della Sala and co-workers (1999) pointed out three aspects of this issue: 1. in healthy subjects, the intercorrelation between visual pattern test and the Corsi Block Test is low, suggesting that the two tests measure different functions; 2. the presence of a double dissociation between the two tasks is found in brain-damage patients. Specifically, two patients who performed normally on the Visual Pattern Test presented an impaired performance on the Corsi Block Test and another patient

presented the opposite performance (Grossi et al., 1993); 3. studies based on the interference paradigm show that participants perform the VPT or the Corsi Blok Test concurrently with activities devised to interfere with either the spatial or the visual component of visual-spatial working memory. The different interference in the two tasks is a powerful evidence that they measure different aspects of visuo-spatial working memory. Another important difference between the VPT and the CBT is the modality of presentation. In the VPT, a simultaneous pattern to remember is showed, whereas the CBT presents an increasing number of cubes and participants have to remember not only the cubes but also the order of sequence. This distinction seems crucial because it demonstrates the presence of a double dissociation between spatial-simultaneous and spatial-sequential working memory in different subtypes of visuospatial (nonverbal) learning disabled children (Mammarella et al., 2006).

4. *Mr. Blobby* (Hamilton, Coates, & Hefferan, 2003). In this test, participants have to memorize the location of a lot of spots presented simultaneously on the body of a puppet. In the recognition phase, they are shown a photo of the puppet and have to decide whether the spots are located in the same places as those presented initially. This task should measure both the visual and the spatial component of VSWM.

5. *Benton Visual Retention Test* (BVRT; Sivan, 1992). The BVRT is a widely used visual recall test with three, parallel, roughly equivalent forms. A three figure-design format is showen for 10 seconds and immediatly recalled by drawing. Six types of error are recognized: omissions, distortions, perseverations, rotations, misplacements, and errors in size. In as much as the errors are tabulated by type, the examiner is able to determine the patient's problem by using the test. The BVRT is also particularly sensitive for detecting the presence of heminattention disorders and of cognitive decline in Alzheimer's disease (Storandt et al., 1986). This test involves many different capacities (i.e., visuomotor response, visuospatial perception, visual and verbal conceptualization - some of the designs can be conceptualized verbally-, and immediate memory span) so its sensitivity to brain disorders is not surprising. Normative data show that a decrease in the number of correct responses is an effect of aging . As to types of errors, older individuals (ages 65 to 89) made mostly distortion errors and fewer rotation and omission errors (Eslinger et al., 1988).

6. *Complex Figure Test: Recall administration* (Rey, 1941; Osterrieth, 1944).
Recall of the Complex Figure is usually given immediately after the copy trial, after a delay, or both. The Rey-Osterrieth figure is the one most commonly used . Due to its popularity, many variations in administration and scoring have been reported. In most administrations, when given the copy instructions subjects are not forewarned that they will have to reproduce the figure from memory. The immediate recall trial is given after a delay of only 30 sec (Loring et al., 1990); but according to Osterrieth's (1944) procedure, some examiners administrer the test after 3 min (short) delay. Significant age effects are reported consistently in recall trials. Spreen and Strauss (1998) found that decline begins when participants are in their 30s and continues rather steadily until they are in their 70s, when a larger score difference appears. Gender differences are also reported, that is, men seem to recall better than women (Bennet-Levy, 1984; Rosselli & Ardila, 1991). The Rey-Osterrieth figure-recall task is sensitive in detecting deficits in a variety of clinical populations (alcoholic patients; traumatic brain-injured patients; Parkinson's disease patients, and

right brain-damaged patients) (Dawson & Grant, 2000; Leininger et al., 1990; Ogden et al., 1990; Lezak et al., 2004).

7. *Visuo-spatial Working Memory Test Battery* (BEMViS; Mammarella, Cornoldi, & Pazzaglia, 2006; Cornoldi & Vecchi, 2003). The battery consists of 13 tasks: 3 assess verbal working memory and 10 VSWM. We will consider only the VSWM tasks, which are based on the continuum model proposed by Cornoldi and Vecchi (2003) and which differentiate between a visual component and spatial (sequential and simultaneous) component on the horizontal continuum and between active and passive processes on the vertical one.

The *Visual* tasks comprise two tests: *The House Recognition Test* (considered a passive task), in which participants have to recognize a complex figure (i.e., a house) shown for 2 seconds in a set of two or more stimuli (from 2 to 6) according to the degree of complexity of the different tasks; and the *Signs Reproduction Test,* which is also considered a passive task (adapted from Cornoldi & Gruppo MT, 1992). Participants have to reproduce a series of signs in the same direction and with the same shape as those they had already studied for 3 seconds. Also in this task, the complexity level is determinate by the number of signs the participants have to remember. Finally, *The Jigsaw Puzzle Task* is classified as an active task (adapted from Vecchi & Richardson, 2000) and based on Snodgrass and Vanderwart's (1980) drawings. It involves solving a puzzle by writing the number corresponding to each piece on the response sheet. All pieces of the puzzle are available throughout the test. As for the others tasks, the number of pieces determines the task complexity.

Three tasks are used to evaluate the *Spatial Sequential* component of VSWM. The *Dynamic Mazes* (adapted from Pickering, Gathercole & Peaker, 1998) is considered a passive task. It consists of remembering a path traced by the experiment in a maze and then successively reproducing it in an identical blank maze. The second task is the *Corsi Block Test* (Corsi, 1972) considered a passive task, which we have already described. Finally, the *Pathway Span Task* is considered an active task. Participants have to mentally visualize a path described by the experimenter in a blank matrix. At the end of the sequence of indications, they have to indicate the goal on the matrix. Task complexity is determined by the size of the matrix and the number of indications specified by the experimenter.

The *Spatial Simultaneous* tasks consist of *The Visual Pattern Test* (adapted from Della Sala et al., 1997), which it is considered a passive task. Participants have to memorize a series of black squares in a matrix within 3 seconds and then to indicate them on an identical blank matrix. *Static Mazes* (adapted from Pickering et al., 1998) is a passive task. Participants have to memorize a path drown on a maze whitin 3 seconds and then have to reproduce it on an identical blank maze. Moreover, *The Dots Reproduction Test* is considered passive. Participants have to reproduce the exact positions of a series of dots already studied for 3 seconds on a blank sheet of paper. Finally, *The Visual Pattern Test* also has an active version (adapted from Della Sala et al., 1997). The difference between this one and the original version, described above, is that here participant has to reproduce the studied pattern in an identical blank matrix.

WAYFINDING AND VISUO-SPATIAL WORKING MEMORY

Wayfinding is the ability to move successfully through the environment. More specifically, it is the ability to learn, recall, and follow a route through the environment (Blades, 1991). Downs and Stea (1973) define four stages in wayfinding: 1) orientation to determine self-location and estimated target location; 2) initial route choice in selecting routes from origin to target location; 3) route monitoring, that is, checking the route taken by estimating self-location and target location as well as reassessing/confirming the route choice; and 4) recognition of the target. Moreover, Golledge (1999) stated that successful wayfinding is determined by the following: 1) identifying origin and destination, 2) determining turn angles, 3) identifying segment lengths and direction of movements, 4) recognizing routes and distant landmarks, and 5) embedding the routes taken into a larger frame of reference.

Usually, there are three different types of wayfinding (Allen, 1999): 1) wayfinding travelling between a known starting point and a known goal along familiar routes (*common type wayfinding*), such as the student's daily trip to the university; 2) exploring different routes to go from a known starting point to reach a known goal (*exploratory wayfinding*); 3) travelling from either a known or unknown starting point to a novel destination (*task-based wayfinding*).

To asses wayfinding ability, experimenters often ask participants to memorize an unfamiliar path and then to repeat it going from the starting point to the goal or, more usually, in reversal order, because it has been shown that backward reconstruction of a route is more difficult than forward reconstruction (Brown, 1976); thus, it is a better measure of wayfinding ability. This task has been performed in different environments, including woods (e.g., Malinowski & Gillespie, 2001; Nori, Grandicelli, & Giusberti, 2009), buildings (e.g., Sadalla & Montello, 1989; Lawton, 1996; Lawton, Charleston, & Zieles, 1996), and university campus (e.g., Kirasic, Allen, & Siegel, 1984; Montello & Pick, 1993; Saucier et al., 2002). This kind of wayfinding, which requires going from one point to another, can be considered basic wayfinding similar to common wayfinding (Reagan & Baldwin, 2006).

As suggested by Denis, Pazzaglia, Cornoldi, and Bertolo (1999), a number of wayfinding measures could be considered (a) *direction errors*: participant walks in the wrong direction at a decision point; (b) *pauses*: participant expresses uncertainty and stops during wayfinding; (c) *travel time*: the time that a participant takes to navigate from the end (start) to the starting (end) point.

Generally, cognitive research deals with the cognitive processes involved in route learning and the strategies adopted to move successfully through the environment. These different measures permit obtaining a complete picture's behavior as they move toward a goal.

With regard to wayfinding ability, cognitive psychologists have investigated the need for route-learning processes and the cognitive structures involved in successful wayfinding (Garden, Cornoldi, & Logie, 2002; Nori, Grandicelli, & Giusberti, 2009). Lindberg and Gärling (1981) conducted one of the first studies in this area. They investigated the role of a limited-capacity cognitive system (Working Memory) in giving directions and estimating distances, abilities considered necessary to reach a goal (Golledge, 1999). Using a dual-task paradigm, Lindberg and Gärling asked participants to walk through alleyways and estimate the direction and distance to reference points when they stopped. In the concurrent task condition, participants had difficulty keeping track of where they were relative to designated reference points along the route, but were able to encode information about the route (distance walked and direction changes). This finding supports the idea that wayfinding requires effective use of a limited-capacity cognitive system. More recently, Garden, Cornoldi and Logie (2002) conducted two experiments to explore the role of working memory and subsequent route retrieval. Specifically, in experiment 1 the authors used a concurrent task paradigm to test the hypothesis that the route learning from a map requires general working memory resources. Results showed that the concurrent spatial task (i.e., spatial tapping) disrupted route recognition more than articulatory suppression. In experiment 2, the authors again used the concurrent task paradigm, but this time in an explored route learning task to analyze wayfinding ability. In particular, they asked the participants to follow an experimenter along a routes in the city center of Padua (Italy).. Results partially confirmed those of the experiment 1: both concurrent tasks (spatial and verbal) interfered with route learning; more specifically, participants with high spatial ability were more affected by the concurrent spatial task than low spatial ability participants who were more affected by the concurrent ariculatory suppression (verbal) task. Therefore, this work supports the hypothesis that VSWM is involved in wayfinding and more specifically that its involvement is determined by the different participants' spatial ability, that is in real environment only performances of people with high spatial ability are based on VSWM. This finding is supported by the work of Nori, Grandicelli and Giusberti (2009) in which participants with high-VSWM ability performed a wayfinding task in a botanical garden better that low-VSWM participants. Specifically, the wayfinding behavior of high-VSWM participants and low-VSWM participants is completely different: the latter pause more often than the former and therefore take longer to reach the goal. As predicted by Nori and co-workers, people with high VSWM compare their mental spatial representation directly with the external environment. This process does not seem to require stopping along the way and could be considered an online updating of spatial information. In fact, walking through an environment entails continually changing perspective, which has to be updated every time a new orientation is presented. The authors also predicted that the moving reference frame would constitute an additional load for the spatial component of VSWM, which individuals with low VSWM are unable to represent.

AGE-RELATED CHANGES IN WAYFINDING AND VISUO-SPATIAL WORKING MEMORY

Wayfinding ability typically declines with age; in fact, older people prefer familiar to novel places and are slower and less accurate in finding their way in new environments (Moffat et al., 2001; Newman & Kasznik, 2000). Elderly individuals self-report deficits in navigation and often avoid unfamiliar routes and places (Burns, 1999).

Evidence suggests that salient cues are important for place learning and developing a cognitive map, especially in aging (Newman & Kaszniak, 2000; Davis et al., 2009). Newman and Kaszniak (2000) observed increased dependence on cues with aging. They reported that older people do not recall previously learned environments as well as younger people when a number of cues are removed after learning trials. Supporting the importance of distinctive landmarks for older people, in a study by Lipman (1991) younger and older participants were asked to remember the most of the critical cues learned during a slide presentation of an environmental route; results showed that older people remember fewer cues and only the most distinctive ones. According to Caduff and Timps (2007), the salience of a landmark is determined by three components: (i) perceptual: the cue's distinctive properties (i.e. the colour); (ii) cognitive: it has personal meaning for the observer related to general knowledge about it or previous experience with it; (iii) contextual: the salience of landmark depends on the navigational task demands, that is, the type of wayfinding task and the cognitive and physical resources necessary to solve it. For example, research has shown that colour may be a critical cue property for place learning in the aging (Fauberty, 2002) and that the use of colour may facilitate recognition of objects in normal aged people and in those with dementia (Cernin, Keller, & Stoner, 2003; Wijk et al., 2002; Wurm, Legge, Isenberg, & Luebker, 1993). Advancing age is associated with decrements in several spatial navigation skills both in place-learning (i.e., learning of salient landmarks) and in action-based navigation (specifically, route learning) (Barrash, 1994; Wilkiness et al., 1997; Moffat et al., 2001; 2006; Driscoll et al., 2003; 2005; Iaria et al., 2009). As mentioned, working memory is involved in attending to, selecting and remembering relevant environmental information that contributes to generating and updating environmental knowledge (Tolman, 1948; Kirasic et al., 1992). Recent studies have also established that visuo-spatial working memory is more age-sensitive than phonological/verbal working memory (e.g., Cornoldi & Vecchi, 2003; Jenkins, Myerson, Joerding, & Hale, 2000a,b). Therefore, most decreased performances in aged people could depend on reduced working memory capacity. Indeed, several studies have reported a decrease in working memory capacity during aging (e.g., Jonides et al., 2000; Reuter-Lorenz et al., 2000; Salthouse et al., 1989; Georgiou-Karistianis et al., 2006) that results in a less detailed and informative environmental knowledge. For instance, Iaria and co-workers (2009) found that older individuals required more time to acquire environmental information and were less efficient in using it to orient themselves then younger individuals. They also reported qualitative performance data indicating that older participants had difficulty in heading in the right direction and in detouring to other landmarks along the way compared to younger participants who generally headed in the right direction and reached the target location following the shortest pathway (Iaria et al., 2009). Decreased ability to focus on or retain nonsalient landmarks could lead to a difficulty in learning new environments and in recognizing previously learned environments (Davis et al., 2009). In a study of place learning and working memory performance in a group of older women, Davis and co-workers (2009) found that place learning in a virtual environment was affected by the type of cues avaible and by working memory capacity. In particular, older women's performances improved in the salient cue condition but were very poor in the nonsalient cue condition. According to Davis and co-workers (2009), when individuals have a decreased working memory capacity they have greater difficulty in learning simple environments without salient cues. These authors also found that verbal working memory, specifically better performance on Digit Span Backward, predicted success on the place learning virtual test. They found no significant effect on spatial working memory (i.e., performance on Corsi Block Test: CBT, Corsi, 1972), in particular, CBT was not a significant predictor of performance for either time to find the target or heading error. They explained this finding by stressing the fact that CBT is a test of small-scale space and may not be related to search strategies in large-scale environments like the CG-Arena, which is a virtual variant of the Morris Water Maze (Morris, 1981) and is used to test place learning humans and animals.

Piccardi et al. (2008) created a large-scale version of CBT, called the Walking Corsi Test (WalCT), in which the platform of CBT is reproduced on the floor (10:1 scale). The participants' task was to reproduce it by walking in sequences of steps, showed by the examiner. The authors proposed this large-scale version because they observed that although the CBT is well-known and extensively used in clinical practice, it is not useful for testing navigational deficits. They found that patients with pervasive topographical disorientation failed on WalCT but not on the CBT (Piccardi et al., 2010; Piccardi et al., submitted). Moreover, they found age-related differences when they compared the younger and older participants; specifically, their results showed a significant difference in working memory and learning performance due to age but no difference for delayed recall. Young participants also had a larger working memory span than older ones on both tests (CBT and WalCT). Nevertheless, learning differences between younger and older individuals emerged only on the WalCT, because younger participants learned significantly faster than older ones. Note also that no significant difference in the ability of older participants to learn supra-span sequences in reaching space (CBT) and in navigational space (WalCT), whereas younger subjects found easier to learn a supra-span sequence in navigational space (WalCT) than in reaching space (CBT). These results can be explained in terms of using of strategies: older participants probably used the same strategy when they had to recall a supra-span sequence in the WalCT and in the CBT, vice versa younger participants probably used selective strategies depending on the type of space (reaching versus navigational). In the delayed recall test, both groups remembered steps more readily than touched cubes (Piccardi et al., submitted). It is generally assumed that normal aging is associated with a decline in many cognitive processes, including episodic memory, attention, working memory, and spatial learning (Evans et al., 1984, Sharps et al., 1987; Kausler, 1994; Rutledge et al., 1997; Driscoll et al., 2005). This decline seems to depend on structural and biochemical changes in the hippocampus and which may underlie the cognitive decay observed in performance (Driscoll et al., 2003). Note that in learning a supra-span sequence the older participants examined in Piccardi and co-workers' study showed no difference between reaching and navigational space and a significant difference compared to the younger subjects' group only in route-memory performance. Again, their finding stresses the presence of different types of visuo-spatial memory, one of which may be more age-dependent than the other. In any case, the presence of topographical disorientation may be one of the early symptoms of mental decay. Thus, it is noteworthy that navigational space is affected more than reaching space also in normal aging. This may depend on changes in the hippocampus, which has a crucial role in place learning (Hartley & Burgess, 2005; Baddeley et al., 1986; Driscoll et al., 2005).

In real-world environments, age-related differences also emerge (for a review see Moffat, 2009). Kirasic (1991) assessed younger and older women's navigational skills in novel and familiar supermarkets and observed that younger women acquired spatial information faster than older ones. Wilkniss and co-workers (1997) asked participants to navigate through the hallways of a hospital after studying the map of it. They found that older participants took longer and made more turning errors than younger ones. Unlike, in studies performed in virtual environment, they found that older participants performed a comparably to younger participants in recalling objects encountered along the way; but, differently from young participants, they had difficulty placing them in the right temporal sequence (Wilkniss et al.,

1997). Moffat and co-workers (2001), used a virtual route learning task, which included several intersecting corridors, found that older people mostly made location errors and tended to revisit corridor which did not lead to the goal.

Besides a global age-related deficit, evidence shows that age effects are apparent in specific component processes of navigation, including critical environmental features (e.g., landmarks), temporally and spatially organizing the relevant features, and in landmark recall, scene recognition, landmark location identification and self-orientation (Wilkniss et al, 1997; Bruce & Herman, 1983; Cushman et al., 2008; Evans et al., 1984). Evidence from studies of route learning (Barash, 1994; Kirasic, 1991, 2000; Lipman, 1991; Lipmann & Caplan, 1992; Wilkniss, Jones, Korol, Gold, & Manning, 1997) and memory for object location (Cooney & Arbuckle, 1997; Evans, Brennan, Skorpanich, & Held, 1984; Uttl & Graf, 1993) indicate an aging-related decrement in integrating information deriving from landmarks and one's position for orientation in the environment, particularly in unfamiliar surroundings.

Other more basic functions involved in navigation also seem be affected by aging. One is the ability to perform simple, return-to origin task. Allen and co-workers (2004) assessed the ability of younger and older participants to perform a so-called "triangle completion task" (a procedure largely used to assess path integration in animals and humans: Etienne et al., 1998; Gallistel, 1990; Loomis et al., 1993; Nico et al., 2002). They also investigated which cognitive resources (i.e., information processing-speed and working memory capability) are involved in path integration skills and affected individual performances. Their results showed that sensitivity to vestibular sources of information regarding acceleration and rotation declines significantly in late adulthood. In fact, Allen and co-workers (2004) found that older adults differed from younger ones in the passive conveyance condition (in which only vestibular information was available) but not in condition in which they were led on foot (in which they had both kinesthetic and vestibular information about locomotion). These findings suggest a deficit in the encoding of body rotation, which is primarily based on vestibular information, leading to a decline in the accuracy of path integration. They also found that although path integration and spatial updating did not require cognitive resources in simple circumstances, they might require them in more demanding task conditions (see for instance, Amorin et al., 1997; Farrell & Thomson, 1998; Garling et al., 1985; Lindberg & Garling, 1983), specifically for encoding successive locations on the basis of kinesthetic or vestibular information requiring a more demanding working memory component. Allen and co-workers (2004) stressed the practical implications of their findings; according to them, the risk of spatial disorientation increases in older adults who are conveyed by passive means from place to place, especially when visual and auditory information is limited.

MENTAL DECAY: VISUO-SPATIAL WORKING MEMORY AND WAYFINDING

Mild cognitive impairment (MCI) and Alzheimer's disease (AD) are associated with wayfinding problems even in the early stages (Chiu et al., 2004; delpolyi et al., 2007; Rowe, 2003). "Getting lost" and "wandering" episodes are a major hints and may serve to indicate that something is wrong (Klein et al., 1999). Around 36,9% of patients with dementia get lost outside their homes and 28,3% get lost inside their homes (Ballard et al., 1991). When we move in the environment, three different types of information are integrated: vestibular information (i.e., awareness of changes in body orientation and motion), proprioceptive information (i.e., awareness of the body and feedback from muscles and joints) and vision (i.e., optic flow, which provides information about visual displacement across the retina). A stronger deficit in optic flow perception was found during navigational tasks in AD patients but not in normally aging individuals; however, the formers were able to perceive simple moving patterns (see Tetewsky & Duffy, 1999; O'Brien et al., 2001; Cushman et al., 2008; Mapstone et al., 2008). Getting lost seems to be more frequent in AD than other types of dementia. A study performed in Taiwan reported that approximatively 71% of mild to severe AD patients showed this behavior (Hwang et al., 1997). Guariglia and Nitrini (2009) found that topographical disorientation is present even in mild stage of AD; similar findings were reported previously (Cherrier et al., 2001; Teri et al., 1989). These authors also found that patients with AD and topographical disorientation were able to perform some visuo-spatial tasks, such as point localization, nonsense drawing, and three-dimensional figure copy when compared to control subjects without dementia, suggesting that topographical disorientation in AD is not the consequence of a more general deficit in spatial and visual functions. In general, a spatial working memory deficit has been described in AD (for a review see Huntley & Howard, 2010); but controversial data have been reported on the presence of visual working memory deficits even in the first stages of the illness (Martin et al., 1985; Grossi et al., 1993; Carlesimo et al., 1994; Trojano et al., 1994; Cherry et al., 1996; Guariglia & Nitrini, 2009; Perry et al., 2000). Huntley and Howard (2010) suggest that conflicting results might be explained by differences in disease severity among subjects. Indeed, examiners who distinguished between "minimal or preclinical" AD and "mild cognitive impairment" found digit spans preserved in minimal and mild AD and impaired in mild and moderate AD (Orsini et al., 1988; Greene et al., 1995; Hodges & Patterson, 1995; Traykov et al., 2007). Failure on digit span tasks has been interpreted as impairment of the phonological loop and central executive as the disease progresses (Backman et al., 2001; Twamley et al., 2006). Differently, spatial memory span assessed by means of Corsi Block Test was impaired in both mild and moderate AD groups compared to both young and elderly healthy people (Corkin, 1982; Orsini et al., 1988; Spinnler et al., 1988; Grossi et al., 1993; Trojano et al., 1994); this deficit was interpreted as impairment of both the visuo-spatial sketchpad and the central executive (Carlesimo et al., 1994). Differently from Guariglia and Nitrini (2009), who observed comparable performance in patients with mild dementia and healthy participants in spatial working memory, and deficits just in: egocentric and allocentric disorientation, landmark recognition, route description, geographic orientation, house drawing, line orientation and mental rotation. Both Monacelli and co-workers (2003) and Uc and co-workers (2005) observed a deficit in landmark recognition even in mild cognitive impairment. The first study evaluated landmark recognition in a hospital hall and the other tested landmark identification during actual driving. Results showed the same difficulty on tasks requiring a strong spatial working memory effort. Hort and co-workers (2006) assessed patients in various stage of mild cognitive impairment (mild to moderate probable AD group; mild cognitive impairment (MCI) group; SMC, in which patients complained about everyday memory problems but did not display any objective memory impairment), AD patients, and healthy elderly participants in four navigational tasks that required locating an invisible goal inside a circular arena. Each task began with an overhead view of the arena on a computer monitor, then real navigation inside the actual space, that is, an enclosed arena 2.9 m in diameter. Depending on the task, the participants could use the starting position and/or cues on the wall for navigation. Thus, they were focused on allocentric and egocentric navigation. The authors found great differences in spatial navigation impairment among the MCI subtypes. The individuals with AD and MCI, who suffered from other subtle semantic and/or attention-executive function deficits, were impaired in all subtests; and those with MCI, who were impaired in non-memory cognitive domains, and SMC groups were similar to controls.

Pure amnesic patients and patients with amnesic problems and attention-executive function deficits differed from each other. The latter were unable to find the goal in any of the tasks. Besides being impaired in the distance error during in all tasks, they were also impaired in recalling the correct side of the arena, suggesting serious impairment in spatial orientation. Differently, the pure amnesic MCI group was impaired only when allocentric navigation depended on two independent cues to reach the starting position and when they had to navigate in real space. Although they have also had problems in remembering the target location for long period, they were able to learn.

Hort and co-workers (2006) interpreted the disorientation observed in MCI in an analogous of Morris Water Maze due to impaired spatial memory. Therefore, they suggested that measuring spatial navigation as predictor of the onset of clinical symptoms might help clinicians to identify patients in the earlier stages of AD and distinguish them from patients with MCI of other etiologies.

NEUROIMAGING STUDIES AND NEUROLOGICAL CORRELATES INVOLVED IN AGE EFFECTS ON NAVIGATION

Neurimaging and brain lesion studies in human and animal research have identified a network of structures involved in navigation, specifically, the hippocampus, the parahippocampal gyrus, the cerebellum, the parietal cortex, the posterior cingulated gyrus, the retrosplenial cortex and the right prefrontal areas (e.g., Aguirre et al., 1996; Barrash, 1998, Aguirre & D'Esposito, 1999; Grön et al. 2000; Katayama et al., 1999; Maguire et al., 1998). In particular, the hippocampus seems to be crucial in allocentric representations of the environment (Feigenbaum & Rolls, 1991; O'Keefe & Nadel, 1978), whereas the posterior parietal cortex is more involved in egocentric representation, that is, body locations with respect to the environment (Thier & Andersen, 1996; Galati et al., 2000; Colby, 1999). Differently, right prefrontal areas (Brodmann areas 9 and 46) are activated by visuospatial working memory tasks and are involved in complex navigational tasks (Owen et al., 1996; Salmon et al., 1996). Ciaramelli (2008) described a patient (L.G.) with a lesion in ventromedial prefrontal and rostral anterior cingulate cortices who was affected by topographical disorientation. The patient's performance improved when he was given the name of the destination or a cue to rehearse destination at regular intervals. This observation suggests that these structures have an important role in maintaining the goal destination in working memory. Indeed, this patient had good general topographical knowledge of his environment but failed when asked to describe a set of routes between locations (Ciaramelli, 2008). Since L.G. was distracted by highly salient landmarks, the author interpreted his performance as inability to suppress irrelevant information, which is usually carried out by the ventromedial prefrontal cortex.

Although human navigation is an extremely complex process, it is possible to observe differences in the brain activation of individuals engaged in performing the same task. For instance, Grön and co-workers (2000) demonstrated a distinct gender-specific brain activation when participants search for an exit a three-dimensional virtual maze. Specifically, in men the left hippocampus was activated whereas and in women the right parietal and right prefrontal cortex . The authors interpreted this distinct functional anatomy of spatial cognition in women versus men as related to differences in the processing of spatial information. Sandstrom and co-workers (1998) showed that women rely predominantly on landmark cues, whereas men use both geometric and landmark cues. Therefore, Grön and co-workers (2000) hypothesised that the activity recorded in the prefrontal area (Brodmann's area 9/46) in the female group reflected the working-memory demand that the landmark cues be held on-line. The left hippocampal activity in the male group represented the neural substrate that enables men to process multiple geometric cues. Alternatively, male-specific hippocampal activity might reflect men's reliance on information from episodic memory in navigation.

The parahyppocampal gyrus seems to have a role in landmark recognition (Aguirre & D'Esposito, 1999), whereas lesions in the retrosplenial cortex are associated with a heading impairment, that is, impaired general sense of direction (Takahashi et al., 1997).

The following studies are also critically involved in the effects of increasing age on navigation: the hippocampus, the parahippocampal gyrus, the posterior cingulated gyrus (retrosplenial cortex), the parietal lobes, and the pre-frontal cortex. For instance, it is well-known that in Alzheimer's disease the medial temporal region is one of the first structure to be affected (e.g., Jack et al., 1997; 1998). Another important structure in spatial memory is the caudate nucleus, which is often activated in young participants during virtual navigation tasks in functional magnetic resonance studies (Maguire et al., 1998; Iaria et al., 2003; Moffat et al., 2006). This structure plays a crucial role because of its connection to the pre-frontal cortex and the hippocampus (Alexander et al., 1986); it is also vulnerable to aging. In fact, Moffat and co-workers (2007) demonstrated that individuals (young and old) with a larger caudate nucleus have better spatial performance. Some studies have reported that the caudate nucleus works with the hippocampal system and has a role in the procedural components of spatial behaviour (e.g., Voermans et al., 2004; Hartley et al., 2003; Iaria et al., 2003). In as much as navigation is a complex cognitive process that depends on the preservation or good functioning of other cognitive domains, such as working memory, attention, and visual perception, it is not surprisingly that a distributed network of brain regions underlies navigational skills. Some structures of this network are particularly sensitive to aging. In particular, the frontostriatal and hippocampal circuits seem to deteriorate with advancing age; and they are associated with place learning behavior and general navigational success (see Raz & Rodrigue, 2006 for a review; Iaria et al., 2009). Reports indicate that route encoding is associated with age-related alterations in neural activity in prefrontal, caudate, parahippocampal, and parietal regions, whereas place learning is associated with age-related reductions in prefrontal, hippocampal, parahippocampal, retrosplenial, and parietal regions (Antonova et al., 2009; Meulenbroek et al., 2004; Moffat et al., 2006). Difficulty in spatial orientation, which is often observed in Alzheimer's disease, has been associated with damage to several brain areas including the medial temporal lobe, the ventral occipitotemporal, the posterior parietal, and the restrosplenial cortex (Aguire & D'Esposito, 1998). The optic flow discrimination deficit, which is also observed in Alzheimer's patients, may reflect posterior parietal cortical dysfunction (Morrone et al., 2000) in integrating multisensory cues for self-movement; instead, selective impairment of allocentric and most real space subtests suggests a hippocampal deficit (Hort et al., 2006). Medial temporal lobe damage has been associated with poor performances in analogues of the Morris Water Maze (e.g., Feugenbaum & Morris, 2004; Holdstock et al., 2000; Bohbot et al., 1998) as well as in a virtual reality shifted-viewpoint spatial memory test (King et al., 2002). Moreover, lesions in the temporal lobe also compromised topographical orientation in a real environment (Maguire et al., 1996). Therefore, impairment of both the allocentric mode of navigation and memory for configurations in the real space is consistent with the medial temporal lobe damage observed both in patients with selective lesions and with mild cognitive impairment.

REFERENCES

[1] Aguirre, G. K. & D'Esposito, M. (1999). Topographical disorientation: A synthesis and taxonomy. *Brain, 122*, 1613-1628.
[2] Aguirre, G. K., Detre, J. A., Alsop, D. C. & D'Esposito, M. (1996). The parahippocampus subserves topographical learning in man. *Cerebral Cortex, 6(6)*, 823–829.
[3] Aguirre, G. K., Zarahn, E. & D'Esposito, M. (1998). Neural components of topographical representation [Review]. *Proc. Natl Acad Sci USA, 95*, 839-46.
[4] Allen, G. L. (1999). Spatial abilities, cognitive maps, and wayfinding. Bases for individual differences in spatial cognition and behavior. In: R. G. Golledge (Ed), *Wayfinding behavior. Cognitive mapping and other spatial processes* (pp. 46-80). Baltimore, MD: Johns Hopkins University Press.
[5] Allen, G. L., Kirasic, K. C. & Rashotte, M. A. (2004). Aging and path integration skill: Kinestetic and vestibular contribution to wayfinding. *Perception & Psychophysics, 66(1)*, 170-179.
[6] Amorim, M. A., Glasauer, S., Corpinot, K. & Berthoz, A. (1997). Updating an object's orientation and location during nonvisual navigation: A comparison between two processing modes. *Perception & Psychophysics, 59*, 404-418.
[7] Antonova, E., Parslow, D., Brammer, M., Dawson, G. R., Jackson, S. H. & Morris, R. G. (2009). Age-related neural activity during allocentric spatial memory. *Memory, 17*, 125-143.
[8] Baddeley, A. D. (2000). Short-Term and Working Memory. In E. Tulving, & F. I. M. Craick (Eds.), *The Oxford Handbook of Memory* (pp. 77-92). Oxford: Oxford University Press.
[9] Baddeley, A. D. (2003). Working memory: looking back and looking forward. *Nature Reviews Neuroscience, 4*, 829-839.
[10] Baddeley, A. D. & Hitch, G. J. L (1974). Working Memory. In G. A. Bower (Ed.), *The psychology of learning and motivation: advances in research and theory* (Vol. 8, pp. 47-89). Academic Press: New York.
[11] Baddeley, A. D., Bressi, S., Della Sala, S., Logie, R. & Spinnler, H. (1986). Dementia and working memory. *Quarterly Journal of Experimental Psychology A, 38*, 603-18.
[12] Ballard, C. G., Mohan, R. N., Handy, C. B. & Patel, A. (1991). Wandering in dementia suffers. *International Journal of Geriatric Psychiatry, 6*, 611-614.

[13] Barrash, J. (1994). Age-related decline in route learning ability. *Developmental Neuropsychology, 10*, 189-201.

[14] Barrash, J. (1998). A historical review of topographical disorientation and its neuroanatomical correlates. *Journal of Clinical and Experimental Neuropsychology, 20(6)*, 807-827.

[15] Bayliss, D. M., Jarrold, C., Gunn, D. M. & Baddeley, A. D. (2003). The complexities of complex span: Explaining individual differences in working memory in children and adults. *Journal of Experimental Psychology: General, 132(1)*, 71-92.

[16] Bennet-Levy, J. (1984). Long term effects of severe head closed injury on memory: evidence from a consecutive series of young adults. *Acta Neurologica Scandinavia, 70*, 285-298.

[17] Berch, D. B., Krikorian, R. & Huha, E. (1998). The Corsi Block-Tapping Task: Methodological and Theoretical Considerations. *Brain & Cognition, 38*, 317-338.

[18] Blades, M. (1991). Wayfinding theory and research: The need for a new approach. In D. M. Mark & A. Y. Franks (Eds.), *Cognitive and Linguistic Aspects of Geographic Space* (pp. 137-165). London: Kluwer Academic.

[19] Bohbot, V., Kalina, M., Stepankova, K., Spackova, N., Petrides, M. & Nadel, L. (1998). Spatial memory deficits in patients with lesions to the right hippocampus and to the right parahippocampal cortex. *Neuropsychologica, 36*, 1217–1238.

[20] Brown, A. L. (1976). The construction of temporal succession by pre-operational children. In A. Pick (Ed.), *Minnesota Symposium on Child Psychology, Vol. 10* (103-152). Minneapolis, MN: University of Minnesota Press.

[21] Bruce P. R., & Herman, J. F. (1983). Spatial knowledge of young and elderly adults: scene recognition from familiar and novel perspectives, *Experimental Aging Research, 9*, 169–173.

[22] Burns, P. C. (1999). Navigation and mobility of older drivers. *Journal of Gerontology: Social Sciences, 54B*, S49–S55.

[23] Caduff, D. & Timpf, S. (2007). A framework for assessing the salience of landmarks for wayfinding tasks. *Cognitive Processing, 7*, 23.

[24] Capitani, E., Laiacona, M., Ciceri, C. & Gruppo Italiano per lo Studio Neuropsicologico dell'Invecchiamento (1991). Sex differences in spatial memory: A reanalysis of block among the very elderly related to visual and cognitive function. *Scandinavian Journal of Caring Sciences, 16*, 91-102.

[25] Carlesimo, G. A., Fadda, L., Lorusso, S., Caltagirone, C. (1994). Verbal and spatial memory spans in Alzheimer's and multi-infarct dementia. *Acta Neurologica Scandinavica, 89*, 132–138.

[26] Carpenter, P. A. & Just, M. A. (1989). The role of working memory in language comprehension. In D. Klahr, & K. Kotovsky, (Eds.). *Complex information processing: The impact of Herbert A. Simon* (pp. 31-68). Hillsdale, NJ, England: Lawrence Erlbaum Associates.

[27] Cavallini, E., Fastame, M. C., Palladino, P., Rossi, S. & Vecchi, T. (2003). Visuo-Spatial Span and Cognitive Functions: A Theoretical Analysis of The "Corsi" Task. *Imagination, Cognition and Personality, 23(2-3)*, 217-224.

[28] Cernin, P., Keller, B. & Stoner, J. (2003). Colour vision in Alzheimer's patients: Can we improve cognition and the human navigation network in AD and MCI. *Neurology, 69*, 986-997.

[29] Cherrier, M. M., Mendez, M. & Perryman, K. (2001). Route learning performance in Alzheimer disease patients. *Neuropsychiatry, Neuropsychology, and Behavioral Neurology, 14*,159-168.

[30] Cherry, B. J., Buckwalter, J. G., Henderson, V. W. (1996). Memory span procedures in Alzheimer's disease. *Neuropsychology, 10*, 286–293.

[31] Ciaramelli, E. (2008). The role of ventromedial prefrontal cortex in navigation: A case of impaired wayfinding and rehabilitation. *Neuropsychologia, 46*, 2099–2105.

[32] Colby, C. (1999). Parietal cortex constructs action-oriented spatial representations In N. Burgess, K. J. Jeffery & J. O'Keefe (Eds.), *The hippocampal and parietal foundations of spatial cognition* (pp. 104–126). Oxford, England: Oxford University Press.

[33] Coluccia, E. & Martello, A. (2004). Il ruolo della memoria di lavoro visuo-spaziale nell'orientamento geografico: Uno studio correlazionale [The role of visuo-spatial working memory in geographical orientation: A correlation study]. *Giornale Italiano di Psicologia, 3*, 523-551.

[34] Corkin, S. (1982). Some relationships between global amnesias and the memory impairments in Alzheimer's disease. In S. Corkin, K. L. Davis, J. H. Growdon, E. Usdin & R. J. Wurtman (Eds). *Alzheimer's Disease: A Report of Progress in Research, Vol. 19*, Raven Press: New York.

[35] Cornoldi, C. (1995). Memoria di lavoro visuospaziale. In F. Marucci (Ed.), *Le immagini mentali* (pp. 145-181). Roma: La Nuova Italia.

[36] Cornoldi, C. & Gruppo, M. T. (1992). *PRCR-2: Prove di prerequisito per la diagnosi delle difficoltà di lettura e scrittura.* Firenze: O. S.

[37] Cornoldi, C. & Vecchi, T. (2000). Mental imagery in blind people: The role of passive and active visuo-spatial processes. In M. Heller (Ed.), *Touch, representation, and blindness* (pp. 143-181). Oxford, UK: Oxford University Press.

[38] Cornoldi, C. & Vecchi, T. (2003). *Visuo-spatial working memory and individual differences.* Hove, UK: Psychology Press.

[39] Cornoldi, C., Rigoni, F., Venneri, A. & Vecchi, T. (2000). Passive and active processes in visuo-spatial memory: Double dissociation in developmental learning disabilities. *Brain and Cognition, 43,* 17-20.

[40] Corsi, P. M. (1972). *Human memory and the medial temporal region of the region of the brain.* Unpublished doctoral dissertation, McGill University, Montreal, Quebec.

[41] Cushman, L. A., Stein, K. & Duffy, C. J. (2008). Detecting navigational deficits in cognitive aging and Alzheimer disease using virtual reality. *Neurology, 71(12),* 888–895.

[42] Davis, R. L., Therrien, B. A. & West, B. T. (2009). Working memory, cues, and wayfinding in older women. *Journal of Applied Gerontology, 28(6),* 743-767.

[43] Dawson, L. K. & Grant, I. (2000). Alcoholics' initial organizational and problem solving skills predict learning and memory performance on the Rey-Osterrieth Complex Figure. *Journal of the International Neuropsychological Society,* 6, 12-19.

[44] De Renzi, E. & Nichelli, P. (1975). Verbal and non-verbal short-term memory impairment following hemispheric damage. *Cortex, 11,* 341–354.

[45] De Renzi, E., Faglioni, P. & Previdi, P. (1977). Spatial memory and hemispheric locus of lesion. *Cortex, 13,* 424–433.

[46] deIpolyi, A. R., Rankin, K. P., Mucke, L., Miller, B. L. & Gorno-Tempini, M. L. (2007). Spatial cognition and the human navigation network in AD and MCI. *Neurology, 69*, 986-997.

[47] Della Sala, S., Gray, C., Baddeley, A. D., Allamano, N. & Wilson, L. (1999). Pattern span: a tool for unwelding visuo-spatial memory. *Neuropsychologia, 37*, 1189-1199.

[48] Della Sala, S., Gray, C., Baddeley, A. D. & Wilson, L. (1997). *Visual Pattern Test*. Bury St Edmunds: Thames Valley Test Company.

[49] Denis, M., Pazzaglia, F., Cornoldi, C. & Bertolo, L. (1999). Spatial discourse and navigation: An analysis of route direction in the city of Venice. *Applied Cognitive Psychology, 13*, 145-174.

[50] Driscoll, I., Derek, A. H., Yeo, R. A., Brooks, W. M. & Sutherland, R. I. (2005). Virtual navigation in humans: the impact of age, sex, and hormones on place learning. *Hormones and Behavior, 47*, 326-355.

[51] Driscoll, I., Hamilton, D. A., Petropoulos, H., Yeo, R. A., Brooks, W. M., Baumgartner, R. N. & Sutherland, R. J. (2003). The aging hippocampus: cognitive, biochemical and structural findings. *Cerebral Cortex, 13*, 1344–1351.

[52] Eslinger, P. J., Pepin, L. & Benton, A. L. (1988). Different patterns of visual memory errors occur with aging and dementia. *Journal of Clinical and Experimental Neuropsychology, 10*, 60-61.

[53] Etienne, A. S., Berlie, J., Georgakopoulos, J. & Maurer, R. (1998). Role of dead reckoning in navigation. In S. Healy (Ed.), *Spatial representation in animals* (pp. 54-68). Oxford: Oxford University Press.

[54] Evans, G. W., Brennan, P. L., Skorpanich, M. A. & Held, D. (1984). Cognitive mapping and elderly adults: verbal and location memory for urban landmarks. *Journal of Gerontology, 39*, 452-457.

[55] Farah, M. J., Levine, D. N., Calvanio, R. (1988). A case study of mental imagery deficit. *Brain and Cognition, 8*, 147-164.

[56] Farrell, M. J. & Thomson, J. A. (1998). Automatic spatial updating during locomotion without vision. *Quarterly Journal of Experimental Psychology, 51A*, 637-654.

[57] Faubert, J. (2002). Visual perception and aging. *Canadian Journal of Experimental Psychology, 56*, 164-176.

[58] Feigenbaum, J. D. & Morris, R. G. (2004). Allocentric versus geocentric spatial memory after unilateral temporal lobectomy in humans. *Neuropsychology, 18*, 462-472.

[59] Feigenbaum, J. D. & Rolls, E. T. (1991). Allocentric and egocentric information processing in the hippocampal formation of the behaving primate. *Psychobiology, 19*, 21–40.

[60] Galati, G., Lobel, E., Vallar, G., Berthoz, A., Pizzamiglio, L. & LeBihan, D. (2000). The neural basis of egocentric and allocentric coding of space in humans: A functional magnetic resonance study. *Experimental Brain Research, 133,* 156–164.

[61] Gallistel, C. R. (1990). *The organization of learning*. Cambridge, MA: MIT Press.

[62] Garden, S., Cornoldi, C. & Logie, R. H. (2002). Visuo-spatial working memory in navigation. *Applied Cognitive Psychology, 16*, 35-50.

[63] Garling, T., Baak, A. & Lindberg, E. (1985). Adults' memory representations of the spatial properties of their everyday physical environment. In R. Cohen (Ed.), *The development of spatial cognition* (pp. 141-184). Hillsdale, NJ: Erlbaum.

[64] Georgiou-Karistianis, N., Tang, J., Mehmedbegovic, F., Farrow, M., Bradshaw, J. & Sheppard, D. (2006). Age-related differences in cognitive function using a global local hierarchical paradigm. *Brain Research, 1124*, 86-95.
[65] Golledge, R. G. (1999). *Wayfinding behavior: Cognitive mapping and other spatial processes.* Baltimore, MD: Johns Hopkins University Press.
[66] Greene, J. D., Hodges, J. R., Baddeley, A. D. (1995). Autobiographical memory and executive function in early dementia of Alzheimer type. *Neuropsychologia, 33*, 1647–1670.
[67] Grön, G., Wunderlich, A. P., Spitzer, M., Tomczak, R. & Riepe, M. W. (2000). Brain activation during human navigation: gender different neural networks as substrate of performance. *Nature Neuroscience, 3(4)*, 404–408.
[68] Grossi, D., Becker, J. T., Smith, C. & Trojano, L. (1993). Memory for visuospatial patterns in Alzheimer's disease. *Psychological Medicine, 23*, 65-70.
[69] Guariglia, C. C. & Nitrini, R. (2009). Topographical disorientation in Alzheimer's disease. *Arq Neuropsiquiatr, 67(4)*, 967-972.
[70] Hamilton, C. H., Coates, R. O. & Hefferan, T. (2003). What develops in visuo-spatial working memory development? *European Journal of Cognitive Psychology, 15*, 43-69.
[71] Hamilton, C. J., Coates, R. O. & Heffernan, T. (2003). What develops in visuo-spatial working memory development? *European Journal of Cognitive Psychology, 15(1)*, 43-69.
[72] Hartley, T. & Burgess, N. (2005). Complementary memory systems: competition, cooperation and compensation. *TRENDS in Neuroscience, 28(4)*, 169-170.
[73] Hartley, T., Maguire, E. A., Spiers, H. J. & Burgess, N. (2003). The well-worn route and the path less travelled: distinct neural bases of route following and wayfinding in humans. *Neuron, 37(5)*, 877–888.
[74] Helstrup, T. (1989). Active and passive memory: States, attitudes, and strategies. *Scandinavian Journal of Psychology, 30(2)*, 113-133.
[75] Hitch, G. J. (1990). Developmental fractionation of working memory. In G. Vallar & T. Shallice (Eds.), *Neuropsychological impairments of short-term memory* (pp. 221-246). New York, NY, US: Cambridge University Press.
[76] Hodges, J. R. & Patterson, K. (1995). Is semantic memory consistently impaired early in the course of Alzheimer's disease? Neuroanatomical and diagnostic implications. *Neuropsychologia, 33*, 441–459.
[77] Holdstock, J. S., Mayes, A. R., Cezayirli, E., Isaac, C. L., Aggleton, J. P. & Roberts, N. (2000). A comparison of egocentric and allocentric spatial memory in a patient with selective hippocampal damage. *Neuropsychologica, 38*, 410–425.
[78] Huntley, J. D. & Howard, R. J. (2010). Working memory in early Alzheimer's disease: A neuropsychological review. *International Journal of geriatric Psychiatry, 25*, 121-132.
[79] Hwang, J., Yang, C., Tsai, S. & Liu, K. (1997). Behavioral disturbances in psychiatric inpatients with dementia of the Alzheimer's types in Taiwan. *International Journal of geriatric Psychiatry, 12*, 902–906.
[80] Iaria, G., Palermo, L., Committeri, G. & Barton, J. J. S. (2009). Age differences in the formation and use of cognitive maps. *Behavioural Brain Research, 196*, 187-191.

[81] Iaria, G., Petrides, M., Dagher, A., Pike, B. & Bohbot, V. D. (2003). Cognitive strategies dependent on the hippocampus and caudate nucleus in human navigation: Variability and change with practice. *Journal of Neuroscience, 23(13)*, 5945–5952.

[82] Isaacs, E. B. & Vargha-Khadem, F. (1989). Differential course of development of spatial and and verbal memory span: A normative study. *British Journal of Developmental Psychology, 7*, 377–380.

[83] Jack, C. R., Jr., Petersen, R. C., Xu, Y. C., Waring, S. C., O'Brien, P. C., Tangalos, E. G., et al. (1997). Medial temporal atrophy on MRI in normal aging and very mild Alzheimer's disease. *Neurology, 49(3)*, 786–794.

[84] Jack, C. R., Jr., Petersen, R. C., Xu, Y., O'Brien, P. C., Smith,G. E., Ivnik, R. J., et al. (1998). Rate of medial temporal lobe atrophy in typical aging and Alzheimer's disease. *Neurology, 51(4)*, 993–999.

[85] McAfoose, J. & Baune, B. T. (2009). Exploring Visual–Spatial Working Memory: A Critical of concepts and models. *Neuropsychology Review, 19(1)*,130-42.

[86] Jones, D., Farrand, P., Stuart, G. & Morris, N. (1995). Functional equivalence of verbal and spatial information in serial short-term memory. *Journal of Experimental Psychology: Learning, Memory, and Cognition, 21*, 1008–1018.

[87] Katayama, K., Takahashi, N., Ogawara, K. & Hattori, T. (1999). Pure topographical disorientation due to right posterior cingulate lesion. *Cortex, 35(2)*, 279–282.

[88] Kausler, D. H. (1994). *Learning and memory in normal aging*. Academic Press, San Diego, CA.

[89] King, J. A., Burgess, N., Hartley, T., Vargha-Khadem, F. & O'Keefe, J. (2002). Human hippocampus and viewpoint dependence in spatial memory. *Hippocampus, 12*, 811–820.

[90] Kirasic, K. C. (1991). Spatial cognition and behavior in young and elderly adults: implications for learning new environments. *Psychology and Aging, 6(1)*, 10–18.

[91] Kirasic, K. C., Allen, G. L. & Siegel, A. W. (1984). Expression of configurational knowledge of large-scale environments: Students' performance of cognitive tasks. *Environment and Behavior, 16(6)*, 687–712.

[92] Klein, D. A., Steinberg, M., Galik, E., Steele, C., Sheppard, J. M., Warren, A., Rosenblatt, A. & Lyketsos, C. G. (1999). Wandering behaviour in community residing persons with dementia. *International Journal of Geriatric Psychiatry, 14(4)*, 272–279.

[93] Lawton, C. A., Charleston, S. I. & Zieles, A. S. (1996). Individual and gender related differences in indoor wayfindings. *Environment and Behavior, 28(2)*, 204–219.

[94] Lawton, C. A. (1996). Strategies for indoor way-finding:the role of orientation. *Journal of Environmental Psychology, 16*, 137–145.

[95] Leininger, B. E., Gramling, S. E., Farrell, A. D. Kreutzer, J. S. & Peck, E. A. 3rd (1990). Neuropsychological deficits in symptomatic minor head injury patients after concussion and mild concussion. *Journal of Neurology, Neurosurgery and Psychiatry, 53*, 293-296.

[96] Levine, D. N., Warach, J. & Farah, M. J. (1985). Two visual systems in mental imagery: Dissociation of "what" and "where" in imagery disorders due to bilateral posterior cerebral lesions. *Neurology, 35(7)*, 1010–1018.

[97] Lezak, M. D., Howieson, D. B., Loring, D. W., Hannay, H. J. & Fisher, J. S. (2004). *Neuropsychological Assessment* (4th ed.). Oxford University Press, New York.

[98] Lindberg, E. & Gärling, T. (1981). Acquisition of locational information about reference points during locomotion with and without a concurrent task: Effects of number of reference points. *Scandinavian Journal of Psychology*, 22, 109-115.
[99] Lindberg, E. & Garling, T. (1983). Acquisition of different types of locational information in cognitive maps: Automatic or effortful processing? *Psychological Research*, 45, 19-38.
[100] Lipman, P. (1991). Age and exposure differences in acquisition of route information. *Psychology and Aging*, 6, 128-133.
[101] Lipman, P. D. & Caplan, L. J. (1992). Adult age differences in memory for routes: effects of instruction and spatial diagram. *Psychology and Aging*, 7, 435–442.
[102] Logie, R. H. (1986). Visuo-spatial processing in working memory. *The Quarterly Journal of Experimental Psychology*, 38A, 229–247.
[103] Logie, R. H. (1989). Characteristics of visual short-term memory. *European Journal of Cognitive Psychology*, 1, 275–284.
[104] Logie, R. H. (1995). *Visuo-spatial working memory*. East Sussex: Erlbaum.
[105] Logie, R. H. (2003). Spatial and visual working memory: A mental workspace. In B. H. Ross & D. E. Irwin (Eds.), *Cognitive vision: The psychology of learning and motivation, Vol. 42*, (pp. 37-78). San Diego, CA: Academic Press.
[106] Logie, R. H. & Marchetti, C. (1991). Visuo-spatial working memory. Visual, spatial or central executive? In R. H. Logie, & M. Denis (Eds.), *Mental Images in Human Cognition* (pp. 105-115). Amsterdam: Elsevier.
[107] Logie, R. H. & Pearson, D. G. (1997). The inner eye and the inner scribe of visuo-spatial working memory: Evidence from developmental fractionation. *European Journal of Cognitive Psychology*, 9, 241-257.
[108] Loomis, J. M., Klatzky, R. L., Golledge, R. G., Cicinelli, J. G., Pellegrino, J. W. & Fry, P. A. (1993). Nonvisual navigation by blind and sighted: Assessment of path integration ability. *Journal of Experimental Psychology: General*, 122, 73-91.
[109] Loring, D. W., Meador, K. J., Lee, G. P. Murro, A. M., Smith, J. R., Flanigin, H. F., Gallagher, B. B. & King, D. W. (1990). Cerebral language lateralization: evidence from intracarotid amobarbital testing. *Neuropsychologia*, 28, 831-838.
[110] Maguire, E. A., Burgess, N., Donnett, J. G., Frackowiak, R. S., Frith, C. D. & O'Keefe, J. (1998). Knowing where and getting there: a human navigation network. *Science, 280* (5365), 921–924.
[111] Maguire, E. A., Burke, T., Phillips, J. & Staunton, H. (1996). Topographical disorientation following unilateral temporal lobe lesions in humans. *Neuropsychologia*, 34, 993–1001.
[112] Mahmood, O., Adamo, D., Briceno, E. & Moffat, S. D. (2009). Age differences in visual path-integration. *Behavioral Brain Research, 205(1)*, 88–95.
[113] Malinowski, J. C. & Gillespie, W. T. (2001). Individual differences in performance on a large scale, real word wayfinding task. *Journal of Environmental Psychology*, 21, 73–82.
[114] Mammarella, I. C. & Cornoldi, C. (2005). Sequence and space. The critical role of back word spatial span in the working memory deficit of visuospatial learning disable children. *Cognitive Neuropsychology*, 22, 1055-1068.
[115] Mammarella, I. C., Cornoldi, C., Pazzaglia F., Toso, C., Grimoldi, M. & Vio C. (2006). Evidence for a double dissociation between spatial-simultaneous and spatial-sequential

working memory in visuospatial (nonverbal) learning disabled children. *Brain and Cognition, 62*, 58-67.

[116] Mammarella, I. C., Pazzaglia, F. & Cornoldi, C. (2006). The assessment of imagery and visuo-spatial working memory functions. In T. Vecchi & G. Bottini (Eds.), *Imagery and Spatial Cognition*, Amsterdam: John Benjamines Publishing Company.

[117] Mapstone, M., Dickerson, K. & Duffy, C. J. (2008). Distinct mechanisms of impairment in cognitive ageing and Alzheimer's disease. *Brain, 131*(Pt 6), 1618–1629.

[118] Martin, A., Brouwers, P., Cox, C. & Fedio, P. (1985). On the nature of the verbal memory deficit in Alzheimer's disease. *Brain & Language, 25*, 323–341.

[119] Meulenbroek, O., Petersson, K. M., Voermans, N., Weber, B. & Fernandez, G. (2004). Age differences in neural correlates of route encoding and route recognition, *NeuroImage, 22*, 1503–1514.

[120] Miller, G., Galanter, E. & Pribram, K. (1960). *Plans and the structure of behavior.* Holt, Rinehart & Wilson: New York.

[121] Milner, B. (1971). Interhemispheric differences in the localization of psychological processes in man. *British Medical Bulletin, 27*, 272-277.

[122] Moffat, S. D., Elkins, W. & Resnick, S. M. (2006). Age differences in the neural systems supporting human allocentric spatial navigation. *Neurobiology of Aging, 27(7)*, 965–972.

[123] Moffat, S. D., Kennedy, K. M., Rodrigue, K. M. & Raz, N. (2007). Extrahippocampal contributions to age differences in human spatial navigation. *Cerebral Cortex, 17(6)*, 1274–1282.

[124] Moffat, S., Zonderman, A. & Resnick, S. (2001). Age differences in spatial memory in a virtual environment navigation task. *Neurobiology of Aging, 22,* 787-796.

[125] Moffat, S. D. (2009). Aging and spatial navigation: what do we know and where do we go? *Neuropsychology Review*, *19*, 478-489.

[126] Moffat, S. D., & Resnick, S. M. (2002). Effects of age on virtual environment place navigation and allocentric cognitive mapping. *Behavioural Neuroscience, 116*, 851–859.

[127] Monacelli, A. M., Cushmagn, L. A., Kavcic, V. &, Duffy, C. J. (2003). Spatial disorientation in Alzheimer's disease. *Neurology, 61*, 1491-1497.

[128] Montello, D. R. & Pick, H. L. (1993). Integrating knowledge of vertically aligned large-scale spaces. *Environment and Behavior, 25*, 457–484.

[129] Morris, R. G. (1981). Spatial localization does not require the presence of local cues. *Learning and Motivation, 12*, 239–260.

[130] Morris, R. G., Downes, J. J., Sahakian, B. J., Evenden, J. L., Heald, A. & Robbins, T. W. (1988). Planning and spatial working memory in Parkinson's disease. *Journal of Neurology, Neurosurgery, and Psychiatry, 51***,** 757–766.

[131] Morrone, M. C., Tosetti, M., Montanaro, D., Fiorentini, A., Cioni, G. & Burr, D. C. (2000). A cortical area that responds specifically to optic flow, revealed by fMRI. *Nature Neuroscience, 3,* 1322-8.

[132] Myerson, J., Jenkins, L., Hale, S. & Sliwinski, M. (2000a). Individual and developmental differences in working memory across the life span: Reply. *Psychonomic Bulletin & Review, 7(4)*, 734-740.

[133] Myerson, J., Jenkins, L., Hale, S. & Sliwinski, M. (2000b). Converging evidence that visuospatial cognition is more age-sensitive than verbal cognition. *Psychology and Aging, 15(1)*, 157-175.

[134] Newman, M. & Kaszniak, A. (2000). Spatial memory and aging: Performance on a human analog of the Morris Water Maze. *Aging, Neuropsychology, and Cognition, 7*, 86-93.

[135] Nico, D., Israël, I. & Berthoz, A. (2002). Interaction of visual and idiothetic information in a path completion task. *Experimental Brain Research*, 146 *(3)*, 379-82.

[136] Nori, R., Grandicelli, S. & Giusberti, F. (2009). Individual differences in visuo-spatial working memory and real-world wayfinding. *Swiss Journal of Psychology, 68 (1)*, 7–16.

[137] O'Brien, H. L., Tetewsky, S. J., Avery, L. M., Cushman, L. A., Makous, W. & Duffy, C. J. (2001). Visual mechanisms of spatial disorientation in Alzheimer's disease. *Cerebral Cortex, 11(11)*, 1083–1092.

[138] O'Keefe, J. & Nadel, L. (1978). *The Hippocampus as a Cognitive Map,* Clarendon, Oxford.

[139] Ogden, J. A., Growdon, J. H. & Corkin, S. (1990). Deficits on visuospatial tests involving forward planning and in high-functioning parkinsonians. *Neuropsychiatry, Neuropsychology and Behavioral Neurology, 3*, 125-139.

[140] Olton, D. S., Walker, J. A., Gage, F. H. (1978). Hippocampal connections and spatial discrimination, *Brain Research, 139(2)*, 295-308.

[141] Orsini, A., Trojano, L., Chiacchio, L. & Grossi, D. (1988). Immediate memory spans in dementia. *Perceptual and Motor Skills, 67,* 267–272.

[142] Orsini, A., Chiacchio, I., Clinque, M., Cocchiaro, C., Schiappa, O. & Grossi, D. (1986). Effects of age, education and sex on two tests of immediate memory: A study of normal subjects from 20 to 99 years of age. *Perceptual and Motor Skills, 63,* 727–732.

[143] Osterrieth, P. A. (1944). Le test de copie d'une figure complexe. *Archives de Psychologie, 30*, 206-356.

[144] Owen, A. M., Evans, A. C. & Petrides, M. (1996) Evidence for a two-stage model of spatial working memory processing within the lateral frontal cortex: a positron emission tomography study. *Cerebral Cortex, 6*, 31–38.

[145] Pazzaglia, F. & Cornoldi, C. (1999). The role of distinct components of visuo-spatial working memory in the processing of texts. *Memory, 7*, 19-41.

[146] Perry, R. J., Watson, P., Hodges, J. R. (2000). The nature and staging of attention dysfunction in early (minimal and mild) Alzheimer's disease: relationship to episodic and semantic memory impairment. *Neuropsychologia, 38*, 252–271.

[147] Piccardi, L., Iaria, G., Ricci, M., Bianchini, F., Zompanti, L. & Guariglia, C. (2008). Walking in the Corsi Test: which type of memory do you need? *Neuroscience Letters, 432*, 127-131.

[148] Piccardi, L., Berthoz, A., Baulac, M., Denos, M., Dupont, S., Samson, S. & Guariglia, C. (2010). Different spatial memory systems are involved in small and large-scale environments: evidence from patients with temporal lobe epilepsy. *Experimental Brain Research, 206* (2), 171-177.

[149] Piccardi, L., Iaria, G., Bianchini, F., Zompanti, L. & Guariglia, C. (submitted). Dissociated deficits of visuo-spatial memory in reaching space and in navigational space: Evidences from brain-damaged patients and healthy older participants.

[150] Pickering, S. J., Gathercole, S. E. & Peaker, M. (1998). Verbal and visuo-spatial short-term memory in children: Evidence for common and distinct mechanisms. *Memory and Cognition, 26,* 1117-1130.

[151] Pickering, S. J., Gathercole, S. E., Hall, M. & Lloyd, S. A. (2001). Development of memory for pattern and path: further evidence for the fractionation of visuo-spatial memory. *The Quarterly Journal of Experimental Psychology, 54A,* 397–420.

[152] Quinn, J. G., McConnell, J. (1996). Irrelevant pictures in visual working memory. *The Quarterly Journal of Experimental Psychology, 49,* 200-215.

[153] Raz, N. & Rodrigue, K. M. (2006). Differential aging of the brain: Patterns, cognitive correlates and modifiers, *Neuroscience and Biobehavioral Reviews, 30,* 730–748.

[154] Reagan, I. & Baldwin, C. L. (2006). Facilitating route memory with auditory route guidance systems. *Journal of Environmental Psychology, 26,* 146-155

[155] Rey, A. (1941). L'examen psychologique dans le cas d'encephalopatie traumatique. *Archives de Psychologie, 28,* 286-340.

[156] Richardson, J. T. E. (1994). Gender differences in mental rotation. *Perceptual and Motor Skills, 78,* 435-448.

[157] Riddoch, M. J., Humphreys, G. W., Blott, W. & Hardy, E. (2003). Visual and spatial short-term memory in integrative agnosia. *Cognitive Neuropsychology, 20(7),* 641–671.

[158] Rosselli, M. & Ardila, A. (1991). Effects of age, education and gender on Rey-Osterrieth Complex Figure. *The Clinical Neuropsychologist, 5,* 370-376.

[159] Rourke, B. P. (1989). *Nonverbal disabilities, the syndrome and the model.* New York: Gulford.

[160] Rowe, M. (2003). Persons with dementia who became lost in the community: Preventing injuries and death. *American Journal of Nursing, 103,* 32-40.

[161] Rutledge, P. C., Hancock, R. A. & Walker, L. (1997). Effects of retention interval length on young and elderly adults' memory for spatial information. *Experimental Aging Research, 23,* 163-177.

[162] Sadalla, E. K. & Montello, D. R. (1989). Remembering changes in direction. *Environment and Behavior, 21,* 346–363.

[163] Salmon, E. Van der Linden, M., Collette, F., Delfiore, G., Maquet, P., Degueldre, C., Luxen, A. & Franck, G. (1996). Regional brain activity during working memory tasks. *Brain, 119,* 1617–1625

[164] Salthouse, T. A. & Mitchell, D. (1989). Structural operational capacities in integrative spatial ability. *Psychology and Aging, 4(1),* 18-25.

[165] Sandstrom, N. J., Kaufman, J. & Huettel, S. A. (1998). Males and females use different distal cues in a virtual environment navigation task. *Cognitive Brain Research, 6,* 351–360.

[166] Saucier, D. M., Green, S. M., Leason, J., MacFadden, A., Bell, S. & Elias, L. J. (2002). Are sex differences in navigation caused by sexually dimorphic strategies or by differences in the ability to use the strategies? *Behavioral Neuroscience, 116(3),* 403–410.

[167] Sharps, M. J. & Gollin, E. S. (1987). Memory for object locations in young and elderly adults. *Journal of Gerontology, 42,* 336-41.

[168] Sivan, A. B. (1992). *Benton Visual Retention Test* (5th ed.). San Antonio, TX: The Psychological Corporation.

[169] Snodgrass, J. G. & Vanderwart, M. (1980). A standardized set of 260 pictures: Norms for name agreement, image agreement, familiarity, and visual complexity. *Journal of Experimental Psychology: Human Learning and Memory, 6*, 174-215.

[170] Spinnler, H., Della Sala, S., Bandera, R. & Baddeley, A. (1988). Dementia, ageing, and the structure of human memory. *Cognitive Neuropsychology, 5*, 193–211.

[171] Storandt, M., Botwinick, J. & Danziger, W. L. (1986). Longitudinal changes: patients with mild SDAT and matched healthy controls. In L. W. Poon (Ed.) *Handbook for clinical memory assessment of older adults.* Washington, D. C.: American Psychological Association.

[172] Takahashi, N., Kawamura, M., Shiota, J., Kasahata, N. & Hirayama, K. (1997). Pure topographic disorientation due to right retrosplenial lesion. *Neurology, 49*, 464-469.

[173] Teri, L., Borson, S., Kiyak, A. & Yamagishi, M. (1989). Behavioral disturbance, cognitive dysfunction, and functional skill: prevalence and relationship in Alzheimer's disease. *Journal of the American Geriatrics Society, 37,*109-116.

[174] Tetewsky, S. J. & Duffy, C. J. (1999). Visual loss and getting lost in Alzheimer's disease. *Neurology, 52(5)*, 958–965.

[175] Thier, P. & Andersen, R. A. (1996). Electrical microstimulation suggests two different forms of representation of head-centered space in the intraparietal sulcus of rhesus monkeys. *Proc. Natl. Acad. Sci. USA, 93*, 4962–4967.

[176] Tolman, E. C. (1948). Cognitive maps in rats and men. *Psychological Review, 73*, 189-208.

[177] Traykov L, Raoux N, Latour F, et al. (2007). Executive functions deficit in mild cognitive impairment. *Cognitive Behavioral and Neurology, 20, 219*–224.

[178] Tresch, M. C., Sinnamon, H. M. & Seamon, J. G. (1993). Double dissociation of spatial and object visual memory: evidence from selective interference in intact human subjects. *Neuropsychologia, 31*, 211-219.

[179] Trojano, L., Chiacchio, L., De Luca, G., Fragassi, N. A. & Grossi, D. (1994). Effect of testing procedure on Corsi's block-tapping task in normal subjects and Alzheimer-type dementia. *Perceptual and Motor Skills, 78*, 859–863.

[180] Tversky, B. (2000). Remembering spaces. In E. Tulving & F. I. M Craik (Eds.), *Handbook of memory* (pp. 363–378). New York: Oxford University Press.

[181] Uc, E. Y., Rizzo, M., Anderson, S. W., Shi, Q., Dawson, J. D. (2005). Driver landmark and traffic sign identification in early Alzheimer's disease. *Journal Neurology, Neurosurgery, and Psychiatry,76,*764-768.

[182] Vandierendonck, A. & Szmalec, A. (2005). An asymmetry in the visuo-spatial demands of forward and backward recall in the Corsi blocks task. *Imagination, Cognition and Personality, 23,* 225-231.

[183] Vandierendonck, A., Kemps, E., Fastame, M. C. & Szmalec, A. (2004). Working memory components of the Corsi block task. *British Journal of Psychology, 95*, 57-79.

[184] Vecchi, T. & Richardson, J. T. E. (2000). Active processing in visuo-spatial working memory. *Cahier de Psychologie Cognitive, 19,* 3-32.

[185] Vecchi, T. (1998). Visuo-spatial limitations in congenitally totally blind people. *Memory, 6,* 91-102.

[186] Vecchi, T. (2001). Visuo-spatial processing in congenitally blind people: Is there a gender-related preference? *Personality and Individual Differences, 29,* 1361-1370.

[187] Vecchi, T. & Richardson, J. T. E. (2001). Measures of visual-spatial short term memory: The Knox cube imitation test and the Corsi blocks test compared. *Brain and Cognition, 46*, 291-294.

[188] Vecchi, T., Phillips, L. H. & Cornoldi, C. (2001). Individual differences in visuo-spatial working memory. In M. Denis, R. H. Logie, C. Cornoldi, M. de Vega & J. Engelkamp (Eds.), *Imagery, language, and visuo-spatial thinking* (pp. 29-58). Hove, UK: Psychology Press.

[189] Voermans, N. C., Petersson, K. M., Daudey, L., Weber, B., Van Spaendonck, K. P., Kremer, H. P. & Fernandez, G. (2004). Interaction between the human hippocampus and the caudate nucleus during route recognition. *Neuron, 43*, 427-435.

[190] Wijk, H., Berg, S., Bergman, B., Hanson, A., Sivik, L. & Steen, B. (2002). Colour perception among the very elderly related to visual and cognitive function. *Scandinavian Journal of Caring Sciences, 16*, 91-102.

[191] Wilkniss, S. M., Jones, M. G., Korol, D. L., Gold, P. E. & Manning, C. A. (1997). Age-related differences in an ecologically based study of route learning. *Psychology and Aging, 12(2)*, 372–375.

[192] Wilson, B. A., Baddeley, A. D., Young, A. W. (1999). LE, a person who lost her 'mind's eye. *Neurocase, 5(2)*, 119-127.

In: Working Memory: Capacity, Developments and… ISBN: 978-1-61761-980-9
Editor: Eden S. Levin © 2011 Nova Science Publishers, Inc.-

Chapter 4

WORKING MEMORY AND PREFRONTAL CORTEX AND THEIR RELATION WITH THE BRAIN REWARD SYSTEM AND DRUG ADDICTION

Ester Miyuki Nakamura-Palacios
Laboratory of Cognitive Sciences and Neuropsychopharmacology,
Department of Physiological Sciences, Health Science Center,
Federal University of Espírito Santo, Vitória-ES, Brazil

ABSTRACT

Cellular and molecular mechanisms involved in learning and memory processes are very similar or the same as those involved in the drug-induced reorganization of neural circuitry that occurs during addiction. Using a classic working memory task in animal learning, the radial maze, we have demonstrated that different drugs of abuse (for instance, ethanol, Δ^9-tetrahydrocanabinol and nicotine) administered into the medial prefrontal cortex (mPFC) affect the performance of a delayed-task, suggesting that these drugs somehow change the spatial working memory processing. These effects may involve dopaminergic and/or glutamatergic mediation in the mPFC because they were prevented by SCH 23390, clozapine or memantine. The mPFC in rodents, which is functionally related to the dorsolateral prefrontal cortex (DLPFC) in primates and human beings, is part of the brain reward circuitry and highly involved in the processing of working memory. Working memory manipulates items in short-term memory to plan, organize, and process information required to generate future thoughts or actions. Its integrity is required in the processing of important cognitive functions such as learning, goal-directed behavior, decision-making, understanding and reasoning, all function that are substantially affected in drug addiction and dependence. In a randomized double-blind placebo-controlled clinical trial we showed that gabapentin, an anticonvulsant drug, reduced alcohol consumption and craving, and also improved frontal cognitive performance involving working memory processing. In a recent study considering different types of alcoholics according to Lesch's typology we found that frontal dysfunction was more seen to a greater extent in Type IV alcoholics, even in those that showed preserved mental function measured by mini-mental status examination.

Considering this pitiful evidence, we started to search for any treatment that would possibly decrease this frontal cortical dysfunction, especially the processing of working memory. We found interesting data showing that transcranial direct current stimulation (tDCS) over the left DLPFC improved the working memory and reduced alcohol craving. Thus, we are currently investigating the effects of tDCS over the left DLPFC in the P3 waveform registered by Event Related Potential (ERP) in alcoholics. So far, in a sample of alcoholics, we have found that tDCS results in a change the P3 waveform in frontal and central region that may be related to changes in brain activity. Completion of this study and adding future investigations that combine pharmacological and non-pharmacological strategies may unravel this intriguing relationship between working memory in the prefrontal cortex and drug addiction, and hopefully establish new therapeutic possibilities.

INTRODUCTION

Drug Addiction and Brain Reward Circuit

Briefly, in a drug dependence cycle, the direct rewarding effects in the brain following drug consumption, reinforces the search for additional drug intake. The seeking behavior is, probably mediated by the mesocortical limbic system via a dopamine (DA) mechanism. This driving drug seeking behavior pursues to maintain the immediate central effects (Figure 1).

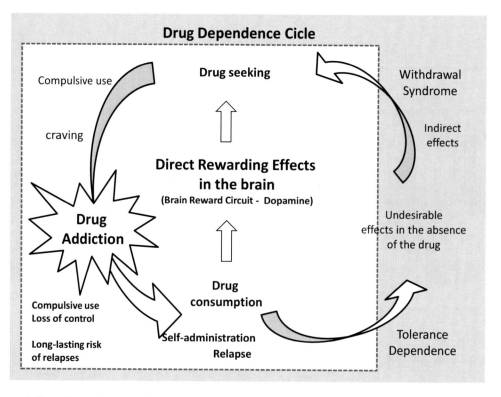

Figure 1. Drug Dependence Cycle, depicting the development of drug addiction and the involvement of the brain reward circuit.

The repetition of drug consumption may induce a more compulsive pattern of drug use, leading eventually to a loss of control and establishing the drug addiction with subsequent long-lasting risk for relapses (Figure 1). This can occur in a small percentage of subjects (not above 10%) experiencing the drug for the first time. [1] Concurrently, neuroadaptive processes take place because of the repetitive presence of the drug in the organism with a subsequent development of tolerance and physiological dependence. Once these changes occur, the drug seeking becomes more driven toward the suppression of undesirable symptoms that emerge in the withdrawal syndrome. Thus, even if the rewarding effects are no longer present because of the tolerance, the ongoing behavior of drug intake is sustained because of the discomfort following drug discontinuation. However, there is evidence that the adaptations occurring in physiological dependence that result in withdrawal symptoms upon drug discontinuation are distinct from those that result in addiction. [2] This notion is reinforced by the observation that they seem to be etiologically unrelated. [1]

Substantial progress has been made in understanding the molecular and cellular mechanisms of tolerance, dependence and withdrawal, but the mechanism underlying compulsive drug use and its persistence is much less understood. [3] Consequently, most treatments of drug dependence focus the managing of the drug intoxication and the immediate treatment of acute withdrawal, and there is no established program to manage the long-lasting symptoms, notably the uncontrolled urge of drug use, that emerges in the late abstinence period.

Drug addiction can be defined behaviorally by a loss of control over drug intake manifesting as a repetitive and compulsive drug use despite treatments for prevention and a knowledge of serious negative consequences associated with chronic substance abuse. [3-6] This condition may account to repetitive relapses, especially after acute withdrawal period, when a highly increased sensitivity to rewarding effects of the drug may trigger compulsion for drug use, [3-6] and in a period that drug users are no longer covered by any specific treatment for their addiction.

The persistence and stability of the behavioral abnormalities has suggested that drug addiction can be considered as a form of drug-induced neural plasticity that might involve a role for gene expression in specific brain regions underlying the behavioral abnormalities seen in drug addicts. [6,7]

Many experimental and clinical studies strongly support the hypothesis that central effects of different types of drugs of abuse are mediated by a central reward system. This system is mainly constituted by the mesocorticolimbic DA pathway, [5-13] joining the ventral tegmental area (VTA) and the nucleus accumbens (NAcc) [11,14,15] and the prefrontal cortex (PFC), that has been finally incorporated as part of this circuit [4,9,10] (Figure 2). This is an evolutionary ancient reward circuit, existing in a rudimentary form in invertebrates. Stimulation of this circuit reinforces natural behaviors needed to the survival of the individual and the species such as hunger, thirst and reproduction. [11,16] Evolutionarily, as the cortical brain area gets progressively larger [17,18] the frontal portion occupies about one third of the whole brain in human beings, [18,19] rendering probably much higher control over several brain functions. When this cortical function fails, the control is weakened and the behavior may be expressed in a more primitive or stimulus-driven form. [4]

It seems that besides the involvement of the subcortical components (VTA and NAcc) of the brain reward circuit, as suggested by many authors, [3,5,20] the drug actions in the central nervous system (CNS) cause a decrease the cortical (top-down) control over these components. [4] It would be like the drug, in some way, decreases the PFC surveillance to seize VTA-NAcc functions.

Drug Addiction and Prefrontal Cortex

Results from animal studies that usually employ paradigms to assess rewarding properties of drugs or the involvement of certain brain areas in reward such as intracranial self-stimulation, drug self-administration, or conditioned place preference, [1,9] have strongly related the compulsive drug intake to VTA-NAcc activity. Indeed, NAcc had been considered as the main reward-related structure involved in drug addiction. [14,15] However, over the last 10 years neuroimaging studies have supported a strong linkage between the prefrontal cortex and drug seeking behavior. [4,12] According to *Kalivas and Volkow* [12] the magnitude of change in metabolic activity in both the orbitofrontal and anterior cingulate cortices correlates with the intensity of the self-reported cue-induced craving. Additionally, these authors [12] suggest that dysfunction of these PFC regions seems to be involved in the difficulty experienced by addicts in cognitive control over drug seeking.

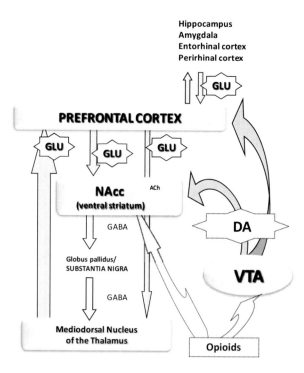

Figure 2. An overview of the neurotransmitters involved in the brain reward circuit. VTA: ventral tegmental area, DA: dopamine, GLU: glutamate, NAcc: nucleus accumbens, GABA: γ-aminobutyric acid. Dopamine mesocorticolimbic pathway emerges from VTA and projects to the NAcc and Prefrontal Cortex (anterior cingulate and orbitofrontal cortex). Prefrontal Cortex receives a massive glutamate projection from Mediodorsal Nucleus of the Thalamus and also from other cortical regions and sends back glutamate projections to these brain structures and to the NAcc. NAcc sends GABA projections to the globus pallidus and substantia nigra that also sends GABA projections to the Mediodorsal Nucleus of the Thalamus. Opioid receptors are present in all extension of this circuit.

In this circuit, DA seems to act either to alert the organism to the appearance of novel salient stimuli, promoting neuroplasticity (learning), or to alert the organism to a cue predicting a familiar motivationally relevant event learned by associations made with environmental stimuli. [12] It has been observed that once a salient stimulus has been associated to a drug effect, DA is no longer release during the drug action but it does when a cue predicting the drug is perceived. [5,20] DA release in the PFC seems to precede the activation of the PFC glutamatergic projection to the NAcc core since preventing cortical DA release prevents glutamate release in the NAcc caused by either a stress or drug prime. In turn, DA released in the Nacc is required for the drug high and for the initiation of addiction. However this action seems to be gradually replaced by a recruitment of the PFC and its glutamatergic projection to the NAcc when repeated use of a drug that causes a reward takes place. [12]

According to *Kalivas and Volkow* [12] the glutamatergic projection emerging from the PFC (more precisely anterior cingulate and orbitofrontal cortex) to the core of the NAcc (Figure 2) is a final common pathway for initiation of drug seeking. They mentioned that the activity of excitatory transmission usually required during the occurrence of learning associated to motivating relevant events also seems to be active when the desire to consume drugs of abuse is established. [12] A dysfunction in excitatory synapses posed by enduring molecular changes, notably in the PFC projection to NAcc, seems highly involved in the uncontrollable desire to take drugs that characterizes drug addiction. [12]

It has also to be considered that activation of the PFC may increase DA release in Nacc. It has been shown that the rewarding effects produced by electrical stimulation of the mPFC may involve glutamatergic projections of the mPFC to the VTA increasing its activity and causing an increase in extracellular DA levels in the NAcc through the mesolimbic dopamine pathway.[9]

Interestingly, *Kalivas and Volkow* [12] observed that functional imaging studies show that prefrontal regulation of behavior is reduced in basal conditions in addicts, probably contributing to the reduced salience of nondrug motivational stimuli and, consequently, impairing the ability for decision-making. However, a profound activation of the PFC and glutamatergic drive to the NAcc occurred when stimuli predicting drug availability was presented. [12] According to these authors, this higher prefrontal drive associated to the drug would contribute to increase the power of the motivational salience related to it and concurrently would trigger the craving and the drug seeking. [12]

Prefrontal Cortex and Working Memory

Prefrontal cortex

Our understanding of the frontal functions, more particularly the functions of the PFC, the most anterior portion of the frontal cortex, has evolved since *Luria*, by observing clinical features in patients with different extents of brain injuries. [21] *Luria* suggested a more broadly high order function for the PFC that would perform a more universal function of general regulation of behavior compared to the posterior associative cortices. [21] It was also referred to as the "organ of civilization" because of its role in monitoring both internal cortical and extrasensory information and thus enabling humans to be "aware" of themselves in relation to the environment. [18]

In fact, according to *Fuster* [22,23] the PFC can be considered as the "top of neural structures involved in sensory-motor integration" and in the charge of "bridging temporal gaps in the perception-action cycle". To mediate this function, the PFC manipulates items in a short-term memory to plan, organize, and processes information required to generate future thoughts or actions. [23,24]

Cummings, [25] by reviewing studies detailing the behavior of patients with degenerative disorders or focal lesions involving frontal lobes or linked subcortical regions, suggested the existence of five parallel segregated circuits linking the frontal lobe and subcortical structures. According to this author, three of these frontal-subcortical circuits originate in PFC: dorsolateral PFC, orbitofrontal cortex, and anterior cingulate cortex (Figure 3). According to this author, each prefrontal circuit has a specific behavioral syndrome: lesions of the dorsolateral prefrontal circuit are related to executive functions, lesions of the orbitofrontal circuit to disinhibition, and injury to the anterior cingulate circuit to apathy. [25]

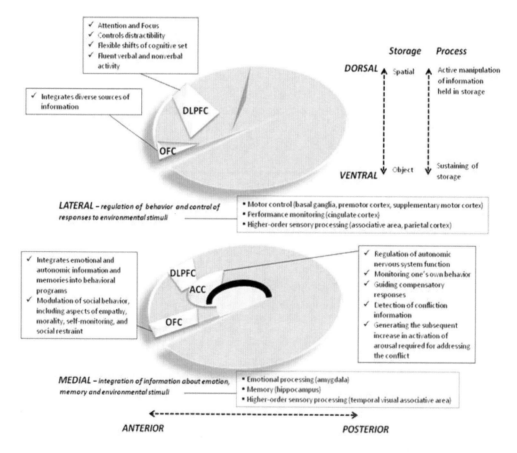

Figure 3. Representation of lateral (upper panel) and medial (bottom panel) view of the brain, summarizing the prefrontal cortex functions divided by regions: [25,26] DLPFC: dorsolateral prefrontal cortex, OFC: orbitofrontal cortex, ACC: anterior cingulate cortex, or between dorsal and ventral considering neuroimagings evidences, [19,29] or lateral and medial functions. [28]

The **dorsolateral prefrontal** area has a central role in the control, regulation, and integration of cognitive activities. It mediates attention, controls distractibility, maintains focus of cognitive set, provides flexible shifts of cognitive set when required, and is involved in generating fluent verbal and nonverbal activity. [26] According to *Fuster* [27] this portion of the PFC is critically involved in all forms of working memory toward a goal, whether in behavior, reasoning, or speech. Therefore, the **dorsolateral prefrontal syndrome** is characterized primarily by "executive function" deficits, such as inability to flexibly maintain or shift sets, showing rigid and perseverative behavior, poor organizational strategies for learning tasks, poor strategies for copying complex designs, and motor programming abnormalities, showing deficiencies in alternating and reciprocal motor tasks and sequential motor tests. [25]

The **orbitofrontal cortex** is considered a part of the limbic system. Its medial part integrates diverse sources of emotional and autonomic information and memories and processes them into various behavioral responses. In this way it is involved in the modulation of social behavior, including aspects of empathy, morality, self-monitoring, and social restraint. [26] The **orbitofrontal syndrome** is characterized by remarkable changes in personality [25] as was well described in the case of Phineas Gage *(see* [26]). Because of the behavioral desinhibition, patients become more outspoken, worriless, more tactless, and because of mood lability they may show fatuous euphoria and irritability. They may present automatic imitation of the gestures and actions of others or utilization of objects in the environment by imitation, reflecting enslavement to environmental cues. [25]

The **anterior cingulate** is also considered as a component of the limbic system that is involved in the regulation of autonomic nervous system function. However, the supracallosal areas are also involved in executive control, divided attention, error detection, response monitoring, the initiation and maintenance of appropriate ongoing behaviors and a central role in attention, arousal, emotion, and motivation. [26] Also it is thought to have a central role in the detection of conflicting information and in generating the subsequent increase in activation of arousal required for addressing the conflict. In this manner it monitors one's own behavior and guides compensatory responses. [26] The **anterior cingulate syndrome** is typically characterized by an akinetic mutism. According to *Cummings*, [25] patients with bilateral lesions are profoundly apathetic: "they typically have their eyes open, do not speak spontaneously, and answer questions in monosyllables if at all; move little, are incontinent, and eat and drink only if fed; display no emotion even when in pain and are indifferent to their dire circumstances".

Multimodality is an important characteristic of the PFC. In this context, it receives information about the external environment from all sensory modalities that have been processed by other primary networks, and also receives information about internal emotional and autonomic status related to relevant memories of previous events that had been consolidated and stored. [26]

Smith and Jonides, [19] reviewed studies utilizing either positron emission tomography or functional magnetic imaging conducted on participants while they were engaged in cognitive tasks. Based on this review they suggested that the PFC is organized by the modality of the information being processed. The spatial information seems to be represented more dorsally than object information (Figure 3). They have noted that verbal storage tasks activate left-hemisphere speech areas, spatial storage activates the right premotor cortex, and object storage activates more ventral regions of the PFC. They also proposed that the PFC would be organized by process (Figure 3), with ventrolateral regions mediating operations needed to sustain storage and dorsolateral regions implementing the active manipulation of information held in storage. They have noted that verbal tasks that require only storage did not activate the dorsolateral PFC, whereas verbal tasks that demand executive processes as well as storage require the activation of this PFC region.

Interestingly, the PFC functions can also be understood by neuronal pathways arising from its medial or lateral sides as well as by connections made by other brain regions to these areas of the PFC. According to *Wood and Grafman* [28] "the ventromedial PFC has reciprocal connections with amygdala associated with emotional processing, hippocampus with memory, and temporal visual associative areas with higher-order sensory processing, as well as with the dorsolateral PFC. The dorsolateral PFC has reciprocal connections with brain regions that are associated with motor control such as basal ganglia, premotor cortex, supplementary motor area, with performance monitoring such as cingulate cortex and with higher-order sensory processing such as associative areas and parietal cortex". According to these authors, the ventromedial PFC and its connections support functions involving the integration of information about emotion, memory and environmental stimuli, and the dorsolateral PFC with its network supports the regulation of behavior and control of responses to environmental stimuli. [28]

Although regions of the PFC seems to have more specific functions alone as mentioned above, they are jointed in order to manage more complex tasks, and they are probably all involved together in order to orchestrate multiple functions in highly complex demands, [29] such as in the processing of the working memory.

Therefore, the prefrontal cortex (PFC) can be considered as a "key cortical substrate of the highest-level mental processes", [30] managing all the necessary processes for short- or long-term goals and to regulate immediate behavior and to plan behavior in the future by exerting a "top-down" control over which information that is relevant and has to be utilized while excluding non-relevant information for the specific task at hand. [26] For all these process, it is implicated in a variety of cognitive and executive processes, including attention, set-shifting, decision-making, inhibitory response control, temporal integration of voluntary behavior, [31] all implicated in working memory processing.

Working memory

The concept of working memory evolved from the older notion of short-term memory of a single unit of memory storage. Working memory is no longer considered as a single unitary memory storage, but rather a system containing multiple cognitive subsystems or a multiple component system. [32]

Although they have differences, working memory models seem to agree that multiple subsystems work together to activate, maintain and manipulate a task-related information during the performance of cognitive tasks. In this manner, the subsystems, shift the state of a simple short-term storage towards a more dynamic and systemic view of working memory. [32] There seems to be a consensus that short-term memory storage is actually a function or one of the components of working memory. [32]

Therefore, working memory has been described as a multi-component system [33,34] (Figure 4) or a collection of distinct cognitive processes [35] that provides active maintenance of trial-selective information of different sensorial modalities in temporary storage. This enables manipulation, processing and retrieval of memories to be converted in a proper and effective action after both short (seconds) and long (minutes to hours) delays [35,36,37] in laboratory tasks and in everyday cognition [38] (Figure 4). Thus, working memory processes the information on a moment to moment basis, and even subtle deficiencies in its machinery can mean substantial deficits in ideation, reasoning and planning. [39]

According to *Smith and Jonides* [19] working memory can be considered as a system divided into two general components, a short-term storage for active maintenance of a limited set of information for a limited period of time (on the order of seconds), and a set of "executive processes" that operates on the content of storage. Thus, goal-directed behavior and essentially the frontal executive functions, such as solving problems, decision making, planning of future action, are highly related to and depend on working memory function.

According to *Rypma* [29] there are results obtained by neuroimaging studies that support the idea of a single framework of PFC function. In this concept, ventral PFC mediates working memory storage whereas dorsal PFC mediates a diverse set of executive processes, possibly including those aimed at optimizing memory performance. This author claimed that in low-demand working memory conditions, the ventral PFC seems to be enough and work alone, but this is a buffer with a limited capacity. Under conditions of high memory demand, in which to-be-remembered information needs to be consolidated or organized, the dorsal PFC function is required. [29]

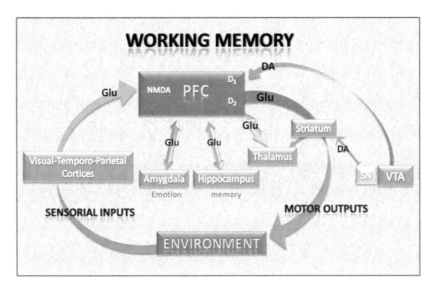

Figure 4. An overview of a hypothetical model of the working memory as a multi-component system processing the representation of multimodal sensorial inputs coming from the environment and pre-processed substantially in associative cortices, and storing them temporarily in a short-term memory as one of the function of the prefrontal cortex (PFC), the top of sensorio-motor integrative structure, which integrates these information with old memories retrieved, for example, from the hippocampus, that are relevant for that specific task, adding emotional content processed by amygdala, and by serving of all executive functions such as solving problems, solving conflicts, decision making, and planning of future action, besides the inhibition of non-relevant stimuli for that moment and correcting errors, it will direct the action to structures of motor system in order to accomplish a goal through motor outputs, delivering the proper behavior back to the environment. SN: substantia nigra, VTA: ventral tegmental area, DA: dopamine, D_1: dopamine D_1 receptor, D_2: dopamine D_2 receptor, Glu: glutamate, NMDA: N-Methyl-D-Aspartate.

Working memory by itself is limited in its capacity of storage that it might be as low as four (± 1) items. [40,41] However, according to *Motes and Rypma*, [41] when the to-be-remembered information exceeds the capacity limit, working memory executive processes can be brought online to optimally reorganize memory codes, allowing the storage and manage of information with larger contents.

Working Memory and Delayed-Tasks

According to *Goldman-Rakic et al*, [39] "the ability to hold an item of information transiently in mind in the service of comprehension, thinking, planning, reasoning, problem-solving and learning, is similar, if not identical, to the process that is measured by delayed-tasks in experimental research", [42] whereby a stimulus is presented then removed during a delay period and the subject must remember the previous stimulus or its location in order to guide later responding. [24] A crucial feature of delayed-response task is the need to update information on every trial. [42]

In the late 1920s investigators established the delayed response task as a paradigm of choice for prefrontal studies. [30] In the early 1970s, electrophysiological studies revealed that neurons in the PFC become activated during the delay period of a delayed-response trial when monkeys recalled a visual stimulus that had been presented at the beginning of a trial. This observation showed that the activity of these prefrontal neurons could be the cellular correlate of a mnemonic event. [43]

In the late 1980s, *Funahashi et al*. [44] found that many neurons in the dorsolateral PFC exhibited mnemonic persistent activity during the delay period in primates, and this cortical area became of a great importance in understanding working memory. [37] The establishment of a brain structure as a site for the processing of working memory allowed the investigation of the cellular and synaptic mechanisms involved in this cognitive function. [42] Many of these investigations have strongly suggested that dopamine activity in this area is highly related to working memory processing, especially through D_1 dopamine receptor activity. [39,45-47]

According to *Rypma*, [29] understanding the role of PFC in delayed-response task performance has been a continuing central focus of neuroimaging research. *Motes and Rypma* [41] have found that only medial and lateral regions of the PFC were differentially responsive to supra- and sub-capacity (six and two letters, respectively) memory sets during encode, maintain, and decide trial periods. A greater activation was seen in lateral regions of the PFC to 6-letter (supra-capacity) set during encode and maintain trial periods.

Working Memory, Drugs of Abuse and Addiction

As we have seen in the beginning of this chapter, plasticity changes and subsequent reorganization of neural circuitry in some specific brain regions occurring during drug addiction may be very similar or even the same as those involved in cellular and molecular mechanisms implicated in learning and memory process. [3,20,48,49]

Therefore, it is reasonable to question if cognitive dysfunctions induced by drugs of abuse involve changes in structures of the brain reward circuit. We will be focusing more specifically in the PFC and working memory.

In rats, the medial portion of the PFC (mPFC) has proven to be analogous to the dorsolateral and medial frontal cortex in the primate. [50,51] The mPFC in rats is constituted by Cg1 and Cg2 areas from anterior and dorsal cingulate cortex, Cg3 area from prelimbic cortex, and Fr2 area from precentral frontal cortex. [10,50,52] According to *Uylings et al.* [50] working memory that is processed in the dorsolateral PFC in primates seems to depend on mPFC integrity in rats, because lesions in these both areas equally produce deficits in this cognitive function.

Experimental procedures in a radial maze have been considered useful to measure working memory in animals [53] by interposing a delayed procedure that has also been called a spatial nonmatching delayed task or spatial win-shift task. Here animals obtain the information concerning the future location of food reward during a discrete acquisition phase (training phase or pre-delay), and the recall of this trial-unique information stored in a short-term memory is used to locate food accurately in a recall test phase (or post-delay), [24,54] carried out after a short (seconds) or a long (1 or more hours) interval of retention.

As already mentioned, neurons in the PFC are activated during the delay period of a delayed-response trial when a subject recalled a stimulus that had been presented at the beginning of a trial. [42,43] According to *Goldman-Rakic*, [42] this activity of prefrontal neurons expands and contracts as the delay is lengthened or shortened and is highly suggestive of a working memory process.

Working memory and drugs of abuse

We have been demonstrated that different drugs of abuse administered into the mPFC affect the delayed-task performance of rats in an 8-arm radial maze. [55,56] Different doses of ethanol (Figure 5 left) or Δ^9-tetrahydrocannabinol (Figure 6 left) administered intracortically disrupted, whereas a low dose of nicotine (Figure 7 left) facilitated, the 1 h post-delay performance, suggesting that these drugs somehow change the spatial working memory processing.

As we have noted before, DA is one of the major neurotransmitter systems involved in PFC functions. The terminal cortical fields of dopaminergic fibers are mainly restricted to the prefrontal areas, comprising a portion of the mesocortical dopamine system, [10] and the entorhinal cortex in rats. However, only the PFC projects back to the dopaminergic neurons in ventral tegmental area and the dopaminergic pars compacta of the substantia nigra (see [50]).

In a delayed task performance in a radial maze, *Phillips et al.* [57] showed that there is a significant increase in DA efflux in the mPFC during the training phase (pre-delay). This increase remained elevated for a further 5 minutes and returned to baseline values for the remaining 25 min of the delay period. DA efflux also increases in the mPFC during the recall test phase (post-delay) when rats have to display an accurate recall. According to *Phillips et al*, [57] DA D_1-like activity in the mPFC seems to be consistent with the increased DA efflux during the pre-delay performance extending to the beginning of the delay component. This is possibly related to the retention of information acquired earlier during the pre-delay performance, and information reacquired after the end of the delay during the post-delay performance [57] when the knowledge of arms already visited during the pre-delay performance has to be retrieved correctly.

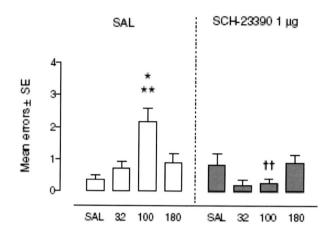

Fgure 5. Ethanol (EtOH) administered bilaterally into the medial prefrontal cortex (0.5 µl in each side at B: +2.5 mmA, +/-1 mmL, -2.7 mmV) impaired the performance (mean errors ± standard error minor (SE)) of 1 h post-delay performance in the 8-arm radial maze (n = 11). Previous bilateral intracortical administration (10 min earlier) of 1 µg SCH 23390, a selective Dopamine D_1 receptor antagonist, prevented the disruptive effect of EtOH on the 1 h post-delay performance. ** $p < 0.01$ as compared to control (saline (SAL)-SAL). * $p < 0.05$ as compared to other doses of EtOH (32 or 180 µg), †† $p < 0.01$ compared to the combination of SAL with 100 µg EtOH (data not published).

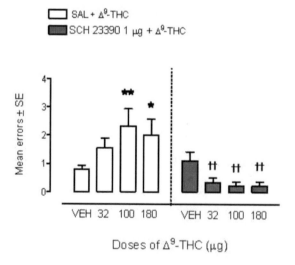

Figure 6. Δ^9-tetrahydrocannabinol (Δ^9-THC) administered bilaterally into the medial prefrontal cortex (0.5 µl in each side at B: +2.5 mmA, +/-1 mmL, -2.7 mmV) impaired the performance of 1 h post-delay performance in the 8-arm radial maze (left). Previous bilateral intracortical administration (10 min earlier) of 1 µg SCH 23390 (n = 9), a selective Dopamine D_1 receptor antagonist (right) prevented the disruptive effect of EtOH on the 1 h post-delay performance. * $p < 0.05$ or ** $p < 0.01$ as compared to control (SAL(saline)-VEH(30% emulphor in DMSO)), †† $p < 0.01$ compared to the respective dose of Δ^9-THC combined with SAL (data not published).

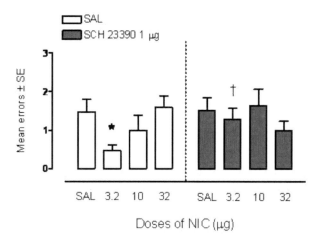

Figure 7. Nicotine (NIC) administered bilaterally into the medial prefrontal cortex (0.5 μl in each side at B: +2.5 mmA, +/-1 mmL, -2.7 mmV) facilitated the 1 h post-delay performance in the 8-arm radial maze at the smallest dose (3.2 μg) (left) (n = 12 to 14). Previous bilateral intracortical administration (10 min earlier) of 1 μg SCH 23390 (right), a selective Dopamine D_1 receptor antagonist prevented this facilitating effect of NIC (right panel). * $p < 0.05$ compared to control (SAL-SAL), † $p < 0.01$ compared to the combination of SAL with 3.2 NIC (data not published).

There is a great possibility that changes in working memory produced by drugs of abuse showed above would involve DA D_1 receptors in the mPFC, because intracortical administration of SCH 23390, a DA D_1 receptor antagonist, prevented the dose-dependent disruptive effect either intracortically administered ethanol (Figure 5 right) or Δ^9-tetrahydrocannabinol (Figure 6 right), as well as the facilitating effect of intracortically administered nicotine (Figure 7 right).

Increasingly, experimental results show that working memory operates optimally within a limited range of DA transmission and D_1 dopamine receptor signaling in the PFC, [39,58] delineating an "inverted U-shaped" (or biphasic, or bell-shaped) relationship between dopamine transmission and the integrity of working memory. [24,43,47,58,59] Thus both an insufficient and an excessive stimulation of dopamine D_1 receptor are disruptive for this cognitive function [39,47,58] (Figure 8 bottom left).

As noted above, the DA system is of a great importance in brain reward mechanisms and its involvement in the development of substance abuse is well established (see [60]). According to *Di Chiara et al*, [61] DA is the brain neurotransmitter that has been more extensively implicated in the mechanism of drug addiction, not only as the substrate of psychostimulant reward but, more generally, as a substrate of drug-related learning and neuroadaptation.

However, our results also suggest that the effects of drugs of abuse on working memory may involve glutamatergic mediation because an intracortical administration of Memantine, a non-competitive N-Methyl-D-Aspartate (NMDA) receptor antagonist, decreased significantly the disruptive effect of 100 μg ethanol (Figure 9 right) administered into the mPFC.

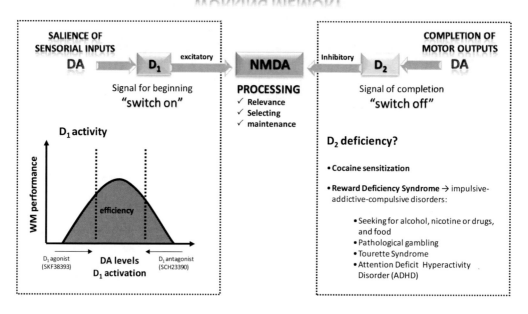

Figure 8. A schematic view of a hypothetical influence of dopamine (DA) D_1-like (detecting the salience of sensorial inputs as a signal for beginning, "switching on" the working memory - WM - process) and D_2-like (providing a signal of the completion of motor response, finishing the working memory process) receptors on N-Methyl-D-Aspartate (NMDA) receptor on processing (by establishing the relevance, selecting, maintaining and organizing the information) of working memory in the prefrontal cortex (PFC). Note the inverted "U" shaped curve related to DA D_1-like receptors activation (left) [24,43,47,58,59] and the possible consequences of the deficiency of D_2-like receptors function (right). [16,73-75]

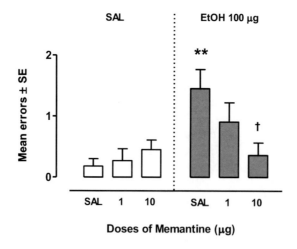

Figure 9. Previous bilateral intracortical administration of Memantine (n = 11), a non-competitive NMDA receptor antagonist, prevented the disruptive effect of 100 μg ethanol (EtOH) administered bilaterally into the medial prefrontal cortex (0.5 μl in each side at B: +2.5 mmA, +/-1 mmL, -2.7 mmV) on the 1 h post-delay performance in the 8-arm radial maze. ** $p < 0.01$ as compared to control saline (SAL)-SAL,† $p < 0.05$ compared to the combination of SAL with 100 μg EtOH (data not published).

NMDA receptors have also a critical role in normal working memory function of the PFC. [62,63] According to *Seamans and Yang* [24] the DA signal would contain no information by itself, but it would provide a processing tone in the PFC and set the gain for PFC networks. These authors suggest that glutamate is the one that actually transmits the information and that limbic glutamatergic inputs would "inform" PFC networks about "when" to initiate persistent activity and "what" type of information has to be held by such activity, while the DA system influences gain of the glutamate-encoded information. [24]

Glutamatergic afferents and dopaminergic terminals are in direct apposition to one another in the PFC, suggesting a presynaptic site of modulation, influencing each other's release. [64,65] It has been also shown that dopaminergic and glutamatergic axon terminals form "synaptic triads" on the postsynaptic dendrites of deep layer PFC pyramidal neurons. [66,67] In fact, *Zheng et al.* [65] provided direct electrophysiological evidence that DA acts postsynaptically to modulate PFC NMDA receptor-mediated glutamate transmission.

To address the dopaminergic-glutamatergic involvement in the delayed task procedures in the 8-arm radial maze, we conducted a study in which we evaluated the effects of a NMDA receptor antagonist on the disruptive effects of a DA D_1-partial agonist. In this study we were able to demonstrate in animals performing 1 h delayed-tasks that the disruptive effect of a small dose of SKF-38393, a partial DA D_1-receptor agonist, was significantly reduced by intracortical administration of a non-competitive NMDA receptor antagonist, MK-801. At the dose used, MK-801 had no significant effects on performance. These results suggest that there is an involvement of dopaminergic–glutamatergic modulation on spatial working memory in the mPFC. [68]

According to *Yang and Chen*, [69] an extended dose range of D_1 agonist produced an inverted "U" shaped dose-dependent D_1 modulation of the synaptically evoked NMDA-excitatory postsynaptic potentials in PFC neurons. As already mentioned, this type of dose-response curve is a characteristic effect of dopamine D_1-like receptors activation on working memory, which raises the possibility that a reciprocal interaction between dopamine D_1 receptors and NMDA receptors exists in the processing of this cognitive function in the PFC.

DA D_2-like receptors seem also to be involved in these effects, considering that intracortical administration of Clozapine, a dopamine D_2/D_4 receptor antagonist, reduced significantly the disruptive effect of different doses of Δ^9-tetrahydrocannabinol (Figure 10) and of 100 µg ethanol (Figure 11) administered into the mPFC.

However, we have also been demonstrated that prior administration of haloperidol, a DA antagonist, into the mPFC in doses that had no effect alone (10 and 32 µg) increased the disruptive effect of 100 µg EtOH also administered intracortically on 1 h delayed tasks in the radial maze. [55]

The involvement of dopamine D_2 receptors in cognitive function, especially working memory, is less clear and controversial. *Sawaguchi and Goldman-Rakic* [46] did not find a clear effect of sulpiride (selective D_2 receptor antagonist) or raclopride (D_2/D_3 receptor antagonist) locally injected into the dorsolateral PFC in monkeys trained to perform an oculomotor delayed-response task, suggesting that neither D_2 nor D_3 receptors seemed to be critical for monkey's performance, at least under their conditions. However, *Von Huben et al.* [70] observed that spatial working memory accuracy, evaluated by a self-ordered spatial search task, was reduced to a greater extent by raclopride than by SCH23390 (D_1 receptor antagonist), and visuo-spatial paired associate learning was impaired by raclopride but not by

SCH23390, suggesting a greater contribution of D_2- over D_1-like receptors to both spatial working memory and object-location associative memory.

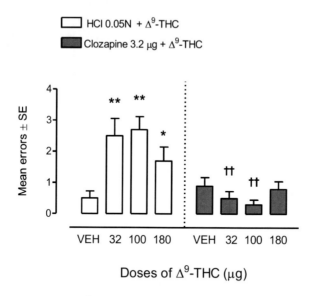

Figure 10. Δ^9-tetrahydrocannabinol (Δ^9-THC) administered bilaterally into the medial prefrontal cortex (0.5 μl in each side at B: +2.5 mmA, +/-1 mmL, -2.7 mmV) impaired the performance of 1 h post-delay performance in the 8-arm radial maze (left). Previous bilateral intracortical administration (10 min earlier) of 3.2 μg Clozapine (n = 10), a Dopamine D_2/D_4 receptor antagonist (right) prevented the disruptive effect of EtOH on the 1 h post-delay performance. * $p < 0.05$ or ** $p < 0.01$ as compared to control (SAL(saline)-VEH(30% emulphor in DMSO)), †† $p < 0.01$ compared to the respective dose of Δ^9-THC combined with HCl 0.05N (data not published).

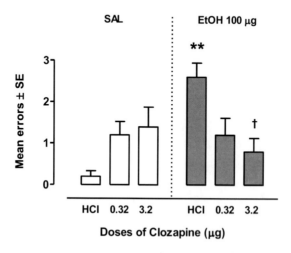

Figure 11. Previous bilateral intracortical administration of Clozapine (n = 10), a Dopamine D_2/D_4 receptor antagonist, prevented the disruptive effect of 100 μg ethanol (EtOH) administered bilaterally into the medial prefrontal cortex (0.5 μl in each side at B: +2.5 mmA, +/-1 mmL, -2.7 mmV) on the 1 h post-delay performance in the 8-arm radial maze. ** $p < 0.01$ as compared to control (HCl (0.05N)-SAL(saline), † $p < 0.05$ compared to the combination of HCl with 100 μg EtOH (data not published).

Wang et al. [71] examined the role of the D_2 family of receptors in the functional properties of prefrontal neurons, by combining single neuron recording in nonhuman primates performing an eight-target spatial oculomotor delayed-response task with iontophoretic application of selective D_2 receptor agonists and antagonists. They found that, in contrast to the D_1 receptor, which alters the delayed-related activity of prefrontal neurons, the D_2 receptor is reliably associated with saccade-related activity at the end of the trial. They suggested that action of dopamine D_1 and D_2 receptors in the PFC differ not only pharmacologically but substantially with respect to cellular circuit and functional specificity, dissociating their action on cortical circuit elements engaged in cognitive function such as working memory. As an attractive possibility, *Wang et al.* [71] suggested in their study that the phasic saccadic responses modulated by D_2 receptors would be a corollary discharge that informs the prefrontal network that a motor command had been completed (Figure 8 upper right).

Albeit dissociated as suggested by *Wang et al*, [71] different dopamine receptors seem to function in an integrated manner in the processing of working memory in the PFC (Figure 8). *Glickstein et al.* [72] using quantitative immunocytochemical studies to analyze prefrontal cortical c-*fos* responses to a systemically administered D_1 receptor agonist on the performance of D_2 and D_3 receptors knock-out mice in a spatial working memory task, showed a significantly blunted D_1 agonist-stimulated c-*fos* responses in the PFC of both mutants which exhibited significant deficits in spatial working memory. They further showed that a single dose of methamphetamine rescued the blunted prefrontal cortical c-*fos* responses and the spatial working memory deficits in D_2 mutants.

Beyer and Steketee [73] showed that quinpirole, an agonist at DA D_2-like receptors, but not a DA D_1-like receptor agonist, administered into the mPFC blocked the initiation and blunted the behavioral (locomotor activity) and neurochemical expression of cocaine-induced sensitization. Furthermore, *Steketee and Walsh* [74] showed that repeated injections of sulpiride, a DA D_2-like receptor antagonist, into the mPFC induced behavioral and neurochemical cross-sensitization to cocaine. These authors suggest that sensitization is associated with a decrease in DA D_2-like receptor function in the mPFC.

These data may be linked to a "*reward deficiency syndrome*" (Figure 8 right). In this case, there is an insensitivity and inefficiency to positive reinforces and/or to the need of escape or avoid negative affect [16] that has been related to a dysfunction of the DA D_2-like receptors in the brain. [75] This leads to aberrant substance seeking behavior and other "impulsive-addictive-compulsive" disorders, including polysubstance abuse, smoking, attention deficit hyperactivity disorder, obesity, and Tourette's syndrome. [75]

Interestingly, there is also evidence that activation of D_2-like receptors on motor cortical plasticity follows an inverted U-shaped pattern, [76] in which high or low dosages of ropinirole (a DA D_2/D_3 receptor agonist) impaired cortical plasticity. However, a moderate dose was ineffective, suggesting, according to the authors, that "modulation of D_2-like receptor activity may exert dose-dependent inhibitory or even facilitatory effects on human cortical neuroplasticity". [76]

Together, these observations suggest that drugs of abuse may influence working memory process by changing DA activity in the PFC. They may disrupt it by overstimulating D_1-like receptors, signaling the effect of the drug as the most salient stimuli to trigger the working memory (Figure 8); or involving D_2-like receptors, in the final input, disturbing the identification of the motor response ending. Both mechanisms may be involved depending on the predominance of the DA activity yielding an imbalance between DA D_1-like and D_2-like receptors in the cortical structure (Figure 8).

Certainly, it is also necessary to consider the importance of the role of NMDA receptors in the PFC in these cognitive processes because they may be involved in the selection, maintenance and organization of the relevant information needed for the proper working memory activity (Figure 8).

Therefore, it is highly suggestive that disturbances in the process of working memory, particularly involving the PFC functions, produced by drugs of abuse may strongly be related to the establishment of drug addiction.

Long-lasting changes in the PFC and addiction

According to *Robinson and Kolb*, [77] "one of the most compelling examples of experience-dependent plasticity, whereby experience at one point in life changes behavior and psychological function for a lifetime, is addiction". The high tendency of addicts to relapse, even months to many years after the discontinuation of drug use, and long after withdrawal symptoms have been treated, provides strong evidence that drug use has long lasting consequences.

Robinson and Kolb [77] recognized that persistent changes in behavior and psychological function, which occur as a consequence of experience, are thought to be mediated by the reorganization or strengthening of synaptic connections in specific neural circuits. They conducted a series of experiments in which they proved that repeated exposure to cocaine, amphetamine, morphine or nicotine, in adult rats, whether administered by an experimenter or self-administered, have long-lasting effects on the structure of dendrites and dendritic spines in brain regions thought to mediate drug-induced changes in incentive motivation and reward (such as the NAcc) and in cognitive function (such as the PFC). They further observed that drug-induced structural plasticity is evident many months after drug discontinuation, suggesting that drugs of abuse produce a persistent reorganization of patterns of synaptic connectivity in these brain regions.

The persistence of molecular changes in the mPFC and NAcc of rats that can occur at the initiation and/or during the abstinence period has also been observed after cocaine self-administration. [78] *Freeman et al.* [78] conducted a whole-genome expression analysis on a rat cocaine binge-abstinence model that had previously been demonstrated to engender increased drug seeking and taking with abstinence. They identified gene expression changes in two mesolimbic terminal fields (mPFC and NAcc) of rats submitted to 10 days of cocaine self-adminstration followed by 1, 10, or 100 days of enforced abstinence and compared to cocaine-naive rats. They found long-lasting changes in gene expression in the mPFC and in a lesser extent in the NAcc and also identified cellular processes that may regulate the development and/or maintenance of incubation of drug-seeking and drug-taking.

According to these authors, changes in the mPFC may be more pronounced than those in the NAcc and involve mostly distinct sets of genes that may indicate different metaplastic processes occurring in these brain regions with the development and expression of abstinence-induced behaviors. [78] Gene expression changes observed in the mPFC were both a result of cocaine self-administration and with the subsequent enforced abstinence. These changes may contribute to the persistent alteration of synaptic plasticity in this structure. Furthermore, they also observed changes in MAPK/ERK and calcium signaling in the mPFC. As this brain structure mediates executive function and decision making processes,

Freeman et al. [78] suggested that it may constitute a key neuroanatomical region in addictive behaviors.

The studies review above show that there are long lasting structural and molecular changes in the PFC induced by drugs of abuse. Along the same line, we know also that some of the long-term behavioral effects and cognitive deficits seen in addicts might be due to drug induced limits on plasticity. [79] Based on these sets of observations, we postulate that addiction may be associated with a long-lasting alteration in the processing of working memory, particularly those pathways involving dopaminergic and glutamatergic modulation in the PFC. Certainly this supposition needs to be evaluated in future investigations.

PFC Function, Working Memory and Alcoholism

As we have seen above, working memory integrity is required in the processing of important cognitive functions such as learning, goal-directed behavior, decision-making, understanding and reasoning. All these function are substantially affected in drug addiction and dependence (see [80]).

Alcoholism has long been considered a complex disease, given its biological, sociological and psychopathological components, and frontal lobe dysfunctions are consistently described in this condition. [81,82] Currently, the literature emphasizes the hypothesis of primary frontal lobe damage in alcoholics. This is also true for chronic alcoholics who appear clinically *'intact'*, because they present with morphological abnormalities in the frontal lobes. [80]

We have studied the effects of an anticonvulsant and analgesic agent, gabapentin, in a randomized, double-blind, placebo-controlled trial performed with 60 male alcohol-dependent subjects with a mean age of 44 years and an average of 27 years of alcohol use, who consumed 17 drinks per day (165 - 170 g/day) over the 90 days prior to entry into the study, We found that gabapentin significantly reduced alcohol consumption and craving in chronic alcoholics over a 28-day of treatment (n = 25) compared to the placebo treated alcoholics (n = 18). [83]

In this study, patients that reached the end of the study in abstinence after 28-day treatment with gabapentin (n = 18), but not those treated with placebo (n = 13), had an improved verbal attention as measured by a Digit Span test in its forward task, and the verbal and visuospatial short-term memory examine by Digit Span and Corsi Block-Tapping test, respectively in their backward tasks. [84] Gabapentin also improved prose recall measured by immediate and delayed tasks in the logical memory test. [84] However it did not change the profound impairment of executive functions found in these alcoholic patients examined by Wisconsin Sorting Card test. [84]

Although executive functions were not ameliorated by gabapentin, this compound improved verbal and visuospatial short-term memories, which are important components of working memory process. In addition, gabapentin also improved the recall of items from short-term memory, another important function involved in the working memory process. These improving effects on short-term memory component of the working memory may be related to the effect of gabapentin on reducing the craving that is a main characteristic of drug addiction.

In another study on the role of frontal functions in alcoholics, we have examined frontal lobe cognitive function in different types of alcohol dependence according to Lesch's typology. [85]

Briefly in Lesch's typology, [86,87] the *Type I* alcoholism is primarily characterized by the development of tolerance with the appearance of early heavy withdrawal symptoms (considered as a *model of allergy*). [88,89] Patients develop meta-alcoholic psychosis, like delirium tremens, and might suffer from withdrawal epileptic seizures. They tend to use alcohol to weaken withdrawal symptoms. [90] *Type II* alcoholics show suicidal intentions, anxiety and pre-morbid conflicts (considered as a *model of anxiety or conflict*). [89] Alcohol seems to be used as a strategy against anxiety, and they frequently become aggressive when intoxicated. [91] *Type III* alcoholics exhibit an aggressive and impulsive behavior with the existence of psychiatric co-morbidity. [89] Alcohol seems to be used as a self-medication to treat an underlying affective disorder (*alcohol as antidepressant*). [88] Finally, *Type IV* alcoholics comprise patients with disturbance or cerebral damage before the conclusion of brain development, [91] associated with behavioral disorders and serious social problems. [88,89] Alcoholic beverages are also used as a means of self-medication to treat symptoms in this group (*alcohol drinking as adaptation*). [85]

Frontal cognitive functions were assessed by a brief instrument developed by *Dubois et al.* [92] The frontal assessment battery (FAB) has been shown to be very sensitive to frontal lobe dysfunction, [92] takes approximately 10 min to administer and can be applied easily at the bedside. [92,93] This battery consists of six subsets that screen global executive dysfunction, including conceptualization, mental flexibility, motor programming, sensitivity to interference, inhibitory control and environmental autonomy. [92]

The study [85] used a sample of 170 alcoholics with a mean age of 46.4 years ± (SD) 9.7, mostly constituted by male (87.1%) heavy drinkers with an average intake of 372.5 ± (SD) 314.2 g of alcohol per day and with a mean age at onset of alcohol use of 14.9 years ± (SD) 4.6. On these subjects, 21.2% were classified as Type I, 29.4% as Type II, 28.8% as Type III and 20.6% as Type IV. [85]

In a global analysis, alcoholics (n = 170) showed significantly lower overall scores on the FAB performance as compared to age, gender, socio-demographic-matched non-alcoholic subjects (n = 40). [85] In a more specific analysis, type IV alcoholics had lower FAB overall scores as compared to non-alcoholic controls and also to all other types of alcoholic subjects. The FAB subsets of motor programming, sensitivity to interference and inhibitory control were significantly reduced in Types II, III and IV alcoholics as compared to non-alcoholic subjects, but only motor programming remained impaired in Type IV alcoholics with preserved mental function (normal range on mini-mental status examination). We concluded that executive dysfunctions in alcohol dependence seem to vary depending upon the type of alcoholism. [85]

Thus, in this sample of alcoholics, Type IV alcoholics showed severe impairments in their executive frontal and general cognitive function. Even in those with a preserved mental function, the executive frontal function was still significantly compromised, notably in the motor programming subset.

Motor programming is a function required for temporal organization and the maintenance and execution of successive actions. [92] This function can be examined by asking the subject to execute motor series in specific orders, such as *Luria*'s [94] 'fist-edge-palm' task used in the FAB. This task assesses the ability to learn novel motor sequences and to engage in purposeful motor output. [95] Therefore, alcoholics with motor programming dysfunction are presumably impaired in their ability to learn new tasks and to engage in successive actions and consequently may show ineffective goal-directed behavior, [85] essentially the main objective of the working memory processing.

There appears to be very few studies on approaches that might improve the PFC function of working memory in alcoholics. A literature search revealed two interesting studies conducted by *Fregni et al.* [96] and *Boggio et al.* [97]. In the first study, they investigated whether a weak anodal transcranial direct current stimulation (tDCS), which was already known to enhance motor cortical excitability in the human brain, would modify the performance of a working memory task (a sequential-letter working memory task) when applied to the left dorsolateral PFC (DLPFC). They tested fifteen healthy college students (19-22 years old, 11 females) in a three-back working memory task based on letters under tDCS (1 mA for 10 min). They observed that anodal stimulation over the left DLPFC increases the accuracy of the task performance when compared with sham stimulation over the same area. They further observed that the effect of the anodal stimulation over the left DLPFC was relatively focal and depended on the polarity of stimulation, because a cathodal stimulation over the left DLPFC and an anodal stimulation over the motor cortex had no such effect.

In other study [97], they showed that a PFC modulation using tDCS reduced alcohol craving. This was a double-blind, sham-controlled study, in which they showed that anodal modulation of DLPFC using tDCS decreased alcohol craving in 13 patients (mean age of 41.3±5.7, two females) with alcohol dependence compared to sham stimulation while being exposed to alcohol visual cues constituted by images of alcoholic beverages and situations that subjects would be more typically exposed to through television commercials and advertisements.

Drug Addiction, ERP and Brain Stimulation

Different types of alcoholics present different degrees of executive dysfunction. Consequently, we wish to determine if different alcoholics also show different patterns of brain activity that could be electrophysiologically measured by evoked-related potential (ERP), especially by the P300 or P3 waveform, as a register from frontal activity. Additionally we wish to determine if brain stimulation either by therapeutic drugs and/or non-pharmacological techniques, such as the tDCS applied over the DLPFC, would improve executive functions, notably the working memory, or change the drug addiction pattern.

To address these questions, we are currently carrying out a collaborative study with Fregni's group to study the effects of anodal tDCS over the left DLPFC on ERP and on executive functions and craving in different types of alcoholics as stratified by Lesch's typology. Some of our preliminary results are presented below. Subjects were recruited from the alcohol dependence unit in the Medical School Hospital of The Federal University of Espirito Santo, Brazil. This study was approved by the Brazilian Institutional Review Board at the Federal University of Espírito Santo, Brazil, which has been conducted in strict adherence to the Declaration of Helsinki and is in accord with ethical standards of the

Committee on Human Experimentation of the Federal University of Espírito Santo, Espírito Santo, Brazil, where this study has been done.

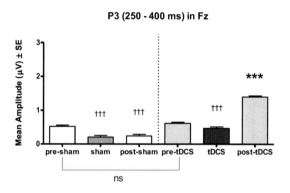

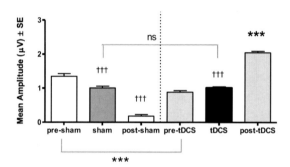

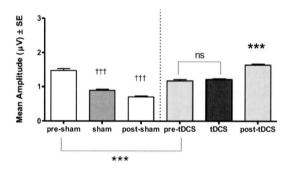

Figure 12. Increase of the mean amplitude of cognitive potential (P3) after the transcranial direct current stimulation (tDCS) (1 mA for 10 min) applied over the left dorsolateral prefrontal cortex (DLPFC) in 16 chronic alcoholics. It was considered a temporal window of 250 to 400 ms in the Evoked-Related Potential (ERP) triggered by sounds related to alcohol drinking mixed randomly with unrelated sounds in the frontal (Fz), central (Cz) and Parietal (Pz) regions of the brain, before, during and after a simulated (sham, pre-sham and post-sham, respectively) or factual brain stimulation (pre-tDCS, tDCS, and post-tDCS, respectively). *** $p < 0.01$ compared to pre-sham in all three electrode position, ††† $p < 0.05$ compared to the respective pre-sham or pre-tDCS condition.

In general the procedures described by *Zago-Gomes and Nakamura-Palacios*, [85] *Fregni et al*, [96] *Luck*, [98] and *Heinze et al*. [99] were used. Prior to study the subjects underwent an average period of forced abstinence of 12 days. ERPs were evoked by sounds delivered via an ear phone that were either associated or not associated with the consumption of alcoholic beverages. [99] Sounds associated with drinking included opening a beer can, pouring the beer into a glass or opening a bottle of champagne, and were considered as significant stimulus. Sounds not associated with drinking alcoholic beverages included opening a door, running water for a shower or typing on a computer keyboard, and were considered as non-significant stimulus.

Preliminary data has been collected from 16 alcoholic. The subjects had a mean age of 48.9 ± 7.7 (3 female), with the mean age at onset of alcohol use of 15.5 ± 4.0, 80% were heavy drinkers drinking above 7 to 10 drinks/day, most of them in the average of 12 days of abstinence in the first experimental session. The mean amplitude (µV) of a temporal window from 250 to 400 milliseconds related to P3 waveform was adjusted for a mean baseline of 200 milliseconds before the beginning of the sounds presentation. For ERP analysis we followed the parameters recommended by *Steven J. Luck*. [98]

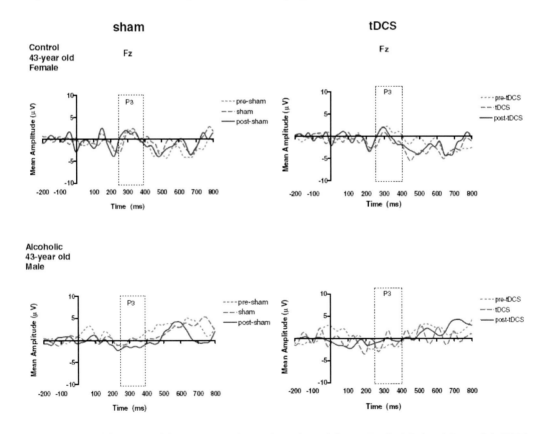

Figure 13. Cognitive potential (P3, 250 - 400 ms) registered in an Evoked-Related Potential (ERP) procedure triggered by sounds related to alcohol drinking mixed randomly with unrelated sounds in the frontal (Fz) site in a non-alcoholic subject (upper) and in a chronic alcoholic subject (bottom), before (pre-tDCS), during (tDCS) and after (post-tDCS) transcranial direct current stimulation (1 mA for 10 min) (right) applied over the left dorsolateral prefrontal cortex (DLPFC) compared to the ERP before, during and after a simulated (sham, pre-sham and post-sham, respectively) procedure (left).

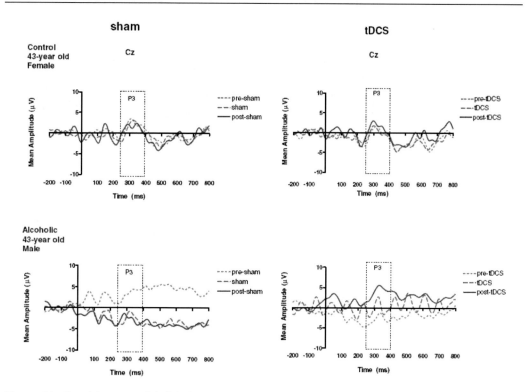

Figure 14. Cognitive potential (P3, 250 - 400 ms) registered in an Evoked-Related Potential (ERP) procedure triggered by sounds related to alcohol drinking mixed randomly with unrelated sounds in the central (Cz) site in a non-alcoholic subject (upper) and in a chronic alcoholic subject (bottom), before (pre-tDCS), during (tDCS) and after (post-tDCS) transcranial direct current stimulation (1 mA for 10 min) (right) applied over the left dorsolateral prefrontal cortex (DLPFC) compared to the ERP before, during and after a simulated (sham, pre-sham and post-sham, respectively) procedure (left).

The data collected from these subjects as the main group as alcoholics is shown in Figure 12. To date, the mean amplitude of the P3 waveform was only increased after tDCS, but not during the tDCS, especially in Fz and Cz sites (Figure 12) as compared to the mean amplitude before the tDCS. The opposite effect was seen in sham procedure, that is, the mean amplitude was decreased during sham and especially after sham procedure, notably in Cz and Pz sites (Figure 12). The 50% area latency has not been changed in both conditions.

So far we can suggest that tDCS does change the P3 waveform in alcoholics and that this might be related to changes in brain activity especially in frontal and central region. Because of the small sample size we are not able to conduct a meaningful analysis to correlate changes in the waveforms with executive function and drug addiction across the different types of alcoholics.

In an individual analysis, there is a remarkable difference in the brain activity between an alcoholic subject and a non-alcoholic subject. In the following figures (13 - 15) we show ERP registers as an example from a non-alcoholic control subject (a 43 year old female), a subject from other specialized service from the same medical school hospital, and one of our alcoholic subjects paired by age (a 43 year old male).

The alcoholic subject shows an unstable brain activity compared to the steadier pattern observed in the non-alcoholic subject (Figures 13 - 15). Note the flattened register during P3 in the alcoholic subject in Fz region (Figure 13 bottom left), suggesting almost the absence of the P3 waveform that was even decreased after sham procedure, but it was slightly increased after tDCS (Figure 13 bottom right). This effect was especially clear in Cz region (Figure 14, bottom left and right).

It seems that the brain activity become a little bit more stable after tDCS at the Pz site in the alcoholic subject (Figure 15 bottom right). Clearly further studies are needed to compare alcoholic and non-alcoholic subjects. These prelimary data offer encouragement. Hopefully, this approach will permit us understand the uses and limits of non-invasive brain stimulation techniques to the development of more advanced protocols and with a more specific examination of working memory.

Future investigations using pharmacological agents, especially those modulating transmission dopaminergic and glutamatergic pathways, and non-pharmacological strategies, such as non-invasive transcranial brain stimulation, may provide a clearer understanding of the intriguing relationship between working memory in the prefrontal cortex and drug addiction, as well as aid in establishing new therapeutic approaches to the treatment of drug abuse.

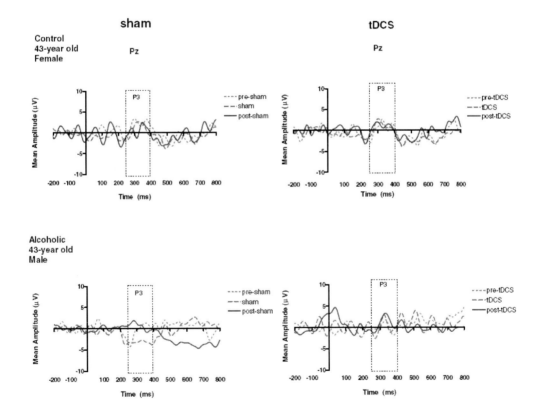

Figure 15. Cognitive potential (P3, 250 - 400 ms) registered in an Evoked-Related Potential (ERP) procedure triggered by sounds related to alcohol drinking mixed randomly with unrelated sounds in the parietal (Pz) site in a non-alcoholic subject (upper) and in a chronic alcoholic subject (bottom), before (pre-tDCS), during (tDCS) and after (post-tDCS) transcranial direct current stimulation (1 mA for 10 min) (right) applied over the left dorsolateral prefrontal cortex (DLPFC) compared to the ERP before, during and after a simulated (sham, pre-sham and post-sham, respectively) procedure (left).

CONCLUSION

According to *Robinson and Kolb*, [77] "drugs and other experiences interact in remodeling synapses". Therefore, it is possible that besides some life experiences, a brain stimulation technique allied by cognitive strategies and medications, could help to decrease the ability of abused drugs to reorganize synaptic connections. Such an action in the PFC could reduce the effects of abused substances on the processing of working memory and mitigate some of the negative neurobehavioral consequences of drug addiction.

We strongly believe that by improving the capacity of working memory by strengthening prefrontal function and subsequently improving new learning will help subjects to relearn and regain at least part of control of their behavior that was lost in the addiction process.

REFERENCES

[1] Sanchis-Segura, C; Spanagel, R. Behavioural assessment of drug reinforcement and addictive features in rodents: an overview. *Addict Biol*, 2006, 11, 2-38.
[2] Volkow, N; Li, TK. The neuroscience of addiction. *Nat Neurosci*, 2005, 8(11), 1429-1430.
[3] Hyman, SE; Malenka, RC. Neurobiology of compulsion and its persistence. *Nat Rev Neurosci*, 2001, 2, 695-703.
[4] Goldstein, RZ; Volkow, ND. Drug addiction and its underlying neurobiological basis: neuroimaging evidence for the involvement of the frontal cortex. *Am J Psychiatry*, 2002 159(10), 1642-1652.
[5] Volkow, ND; Fowler, JS; Wang, GJ; Swanson, JM. Dopamine in drug abuse and addiction: results from imaging studies and treatment implications. *Mol Psychiatry*, 2004, 9, 557-569.
[6] Nestler, EJ. Molecular mechanisms of drug addiction. *Neuropharmacology*, 2004, 47, 24-32.
[7] Nestler, EJ. Molecular basis of long-term plasticity underlying addiction. *Nat Rev Neurosci*, 2001 2, 119-128.
[8] Koob, GF. The role of the striatopallidal and extended amygdala systems in drug addiction. *Ann N Y Acad Sci*, 1999, 877, 445-460.
[9] Tzchentke, TM. The medial prefrontal cortex as a part of the brain reward system. *Amino Acids*, 2000, 19, 211-219.
[10] Steketee, JD. Neurotransmitter systems of the medial prefrontal cortex: potential role in sensitization to psychostimulants. *Brain Res Brain Res Rev*, 2003, 41, 203-228.
[11] Nestler, EJ. Is there a common molecular pathway for addiction? *Nat Neurosci,* 2005, 8(11), 1445-1449.
[12] Kalivas, PW; Volkow, ND. The neural basis of addiction: a pathology of motivation and choice. *Am J Psychiatry*, 2005, 162, 1403-1413.
[13] Everitt, BJ; Robbins, TW. Neural system of reinforcement for drug addiction: from action to habits to compulsion. *Nature Neurosci*, 2005 8(11), 1481-1489.
[14] Koob, GF. Drugs of abuse: anatomy, pharmacology and function of reward pathways. *Trends Pharmacol Sci*, 1992, 13, 177-184.

[15] Koob, GF; Le Moal, M. Drug addiction, dysregulation of reward, and allostasis. *Neuropsychopharmacology*, 2001, 24, 97-129.
[16] Bowirrat, A; Oscar-Berman, M. Relationship between dopaminergic neurotransmission, alcoholism, and reward deficiency syndrome. *Am J Med Genet*, 2005, 132B, 29-37.
[17] Fuster, JM. *The prefrontal cortex*. 4th edition. London: Academic Press; 2008.
[18] McBride, T; Arnold, SE; Gur, RC. A comparative volumetric analysis of the prefrontal cortex in human and baboon MRI. *Brain Behav Evol*, 1999, 54, 159-166.
[19] Smith, ED; Jonides, J. Storage and executive processes in the frontal lobes. *Sci*, 1999, 283, 1657-1661.
[20] Hyman, SE. Addiction: A Disease of Learning and Memory. *Am J Psychiatry*, 2005, 162, 1414-1422.
[21] Thompson-Schill, SL; Bedny, M; Goldberg RF. The frontal lobes and the regulation of mental activity. *Curr Opin Neurobiol*, 2005, 15, 219-224.
[22] Fuster, JM. The prefrontal cortex and its relation to behavior. *Prog Brain Res*, 1991, 87, 201-211.
[23] Fuster, JM. The prefrontal cortex - an update: time is of the essence. *Neuron*, 2001, 30, 319-333.
[24] Seamans, JK; Yang, CR. The principal features and mechanisms of dopamine modulation in the prefrontal cortex. *Prog Neurobiol*, 2004 74, 1-57.
[25] Cummings, JL. Frontal-subcortical circuits and human behavior. *Arch Neurol*, 1993, 50, 873-880.
[26] Powell, KB; Voeller, KS. Prefrontal executive function syndromes in children. *J Child Neurol*, 2004, 19, 785-797.
[27] Fuster, JM. Executive frontal functions. *Exp Brain Res*, 2000, 133, 66-70.
[28] Wood, JN; Grafman, J. Human prefrontal cortex: processing and representational perspectives. *Nat Rev Neurosci*, 2003, 4, 139-147.
[29] Rypma, B. Factors controlling neural activity during delayed-response task performance: testing a memory organization hypothesis of prefrontal function. *Neuroscience*, 2006, 139, 223-235.
[30] Wang, XJ. Discovering spatial working memory fields in prefrontal cortex. *J Neurophysiol*, 2005, 93, 3027-3028.
[31] Dalley, JW; Cardinal, RN; Robbins, TW. Prefrontal executive and cognitive functions in rodents: neural and neurochemical substrates. *Neurosci Biobehav Rev*, 2004, 28, 771-784.
[32] Yuan, K; Steedle, J; Shavelson, R; Alonzo, A; Oppezzo, M. Working memory, fluid intelligence, and science learning. *Educ Res Rev*, 2006, 1, 83-98.
[33] Baddeley, A. Working memory: looking back and looking forward. *Nat Rev Neurosci*, 2003, 4, 829-839.
[34] Repovš, G; Baddeley, A. The multi-component model of working memory: explorations in experimental cognitive psychology. *Neuroscience*, 2006, 139, 5-21.
[35] Floresco, SB; Phillips, AG. Delay-dependent modulation of memory retrieval by infusion of a dopamine D_1 agonist into the rat medial prefrontal cortex. *Behav Neurosci*, 2001 115(4), 934-939.
[36] Fuster, JM. Network memory. *Trends Neurosci*, 1997, 20, 451-459.
[37] Funahashi, S. Prefrontal cortex and working memory processes. *Neuroscience*, 2006, 139, 251-261.

[38] Baddeley, AD; Logie, RH. Working memory: the multiplecomponent model. In: Miyake A, Shah P editors. Models of working memory. *Mechanism of active maintenance and executive control.* New York: Cambridge University Press; 1999, 28-61.
[39] Goldman-Rakic, PS; Muly, EC; Williams, GV. D_1 receptors in prefrontal cells and circuits. *Brain Res Rev*, 2000, 31, 295-301.
[40] Cowan, N. The magical number 4 in short-term memory: a reconsideration of mental storage capacity. *Behav Brain Sci*, 2000 24, 87-185.
[41] Motes, MA; Rypma, B. Working memory component processes: isolating BOLD signal changes. *Neuroimage*, 2010, 49, 1933-1941.
[42] Goldman-Rakic, PS. Cortical localization of working memory. In: McGaugh JL, Weinberger NM, Linch G editors. Brain organization and memory. *Cells, systems and circuits.* New York: Oxford Science Publications; 1990, 285-298.
[43] Goldman-Rakic, PS. Regional and cellular fractionation of working memory. *Proc Natl Acad Sci*, 1996, 93, 13473-13480.
[44] Funahashi, S; Bruce, CJ; Goldman-Rakic, PS. Mnemonic coding of visual space in the monkey's dorsolateral prefrontal cortex. *J Neurophysiol*, 1989, 61(2), 331-349.
[45] Sawaguchi, T; Goldman-Rakic, PS. D1 dopamine receptors in prefrontal cortex: involvement in working memory. *Sci*, 1991, 251(4996), 947-950.
[46] Sawaguchi, T; Goldman-Rakic, PS. The role of D1-dopamine receptor in working memory: local injections of dopamine antagonists into the prefrontal cortex of rhesus monkeys performing an oculomotor delayed-response task. *J Neurophysiol*, 1994, 71(2), 515-528.
[47] Zahrt, J; Taylor, JR; Mathew, RG; Arnsten, AFT. Supranormal stimulation of D1 dopamine receptors in the rodent prefrontal cortex impairs spatial working memory performance. *J Neurosci*, 1997, 17(21), 8528-8535.
[48] Nestler, EJ. Common molecular and cellular substrates of addiction and memory. *Neurobiol Learn Mem*, 2002 78, 637-647.
[49] Everitt, BJ; Wolf, ME. Psychomotor stimulant addiction: a neural system perspective. *J Neurosci*, 2002 22, 3312–3320.
[50] Uylings, HBM; Groenewegen, HJ; Kolb, B. Do rats have a prefrontal cortex? *Behav Brain Res*, 2003, 146, 3-17.
[51] Kolb, B; Pellis, S; Robinson, TE. Plasticity and functions of the orbital frontal cortex. *Brain Cognition*, 2004, 55, 104-115.
[52] Zilles, K; Wree, A. Cortex: Areal and laminar structure. In: Paxinos, G editor. The rat nervous system – forebrain and midbrain. San Diego: *Academic Press, Inc*, 1985, 374-415.
[53] Shah, P; Miyake, A. Models of working memory. An introduction. In: Miyake A, Shah P editors. Models of working memory. *Mechanisms of active maintenance and executive control.* New York: Cambridge University Press; 1999, 1-27.
[54] Seamans, JK; Floresco, SB; Phillips, AG. D_1 receptor modulation of hippocampal-prefrontal cortical circuits integrating spatial memory with executive functions in the rat. *J Neurosci*, 1998, 18(4), 1613-1621.
[55] Oliveira, RW; Nakamura-Palacios, EM. Haloperidol increases the disruptive effect of alcohol on spatial working memory in rats: a dopaminergic modulation in the medial prefrontal cortex. Psychopharmacology (Berl), 2003 170, 51-61.

[56] Silva de Melo, LC; Cruz, AP; Rios Valentim Jr, SJ; Marinho, AR; Mendonça, JB; Nakamura-Palacios, EM. Δ^9-THC administered into the medial prefrontal cortex disrupts the spatial working memory. *Psychopharmacology* (Berl), 2005 183, 54-64.

[57] Phillips, AG; Ahn, S; Floresco, SB. Magnitude of dopamine release in medial prefrontal cortex predicts accuracy of memory on a delayed response task. *J Neurosci*, 2004, 24(2), 553-547.

[58] Williams, GV; Castner, SA. Under the curve: critical issues for elucidating D1 receptor function in working memory. *Neuroscience*, 2006, 139, 263-276.

[59] Arnsten, AFT. Cathecolamine modulation of prefrontal cortical cognitive function. *Trends Cogn Sci*, 1998, 2, 436-447.

[60] Tupala, E; Tiihonen, J. Dopamine and alcoholism: neurobiological basis of ethanol abuse. *Prog Neuro-Psychoph*, 2004, 28, 1221-1247.

[61] Di Chiara, G; Bassareo, V; Fenu, S; De Luca, MA; Spina, L; Cadoni, C; Acquas, E; Carboni, E; Valentini, V; Lecca, D. Dopamine and drug addiction: the nucleus accumbens Shell connection. *Neuropharmacology*, 2004, 47, 227-241.

[62] Lisman, JE; Fellous, JM; Wang, XJ. A role for NMDA-receptor channels in working memory. *Nat Neurosci*, 1998, 1(4), 273-275.

[63] Wang, XJ. Synaptic basis of cortical persistent activity: the importance of NMDA receptors to working memory. *J Neurosci*, 1999, 19(21), 9587-9603.

[64] Feenstra, MGP; van der Weij, W; Botterblom, MHA. Concentration-dependent dual action of locally applied N-methyl-D-aspartate on extracellular dopamine in the rat prefrontal cortex in vivo. *Neurosci Lett*, 1995, 201, 175-178.

[65] Zheng, P; Zhang, XX; Bunney, BS; Shi, WX. Opposite modulation of cortical N-methyl-d-aspartate receptor-mediated responses by low and high concentrations of dopamine. *Neuroscience*, 1999, 91, 527-535.

[66] Krimer, LS; Jakab, RL; Goldman-Rakic, PS. Quantitative three-dimensional analysis of the catecholaminergic innervation of identified neurons in the macaque prefrontal cortex. *J Neurosci*, 1997, 17(19), 7450-7461.

[67] Seamans, JK; Gorelova, N; Durstewitz, D; Yang, CR. Bidirectional dopamine modulation of GABAergic inhibition in prefrontal cortical pyramidal neurons. *J Neurosci*, 2001, 21(10), 3628-3638.

[68] Rios Valentim Jr, SJ; Gontijo, AVL; Peres, MD; Rodrigues, LCM; Nakamura-Palacios, EM. D1 dopamine and NMDA receptors interactions in the medial prefrontal cortex: Modulation of spatial working memory in rats. *Behav Brain Res*, 2009, 204, 124-128.

[69] Yang, CR; Chen, L. Targeting prefrontal cortical dopamine D1 and N-Methyl-D-Aspartate receptor interactions in schizophrenia treatment. *Neuroscientist*, 2005, 11, 452-470.

[70] Von Huben, SN; Davis, SA; Lay, CC; Katner, SN; Crean, RD; Taffe, MA. Differential contributions of dopaminergic D_1- and D_2-like receptors to cognitive function in rhesus monkeys. *Psychopharmacology*, 2006 188, 586-596.

[71] Wang, M; Vijayraghavan, S; Goldman-Rakic, PS. Selective D2 receptor actions on the functional circuitry of working memory. *Sci*, 2004 303, 853-856.

[72] Glickstein, SB; Hof, PR; Schmauss, C. Mice lacking dopamine D_2 and D_3 receptors have spatial working memory deficits. *J Neurosci*, 2002 22(13), 5619-5629.

[73] Beyer, CE; Steketee, JD. Cocaine sensitization: modulation by dopamine D_2 receptors. *Cereb Cortex*, 2002 12, 526-535.

[74] Steketee, JD; Walsh, TJ. Repeated injections of sulpiride into the medial prefrontal cortex induces sensitization to cocaine in rats. *Psychopharmacology*, 2005 179, 753-760.

[75] Blum, K; Sheridan, PJ; Wood, RC; Braverman, ER; Chen, TJH; Cull, JG; Comings, DE. The D_2 dopamine receptor gene as a determinant of reward deficiency syndrome. *J Roy Soc Med*, 1996, 89, 396-400.

[76] Monte-Silva, K; Kuo, M-F; Thirugnanasambandam, N; Liebetanz, D; Paulus, W; Nitsche, MA. *J Neurosci*, 2009, 29(19), 6124-6131.

[77] Robinson, TE; Kolb, B. Structural plasticity associated with exposure to drugs of abuse. *Neuropharmacology*, 2004, 47, 33-46.

[78] Freeman, WM; Lull, ME; Patel, KM; Brucklacher, RM; Morgan, D; Roberts, DCS; Vrana, KE. Gene explression changes in the medial prefrontal cortex and nucleus accumbens following abstinence from cocaine self-administration, *BMC Neuroscience*, 2010, 11, 29-41.

[79] Kolb, B; Gorny, G; Li, Y; Samaha, AN; Robinson, TE. Amphetamine or cocaine limits the ability of later experience to promote structural plasticity in the neocortex and nucleus accumbens. *PNAS*, 2003, 100(18), 10523-10528.

[80] Moselhy, HF; Georgiou, G; Kahn, A. Frontal lobe changes in alcoholism: a review of the literature. *Alcohol Alcohol*, 2001, 36, 357-368.

[81] Ihara, H; Berrios, GE; London, M. Group and case study of the dysexecutive syndrome in alcoholism without amnesia. *J Neurol Neurosurg Psychiatry*, 2000, 68, 731-737.

[82] Munro, CA; Saxton, J; Butters, MA. The neuropsychological consequences of abstinence among older alcoholics: a cross-sectional study. *Alcohol Clin Exp Res*, 2000, 24(10), 1510-1516.

[83] Furieri, FA; Nakamura-Palacios, EM. Gabapentin Reduces Alcohol Consumption and Craving: A Randomized, Double-blind, Placebo Controlled Trial. *J Clin Psychiatry*, 2007, 68, 1691-1700.

[84] Furieri, F; de Oliveira, R; Nakamura-Palacios, E. Gabapentin Enhances the Recovery of Attention and Short-Term Memory in Alcoholics. Mind & Brain, the *Journal of Psychiatry*, 2010, 1(1), 1-9.

[85] Zago-Gomes, MP; Nakamura-Palacios, EM. Cognitive Components of Frontal Lobe Function in Alcoholics Classified According to Lesch's Typology. *Alcohol Alcohol*, 2009, 44(5), 449-457.

[86] Lesch, OM; Dietzel, M; Musalek, M; Walter, H; Zeiler, K.The course of alcoholism, long-term prognosis in different types. *Forensic Sci Int*, 1988, 36, 121-38.

[87] Lesch, OM; Kefer, J; Lentner, S; Mader, R; Marx, B; Musalek, M; Nimmerrichter, A; Preinsberger, H; Puchinger, H; Rustembegovic, A; Walter, H; Zach, E. Diagnosis of chronic alcoholism-classificatory problems. *Psychopathology*, 1990, 23, 88-96.

[88] Hillemacher, T; Bleich, S. Neurobiology and treatment in alcoholism - recent findings regarding Lesch's typology of alcohol dependence. *Alcohol Alcohol*, 2008, 43, 341-346.

[89] Pombo, S; Lesch, OM. The alcoholic phenotypes among different multidimensional typologies: similarities and their classification procedures. *Alcohol Alcohol*, 2009, 44, 46-54.

[90] Bönsch, D; Bayerlein, K; Reulbach, U; Fiszer, R; Hillemacher, T; Sperling, W; Kornhuber, J; Bleich, S. Different alleledistribution of MTHFR 677 C → T MTHFR-

393 C → A in patients classified according to subtypes of Lesch's typology. *Alcohol Alcohol*, 2006, 41, 364-367.

[91] Walter, H; Ramskogler-Skala, K; Dvorak, A; Gutierrez-Lobos, K; Hartl, D; Hertling, I; Munda, P; Thau, K; Lesch, OM; De Witte, P. Glutamic acid in withdrawal and weaning in patients classified according to Cloninger's and Lesch's typologies. *Alcohol Alcohol*, 2006, 41, 505-511.

[92] Dubois, B; Slachevsky, A; Litvan, I; Pillon, B. The FAB. A frontal assessment battery at bedside. *Neurology*, 2000, 55, 1621-1626.

[93] Appollonio, I; Leone, M; Isella, V; Piamarta, F; Consoli, T; Villa, ML; Forapani, E; Russo, A; Nichelli, P. The frontal assessment battery (FAB): normative values in an Italian population sample. *Neurol Sci*, 2005 26, 108-116.

[94] Luria, AR. *Higher Cortical Functions in Man.* NewYork: Basic Books; 1966.

[95] Suchy, Y; Kraybill, M. The relationship between motor programming and executive abilities: constructs measured by the Push-Turn-Taptap task from the Behavioral Dyscontrol Scale-Electronic Version. *J Clin Exp Neuropsychol*, 2007 29, 648-659.

[96] Fregni, F; Boggio, OS; Nitsche, M; Bermpohl, F; Antal, A; Feredoes, E; Marcolin, MA; Rigonatti, SP; Silva, MTA; Paulus, W; Pascual-Leone, A. Anodal transcranial direct current stimulation of prefrontal cortex enhances working memory. *Exp Brain Res*, 2005, 166, 23-30.

[97] Boggio, PS; Sultani, N; Fecteau, S; Merabet, L; Mecca, T; Pascual-Leone, A; Basaglia, A; Fregni, F. Prefrontal cortex modulation using transcranial DC stimulation reduces alcohol craving: A double-blind, sham-controlled study. *Drug Alcohol Depend*, 2008, 92, 55-60.

[98] Luck, SJ. An introduction to the event-related potential technique. Cambridge: *The MIT Press*; 2005.

[99] Heinze, M; Wölfling, K; Grüsser, SB. Cue-induced auditory evoked potentials in alcoholism. *Clin Neurophysiol*, 2007, 118, 856–862.

In: Working Memory: Capacity, Developments and…
Editor: Eden S. Levin

ISBN: 978-1-61761-980-9
© 2011 Nova Science Publishers, Inc.-

Chapter 5

WORKING MEMORY IN THE SERVICE OF VERBAL EPISODIC ENCODING: A COGNITIVE NEUROPSYCHOLOGICAL PERSPECTIVE

Matthew J. Wright[1], Peter Bachman[2] and Ellen Woo[3]

[1] Psychology Division, Department of Psychiatry, Harbor-UCLA Medical Center, Torrance, CA, USA

[2] Semel Institute for Neuroscience and Human Behavior, Department of Psychiatry and Biobehavioral Sciences, UCLA David Geffen School of Medicine, Los Angeles, CA, USA

[3] Mary S. Easton Center for Alzheimer's Disease Research, Department of Neurology, UCLA David Geffen School of Medicine, Los Angeles, CA, USA

ABSTRACT

While dissociations between working memory and episodic memory have been shown, both of these processes appear to partially overlap at the behavioral and neuroanontomical levels. Episodic encoding and working memory both appear to depend on the integrity and integration of processes carried out within the lateral prefrontal cortex and both appear to be related to effective verbal learning. The neuroanatomic substrate of semantic memory also appears to overlap with these processes in the prefrontal cortex. In the current chapter, we review interactions between verbal working memory, semantic memory, and episodic memory in individuals suffering from closed head injury, human immunodeficiency virus/acquired immunodeficiency syndrome, Alzheimer's disease, and Schizophrenia in an attempt to elucidate the cognitive neuropsychology of verbal memory encoding. Our review suggests that working memory enhances encoding, but not retention, of verbal episodic memories across these memory-disordered populations.

INTRODUCTION

The notion of separable memory systems or stores for current and past experiences has a long history. For example, William James (1890) discussed primary and secondary memory, the awareness for current and past events, respectively. Much of the research regarding the distinction between short-term memory (STM) and long-term memory (LTM) was fueled by Atkinson and Shiffrin's (1968) modal model of memory. This model stated that: (1) information is initially held in a sensory register; (2) some information held in sensory register, if selected via attentional processes, is transferred to STM, where it is briefly retained (for seconds to minutes); (3) through the process of rehearsal in STM, information can be transferred to LTM, where it is stored indefinitely. While a number of studies showed that to-be-learned information did not have to be filtered through STM prior to being acted upon by LTM, the journey to this conclusion spawned a host of theories and models designed to support or refute STM-LTM distinctions (see Thorn & Page, 2009). Some investigators deny the necessity of separate STM and LTM systems/stores and provide some fairly compelling arguments for a unitary memory system (e.g., Fuster 2003, 2009; Surprenant & Neath, 2009), although this position is not uniformly held (see Thorn & Page, 2009; Tulving & Craik, 2005). Many major advances in cognitive science resulted from the study of the relationship between STM and LTM; chief among these was the concept of working memory (WM).

WM refers to the ability to briefly hold and actively manipulate information from exogenous and endogenous sources. The concept of WM helped to overcome many of the difficulties the modal memory model had in dealing with STM-LTM interactions. Moreover, the concept of WM obviates the need to distinguish between STM and LTM systems, as WM can be viewed either as a separate system or as a special case of LTM activated by attention in the service of goal directed activity (Fuster, 2000, 2003, 2009). Baddeley and Hitch's (1974) model of WM is among the most influential in the field. They proposed a three component model that contained a primary control mechanism, the *central executive*, and two subordinate systems, the *phonological loop* and the *visuospatial sketch pad*. The *phonological loop* was hypothesized to house mechanisms for briefly maintaining and rehearsing verbal material. The *visuospatial sketch pad* was hypothesized to contain mechanisms for briefly maintaining and rehearsing visual (nonverbal) material. The *central executive*, an attentional control system, was purported to govern the interactions of the two subordinate systems and LTM. More recently, Baddeley et al. (2000) fractionated the central executive to create a fourth component, the *episodic buffer*, to deal with the old model's difficulty with explaining how large strings of relational information (e.g., sentences, prose) could be held in the phonological loop, given its relatively small temporal capacity (a few seconds). The *episodic buffer* is said to be a limited capacity, modality nonspecific store with the ability to bind information from the phonological loop and visuospatial sketch pad within LTM to form integrated episodic memories. Additionally, the actions of the episodic buffer are said to be resource demanding. Allen and Baddeley (2009) further elaborated on the model by adding direct connections between LTM and the phonological loop for automatic binding as well as syntactic and semantic processing of words presented in sentential structure, as they found that sentence processing did not appear to utilize significant WM resources in healthy individuals.

Episodic Memory

A long and rich history of LTM research has elucidated many forms that memory can take; including, but not limited to, declarative memory (consciously available memory for episodes; e.g., "I changed a flat tire yesterday") and non-declarative memory (memory that can be formed and utilized without conscious awareness; e.g., the well-learned procedures involved in changing a tire; for a thorough discussion of memory, see Tulving & Craik, 2005). With regard to declarative memory, one particularly useful distinction was made by Endel Tulving (1972, 1985). He distinguished *episodic memory* (EM) from *semantic memory* (SM). He likened EM to mental time travel, in that it allows an individual to re-experience previous events. In that sense, EM is our repository of past experiences. On the other hand, SM is our fund of knowledge about the world, regardless of what event provided that knowledge to us; we do not need to recollect where we first learned about chimpanzees to recognize one at the zoo. Some investigators argue that the very nature of memory is associative at both the neural and phenomenological levels (Fuster, 2000, 2003, 2009; Hebb, 1949; Kandel, 1991), so that all memories are integrated into one's fund of knowledge and perceptual experience such that declarative verbal material would be associated with higher order semantic and conceptual representations (Fuster, 2000, 2003, 2009). Further, Joaquín Fuster (2000, 2003, 2009) has postulated that the apparent associative nature of memory makes distinctions between memory systems (e.g., declarative vs. non-declarative) unnecessary, as different memory phenomena more likely reflect the degree of cortical distribution and hierarchical associative strength rather separate systems (with phyletic motor and sensory memory associations at the lowest levels and semantic and conceptual memory associations at the highest). While debates over unitary and multiple systems approaches to memory continue, it is clear that the formation of EM is a relational process. Indeed, new memories do appear to be related to (and modified by) previously stored experiences (Ahlberg & Sharps, 2002; Bartlett, 1932) and enhancing relations to SM strengthens recall of new verbal information (Craik, 2002; Craik & Lockhart, 1972; Craik & Tulving, 1975).

Psychologists often employ a three-process model when discussing EM (Ellis & Hunt, 1983; but see Howe, 1988). The first stage is *encoding*, where information is taken in and transformed into a format that can be stored in the brain. The second stage is *consolidation*, where the transformed information is stored for later use. The third stage is *retrieval*, or extraction of the stored information for use. While both cognitive and neuropsychological studies have shown that the encoding, consolidation, and retrieval processes overlap, there is evidence that distinctions do exist among them (e.g., Bernard, Desgranges, Platel, Baron, & Eustache, 2001; Nyberg, Cabeza, & Tulving, 1996; Greicius et al., 2003; Nyberg et al., 1996; Tulving & Markowitsch, 1997; Tulving & Osler, 1968; Tulving & Thompson, 1973). Therefore, the terms encoding, consolidation, and retrieval are useful for discussing temporally graded EM processes that are partially subserved by different neuroanatomical regions (see Bernard et al., 2001; Fuster, 2000; Greicius et al., 2003; Nielsen-Bohlman & Knight, 1994; Nyberg et al., 1996; Nyberg, Forkstam, Petersson, Cabeza, & Ingvar, 2002).

WORKING MEMORY AND EPISODIC ENCODING: CONTRASTS AND COMMUNALITIES

Case studies of individuals with relatively focal brain injuries are often cited as evidence for a distinction between WM and EM, although this evidence is not universally accepted (e.g., Surprenant & Neath, 2009). The most recognized case study of amnesia is that of H.M. (see Corkin, 2002), who underwent neurosurgery to treat intractable epilepsy. Following bilateral resection of his hippocampus and some adjacent tissue, he was unable to form new LTMs, although he was able to retain and manipulate information for brief periods of time. Another famous case report is that of E.E., who underwent resection of a tumor centered on his left angular gyrus (see Markowitsch, et al., 1999). Unlike H.M., E.E. could form new EMs following surgery, but he had deficits in short-term retention and manipulation of verbal and numeric information. Taken together, data from H.M. and E.E. suggest a double dissociation between EM and WM. However, the functional and neuroanatomical relationship between WM and EM is far more complex than suggested by these case studies.

Functional Neuroanatomy of Working Memory and Episodic Memory

Numerous studies have been conducted to determine the functional neuroanatomy of EM. Functional imaging and lesion studies have implicated the left lateral prefrontal cortex [PFC; Brodman (BA) 44, 45, 46, 47] and left medial-temporal lobe (MTL) regions (primarily the parahippocampal gyrus; BA 27, 28, 34, 35, 36) in the encoding of verbal memories (Alessio et al., 2004; Ariza et al., 2006; Bor, Cumming, Scott, & Owen, 2004; Buckner, Kelly, & Petersen, 1999; Dolan & Fletcher, 1999; Fernandez et al., 1998; Gimranov & Mal'tseva, 2005; Habib, Nyberg, & Tulving, 2003; Karlsgodt, Shirinyan, van Erp, Cohen, & Cannon, 2005; Nyberg et al., 1996; Strange, Otten, Josephs, Rugg, & Dolan, 2002; Vingerhoets, Miatton, Vonck, Seurinck, & Boon, 2006); the right PFC is also involved, but to a lesser degree than the left PFC (Tulving et al., 1994; Nyberg et al., 1996; Habib et al., 2003). A large body of work indicates that MTL structures—namely, the hippocampus—orchestrate the consolidation of memories, although with the passage of time, memory storage appears to come under the control of the neocortex (Squire, 1980, 1994; Squire & Zola, 1998; Tulving & Markowitsch, 1998). Data from a number of studies indicate that verbal memory consolidation tends to be controlled by the left hemisphere (Alessio et al., 2004; Ariza et al., 2006; Gimranov & Mal'tseva, 2005; Vingerhoets et al., 2006). While encoding of verbal memories appears to be primarily supported by the left PFC and hippocampus, research suggests that the retrieval of verbal memories is primarily under the control of the right PFC (BA 44, 45, 46, 47; although the left PFC is involved to a lesser degree) and, in some cases, the hippocampus (Dolan & Fletcher, 1999; Greicius et al., 2003; Habib et al., 2003; Karlsgodt et al., 2005; Nyberg et al., 1996).

Neuroimaging studies have consistently highlighted the role of the frontal lobes in verbal WM. Meta-analyses of positron emission tomography (PET) and functional magnetic resonance imaging (fMRI) studies suggest that maintenance of verbal material in WM is associated with activations in the left lateral PFC (BA 44, 45, 46) and the premotor cortex (BA 6), while manipulation of material in WM is related to activity in the right lateral PFC

(BA 46, 47) and the anterior PFC (BA 10; Chein, Fissell, & Fiez, 2002; Wager & Smith, 2003). It should be noted that this pattern of activations is not in perfect agreement with all large scale neuroimaging studies or reviews of WM (e.g., Jennings, van der Veen, & Meltzer, 2006), possibly for methodological reasons[1]. Also, manipulation of verbal WM load is associated with activations in the left inferior dorsal parietal lobe (Jennings et al., 2006), consistent the WM deficits displayed by E.E. following the resection of his left angular gyrus and adjacent white matter (Markowitsch et al., 1999). Comparison of common areas implicated in EM and WM shows significant overlap between EM encoding and WM maintenance in the left lateral PFC (BA 44, 45, 46) and also EM retrieval and WM manipulation in the right PFC (BA 46, 47). Moreover, a number of investigators have demonstrated compelling evidence for a common PFC network involved in EM, WM, and SM (Cabeza & Nyberg, 2000; Christoff & Gabrieli, 2000; Duncan & Owen, 2000; Nyberg et al., 2003; Nyberg, Forkstam, Peterson, Cabeza, & Ingvar, 2002; Ranganath, Johnson, & D'Esposito, 2003). Activations in the dorsolateral and ventrolateral PFC (BA 9, 46; BA 44, 45, 47, respectively) are frequently observed across EM, SM, and WM tasks and these common activations tend occur in the left hemisphere more than the right (Nyberg et al., 1996; Nyberg et al., 2003; Ranganath et al., 2003; Cabeza & Nyberg, 2000)[2]. Accordingly, this network could be conceptualized as a nexus for holding (WM maintenance), evaluating (WM manipulation), and imparting meaning (semantic association) to incoming verbal material so that it can be encoded and consolidated (via interactions with MTL structures) in an efficient manner.

WORKING MEMORY AND EPISODIC MEMORY INTERACTIONS IN NEUROLOGICALLY COMPROMISED POPULATIONS

Although WM and EM processes can be dissociated at the behavioral and neuroanatomic levels, the lateral PFC networks involved in WM, EM encoding, and SM likely work together to code and store new verbal memories through coordinated interactions with MTL structures. If this is indeed the case, data from neuropsychologically impaired populations should be able to show (1) that reduced (but not absent) connectivity between generally intact PFC and MTL structures should interfere with efficient acquisition and recall of new verbal information under normal learning conditions, but recall should improve under modified encoding conditions where information is meaningfully organized at learning (reducing WM and semantic network requirements necessary for efficient encoding and initial consolidation); (2) verbal WM ability should have little or no impact on delayed recall of verbal material in cases of gross MTL injury (new material, organized or not, should fail to be consolidated); (3) significant PFC dysfunction should impact learning and recall even under modified encoding conditions where to-be-learned information is meaningfully organized at learning (pre-organized material may not be properly maintained or may be bound to poorly organized

---

[1] Jennings et al. (2006) conducted a large scale study (*n*=89) with older adults (50-70 years of age), whereas Wager and Smith (2003) included data from studies of both younger and older adults in their meta-analysis.
[2] It is important to note that EM, WM and semantic memory are also associated with different areas of activation (see Nyberg et al., 2003; Ranganath et al., 2003; Cabeza & Nyberg, 2000).

semantic networks), although retention of the information learned in these cases should not be overly affected by the degree of PFC pathology.

Diffuse White Matter Pathology

To determine if reduced connectivity between grossly intact PFC and MTL structures differentially interferes with acquisition and recall of new verbal information, we surveyed the verbal memory literature on populations with diffuse white matter pathology. Stephen Rao (1996) reviewed literature relevant to neurobehavioral functioning in populations with diffuse white matter pathology, namely multiple sclerosis (MS), human immunodeficiency virus/acquired immunodeficiency syndrome (HIV/AIDS), Binswanger's disease, and closed head injury (CHI). He noted that these etiologically different groups exhibited a similar neuropsychological profile consisting of deficits in attention and speed of processing, memory, and executive functioning in the absence of aphasia or apraxia. While slowed processing in conjunction with intact language abilities is often cited as a feature of subcortical dementia (Cummings & Benson, 1984), diffuse white matter pathology can be distinguished from subcortical dementias via the presence of intact non-declarative/procedural memory (Jones & Tranel, 1991; Lafosse et al., 2007; Rao et al., 1993; Timmerman & Brouwer, 1999; but also see Gonzalez et al., 2008), which is routinely impaired in cases of subcortical (grey matter) disease (Heindel, Butters, & Salmon, 1988; Heindel, Salmon, Shults, Walicke, & Butters, 1989; Lafosse et al., 2007).

The literature is somewhat mixed with regard to the nature of verbal EM deficits in white matter populations. However, it has been suggested that much of this is due to the use of imprecise or invalid methods for parsing the contributions of encoding, consolidation, and retrieval to verbal memory performances (Wilde, Boake, & Sherer, 1995; Wiegner & Donders, 1999; Wright et al., 2009; Wright, Schmitter-Edgecombe, & Woo, 2010a). However, when psychometrically sound methods or properly controlled experimental procedures are utilized, individuals with CHI, MS, and HIV/AIDS primarily demonstrate encoding deficits for verbal material[3][4] (Arnett et al., 1997; Basso et al., 2006; Basso et al., 2008; Blachstein, Vakil, & Hoofien, 1993; Chiaravalloti & DeLuca, 2002; DeLuca et al., 2000; Gongvatana et al., 2007; Levin & Goldstein, 1986; Schmitter-Edgecombe, Marks, Wright, & Ventura, 2004; Scott et al., 2006; Stallings, Boake, & Sherer, 1995; Thornton, Raz, & Tucker, 2002; Waldrop, Ownby, & Kumar, 2004; Wright et al., 2010b; Wright et al., 2010a).

Research has consistently indicated that individuals with CHI, MS, and HIV/AIDS suffer from WM deficits, particularly with regard to the executive components of WM (Asloun et al., 2008; Chang et al., 2001; Hinkin et al., 2002; Lengenfelder et al., 2006; Parmenter, Shucard, Benedict, & Shucard, 2006; Sánchez-Carrión et al., 2008; Sepulcre et al., 2009; Sweet, Rao, Primeau, Durgerian, & Cohen, 2006; Vallat-Azouvi, Weber, Legrand, & Azouvi, 2007;York, Franks, Henry, & Hamilton, 2001). We will review the relationship between

---

[3] Literature regarding the memory profile of Binswanger's disease is relatively sparse.
[4] The term "acquisition" is used in some of the studies cited as a way to group encoding and consolidation into one process, as these tend to be difficult to dissociate. We only included studies here that had methods that appeared to parse encoding abilities from consolidation.

verbal EM encoding and WM in CHI below, followed by a brief discussion of this topic in HIV/AIDS.

CHI. While there is great heterogeneity in the etiology and neuropathological consequences of traumatic brain injury [National Institutes of Health (NIH), 1999; Williamson, Scott, & Adams, 1996], most cases of CHI are due to acceleration-deceleration events (e.g., motor-vehicle accidents; Esselman & Uomoto, 1995; King, 1997; NIH, 1999; Williamson et al., 1996) and result in diffuse axonal injury (DAI; Abou-Hamden et al., 1997; Adams et al., 1989; Adams & Jennett, 2001), although lesions to the ventral frontal and ventral anterior MTL areas also occur with a fair degree of regularity (Williamson et al., 1996; Wilson, Hadlet, Wiedmann, & Teasdale, 1995). That said, data from studies of moderate to severe[5] CHI likely reflect deficits associated with DAI (Hattori et al., 2003).

As mentioned above, several studies have provided compelling evidence for EM encoding deficits in CHI. Specifically, CHI participants show a decreased learning curve (Blachstein et al., 1993), reduced semantic clustering (Stallings et al., 1995), and lack of spontaneous strategy use during list-learning (Levin & Goldstein, 1986) compared to controls. Furthermore, presenting CHI participants with verbal material that is organized by semantic category at learning greatly enhances their acquisition and recall of that material compared to disorganized verbal material (Levin & Goldstein, 1986). DeLuca et al. (2000) provided convincing evidence for a verbal memory acquisition[6] deficit following CHI. In this study, moderate-to-severe CHI participants and demographically matched controls were administered a modified version of the Selective Reminding Test (SRT; Buschke, 1973), where a list of 10 semantically related words were utilized. Unrecalled items were presented until all of the words were recalled on two consecutive trials over a maximum of 15 trials. Seventy percent of the CHI participants were able to meet acquisition criteria. This group did not differ in delayed recall or recognition scores from controls but required more learning trials to learn the list of words. Deluca and colleagues interpreted these results as reflecting a CHI-related acquisition deficit. We feel that their data more specifically suggest that CHI-associated memory dysfunction results from an encoding deficit, as the support during the encoding phase improved CHI participants' later recall and recognition.

We recently conducted a study to further elucidate the nature of verbal memory deficits exhibited by severe CHI survivors (Wright et al., 2010a). In this study we applied the Item Specific Deficit Approach, ISDA, a psychometrically sound item-analytic method to quantify deficits of encoding, consolidation, and retrieval (Wright et al., 2009), to California Verbal Learning Test (CVLT; Delis, Kramer, Kaplan, & Ober, 1987) performances. We only included severe CHI participants (*n*= 56) that acquired their head injuries as the result of significant acceleration-deceleration forces to control for confounding etiological factors and to provide some clues as to the impact of DAI on verbal memory. Finally, we compared CHI participants' performances against those of healthy controls (*n*= 62); these groups were matched on age, education, premorbid estimated intelligence, and sex.

As would be expected, the CHI participants exhibited markedly worse learning and delayed recall performances on the CVLT in comparison to the controls. Additionally, in

---

[5] Moderate to severe CHI is often indexed by an injury related loss of conscious of more than 30min., a Glasgow Coma Scale of 12 or less (Teasdale & Jennet, 1974), and/or posttraumatic amnesia of more than one hour (Lucas & Addeo, 2006).

[6] Deluca and colleagues use the term "acquisition" to refer to the encoding/consolidation process.

comparison to the controls, the CHI participants evidenced deficits on the ISDA indices of encoding, consolidation, and retrieval. However, hierarchical regression[7] analysis revealed that encoding deficits accounted for the majority of the variance (63%) in the CHI participants delayed recall. Consolidation deficits also added significant predictive value to the model, accounting for 14% more variance and retrieval deficits were a significant, but negligible predictor, accounting for an additional 2% of the variance. Further analyses confirmed that the CHI participants exhibited minor consolidation difficulties above and beyond their encoding deficits.

We also investigated strategic processing of the CVLT list items over the five learning trials via list-based semantic clustering calculations (Stricker, Brown, Wixted, Baldo, and Delis, 2002). Semantic clustering of words (grouping items by category) during learning reflects the ability to reorganize to-be-learned information into a more meaningful and chunkable format that is associated with improved recall (Forrester & King, 1971; Craik & Tulving, 1975; Delis et al., 1987). Also, while semantic clustering is assessed by analyzing recall patterns, it appears to be the product of elaborate processes carried out during encoding (Cinan, 2003; Mori, 1975). Thus, semantic clustering appears to represent an instance when EM encoding, WM, and SM interact, as the to-be-learned words need to be maintained, manipulated, and associated with semantic representations. Although we did not investigate the WM components that might be involved in this process, it is possible that the central executive, phonological loop and episodic buffer are involved in semantic clustering during list learning trials. As discussed above, the interaction of EM encoding, SM, and WM would require coordinated interaction between the lateral PFC and MTLs, among other widespread neural networks (Fuster, 2000, 2003, 2009).

We found that the CHI participants exhibited significantly poorer semantic clustering during list learning in comparison to the controls. Moreover, they showed a retarded rate of semantic clustering over learning trials; the CHI participants only improved between trials 3 and 4, where the controls showed improvements between trials 1 and 2, 2 and 3, and 3 and 4. Finally, regression analyses showed that average semantic clustering significantly predicted encoding deficits in the CHI participants, accounting for 48% of the variance.

Our study (Wright et al., 2010a) in conjunction with previous research on list-learning (Levin & Goldstein, 1986; Blachstein et al., 1993; Stallings et al., 1995; DeLuca et al., 2000) and working memory (Asloun et al., 2008; Sánchez-Carrión et al.; Vallat-Azouvi et al., 2007) following traumatic brain injury suggests that moderate-to-severe CHI results in encoding deficits characterized by inefficient organization and binding of to-be-learned information to SM. In other words, verbal memory deficits in moderate-to-severe CHI appear to be related to deficits in WM-driven encoding processes. Additionally, when to-be-learned verbal material is presented to CHI survivors in a semantically organized fashion, their acquisition and recall improve (Levin & Goldstein, 1986; DeLuca et al., 2000), suggesting that they have a reduced capacity for PFC-MTL interaction, but that they can make use of the PFC and MTL structures involved in acquisition and recall of new verbal information given reduced network/associative processing requirements. Moreover, neuroimaging studies have shown that DAI plays a significant role in verbal EM and WM deficits observed in CHI participants (Fork et al., 2005; Sánchez-Carrión et al., 2008; Turner & Levine, 2008), providing some

---

[7] The ISDA indices were entered into the regression based on their natural temporal relationship (i.e., 1. encoding, 2. consolidation, 3. retrieval). Changing the order of predictors did not significantly influence the results.

additional support for the idea that diffuse white matter injury disrupts WM, EM encoding, and SM interactions in the lateral PFC that are likely involved in the coding and storage of new verbal memories through coordinated interactions with MTL structures, at least in cases of moderate-to-severe CHI. That said, do other populations with diffuse white matter pathology show similar patterns of EM encoding and WM deficits?

HIV/AIDS. Diffuse white matter and striatal pathology have been repeatedly demonstrated in HIV infection (Archibald et al., 2004; Cohen et al., 2010; Vehmas et al., 2004; Giometto et al., 1997). Further, white matter compromise is one of the most common central nervous system (CNS) disturbances associated with HIV disease, which has led some investigators to postulate that it may be an important neuropathological manifestation of the disease and a possible cause for many of the observed cognitive deficits (Giometto et al., 1997; Gongvatana et al., 2009; Medana & Esiri, 2003). White matter abnormalities in HIV have been associated with dendritic injury, suggesting that white and gray matter pathologies are closely linked (Archibald et al., 2004). Additionally, hippocampal and neostriatal volumes are predictive of neuropsychological impairment in HIV-infected individuals (Moore et al., 2006; for a review see Paul, Cohen, Navia, & Tashima, 2002). Since the advent of highly active antiretroviral therapy (HAART) the neuropathological expression of chronic HIV-infection his evolved to resemble more of a cortical pathology as opposed to subcortical disease (Cohen et al., 2010). Also, HIV-related white matter pathology appears to continue despite the use of successful antiretroviral regimes as does HIV-associated cognitive dysfunction (Gongvatana et al., 2009), although the neurocognitive sequelae of HIV has lessened in severity (Baldewicz et al., 2004; Ferrando et al., 2003; McCutchan et al., 2007; Robertson et al., 2007; Robinson-Papp, Elliott, & Simpson, 2009; Sacktor et al., 2006) and become somewhat more variable in expression (Bandaru et al., 2007).

Historically, HIV infection has been thought to produce EM retrieval deficits similar to the subcortical dementias observed in cases of Huntington's disease or Parkinson's disease (Delis et al., 1995; Peavy et al., 1994). This assertion was primarily based on discrepancies in verbal EM performances, where participants show reduced free recall relative to recognition for a list of words. The underlying concept is that cues provided by recognition testing improve memory retrieval. The validity of recognition-recall discrepancies as markers of verbal memory retrieval have been called into question due to mixed results in various populations, in addition to disagreement with other hypothesized indicators of retrieval ability (Wilde et al., 1995; Wright et al., 2009). Additionally, recall and recognition are now thought to reflect different cognitive processes; recall relies on recollective abilities, and recognition depends on both recollection and familiarity (Aggleton & Brown, 2006). More recent investigations that made use of alternative approaches to assessing memory disruptions suggest that HIV-associated verbal memory dysfunction may be due to encoding deficits (Scott et al., 2006; Gongvatana et al., 2007).

Another possible reason for the mixed literature on HIV-related EM impairment is the advent of HAART. Post-HAART data on EM impairment suggest a primary encoding deficit (Waldrop et al., 2004; Scott et al., 2006; Gongvatana et al., 2007), while the pre-HAART data indicate both retrieval and encoding deficits (Delis et al., 1995; White et al., 1997; Murji et al., 2003). More recent studies that support the EM encoding deficit hypothesis were based on the examination of list learning characteristics. Specifically, these studies found that HIV-infected participants exhibited poor semantic clustering (Gongvatana et al., 2007) and lower primacy effects[8] (Waldrop et al., 2004; Scott et al., 2006) in contrast to HIV- controls.

We recently collected verbal memory and medication adherence data to determine the role that HAART played in HIV-related EM impairment (Wright et al., 2010b). In this study we utilized Medication Event Monitoring System (MEMS) caps to track HIV+ participants' adherence to one of their HAART medications (protease inhibitors for most of the participants) and the CVLT in conjunction with the ISDA to assess verbal memory. Evaluation of HAART adherence data indicated that 33 of the HIV+ participants demonstrated good adherence (90% or better) while the remaining 42 had poor adherence (< 90%). We also collected CVLT and ISDA data from HIV- controls ($n= 25$). Both adherence groups evidenced greater EM encoding difficulties in comparison to the control participants, while the poor antiretroviral adherence group showed greater retrieval deficits in contrast to the control participants. No significant differences were found between the two adherence groups with regard to the ISDA indices of EM encoding, consolidation, and retrieval.

To determine the impact of verbal EM encoding and retrieval deficits on the delayed recall abilities of the two adherence groups, we conducted two hierarchical regressions[9]. Both regression models were significant and accounted for a sizable amount of the variance in HIV+ participants' long-delay free recall. Encoding deficits accounted for the majority of the variance in both models (50% for good adherers; 43% for poor adherers). Retrieval deficits accounted for a greater degree of additional variance for the poor adherers (22%) in contrast to good adherers (9%).

Our findings of a primary encoding deficit in conjunction with studies showing WM impairment (Chang et al., 2001; Hinkin et al., 2002; York et al., 2001), reduced strategic processing during list-learning [i.e., poor semantic clustering (Gongvatana et al., 2007), and reduced primacy effects (Waldrop et al., 2004; Scott et al., 2006)] in HIV/AIDS is similar to that observed in CHI. Thus, episodic verbal memory impairment in HIV/AIDS appears to be related to deficits in WM-driven encoding processes. Additionally, research has indicated that white matter compromise is associated with cognitive deficits in HIV/AIDS (Pfefferbaum, Rosenbloom, Adalsteinsson, & Sullivan, 2007; Ragin, Storey, Cohen, Edelman, & Epstein, 2004; Ragin et al., 2005) and, more importantly, that white matter injury in the frontal lobes is associated with reduced EM in HIV/AIDS participants (Wu et al., 2006).

Taken together, the literature on CHI and HIV/AIDS suggests that reduced connectivity between grossly intact PFC and MTL lobe structures differentially interferes with acquisition and recall of new verbal information. Additionally, these studies suggest that that to-be-learned material that requires greater WM processing (e.g., list learning) results in poorer acquisition and recall performances. Thus, verbal EM deficits associated with diffuse white matter pathology may be due to inefficient coordination of WM, EM encoding, and SM processes in the lateral PFC and MTL structures. That said, these observations are retrospective in nature and prospective studies are needed to confirm or deny their validity.

---

[8] During list-learning, individuals typically show better recall of list items at the beginning (primacy effect) and end (recency effect) of the list (Glanzer & Cunitz, 1966; Glanzer, 1972). The recency effect reflects short-term retention (STM/WM maintenance) of the last several list items and the primacy effect reflects rehearsal and retention (i.e., encoding and storage) of the first several list items. Therefore, primacy deficits suggest difficulties with encoding and/or storage.

[9] The ISDA indices were entered into the regression based on their natural temporal relationship (i.e., 1. encoding, 2. retrieval). Changing the order of predictors did not significantly influence the results.

Medial-Temporal Pathology

While a host of conditions have been shown to affect MTL structures, Alzheimer's disease (AD) is arguably the most studied condition with significant MTL impact (Braak & Braak, 1991; Head, Snyder, Girton, Morris, & Buckner, 2005; Holland et al., 2009). The National Institute of Neurological and Communicative Disorders and Stroke and the Alzheimer's Disease and Related Disorders Association (NINCDS-ADRDA) diagnostic criteria (McKhann et al., 1984) for probable AD[10] are: (1) onset of dementia between 40 and 80 years of age, typically after 65; (2) dementia diagnosis established by clinical examination and confirmed by an objective measure of gross cognitive ability (e.g., Mini-Mental State Exam) in addition to disturbed memory and one or more other cognitive deficits shown by a neuropsychological assessment; (3) progressive decline in memory and other cognitive abilities; (4) no impairment in consciousness; and (5) absence of other disorders that may account for progressive deficits in memory and cognition. Furthermore, the diagnosis of probable AD is supported by: (1) progressive decline in specific cognitive abilities; (2) impairments in activities of daily living and alterations in typical behavior; (3) familial history of similar disorders; (4) laboratory results indicating normal lumbar puncture findings, normal or nonspecific electroencephalogram results (e.g., increased slow-wave activity), and structural neuroimaging studies suggestive of progressive cerebral atrophy.

While progressive MTL pathology and EM impairment are key features of AD[11] (e.g, Dickerson et al., 2009), these clearly are not the only neurocognitive consequences of AD (Braak & Braak, 1991; Salmon & Bondi, 1999). Specifically, the neuropathological changes associated with AD (neuronal atrophy, synapse loss, marked accumulation of neuritic plaques and neurofibrillary tangles) primarily start in the MTL, but they spread to other areas in the temporal, frontal, and parietal lobes as the disease progresses (Braak & Braak, 1991). Also, beyond EM impairment, and consistent with the neuropathology of the disease, AD is associated with deficits in attention, language, SM, executive abilities (including WM), and constructional and visuospatial functions (for reviews, see Salmon & Bondi, 1999; Bondi, Salmon, & Kaszniak, 2009). So, while MTL pathology is associated with verbal memory impairment in mild to moderate AD (Venneri et al., 2008; Dickerson et al., 2009), functional and structural neuroimaging studies also suggest that PFC abnormalities play a role in the memory deficits observed in mild to moderate AD (Balthazar, Yasuda, Cendes, & Damasceno, 2010; Desgranges et al., 1998). That said, some investigators have shown that participants with mild AD recruit the PFC cortices during memory tests more than healthy controls (Grady et al., 2003; Schwindt & Black, 2009). Also, these increased areas of activity in the dorsal lateral PFC (primarily in the right hemisphere) and ventrolateral PFC (primarily in the left hemisphere) appear to provide compensation for reduced MTL function in mild AD (Grady et al., 2003; Schwindt & Black, 2009).

---

[10] A diagnosis of definite AD requires histopathological findings from biopsy or autopsy (McKhann et al., 1984).
[11] AD is used to refer to probable AD in the follow discussion. Also, as a matter of convention, severity levels of AD discussed herein are roughly based on Mini Mental Status Exam scores (Folstein, Folstein, & McHugh, 1975), where scores of 19-24/30 indicate mild AD, scores of 10-18/30 indicate moderate AD, and scores of 17/30 or less indicate severe AD. Such MMSE score ranges have been shown to be useful for tracking the progression of AD (Han, Cole, Bellavance, McCusker, & Primeau, 2000; Ward, Caro, Kelly, Eggleston, Molloy, 2002).

WM, EM and AD. Given the hypothetical framework we have outlined regarding the interaction between EM encoding, WM, and SM, the characteristic MTL pathology of AD should interfere with the acquisition (i.e., encoding and storage) of new EMs even in the presence of procedures that aid PFC networks involved in the three processes. That said, AD is known to impact WM and SM in addition to EM (Berlingeri et al., 2008; Carlesimo et al., 1998; Panegyres, 2004; Venneri et al., 2008). With regard to WM, there has been some debate as to which components of WM (e.g., central executive, phonological loop, episodic buffer) might be involved in EM impairment among AD participants. In a comprehensive review of EM and WM in AD, Della Sala, Logie, and Spinnler (1992) presented compelling data and arguments that rule out the phonological loop and suggest that a central executive impairment is responsible for AD-related EM deficits, based largely on the results of a number of dual-task performance studies. However, in a sample of 71 mild AD participants, Becker (1988) demonstrated that EM and WM could be dissociated analytically based on neuropsychological test performances and also via the identification of participants with isolated EM or WM deficits. Additionally, Becker and colleagues (Becker, Bajulaiye, & Smith, 1992) showed that AD participants with isolated EM or WM impairments tend to develop deficits in both of these functions over time, suggesting that AD leads to a multifactorial memory loss. Della Sala and colleagues (1992) argue that the existence of AD participants with isolated WM and EM deficits does not rule out the possibility that a central executive impairment may be responsible for EM problems, as they report that there is heterogeneity in the memory profiles exhibited by participants with AD. Nevertheless, the demonstration of isolated WM and EM deficits in some cases of AD does strongly imply that an impairment in WM is not solely responsible for the EM deficit in AD. That is not to say that WM deficits do not have any impact on EM.

WM deficits do appear to be related to EM acquisition in AD (Germano & Kinsella, 2005). One novel study that addressed this issue was conducted by Castel, Balota, and McCabe (2009). They completed a list-learning experiment where participants (younger adults, older adults, very mild AD, and mild AD) were given point values (1-12) for to-be-learned words and instructed to maximize the point value of the items in their learning and recall of the list. Having participants focus their efforts on learning items by point value was thought to invoke greater WM demands during list acquisition, as participants had to judge and react to the relative value of each word. As expected, the AD groups demonstrated significantly lower recall and selectivity than the older and younger adults groups; all the groups differed with respect to recall (younger adults > older adults > very mild AD > mild AD), but not selectivity (younger adults & older adults > very mild AD & mild AD). Additionally, all of the groups appeared to focus their efforts on learning and recall of items with higher point values and their selectivity scores showed an increase between the first and last four lists with which they were presented. Interestingly, while the younger adults, older adults, and very mild AD participants showed an increase in recall between the first and last four lists, the mild AD group showed no increase in recall despite demonstrating increased selectivity. The performance of the mild AD group suggests that EM (recall) and WM (selectivity) may be dissociable. However, a WM composite score derived from reading span and computation span[12] performances correlated with the recall of words with higher point

---

[12] The reading span task required participants to read sentences of increasing length over trials and decide if they were false or true statements in addition to committing the last word of each sentence to memory. The

values in the older adult and AD groups, although selectivity scores were not associated with the WM composite score in any of the groups. Castel and colleagues (2009) interpreted this finding as suggesting that impairments in central executive/selective control abilities of AD participants might interfere with their EM encoding abilities and the selectivity during encoding may be associated with other executive or metacognitive processes. Given that Castel and colleagues' (2009) WM composite was comprised of reading and computation span scores, it possible that the association between selective recall and WM may have been due to reductions in either the central executive and/or the episodic buffer components of WM, as participants had to monitor the correctness of- and remember a specified item from each span (presumably requiring executive control) in a set of spans that increased in length over trials (possibly requiring the episodic buffer).

As reviewed earlier, Baddeley et al. (2000) proposed the concept of the episodic buffer as a limited capacity, modality nonspecific WM store that could handle large strings of relational information (e.g., sentences, prose) that could not be accommodated by the phonological loop. Interestingly, a recent study utilizing voxel-based morphometry and a battery of neuropsychological tests found evidence that the episodic buffer is associated grey matter density in the left anterior hippocampus in mild to moderate AD participants (Berlingeri et al., 2008). Thus, the early MTL involvement in AD may disrupt the episodic buffer, which might impact EM acquisition. However, our review of the literature does not clarify whether or not the episodic buffer, central executive, or both of these WM components are involved in reduced strategic encoding in AD. Nevertheless, while WM and EM are dissociable in cases of mild AD, WM deficits appear to reduce strategic EM encoding in this population.

SM in AD. SM impairments are common in AD (Fink & Randolph, 1998; Spaan, Raaijmakers, & Jonker, 2003). In fact, a detailed analysis of the SM abilities of AD participants, particularly on confrontation naming and semantic fluency tasks, suggests that the disease creates a breakdown of the semantic network rather than just reduced semantic access (Fink & Randolph, 1998; Sailor, Bramwell, & Griesing, 1998; Spaan et al., 2003). The SM breakdown in AD appears to occur from the "bottom-up," as subordinate distinctions (e.g., terriers vs. hounds) are disrupted prior to the deterioration of superordinate divisions (e.g., dogs or animals; Fink & Randolph, 1998; Spaan et al., 2003). Furthermore, research on the category sorting performances of AD participants indicates that they tend to categorize objects on perceptual features rather than abstract features, and that they are inconsistent in their use of object qualities/features when categorizing in comparison to healthy older adults (Chan, Butters, Salmon, & McGuire, 1993). These findings suggest that the semantic network disruption in AD may result in the development of atypical, less defined semantic associations. Structural neuroimaging studies indicate that the SM deficits in mild AD are associated with reduced grey matter densities in the PFC and temporal lobes (including the MTL) in both hemispheres, although volumetric reductions in the left hemisphere are observed more frequently (Venneri et al., 2008; Joubert et al., 2010).

The impact of WM and SM on EM in AD. Several studies have been conducted to determine if inducing SM processing at encoding improves EM in AD participants. While SM and EM are disrupted in AD, Martin, Brouwers, Cox, and Fedio (1985) showed that AD

---

computation span task required participants to read simple addition and subtraction problems of increasing length over trials and decide if the answers presented for each problem were correct or not in addition to committing the middle number in the problem to memory. Both span tasks were scored in terms of immediate recall of the to-be-remembered items.

participants do appear to engage some level of SM processing during list-learning in a series of two experiments. In their first experiment, AD participants demonstrated poorer learning and immediate recognition in comparisons to controls. However, a fine grained analysis of recognition errors showed that the AD participants chose more semantic foils in comparison to phonetic and unrelated foils, suggesting that they partially encoded the to-be-remembered items. In the second experiment, healthy older adults and AD participants were presented with unrelated word lists in four different encoding conditions. The first condition was a "free" encoding condition where participants were presented a list without any encoding manipulation. The remaining three conditions were then presented in a counterbalanced fashion across participants. These included a "rhyme" condition, a "where" condition, and "pantomime" condition. In the *rhyme* condition, participants produced a word that rhymed with each to-be-learned word. In the *where* condition, participants stated where each list member could be found. In the *pantomime* condition, participants mimicked actions associated with each list member. The *where* and *pantomime* conditions were designed to enhance semantic processing. In all conditions, recall was tested immediately after a single list presentation. No group differences were found, but both groups' recall was reduced in the *rhyme* condition relative to the other conditions. The semantically cued conditions may have not improved recall in the healthy older adult group due to the fact that only one learning trial was presented. However, the fact that both groups had similar recall in the *free*, *where*, and *pantomime* conditions and that their recall was uniformly reduced in the *rhyme* condition suggests that they may have both had similar levels of initial SM engagement during list acquisition.

Other list-learning studies that utilized a greater number of learning trials and active semantic processing manipulations at encoding (e.g., semantic judgments, pantomime) similar to those utilized by Martin et al. (1985) have shown that SM processing during EM encoding shows a gradient effect in AD (Diesfeldt, 1984; Herlitz, Adolfsson, Bäckman, & Nilsson, 1991). That is, greater SM encoding in EM tasks improves recall in mild AD, but moderate AD recall only improves with both increased SM processing at encoding and retrieval (Diesfeldt, 1984; Herlitz et al., 1991). However, such cued verbal EM performances remain markedly reduced in AD participants relative to healthy older adults (Herlitz et al., 1991). One could argue that such active semantic processing manipulations might tax WM abilities, as participants have completed the semantic processing task (e.g., category judgment) while also focusing their attention on learning the to-be-remembered list items.

That said, similar results have been shown in AD samples when relatively passive SM processing manipulations (e.g., category blocking) that make few, if any, demands on WM have been used in list-learning studies (Au, Chan, Chiu, 2003; Gaines, Shapiro, Alt, & Benedict, 2006; Germano, Kinsella, Storey, Ong, & Ames, 2008). AD participants appear to show some initial benefits from the presentation of category blocked lists during verbal learning, as they show greater semantic clustering (compared to unblocked list conditions; Au et al., Germano et al., 2008) and slight reductions in rapid forgetting (word loss in recall between the last learning trial and a short-delay recall trial; Au et al., 2003). However, these effects are observed more in milder cases of AD as opposed to moderate AD and do not appear to significantly impact learning trials or delayed recall (Au et al., 2003; Germano et al., 2008[13]). Also, the semantic clustering of mild AD participants under blocked list conditions is significantly lower than healthy older controls (Au et el., 2003; Gaines et al., 2006; Germano et al., 2008) and it deteriorates precipitously between learning and delayed recall, unlike the semantic clustering of healthy older adults (Gaines et al., 2006).

To summarize, EM impairment and MTL pathology are characteristic features of AD (Braak & Braak, 1991; Salmon & Bondi, 1999; Head, Snyder, Girton, Morris, & Buckner, 2005; Holland et al., 2009; Dickerson et al., 2009; Bondi, Salmon, & Kaszniak, 2009), although AD is also associated with deficits in attention, language, SM, executive functions (including WM), and constructional and visuospatial skills (Salmon & Bondi, 1999; Bondi, Salmon, & Kaszniak, 2009), along with neurodegeneration that spreads from the MTLs to other areas in the temporal, frontal, and partial lobes over time (Braak & Braak, 1991). Research has shown that WM and EM are dissociable in cases of AD (Becker, 1988; Becker, Bajulaiye, & Smith, 1992), but that WM decrements may be responsible for reduced strategic encoding of verbal EM in this population (Castel et al., 2009). When WM and SM are enhanced via encoding manipulations (i.e., category blocking during list learning), mild AD participants show some improvements in clustering during learning and reductions in rapid forgetting, but their learning and delayed recall performances show no discernable improvement and their clustering of list items quickly breaks down over time (Au et al., 2003; Gaines et al., 2006; Germano et al., 2008). In sum, research on WM, SM, and EM encoding in AD appears to support the notion that interactions between these processes may facilitate acquisition of verbal EM, but at the same time indicate that WM, SM, and EM encoding are separable, as enhancing these abilities does not overcome the marked LTM deficits produced by significant MTL pathology.

Prefrontal Cortex Pathology

In its earliest modern-era descriptions, schizophrenia (SZ), like Alzheimer's disease, was classified as a dementia, albeit one with its modal age of onset during early adulthood (Kraeplin, 1971/1919/1913). Indeed, the profoundly compromised reality testing, the emotional dysregulation, and the substantial level of functional impairment characteristic of SZ are associated with a range of moderate cognitive impairments (Heinrichs and Zakzanis, 1998). The demonstration that SZ participants' impairments tend to remain stable in nature and severity over their lifespan (e.g., Harvey et al., 1995; Nopoulos et al., 1994), after an initial insult coinciding with illness onset (Mesholam-Gately, et al., 2009), suggest that SZ may be more fruitfully compared to the sequelae of CHI. Given that SZ remains a syndrome with unknown etiology, however, any mechanistic links to other disorders are speculative. Nevertheless, clinical research has shown that SZ participants display substantial impairments in WM (Lee & Park, 2005) and EM (Aleman et al., 1999), and that, as in the cases of the other disorders reviewed in this chapter, these behavioral impairments are associated with abnormal structure-function relationships in a PFC-MTL and memory system (Cirillo &

---

[13] Germano et al. (2008) utilized a healthy older adult group, a "very mild AD" group, and a mild AD group. Both the healthy older adult and the very mild AD groups showed a recall advantage for blocked as opposed to unblocked lists during learning and at a delayed recall trial, but the mild AD group did not. Upon closer inspection, the very mild AD group appeared to be comprise of participants with mild cognitive impairment rather than AD, as the groups mean MMSE score was 26.39 (SD=1.79).

Seidman, 2003; Glahn, et al., 2005; Weiss & Heckers, 2001). Furthermore, the nature of SZ participants' mnemonic deficits and the preponderance of physiological data point to the prefrontal nodes of this system as disproportionately responsible for participants' compromised information processing (Barch, 2005; Ragland, et al., 2009).

The profile of cognitive abilities associated with SZ diagnosis includes a broad, generalized deficit exhibited in response to nearly all information processing demands (e.g., Bilder, et al., 2000; Blanchard and Neale, 1994; Mohamed et al., 1999; but also see, Saykin, et al., 1994). Superimposed on this generalized deficit are more severe, focal impairments in executive function, cognitive processing speed, and verbal memory (Aleman, et al., 1999; Rajji et al., 2009).

Neuropathology of WM and EM in SZ. A large and still growing body of work has sought to map many of these behavioral deficits onto neurophysiological findings in SZ. Regarding SZ-associated WM impairment, functional neuroimaging research has highlighted SZ participants' failure to activate dorsolateral PFC (especially when manipulation or inhibition demands are great), but has also provided evidence for hyperactivity in other areas of the PFC among participants, as well as relatively normal levels of activation in inferior sections of the parietal lobe and task-relevant sensory cortex (Glahn et al., 2005). Interestingly, this pattern of increased and decreased activation across the PFC, and depending on the study, sometimes even within the dorsolateral PFC itself (Callicott, et al., 2003; Manoach, et al., 2003) appears to be moderated by the task performance achieved (Karlsgodt, et al., 2007; Van Snellenberg, et al., 2006). These findings confirm the critical relationship between the PFC, a network of task-relevant posterior regions, and goal-directed behavioral performance; however, they do not clarify the actual cause of SZ participants' neurocognitive inefficiency.

An alternate approach to identifying a locus of abnormality is to identify a point in time where participants begin to show abnormal activity in tasks that temporally segregate stimulus encoding and retrieval (i.e., using a Sternberg-like, delayed match-to-sample task, rather than an n-back task requiring constant memory set updating). Although this differentiation is possible to accomplish using fMRI (see Johnson et al., 2006), measurement of task-sensitive event-related potentials (ERPs) from the ongoing electroencephalogram (EEG) has provided evidence of substantial temporal specificity in participants' WM deficits. When one of us examined ERP data recorded while SZ participants and matched controls performed a spatial delayed match-to-sample task, the SZ group showed a hypersensitivity to task load that began during the late encoding/stimulus representation consolidation phase of task performance (Bachman et al., 2009). Furthermore, a combined ERP and fMRI study of visual object WM in SZ participants demonstrated that memory for novel, difficult to discriminate stimuli places an even greater burden on participants' impaired encoding ability, showing that abnormal visual system activation appearing in the 200ms post-stimulus-onset may account for SZ participants' memory impairments, under some circumstances (Haenschel, et al., 2007). In this instance, Haenschel and colleagues presented a very compelling demonstration of stimulus encoding deficits - perhaps even at the perceptual stage - constraining SZ participants' subsequent WM performance.

The body of investigations of the physiology of SZ participants' episodic memory deficits has been reviewed recently (Ranganath et al., 2008), with the conclusion that although an extensive fronto-temporal network (also extending into parietal and cerebellar regions) is engaged by EM encoding and retrieval, participants' impairments appear to be driven by PFC activation differences (for meta-analysis, see Ragland et al., 2009). This primarily PFC abnormality is consistent with the suggestion that stimulus encoding deficits may be tightly intertwined with executive functioning among participants (Leeson et al., 2009) and may be disproportionately responsible for participants' EM impairment; by this formulation, SZ participants' retrieval deficits play a relatively reduced role in explaining mnemonic impairment (e.g., Cirilo & Seidman, 2003).

In fact, Ragland and colleagues' (2009) meta-analysis showed that the most reliable activation differences associated with stimulus encoding appeared in left polar PFC, dorsolateral PFC, and ventrolateral PFC. They also noted that when participants were explicitly provided with memory encoding strategies, such as semantic organization of word lists to be memorized, the group-wise deficits in ventrolateral PFC activation disappeared (Bonner-Jackson et al., 2005; Ragland et al., 2005), which they attributed to the region's role in semantic elaboration and binding stimuli into an episodic context (Blumenfeld & Ranganath, 2007). Moreover, although activation in the hippocampus proper did not differentiate between the groups (Ragland, et al., 2009), at least one group has found an association between integrity of the left fornix, a white matter bundle linking the hippocampus to ventrolateral PFC via the septal nucleus, and use of semantic clustering during a verbal learning task (Takei, et al., 2008). This finding suggests a pathway by which the PFC implements a strategy to facilitate memory encoding, something SZ participants tends not to do spontaneously (e.g., Iddon et al., 1998).

EM and WM in SZ. In light of the functional overlap between prefrontal stimulus encoding and organization mechanisms in WM and in EM (e.g., Cowan, 1999), as well as the overlapping locus of dysregulated PFC activation detected when SZ participants perform these tasks (Barch et al., 2002), it is reasonable to ask whether these deficits reflect the same fundamental pathology. As Van Snellenberg (2009) addresses in a recent commentary, very little available data address this question directly, yet the neuroscience research delineated in the introduction to this chapter and SZ research discussed above suggest that a unitary deficit may be the most parsimonious explanation. In contrast to clinical syndromes in which information is registered in mind and then lost, in SZ, the PFC may fail to guide selective attention to encode stimulus features into an episodic context (e.g., Talamini, et al., 2010) or to reactivate an already-bound, consolidated representation, hindering the efficient retrieval of target information, especially in the face of competition from associated but task-irrelevant information.

A few conclusions can be drawn regarding SZ participants' mnemonic impairment in particular. Participants consistently show impairment on a range of WM tasks, employing a range of different types of target information (e.g., verbal, visual, tactile; Lee & Park, 2005). The impairment is relatively insensitive to the length of time over which representations must be maintained (Lee & Park, 2005), but it tends to increase when WM manipulation demands increase (Kim, Glahn, et al., 2004). Accumulating evidence suggests an information encoding and storage deficit contributes substantially to the WM impairment (Fuller et al., 2009), but WM encoding and/or consolidation deficits alone cannot account for all findings (Tek, Gold, et al., 2002).

Shifting to LTM impairment, SZ participants' robust EM deficit is considered distinct from a more "forgetful" type of impairment seen in AD (Heaton et al., 1994; Paulsen et al., 1995). In one recent investigation, when cognitive performance in older SZ participants was contrasted directly against performance in participants with probable AD, the SZ participants showed comparable difficulty in list learning; however, the SZ participants were significantly better than the AD participants in delayed recall (Ting et al., 2010). Findings such as these support the contention that SZ participants' memory difficulties result from inefficient or inadequate acquisition of information during the learning episode (Cirillo & Seidman, 2003). Additionally, this decrement appears insensitive to the type of material presented for memorization (Aleman, et al., 1999), although the few studies that find a difference consistently report that memory for verbal information is especially compromised (e.g., Bilder, et al., 2000).

Interestingly, a number of investigations focusing on putative impairments in SZ participants' memory acquisition have provided compelling evidence that they do not spontaneously engage in normative strategies to organize or elaborate upon target information; however, when those strategies are provided explicitly, SZ participants do appear to benefit from them (see Ranganath, et al., 2008). In one instance, Ragland and colleagues (2003) discovered that using a standard levels-of-processing encoding task to force SZ participants to engage in a semantic elaboration with a given set of words substantially improved their delayed memory for the words. In fact, when compared with controls, SZ participants showed an entirely intact depth of processing effect (Craik and Lockhart, 1972), despite starting with a reduced level of semantic knowledge.

The impact of WM and SM on EM in SZ. That said, while several list-learning studies suggest that SZ participants' learning and recall may benefit from increased opportunities for semantic processing, their recall performances remain deficient in contrast to healthy control participants (Brébion, David, Jones, & Pilowsky, 2004; Chan et al., 2000; Christensen, Girard, Benjamin, & Vidailhet, 2006; Lutz & Marsh, 1981; Matsui, Yuuki, Kato, & Kurachi, 2006; Matsui et al., 2008). This effect appears to be driven by disturbances in the semantic network organization of SZ participants (Bozikas, Kosmidis, & Karavatos, 2004; Moelter et al., 2005) that appears to contribute to EM encoding deficits frequently observed in SZ (Cirillo & Seidman, 2003). Interestingly, SZ participants do show increased recall for organizable word lists where semantic associates are in noncontiguous positions in contrast to word lists comprised of unrelated words (Brébion et al., 2004; Lutz & Marsh, 1981). However, they continue to show recall decrements and less semantic clustering for organizable lists in comparison to healthy controls (Matsui et al., 2006; Brébion et al., 2004; Lutz & Marsh, 1981), possibly due to differences in left PFC volumes (Matsui et al., 2008). Also, unlike healthy controls, SZ participants' spontaneous semantic clustering for organizable lists appears to be minimally associated with or unrelated to their recall performances (Lutz & Marsh, 1981). That said, SZ participants, like healthy controls, show increased learning and delayed recall performances for word lists that are blocked by category in contrast to unblocked, organizable lists (Christensen et al., 2006; Chan et al., 2000). Nevertheless, while SZ participants benefit from category blocking, they continue to show impaired recall and depressed semantic clustering in contrast to controls (Christensen et al., 2006; Chan et al., 2000).

Overall, deficits in EM encoding, WM, and SM organization appear to interact and impact verbal learning and recall in SZ (Ranganath, et al., 2008; Christensen et al., 2006; Chan et al., 2000; Brébion et al., 2004; Lutz & Marsh, 1981; Bozikas, Kosmidis, & Karavatos, 2004; Moelter et al., 2005; Cirilo & Seidman, 2003 Leeson et al., 2009). These deficits seem to correlate with PFC pathology in this population (Ragland et al., 2009; Cirillo

& Seidman, 2003; Matsui et al., 2008), although other brain areas are clearly involved as well (Ragland et al., 2009; Cirillo & Seidman, 2003). When WM and SM are supported during encoding via category blocking, SZ participants show increased learning, delayed recall, and semantic clustering, but their performances remain significantly lower than healthy control participants (Christensen et al., 2006; Chan et al., 2000). The literature reviewed provides partial support for the assertion that significant PFC dysfunction impacts learning and recall even under modified encoding conditions where to-be-learned information is meaningfully organized at learning. However, SZ participants' learning and recall does seem to show some benefit from meaningful organization of to-be-learned information, suggesting we may have under estimated the role of the MTL in EM encoding, WM, and SM interactions.

CONCLUSION

As reviewed above, a large body of work suggests that EM, SM, and WM show a significant degree of overlap in the PFC, although these processes also have partially separable neural substrates. Thus, the PFC could be argued to be a nexus for holding (WM maintenance), evaluating (WM manipulation), and imparting meaning (semantic association) to incoming verbal material so that it can be efficiently encoded and consolidated (via interactions with MTL structures). Specifically, verbal EM encoding appears to engage the lateral PFC (left hemisphere > right hemisphere) and MTL structures, while verbal WM tasks often elicits activity in the lateral PFC, with left hemisphere activations associated with the maintenance of information and right hemisphere activations correlating with manipulation of information. Also, verbal list learning studies seem to be ideal for studying the interactions between these memory processes, as semantic clustering during list acquisition appears to represent an instance when EM encoding, WM, and SM interact; presented words need to be maintained, manipulated, and associated with semantic representations in order for efficient list learning. To explore the plausibility of a EM encoding-WM-SM processing nexus in the PFC, we reviewed the verbal memory literature regarding CHI, HIV/AIDS, AD, and SZ. We posited (1) that reduced connectivity between generally intact PFC and MTL structures (via diffuse white matter pathology in CHI and HIV/AIDS) should interfere with efficient acquisition and recall of new verbal information under normal learning conditions, but recall should improve under modified encoding conditions where information is meaningfully organized at learning (reducing the network/associative requirements necessary for efficient acquisition); (2) WM ability should have little or no impact on delayed recall of verbal material in cases of gross MTL injury (as observed in AD; new material, organized or not, should fail to be consolidated); (3) significant PFC dysfunction (as observed in SZ) should impact learning and recall even under modified encoding conditions where to-be-learned information is meaningfully organized at learning (pre-organized material may not be properly maintained or may be bound to poorly organized semantic networks), although retention of the information learned in these cases should not be overly affected by the degree of PFC pathology.

While all of the groups considered in this review are known to suffer from some degree of PFC and MTL pathology, in addition to deficits in both EM and WM (and AD and SZ participants have been shown to exhibit semantic network disruptions), our review of the literature generally supports the notion of PFC EM encoding-WM-SM processing nexus. Research on verbal memory in CHI and HIV/AIDS suggests that reduced connectivity between grossly intact PFC and MTL lobe structures differentially interferes with acquisition and recall of new verbal information. Specifically, these studies imply that that to-be-learned material that requires greater WM processing (e.g., word lists) results in reduced acquisition and recall performances and that these decrements can be largely negated by providing WM and SM support (e.g., category blocking of list items). As such, verbal EM deficits associated with diffuse white matter pathology appear to be due to inefficient coordination of WM, EM encoding, and SM processes in the lateral PFC and MTL structures. With regard to MTL pathology, when mild AD participants' WM and SM are enhanced via category blocking during list learning, they show some improvements in clustering during learning and reductions in rapid forgetting, but their learning and delayed recall performances show no discernable improvement. Additionally, their clustering of list items quickly breaks down during the retention interval between learning and delayed recall. These finding suggest that gross MTL pathology results in EM deficits that cannot be overcome by improving EM encoding, WM, and SM interactions during verbal learning. Finally, PFC pathology, as evidenced by studies of SZ, showed that enhancing WM and SM via category blocking at learning improved SZ participants' learning, delayed recall, and semantic clustering, but that these performances remain significantly lower than healthy control participants. Thus, PFC pathology partially attenuates the benefits of WM and SM support during EM encoding, suggesting that MTL processing may also contribute to interactions between WM, SM, and EM during the encoding of verbal material.

In sum, verbal EM encoding, WM, and SM appear to be functionally dissociable across a wide span of neurologically compromised populations. However, the neural substrates of these processes appear to overlap in the PFC. Improving EM encoding by supporting WM and SM during learning can enhance LTM in populations with PFC pathology and reduced PFC-MTL connectivity, but not in those with gross MTL injury. Our review also suggested that the MTL may play a significant role in the interactions between EM encoding, WM, and SM. Future studies contrasting the verbal memory performances of participants with injuries to the PFC, MTL, and PFC-MTL connections may help to better illuminate how coordinated interactions between WM, SM, and EM encoding give rise to improved LTM and may ultimately provide clues to effective neuropsychological rehabilitation methods for patients with memory disorders due to different patterns of neuropathology.

REFERENCES

Abou-Hamde, A., Blumbergs, P.C., Scott G., Manavis, J., Wainwright, H., Jones, N., et al. (1997). Axonal injury in falls. *Journal of Neurotrauma, 14,* 699-713.

Adams J. H., & Jennett D. I. G. (2001). The structural basis of moderate disability after traumatic brain injury. *Journal of Neurology, Neurosurgery & Psychiatry, 71,* 521-524.

Adams, J. H., Doyle, D., Ford I., Gennarelli, T. A., Graham, D. I., & McLellan, D. R. (1989). Diffuse axonal injury in head injury: Definition, diagnosis, and grading. *Histopathology, 15,* 49-59.

Aggleton, J. P., & Brown, M. W. (2006). Interleaving brain systems for episodic and recognition memory. *Trends in Cognitive Sciences, 10,* 455-463.

Ahlberg, S. W., & Sharps, M. J. (2002). Bartlett revisited: Reconfiguration of long-trem memory in young and older adults. *The Journal of Genetic Psychology, 163,* 211-218.

Aleman, A., Hijman, R., de Haan, E. H. F., & Kahn, R. S. (1999). Memory impairment in schizophrenia: A meta-analysis. *The American Journal of Psychiatry, 156,* 1358-1366.

Alessio, A., Damasceno, B. P., Camargo, C. H. P., Kobayashi, E., Guerreiro, C. A. M., & Cendes, F. (2004). Differences in memory performance and other clinical characteristics in patients with mesial temporal lobe epilepsy with and without hippocampal atrophy. *Epilepsy & Behavior, 5,* 22-27.

Allen, R. J., & Baddeley, A. D. (2009). Working memory and sentence recall. In A. S. C. Thorn, & M. P. A. Page (Eds.), *Interactions between short-term and long-term memory in the verbal domain.* (pp. 63-85). New York, NY, US: Psychology Press.

Archibald, S. L., Masliah, E., Fennema-Notestine, C., Marcotte, T. D.,Ellis, R. J., McCutchan, J. A. et al. (2004). Correlation of in vivo neuroimaging abnormalities with postmortem human immunodeficiency virus encephalitis and dendritic loss. *Archives of Neurology, 61,* 369-376.

Ariza, M., Pueyo, R., Junqué, C., Mataró, M., Poca, M. A., & Mena, M. P. et al. (2006). Differences in visual vs. verbal memory impairments as a result of focal temporal lobe damage in patients with traumatic brain injury. *Brain Injury, 20,* 1053-1059.

Arnett, P. A., Rao, S. M., Grafman, J., Bernardin, L., Luchetta, T., Binder, J. R., et al. (1997). Executive functions in multiple sclerosis: An analysis of temporal ordering, semantic encoding, and planning abilities. *Neuropsychology, 11,* 535-544.

Asloun, S., Soury, S., Couillet, J., Giroire, J., Joseph, P., Mazaux, J., & Azouvi, P. (2008). Interactions between divided attention and working-memory load in patients with severe traumatic brain injury. *Journal of Clinical and Experimental Neuropsychology, 30,* 481-490.

Atkinson, R. C., & Shiffrin, R. M. (1968). Human memory: A proposed system and its control processes. In *The psychology of learning and motivation*: II. Oxford, England: Academic Press.

Au, A., Chan, A. S., & Chiu, H. (2003). Verbal learning in Alzheimer's dementia. *Journal of the International Neuropsychological Society, 9,* 363-375.

Bachman, P., Kim, J., Yee, C. M., Therman, S., Manninen, M., Lönnqvist, J., Kaprio, J., Huttunen, M. O., Näätänen, R., & Cannon, T. D. (2009). Efficiency of working memory encoding in twins discordant for schizophrenia. *Psychiatry Research: Neuroimaging, 174,* 97-104.

Baddeley, A. (2000). The episodic buffer: A new component of working memory? *Trends in Cognitive Sciences, 4,* 417-423.

Baddeley, A. and Hitch, G. (1974). Working memory. In G. Bower (Ed.), *The Psychology of Learning and Motivation* (pp. 47–89). New York: Academic Press.

Baldewicz, T. T., Leserman, J., Silva, S. G., Petitto, J. M., Golden, R. N., Perkins, D. O., Barroso, J., & Evans, D. L. (2004). Changes in neuropsychological functioning with progression of HIV-1 infection: Results of an 8-year longitudinal investigation. *AIDS and Behavior, 8,* 345-355.

Balthazar, M. L. F., Yasuda, C. L., Cendes, F., & Damasceno, B. P. (2010). Learning, retrieval, and recognition are compromised in aMCI and mild AD: Are distinct episodic memory processes mediated by the same anatomical structures? *Journal of the International Neuropsychological Society, 16,* 205-209.

Bandaru, V. V. R., McArthur, J. C., Sacktor, N., Cutler, R. G., Knapp, E. L., Mattson, M. P., & Haughey, N. J. (2007). Associative and predictive biomarkers of dementia in HIV-1-infected patients. *Neurology, 68,* 1481-1487.

Barch, D. M. (2005). The cognitive neuroscience of schizophrenia. *Annual Review of Clinical Psychology, 1,* 321-353.

Barch, D. M., Csernansky, J. G., Conturo, T., & Snyder, A. Z. (2002). Working and long-term memory deficits in schizophrenia: Is there a common prefrontal mechanism? *Journal of Abnormal Psychology, 111,* 478-494.

Bartlett, F. C. (1932). *Remembering: A study in experimental and social psychology.* Oxford, England: Macmillan.

Basso, M. R., Ghormley, C., Lowery, N., Combs, D., & Bornstein, R. A. (2008). Self-generated learning in people with multiple sclerosis: An extension of Chiaravalloti and DeLuca (2002). *Journal of Clinical and Experimental Neuropsychology, 30,* 63-69.

Basso, M. R., Lowery, N., Ghormley, C., Combs, D., & Johnson, J. (2006). Self-generated learning in people with multiple sclerosis. *Journal of the International Neuropsychological Society, 12,* 640-648.

Becker, J. T. (1988). Working memory and secondary memory deficits in Alzheimer's disease. *Journal of Clinical and Experimental Neuropsychology, 10,* 739-753.

Becker, J. T., Bajulaiye, O., & Smith, C. (1992). Longitudinal analysis of a two-component model of the memory deficit in Alzheimer's disease. *Psychological Medicine, 22,* 437-445.

Berlingeri, M., Bottini, G., Basilico, S., Silani, G., Zanardi, G., Sberna, M., Colombo, N., Sterzi, R., Scialfa, G., & Paulesu, E. (2008). Anatomy of the episodic buffer: A voxel-based morphometry study in patients with dementia. *Behavioural Neurology, 19,* 29-34.

Bernard, F., Desgranges, B., Platel, H., Baron, J., & Eustache, F. (2001). Contributions of frontal and medial temporal regions to verbal episodic memory: A PET study. *NeuroReport, 12,* 1737-1741.

Bilder, R. M., Goldman, R. S., Robinson, D., Reiter, G., Bell, L., Bates, J. A., Pappadopulos, E., Willson, D. F., Alvir, J. M. J., Woerner, M. G., Geisler, S., Kane, J. M., & Lieberman, J. A. (2000). Neuropsychology of first-episode schizophrenia: Initial characterization and clinical correlates. *The American Journal of Psychiatry, 157,* 549-559.

Blachstein, H., Vakil, E., & Hoofien, D. (1993). Impaired learning in patients with closed-head injuries: An analysis of components of the acquisition process. *Neuropsychology, 7,* 530-535.

Blanchard, J. J., & Neale, J. M. (1994). The neuropsychological signature of schizophrenia: Generalized or differential deficit? *The American Journal of Psychiatry, 151,* 40-48.

Blumenfeld, R. S., & Ranganath, C. (2006). Dorsolateral prefrontal cortex promotes long-term memory formation through its role in working memory organization. *The Journal of Neuroscience, 26,* 916-925.

Bondi, M. W., Salmon, D. P., & Kasvniak, A. W. (2009). The neuropsychology of Dementia. In K. M. Adams & I. Grant (Eds.), *Neuropsychological assessment of neuropsychiatric and neuromedical disorders,* 3rd edition (pp. 159-198). New York: Oxford University Press, Inc.

Bonner-Jackson, A., Haul, K., Csernansky, J. G., & Barch, D. M. (2005). The influence of encoding strategy on episodic memory and cortical activity in schizophrenia. *Biological Psychiatry, 58,* 47-55.

Bor, D., Cumming, N., Scott, C. E. L., & Owen, A. M. (2004). Prefrontal cortical involvement in verbal encoding strategies. *European Journal of Neuroscience, 19,* 3365-3370.

Bozikas, V., Kosmidis, M. H., & Karavatos, A. (2004). Disproportionate impairment in semantic verbal fluency in schizophrenia: differential deficit in clustering. *Schizophrenia Research, 74,* 51-59.

Braak, H., & Braak, E. (1991). Neuropathological stageing [sic] of Alzheimer-related changes. *Acta Neuropathologica, 82,* 239–259,

Brébion, G., David, A. S., Jones, H., & Pilowsky, L. S. (2004). Semantic organization and verbal memory efficiency in patients with schizophrenia. *Neuropsychology, 18,* 378-383.

Buckner, R. L., Kelley, W. M., & Petersen, S. E. (1999). Frontal cortex contributes to human memory formation. *Nature Neuroscience, 2,* 311-314.

Buschke, H. (1973). Selective reminding for the analysis of memory and learning. *Journal of Verbal Learning & Verbal Behavior, 12,* 543-550.

Cabeza, R., & Nyberg, L. (2000). Imaging cognition II: An empirical review of 275 PET and fMRI studies. *Journal of Cognitive Neuroscience, 12,* 1-47.

Callicott, J. H., Mattay, V. S., Verchinski, B. A., Marenco, S., Egan, M. F., & Weinberger, D. R. (2003). Complexity of prefrontal cortical dysfunction in schizophrenia: More than up or down. *The American Journal of Psychiatry, 160,* 2209-2215.

Carlesimo, G. A., Mauri, M., Graceffa, A. M. S., Fadda, L., Loasses, A., Lorusso, S., & Caltagirone, C. (1998). Memory performances in young, elderly, and very old healthy individuals versus patients with Alzheimer's disease: Evidence for discontinuity between normal and pathological aging. *Journal of Clinical and Experimental Neuropsychology, 20,* 14-29.

Castel, A. D., Balota, D. A., & McCabe, D. P. (2009). Memory efficiency and the strategic control of attention at encoding: Impairments of value-directed remembering in Alzheimer's disease. *Neuropsychology, 23,* 297-306.

Chan, A. S., Butters, N., Salmon, D. P., & McGuire, K. A. (1993). Dimensionality and clustering in the semantic network of patients with Alzheimer's disease. *Psychology and Aging, 8,* 411-419.

Chan, A. S., Kwok, I. C., Chiu, H., Lam, L., Pang, A., & Chow, L. (2000). Memory and organizational strategies in chronic and acute schizophrenic patients. *Schizophrenia Research, 41,* 431-445.

Chang, L., Speck, O., Miller, E. N., Braun, J., Jovicich, J., Koch, C., Itti, L., & Ernst, T. (2001). Neural correlates of attention and working memory deficits in HIV patients. *Neurology, 57,* 1001-1007.

Chein, J. M., Fissell, K., Jacobs, S., & Fiez, J. A. (2002). Functional heterogeneity within Broca's area during verbal working memory. *Physiology & Behavior, Special Issue: The Pittsburgh Special Issue, 77,* 635-639.

Chiaravalloti, N. D., & DeLuca, J. (2002). Self-generation as a means of maximizing learning in multiple sclerosis: An application of the generation effect. *Archives of Physical Medicine and Rehabilitation, 83,* 1070–1079.

Christensen, B. K., Girard, T. A., Benjamin, A. S., & Vidailhet, P. (2006). Evidence for impaired mnemonic strategy use among patients with schizophrenia using the part-list cuing paradigm. *Schizophrenia Research, 85,* 1-11.

Christoff, K., & Gabrieli, J. D. E. (2000). The frontopolar cortex and human cognition: Evidence for a rostrocaudal hierarchical organization within the human prefrontal cortex. *Psychobiology.Special Issue: Subregional Analysis of Prefrontal Cortex Mediation of Cognitive Functions in Rats, Monkeys, and Humans, 28,* 168-186.

Cinan, S. (2003). Executive processing in free recall of categorized lists. *Learning & Motivation, 34,* 240-261.

Cirillo, M. A., & Seidman, L. J. (2003). Verbal declarative memory dysfunction in schizophrenia: From clinical assessment to genetics and brain mechanisms. *Neuropsychology Review, 13,* 43-77.

Cohen, R. A., Harezlak, J., Schifitto, G., Hana, G., Clark, U., Gongvatana, A., ... & HIV Neuroimaging Consortium. (2010). Effects of nadir CD4 count and duration of human immunodeficiency virus infection on brain volumes in the highly active antiretroviral therapy era. *Journal of Neurovirology, 16,* 25-32.

Corkin, S. (2002). "What's new with the amnesic patient H.M.?" *Nature Reviews Neuroscience, 3,* 153–160.

Cowan, N. (1999). An embedded-processes model of working memory. In A. Miyake, & P. Shah (Eds.), *Models of working memory: Mechanisms of active maintenance and executive control.* (pp. 62-101). New York, NY, US: Cambridge University Press.

Craik, F. I. M. & Tulving, E. (1975). Depth of processing and the retention of words in episodic memory. *Journal of Experimental Psychology: General, 104,* 268-294.

Craik, F. I. M. (2002). Levels of processing: Past, present, ...and future? *Memory, 10,* 305-318.

Craik, F. I. M., & Lockhart, R. S. (1972). Levels of processing: A framework for memory research. *Journal of Verbal Learning & Verbal Behavior, 11,* 671-684.

Delis, D. C., Kramer, J. H., Kaplan, E., & Ober, E. (1987). *California Verbal Learning Test.* San Antonio, TX: Psychological Corporation.

Delis, D. C., Peavy, G., Heaton, R., & Butters, N. (1995). Do patients with HIV-associated minor Cognitive/Motor disorder exhibit a "subcortical" memory profile? Evidence using the California Verbal Learning Test. *Assessment, 2,* 151-165.

Della Sala, S., Logie, R. H., & Spinnler, H. (1992). Is primary memory deficit of Alzheimer's patients due to a "central executive" impairment? *Journal of Neurolinguistics.Special Issue: Systemic–functional Analysis of Pathological Discourse and Non-Systemic Accounts of Brain Function in Language Behavior, 7,* 325-346.

DeLuca, J., Schultheis, M. T., Madigan, N. K., Christodoulou, C., & Averill, A. (2000). Acquisition vs. retrieval deficits in traumatic brain injury: Implications for memory rehabilitation. *Archives of Physical Medicine and Rehabilitation, 81,* 1327-1333.

Desgranges, B., Baron, J., de la Sayette, V., Petit-Taboué, M., Benali, K., Landeau, B., Lechevalier, B., & Eustache, F. (1998). The neural substrates of memory systems impairment in Alzheimer's disease: A PET study of resting brain glucose utilization. *Brain, 121,* 611-631.

Dickerson, B. C., Feczko, E., Augustinack, J. C., Pacheco, J., Morris, J. C., Fischl, B., & Buckner, R. L. (2009). Differential effects of aging and Alzheimer's disease on medial temporal lobe cortical thickness and surface area. *Neurobiology of Aging, 30,* 432-440.

Diesfeldt, H. F. (1984). The importance of encoding instructions and retrieval cues in the assessment of memory in senile dementia. *Archives of Gerontology and Geriatrics, 3,* 51-57.

Dolan, R. J., & Fletcher, P. F. (1999). Encoding and retrieval in human medial temporal lobes: An empirical investigation using functional magnetic resonance imaging (fMRI). *Hippocampus, 9,* 25-34.

Duncan, J., & Owen, A. M. (2000). Common regions of the human frontal lobe recruited by diverse cognitive demands. *Trends in Neurosciences, 23,* 475-483.

Ellis, H. C., & Hunt, R. R. (1983). *Fundamentals of human memory and cognition*, 3rd edition (pp. 84–130). Dubque, IA: Wm. C. Brown Company Publishers.

Esselman, P. C., & Uomoto, J. M. (1995). Classification of the spectrum of mild traumatic brain injury. *Brain Injury, 9,* 417-424.

Fernandez, G., Weyerts, H., Schrader-Bolsche, M., Tendolkar, I., Smid, H. G. O. M., Tempelmann, C., et al. (1998). Successful verbal encoding into episodic memory engages the posterior hippocampus: a parametrically analyzed functional magnetic resonance imaging study. *The Journal of Neuroscience, 18,* 1841–1847.

Ferrando, S. J., Rabkin, J. G., van Gorp, W., & McElhiney, M. (2003). Longitudinal improvement in psychomotor processing speed is associated with potent combination antiretroviral therapy in HIV-1 infection. *The Journal of Neuropsychiatry and Clinical Neurosciences, 15,* 208-214.

Fink, J. W., & Randolph, C. (1998). Semantic memory in neurodegenerative disease. In A. I. Tröster (Ed.), *Memory in neurodegenerative disease: Biological, cognitive, and clinical perspectives.* (pp. 197-209). New York, NY, US: Cambridge University Press.

Folstein, M. F., Folstein, S. E., & McHugh, P. R. (1975). Mini-mental state: A practical method for grading the cognitive state of patients for the clinician. *Journal of Psychiatric Research, 12,* 189-198.

Fork, M., Bartels, C., Ebert, A. D., Grubich, C., Synowitz, H., & Wallesch, C. (2005). Neuropsychological sequelae of diffuse traumatic brain injury. *Brain Injury, 19,* 101-108.

Forrester, W. E., & King, D. J. (1971). Effects of semantic and acoustic relatedness on free recall and clustering. *Journal of Experimental Psychology, 88,* 16-19.

Fuller, R. L., Luck, S. J., Braun, E. L., Robinson, B. M., McMahon, R. P., & Gold, J. M. (2009). Impaired visual working memory consolidation in schizophrenia. *Neuropsychology, 23,* 71-80.

Fuster, J. M. (2000). Cortical dynamics of memory. *International Journal of Psychophysiology, 35,* 155-164.

Fuster, J. M. (2003). *Cortex and mind: Unifying cognition* (pp.111-142). New York, NY, US: Oxford University Press.

Fuster, J. M. (2009). Cortex and memory: Emergence of a new paradigm. *Journal of Cognitive Neuroscience, 21,* 2047-2072.

Gaines, J. J., Shapiro, A., Alt, M., & Benedict, R. H. B. (2006). Semantic clustering indexes for the Hopkins Verbal Learning Test-revised: Initial exploration in elder control and dementia groups. *Applied Neuropsychology, 13,* 213-222.

Germano, C., & Kinsella, G. J. (2005). Working memory and learning in early Alzheimer's disease. *Neuropsychology Review, 15,* 1-10.

Germano, C., Kinsella, G. J., Storey, E., Ong, B., & Ames, D. (2008). The episodic buffer and learning in early Alzheimer's disease. *Journal of Clinical and Experimental Neuropsychology, 30,* 613-638.

Gimranov, R. F., & Mal'tseva, E. A. (2005). Effect of transcranial magnetic stimulation on short- and long-term memory in healthy subjects and patients with Parkinson's disease. *Human Physiology, 31,* 398-401.

Giometto, B., An, S. F., Groves, M., Scaravilli, T., Geddes, J. F., Miller, R., Tavolato, B., Beckett, A. A. J., & Scaravilli, F. (1997). Accumulation of β-amyloid precursor protein in HIV encephalitis: Relationship with neuropsychological abnormalities. *Annals of Neurology, 42,* 34-40.

Glahn, D. C., Ragland, J. D., Abramoff, A., Barrett, J., Laird, A. R., Bearden, C. E., & Velligan, D. I. (2005). Beyond hypofrontality: A quantitative meta-analysis of functional neuroimaging studies of working memory in schizophrenia. *Human Brain Mapping.Special Issue: Meta-Analysis in Functional Brain Mapping, 25,* 60-69.

Glanzer, M. (1971). Short-term storage and long-term storage in recall. *Journal of Psychiatric Research, 8,* 423-438.

Glanzer, M., & Cunitz, A. R. (1966). Two storage mechanisms in free recall. *Journal of Verbal Learning & Verbal Behavior, 5,* 351-360.

Gongvatana, A., Schweinsburg, B. C., Taylor, M. J., Theilmann, R. J., Letendre, S. L., Alhassoon, O. M., ... CHARTER Group. (2009). White matter tract injury and cognitive impairment in human immunodeficiency virus-infected individuals. *Journal of Neurovirology, 15,* 187-195.

Gongvatana, A., Woods, S. P., Taylor, M. J., Vigil, O., Grant, I., & the HNRC Group. (2007). Semantic clustering inefficiency in HIV-associated dementia. *The Journal of Neuropsychiatry and Clinical Neurosciences, 19,* 36-42

Gonzalez, R., Jacobus, J., Amatya, A. K., Quartana, P. J., Vassileva, J., & Martin, E. M. (2008). Deficits in complex motor functions, despite no evidence of procedural learning deficits, among HIV+ individuals with history of substance dependence. *Neuropsychology, 22,* 776-786.

Grady, C. L., McIntosh, A. R., Beig, S., Keightley, M. L., Burian, H., & Black, S. E. (2003). Evidence from functional neuroimaging of a compensatory prefrontal network in Alzheimer's disease. *The Journal of Neuroscience, 23,* 986-993.

Greicius, M. D., Krasnow, B., Boyett-Anderson, Stephan, E., Schatzberg, A. F., Reiss, A. L., et al. (2003). Regional analysis of hippocampal activation during memory encoding and retrieval: fMRI study. *Hippocampus, 13,* 164-174

Habib, R., Nyberg, L., & Tulving, E. (2003). Hemispheric asymmetries of memory: The HERA model revisited. *Trends in Cognitive Sciences, 7,* 241-245.

Haenschel, C., Bittner, R. A., Haertling, F., Rotarska-Jagiela, A., Maurer, K., Singer, W., & Linden, D. E. J. (2007). Contribution of impaired early-stage visual processing to working memory dysfunction in adolescents with schizophrenia: Study with event-related potentials and functional magnetic resonance imaging. *Archives of General Psychiatry, 64,* 1229-1240.

Han, L., Cole, M., Bellavance, F., McCusker, J., & Primeau, F. (2000). Tracking cognitive decline in Alzheimer's disease using the mini-mental state examination: A meta-analysis. *International Psychogeriatrics, 12,* 231-247.

Harvey, P. D., White, L., Parrella, M., & Putnam, K. M. (1995). The longitudinal stability of cognitive impairment in schizophrenia: Mini-mental state scores at one- and two-year follow-ups in geriatric in-patients. *British Journal of Psychiatry, 166,* 630-633.

Hattori, N., Hung, S. C., Wu, H. M., Yeh, E., Glenn, T. C., Vespa, P. M., ...Bergsneider, M. (2003). Correlation of regional metabolic rates of glucose with Glasgow Coma Scale after traumatic brain injury. *The Journal of Nuclear Medicine, 44,* 1709-1716.

Head, D., Snyder, A. Z., Girton, L. E., Morris, J. C., & Buckner, R. L. (2005). Frontal-hippocampal double dissociation between normal aging and Alzheimer's disease. *Cerebral Cortex, 15,* 732-739.

Heaton, R., Paulsen, J. S., McAdams, L. A., & Kuck, J. (1994). Neuropsychological deficits in schizophrenics: Relationship to age, chronicity, and dementia. *Archives of General Psychiatry, 51,* 469-476.

Hebb, D. O. (1949). *The organization of behavior; a neuropsychological theory.* Oxford, England: Wiley.

Heindel, W. C., Butters, N., & Salmon, D. P. (1988). Impaired learning of a motor skill in patients with Huntington's disease. *Behavioral Neuroscience, 102,* 141-147.

Heindel, W. C., Salmon, D. P., Shults, C. W., Walicke, P. A., & Butters, N. (1989). Neuropsychological evidence for multiple implicit memory systems: A comparison of Alzheimer's, Huntington's, and Parkinson's disease patients. *The Journal of Neuroscience, 9,* 582-587.

Heinrichs, R. W., & Zakzanis, K. K. (1998). Neurocognitive deficit in schizophrenia: A quantitative review of the evidence. *Neuropsychology, 12,* 426-445.

Herlitz, A., Adolfsson, R., Bäckman, L., & Nilsson, L. (1991). Cue utilization following different forms of encoding in mildly, moderately, and severely demented patients with Alzheimer's disease. *Brain and Cognition, 15,* 119-130.

Hinkin, C. H., Hardy, D. J., Mason, K. I., Castellon, S. A., Lam, M. N., Stefaniak, M., & Zolnikov, B. (2002). Verbal and spatial working memory performance among HIV-infected adults. *Journal of the International Neuropsychological Society, 8,* 532-538.

Holland, D., Brewer, J. B., Hagler, D. J., Fenema-Notestine, C., Dale, A. M., & Alzheimer's Disease Neuroimaging Initiative. (2009). Subregional neuroanatomical change as a biomarker for Alzheimer's disease. *Proceedings of the National Academy of Sciences of the United States of America, 106,* 20954-20959.

Howe, M. L. (1988). Measuring memory development in adulthood: A model-based approach to disentangling storage-retrieval contributions. In M. L. Howe & C. J. Brainerd (Eds.), *Cognitive development in adulthood* (pp. 39-64). New York, NY: Springer-Verlag.

Iddon, J. L., McKenna, P. J., Sahakian, B. J., & Robbins, T. W. (1998). Impaired generation and use of strategy in schizophrenia: Evidence from visuospatial and verbal tasks. *Psychological Medicine, 28,* 1049-1062.

James, W. (1890). *Memory.* New York, NY, US: Henry Holt and Co.

Jennings, J. R., van der Veen,Frederik M., & Meltzer, C. C. (2006). Verbal and spatial working memory in older individuals: A positron emission tomography study. *Brain Research, 1092,* 177-189.

Johnson, M. R., Morris, N. A., Astur, R. S., Calhoun, V. D., Mathalon, D. H., Kiehl, K. A., & Pearlson, G. D. (2006). A functional magnetic resonance imaging study of working memory abnormalities in schizophrenia. *Biological Psychiatry, 60,* 11-21.

Jones, R. D., & Tranel, D. 1991. Preservation of procedural memory in HIV-positive patients with subcortical dementia. *Journal of Clinical and Experimental Neuropsychology, 13,* 74.

Joubert, S., Brambati, S. M., Ansado, J., Barbeau, E. J., Felician, O., Didic, M., Lacombe, J., Goldstein, R., Chayer, C., & Kergoat, M. (2010). The cognitive and neural expression of semantic memory impairment in mild cognitive impairment and early Alzheimer's disease. *Neuropsychologia, 48,* 978-988.

Kandel, E. R. Cellular mechanisms of learning and the biological basis of individuality. In: E. R. Kandel, J. H. Schwartz, & T. M. Jessell (Eds.), *Principles of neural science* (1009-1031). Norwalk, CT: Appleton & Lange.

Karlsgodt, K. H., Glahn, D. C., van Erp, T. G. M., Therman, S., Huttunen, M., Manninen, M., Kaprio, J., Cohen, M. S., Lönnqvist, J., & Cannon, T. D. (2007). The relationship between performance and fMRI signal during working memory in patients with schizophrenia, unaffected co-twins, and control subjects. *Schizophrenia Research, 89,* 191-197.

Karlsgodt, K. H., Shirinyan, D., van Erp, T. D., Cohen, M. S., & Cannon, T. D. (2005). Hippocampal activations during encoding and retrieval in a verbal working memory paradigm. *NeuroImage, 25,* 1224-1231.

Kim, J., Glahn, D. C., Nuechterlein, K. H., & Cannon, T. D. (2004). Maintenance and manipulation of information in schizophrenia: Further evidence for impairment in the central executive component of working memory. *Schizophrenia Research, 68,* 173-187.

King, N. (1997). Mild head injury: Neuropathology, sequelae, measurement and recovery. *British Journal of Clinical Psychology, 36,* 161-184.

Kraepelin, E. (1971). *Dementia praecox and paraphrenia.* (R.M. Barclay, trans.). Huntington, NY: Robert E. Krieger Publishing Company. (Original work published 1919).

Lafosse, J. M., Corboy, J. R., Leehey, M. A., Seeberger, L. C., & Filley, C. M. (2007). MS vs. HD: Can white matter and subcortical gray matter pathology be distinguished neuropsychologically? *Journal of Clinical and Experimental Neuropsychology, 29,* 142-154.

Lee, J., & Park, S. (2005). Working memory impairments in schizophrenia: A meta-analysis. *Journal of Abnormal Psychology.Special Issue: Toward a Dimensionally Based Taxonomy of Psychopathology, 114,* 599-611.

Leeson, V. C., Robbins, T. W., Franklin, C., Harrison, M., Harrison, I., Ron, M. A., Barnes, T. R. E., & Joyce, E. M. (2009). Dissociation of long-term verbal memory and fronto-executive impairment in first-episode psychosis. *Psychological Medicine, 39,* 1799-1808.

Lengenfelder, J., Bryant, D., Diamond, B. J., Kalmar, J. H., Moore, N. B., & DeLuca, J. (2006). Processing speed interacts with working memory efficiency in multiple sclerosis. *Archives of Clinical Neuropsychology, 21,* 229-238.

Levin, H. S., & Goldstein, F. C. (1986). Organization of verbal memory after severe closed-head injury. *Journal of Clinical & Experimental Neuropsychology, 8,* 643-656.

Lucas, J. A., & Addeo, R. (2006). Traumatic brain injury and postconcussion syndrome. In P. J. Snyder, P. D. Nussbaum & D. L. Robins (Eds.), *Clinical neuropsychology: A pocket handbook for assessment,* 2nd ed. (pp. 351-380). Washington, DC, US: American Psychological Association.

Lutz, J., & Marsh, T. K. (1981). The effect of a dual level word list on schizophrenic free recall. *Schizophrenia Bulletin, 7,* 509-515.

Manoach, D. S. (2003). Prefrontal cortex dysfunction during working memory performance in schizophrenia: Reconciling discrepant findings. *Schizophrenia Research, 60,* 285-298.

Markowitsch, H. J., Kalbe, E., Kessler, J., von Stockhausen, H., Ghaemi, M., & Heiss, W. (1999). Short-term memory deficit after focal parietal damage. *Journal of Clinical and Experimental Neuropsychology, 21,* 784-797.

Martin, A., Brouwers, P., Cox, C., & Fedio, P. (1985). On the nature of the verbal memory deficit in Alzheimer's disease. *Brain & Language, 25,* 323-341.

Matsui, M., Suzuki, M., Zhou, S., Takahashi, T., Kawasaki, Y., Yuuki, H., Kato, K., & Kurachi, M. (2008). The relationship between prefrontal brain volume and characteristics of memory strategy in schizophrenia spectrum disorders. *Progress in Neuro-Psychopharmacology & Biological Psychiatry, 32,* 1854-1862.

Matsui, M., Yuuki, H., Kato, K., & Kurachi, M. (2006). Impairment of memory organization in patients with schizophrenia or schizotypal disorder. *Journal of the International Neuropsychological Society, 12,* 750-754.

McCutchan, J. A., Wu, J. W., Robertson, K., Koletar, S. L., Ellis, R. J., Cohn, S., Taylor, M., Woods, S., Heaton, R., Currier, J., & Williams, P. L. (2007). HIV suppression by HAART preserves cognitive function in advanced, immune-reconstituted AIDS patients. *AIDS, 21,* 1109-1117.

McKhann, G., Drachman, D., Folstein, M., Katzman, R., Price, D., & Stadlan, E. M. (1984). Clinical diagnosis of Alzheimer's disease: Report of the NINCDS-ADRDA Work Group under the auspices of Department of Health and Human Services Task Force on Alzheimer's Disease. *Neurology, 34,* 939-944.

Medana, I. M., & Esiri, M. M. (2003). Axonal damage: a key predictor of outcome in the human CNS diseases. *Brain, 126,* 515-530.

Mesholam-Gately, R. I., Giuliano, A. J., Goff, K. P., Faraone, S. V., & Seidman, L. J. (2009). Neurocognition in first-episode schizophrenia: A meta-analytic review. *Neuropsychology, 23,* 315-336.

Moelter, S. T., Hill, S. K., Hughet, P., Gur, R. C., Gur, R. E., & Ragland, J. D. (2005). Organization of semantic category exemplars in schizophrenia. *Schizophrenia Research, 78,* 209-217.

Mohamed, S., Paulsen, J. S., O'Leary, D., Arndt, S., & Andreasen, N. (1999). Generalized cognitive deficits in schizophrenia: A study of first-episode patients. *Archives of General Psychiatry, 56,* 749-754.

Moore, D. J., Masliah, E., Rippeth, J. D., Gonzalez, R., Carey, C. L., Cherner, M., Ellis, R. J., Achim, C. L., Marcotte, T. D., Heaton, R. K., Grant, I., & HNRC Group. (2006). Cortical and subcortical neurodegeneration is associated with HIV neurocognitive impairment. *AIDS, 20,* 879-887.

Mori, T. (1975). Processes underlying clustering in free recall. *Hiroshima Forum for Psychology, 2,* 25-30.

Murji, S., Rourke, S. B., Donders, J., Carter, S. L., Shore, D., & Rourke, B. P. (2003). Theoretically derived CVLT subtypes in HIV-1 infection: Internal and external validation. *Journal of the International Neuropsychological Society, 9,* 1-16.

National Institutes of Health (1999). NIH consensus development panel on rehabilitation of persons with traumatic brain injury. *Journal of the American Medical Association, 282,* 974-983.

Nielsen-Bohlman, L., & Knight, R. T. (1994). Electrophysiological dissociation of rapid memory mechanisms in humans. *NeuroReport, 5,* 1517-1521.

Nopoulos, P., Flashman, L., Flaum, M., & Arndt, S. (1994). Stability of cognitive functioning early in the course of schizophrenia. *Schizophrenia Research, 14,* 29-37.

Nyberg, L., Cabeza, R., & Tulving, E. (1996). PET studies of encoding and retrieval: The HERA model. *Psychonomic Bulletin & Review, 3,* 135-148.

Nyberg, L., Forkstam, C., Petersson, K. M., Cabeza, R., & Ingvar, M. (2002). Brain inmaging of human memory systems: between-systems similarities and within-system differences. *Cognitive Brain Research, 13,* 281-292.

Nyberg, L., Marklund, P., Persson, J., Cabeza, R., Forkstam, C., Petersson, K. M., & Ingvar, M. (2003). Common prefrontal activations during working memory, episodic memory, and semantic memory. *Neuropsychologia.Special Issue: Functional Neuroimaging of Memory, 41,* 371-377.

Panegyres, P. K. (2004). The contribution of the study of neurodegenerative disorders to the understanding of human memory. *QJM: An International Journal of Medicine, 97,* 555-567.

Parmenter, B. A., Shucard, J. L., Benedict, R. H. B., & Shucard, D. W. (2006). Working memory deficits in multiple sclerosis: Comparison between the n-back task and the paced auditory serial addition test. *Journal of the International Neuropsychological Society, 12,* 677-687.

Paul, R., Cohen, R., Navia, B., & Tashima, K. (2002). Relationships between cognition and structural neuroimaging findings in adults with human immunodeficiency virus type-1. *Neuroscience and Biobehavioral Reviews, 26,* 353-359.

Paulsen, J. S., Heaton, R. K., Sadek, J. R., & Perry, W. (1995). The nature of learning and memory impairments in schizophrenia. *Journal of the International Neuropsychological Society, 1,* 88-99.

Peavy, G., Jacobs, D., Salmon, D. P., & Butters, N. (1994). Verbal memory performance of patients with human immunodeficiency virus infection: Evidence of subcortical dysfunction. *Journal of Clinical and Experimental Neuropsychology, 16,* 508-523.

Pfefferbaum, A., Rosenbloom, M. J., Adalsteinsson, E., & Sullivan, E. V. (2007). Diffusion tensor imaging with quantitative fibre tracking in HIV infection and alcoholism comorbidity: Synergistic white matter damage. *Brain, 130,* 48-64.

Ragin, A. B., Storey, P., Cohen, B. A., Edelman, R. R., & Epstein, L. G. (2004). Disease burden in HIV-associated cognitive impairment: A study of whole-brain imaging measures. *Neurology, 63,* 2293-2297.

Ragin, A. B., Wu, Y., Storey, P., Cohen, B. A., Edelman, R. R., & Epstein, L. G. (2005). Diffusion tensor imaging of subcortical brain injury in patients infected with human immunodeficiency virus. *Journal of NeuroVirology, 11,* 292-298.

Ragland, J. D., Gur, R. C., Valdez, J. N., Loughead, J., Elliott, M., Kohler, C., …Gur, R. E. (2005). Levels-of-processing effect on frontotemporal function in schizophrenia during word encoding and recognition. *The American Journal of Psychiatry, 162,* 1840-1848.

Ragland, J. D., Laird, A. R., Ranganath, C., Blumenfeld, R. S., Gonzales, S. M., & Glahn, D. C. (2009). Prefrontal activation deficits during episodic memory in schizophrenia. *The American Journal of Psychiatry, 166,* 863-874.

Ragland, J. D., Moelter, S. T., McGrath, C., Hill, S. K., Gur, R. E., Bilker, W. B., ... Gur, R. C. (2003). Levels-of-processing effect on word recognition in schizophrenia. *Biological Psychiatry, 54,* 1154-1161.

Rajji, T. K., Ismail, Z., & Mulsant, B. H. (2009). Age at onset and cognition in schizophrenia: Meta-analysis. *British Journal of Psychiatry, 195,* 286-293.

Ranganath, C., Johnson, M. K., & D'Esposito, M. (2003). Prefrontal activity associated with working memory and episodic long-term memory. *Neuropsychologia, 41,* 378–389.

Ranganath, C., Minzenberg, M. J., & Ragland, J. D. (2008). The cognitive neuroscience of memory function and dysfunction in schizophrenia. *Biological Psychiatry, 64,* 18-25.

Rao, S. M. (1996). White matter disease and dementia. *Brain & Cognition, 31,* 250-268.

Rao, S. M., Grafman, J., DiGiulio, D., Mittenberg, W., Bernardin, L., Leo, G. J., Luchetta, T., & Unverzagt, F. (1993). Memory dysfunction in multiple sclerosis: Its relation to working memory, semantic encoding, and implicit learning. *Neuropsychology, 7,* 364-374.

Robertson, K. R., Smurzynski, M., Parsons, T. D., Wu, K., Bosch, R. J., Wu, J., McArthur, J. C., Collier, A. C., Evans, S. R., & Ellis, R. J. (2007). The prevalence and incidence of neurocognitive impairment in the HAART era. *AIDS, 21,* 1915-1921.

Robinson-Papp, J., Elliott, K. J., & Simpson, D. M. (2009). HIV-related neurocognitive impairment in the HAART era. *Current HIV/AIDS Reports, 6,* 146-152.

Sacktor, N., Nakasujja, N., Skolasky, R., Robertson, K., Wong, M., Musisi, S., Ronald, A., & Katabira, E. (2006). Antiretroviral therapy improves cognitive impairment in HIV + individuals in sub-Saharan Africa. *Neurology, 67,* 311-314.

Sailor, K. M., Bramwell, A., & Griesing, T. A. (1998). Evidence for an impaired ability to determine semantic relations in Alzheimer's disease patients. *Neuropsychology, 12,* 555-564.

Salmon, D. P., & Bondi, M. W. (1999). Neuropsychology of Alzheimer disease. In: R. D. Terry, R. Katzman, K. L. Bick, S. S. Sisodia (Eds.), *Alzheimer disease* (pp. 39–56), 2nd ed. Philadelphia: Lippincott Williams & Wilkins.

Sánchez-Carrión, R., Gómez, P. V., Junqué, C., Fernández-Espejo, D., Falcon, C., Bargalló, N., Roig-Rovira, T., Enseñat-Cantallops, A., & Bernabeu, M. (2008). Frontal hypoactivation on functional magnetic resonance imaging in working memory after severe diffuse traumatic brain injury. *Journal of Neurotrauma, 25,* 479-494.

Saykin, A. J., Shtasel, D. L., Gur, R. E., & Kester, D. B. (1994). Neuropsychological deficits in neuroleptic naive patients with first-episode schizophrenia. *Archives of General Psychiatry, 51,* 124-131.

Schmitter-Edgecombe, M., Marks, W., Wright, M. J., & Ventura, M. (2004). Retrieval inhibition in directed forgetting following severe closed-head injury. *Neuropsychology, 18,* 104-114.

Schwindt, G. C., & Black, S. E. (2009). Functional imaging studies of episodic memory in Alzheimer's disease: A quantitative meta-analysis. *NeuroImage, 45,* 181-190.

Scott, J. C., Woods, S. P., Patterson, K. A., Morgan, E. E., Heaton, R. K., & Grant, I. et al. (2006). Recency effects in HIV-associated dementia are characterized by deficient encoding. *Neuropsychologia, 44,* 1336-1343.

Sepulcre, J., Masdeu, J. C., Pastor, M. A., Goñi, J., Barbosa, C., Bejarano, B., & Villoslada, P. (2009). Brain pathways of verbal working memory: A lesion–function correlation study. *NeuroImage, 47,* 773-778.

Spaan, P. E. J., Raaijmakers, J. G. W., & Jonker, C. (2003). Alzheimer's disease versus normal ageing: A review of the efficiency of clinical and experimental memory measures. *Journal of Clinical and Experimental Neuropsychology, 25,* 216-230.

Squire, L. R. (1994). Memory and forgetting: Long-term and gradual changes in memory storage. *International Review of Neurobiology, 37,* 243-269.

Squire, L. R. (1980). Specifying the defect in human amnesia: Storage, retrieval, and semantics. *Neuropsychologia, 18,* 369-372.

Squire, L. R., & Zola, S. M. (1998). Episodic memory, semantic memory, and amnesia. *Hippocampus, 8,* 205-211.

Stallings, G., Boake, C., & Sherer, M. (1995). Comparison of the California Verbal Learning Test and the Rey Auditory Verbal Learning Test in head-injured patients. *Journal of Clinical and Experimental Neuropsychology, 17,* 706-712.

Strange, B. A., Otten, L. J., Josephs, O., Rugg, M. D., & Dolan, R. J. (2002). Dissociable human perirhinal, hippocampal, and parahippocampal roles during verbal encoding. *Journal of Neuroscience, 15,* 523-528.

Stricker, J. L., Brown, G. G., Wixted, J., Baldo, J. V., & Delis, D. C. (2002). New semantic clustering indices for the California Verbal Learning Test-second edition: Background, rational, and formulae. *Journal of the International Neuropsychological Society, 8,* 425-435.

Surprenant, A. M., & Neath, I. (2009). The nine lives of short-term memory. In A. S. C. Thorn, & M. P. A. Page (Eds.), *Interactions between short-term and long-term memory in the verbal domain.* (pp. 16-43). New York, NY, US: Psychology Press.

Sweet, L. H., Rao, S. M., Primeau, M., Durgerian, S., & Cohen, R. A. (2006). Functional magnetic resonance imaging response to increased verbal working memory demands among patients with multiple sclerosis. *Human Brain Mapping, 27,* 28-36.

Takei, K., Yamasue, H., Abe, O., Yamada, H., Inoue, H., Suga, M., Sekita, K., Sasaki, H., Rogers, M., Aoki, S., & Kasai, K. (2008). Disrupted integrity of the fornix is associated with impaired memory organization in schizophrenia. *Schizophrenia Research, 103,* 52-61.

Talamini, L. M., de Haan, L., Nieman, D. H., Linszen, D. H., & Meeter, M. (2010). Reduced context effects on retrieval in first-episode Schizophrenia. *PLoS ONE, 5,* e10356. Retrieved from: http://www.plosone.org/article/info%3Adoi%2F10.1371%2Fjournal.pone.0010356.

Teasdale, G., & Jennett, B. (1974). Assessment of coma and impaired consciousness: A practical scale. *Lancet, 1,* 81-84.

Tek, C., Gold, J., Blaxton, T., Wilk, C., McMahon, R. P., & Buchanan, R. W. (2002). Visual perceptual and working memory impairments in schizophrenia. *Archives of General Psychiatry, 59,* 146-153.

Thorn, A. S. C., & Page, M. P. A. (2009). Current issues in understanding interactions between short-term and long-term memory. In A. S. C. Thorn, & M. P. A. Page (Eds.), *Interactions between short-term and long-term memory in the verbal domain.* (pp. 1-15). New York, NY, US: Psychology Press.

Thornton, A. E., Raz, N., & Tucker, K. A. (2002). Memory in multiple sclerosis: Contextual encoding deficits. *Journal of the International Neuropsychological Society, 8,* 395-409.

Timmerman, M. E., & Brouwer, W. H. (1999). Slow information processing after very severe closed head injury: Impaired access to declarative knowledge and intact application and acquisition of procedural knowledge. *Neuropsychologia, 37,* 467-478.

Ting, C., Rajji, T. K., Ismail, Z., Tang-Wai, D. F., Apanasiewicz, N., Miranda, D., ... Mulsant, B. H. (2010). Differentiating the cognitive profile of Schizophrenia from that of Alzheimer disease and depression in late life. *PLoS ONE, 5*: e10151. Retrieved from: http://www.plosone.org/article/info:doi/10.1371/journal.pone.0010151

Tulving, E. & Markowitsch, H. J. (1997). Memory beyond the hippocampus. *Current Opinion in Neurobiology, 7,* 209-216.

Tulving, E. (1972). Episodic and semantic memory. In E. Tulving & W. Donaldson (Eds.), *Organization of Memory* (pp. 381-402). New York: Academic Press.

Tulving, E. (1985). How many memory systems are there? *American Psychologist, 40,* 385-398.

Tulving, E., & Craik, F. (2005). *The Oxford handbook of memory.* Oxford: Oxford University Press.

Tulving, E., & Markowitsch, H. J. (1998). Episodic and declarative memory: Role of the hippocampus. *Hippocampus, 8,* 198-204.

Tulving, E., & Osler, S. (1968). Effectiveness of retrieval cues in memory for words. *Journal of Experimental Psychology, 77,* 593-601.

Tulving, E., & Thompson, D. M. (1973). Encoding specificity and retrieval processes in episodic memory. *Psychological Review, 80,* 352-373.

Turner, G. R., & Levine, B. (2008). Augmented neural activity during executive control processing following diffuse axonal injury. *Neurology, 71,* 812-818.

Vallat-Azouvi, C., Weber, T., Legrand, L., & Azouvi, P. (2007). Working memory after severe traumatic brain injury. *Journal of the International Neuropsychological Society. Special Issue: Reviews, 13,* 770-780.

Van Snellenberg, J. X. (2009). Working memory and long-term memory deficits in schizophrenia: Is there a common substrate? *Psychiatry Research: Neuroimaging, 174,* 89-96.

Van Snellenberg, J. X., Torres, I. J., & Thornton, A. E. (2006). Functional Neuroimaging of Working Memory in Schizophrenia: Task Performance as a Moderating Variable. *Neuropsychology, 20,* 497-510.

Vehmas, A., Lieu, J., Pardo, C. A., McArthur, J. C., & Gartner, S. (2004). Amyloid precursor protein expression in circulating monocytes and brain macrophages from patients with HIV-associated cognitive impairment. *Journal of Neuroimmunology.Special Issue: Molecular Markers and Mechanisms of HIV-Induced Nervous System Disease, 157,* 99-110.

Venneri, A., McGeown, W. J., Hietanen, H. M., Guerrini, C., Ellis, A. W., & Shanks, M. F. (2008). The anatomical bases of semantic retrieval deficits in early Alzheimer's disease. *Neuropsychologia, 46,* 497-510.

Vingerhoets, G., Miatton, M., Vonck, K., Seurinck, R., & Boon, P. (2006). Memory performance during the intracarotid amobarbital procedure and neuropsychological assessment in medial temporal lobe epilepsy: The limits of material specificity. *Epilepsy & Behavior, 8,* 422-428.

Wager, T. D., & Smith, E. E. (2003). Neuroimaging studies of working memory: A meta-analysis. *Cognitive, Affective & Behavioral Neuroscience, 3,* 255-274.

Waldrop, D., Ownby, R. L., & Kumar, M. (2004). Serial position effects in HIV-infected injecting drug users. *International Journal of Neuroscience, 114,* 493-516.

Ward, A., Caro, J. J., Kelley, H., Eggleston, A., & Molloy, W. (2002). Describing cognitive decline of patients at the mild or moderate stages of Alzheimer's disease using the standardized MMSE. *International Psychogeriatrics, 14,* 249-258.

Weiss, A. P., & Heckers, S. (2001). Neuroimaging of declarative memory in schizophrenia. *Scandinavian Journal of Psychology, 42,* 239-250.

White, D. A., Taylor, M. J., Butters, N., Mack, C., Salmon, D. P., Peavy, G., et al. (1997). Memory for verbal information in individuals with HIV-Associated Dementia Complex. *Journal of Clinical and Experimental Neuropsychology, 19,* 357-366.

Wiegner, S., & Donders, J. (1999). Performance on the California Verbal Learning Test after traumatic brain injury. *Journal of Clinical and Experimental Neuropsychology, 21,* 159-170.

Wilde, M. C., Boake, C., & Sherer, M. (1995). Do recognition-free recall discrepancies detect retrieval deficits in closed-head injury? An exploratory analysis with the California Verbal Learning Test. *Journal of Clinical and Experimental Neuropsychology, 17,* 849-855.

Williamson, D. J. G., Scott, J. G., & Adams, R. L. (1996). Traumatic brain injury. In R. L. Adams, O. A. Parsons, J. L. Culbertson, & S. J. Nixon (Eds.), *Neuropsychology for clinical practice: Etiology, assessment, and treatment of common neurological disorders* (pp. 9-64). Washington, DC, US: American Psychological Association.

Wilson, J. T. L., Hadley, D. M., Wiedmann, K. D., & Teasdale, G. M. (1995). Neuropsychological consequences of two patterns of brain damage shown by MRI in survivors of severe head injury. *Journal of Neurology, Neurosurgery & Psychiatry, 59,* 328-331.

Wright, M. J., Schmitter-Edgecombe, M., & Woo, E. (2010a). Verbal memory impairment in severe closed-head injury: The role of encoding and consolidation. *Journal of Clinical and Experimental Neuropsychology, 32,* 728-736.

Wright, M. J., Woo, E., Foley, J., Ettenhofer, M. L., Cottingham, M. E., Gooding, A. L., Jang, J., Kim, M. S., Castellon, S. A., Miller, E. N., & Hinkin, C. H. (March, 2010b). *HAART adherence and the expression of verbal memory impairment in HIV.* Poster presentation at the 21st annual meeting of the American Neuropsychiatric Association, Tampa, FL.

Wright, M. J., Woo, E., Schmitter-Edgecombe, M., Hinkin, C. H., Miller, E. N., & Gooding, A. L. (2009). The Item-Specific Deficit Approach (ISDA) to evaluating verbal memory dysfunction: Rationale, psychometrics, and application. *Journal of Clinical and Experimental Neuropsychology, 31,* 790-802.

York, M. K., Franks, J. J., Henry, R. R., & Hamilton, W. J. (2001). Verbal working memory storage and processing deficits in HIV-1 asymptomatic and symptomatic individuals. *Psychological Medicine, 31,* 1279-1291.

In: Working Memory: Capacity, Developments and... ISBN: 978-1-61761-980-9
Editor: Eden S. Levin © 2011 Nova Science Publishers, Inc.-

Chapter 6

WORKING MEMORY IN PRETERM AND FULL-TERM INFANTS

Jing Sun[1]* *and Nicholas Buys*[1]
[1] Griffith Health Institute, Griffith University, Australia

ABSTRACT

Introduction

This study investigated working memory in preterm and full-term infants at 8 months after expected date of delivery. Working memory is defined as "the ability to maintain an appropriate problem solving set for the attainment of a future goal" [1, p. 201]. An important characteristic of working memory is that it is prospective, that is, its purpose is to attain a goal, and it not only enables information to be held in mind but also to be manipulated. Working memory emerges in infancy and continues to develop throughout childhood. Working memory is believed to underlie some learning problems in children at school age. Although numerous studies have reported that the overall development of preterm infants is comparable to that of full-term infants at the same corrected age, it is unclear to what extent the development of specific cognitive abilities is affected by prematurity and/or other factors such as medical complications. As preterm infants have a high rate of learning difficulties, it is possible that factors associated with prematurity specifically affect the development of some regions of the brain associated with the regulation of working memory.

Methods

The current study aimed to examine the effects of maturation and length of exposure to extrauterine environmental stimuli on the development of working memory, by comparing the development of preterm infants with that of full-term infants at both the

---

[*] Corresponding author: j.sun@griffith.edu.au; School of Public Health, Griffith University, & Griffith Health Institute, Griffith University Meadowbrook Q4131 Australia.

same corrected age and the same chronological age. A case-control study design was used for the study. Thirty-seven preterm infants without identified disabilities and 74 full-term and gender matched healthy full-term infants participated in the study. The preterm infants were all less than 32 weeks gestation and less than 1500 grams birthweight. All infants were assessed on working memory tasks at 8 months after the expected date of delivery (when preterm infants were actually 10-11 months chronological age).

Results

The findings of the study showed that preterm infants performed significantly more poorly than full-term infants at 8 months after the expected date of delivery on measures of working memory. The results suggest that the effects of maturation are greater than the effects of exposure to extrauterine environmental stimuli on the development of working memory. Furthermore, the preterm infants were divided into two subgroups on the basis of (a) low or high medical risk factors, (b) birthweight of < 1000 g versus 1000-1500 g, and (c) gestation age of < 28 weeks versus 28-32 weeks, in order to assess the effects of these variables on the performance of working memory. Medical risk, lower birthweight and lower gestation age were all found to adversely affect performance on working memory.

Discussions and Conclusions

It is argued that medical risk, lower birthweight and lower gestation factors may influence the development of specific areas of the brain which govern working memory, and given that the prefrontal regions are particularly immature they may be especially vulnerable to damage or disruption. The present study provides further insights into the emergence of working memory in infants and the feasibility of evaluating these abilities in infants who are at risk for further learning difficulties and attention deficits.

INTRODUCTION

Advances in medical technology continue to improve the survival rate of preterm infants, so that increasing numbers of children who weigh < 1000 g at birth are surviving and entering the school system [2, 3]. These at-risk children have been the focus of much research and many follow-up studies have identified a strong relationship between birthweight and learning development at school age [4-6]. Confounding this relationship, however, is the fact that as birthweight declines, the number and severity of perinatal complications experienced by infants is likely to increase [7].

Extensive attempts have been made to identify sensitive predictors of later learning problems in both term and preterm children [8-10]. It has been accepted that learning problems have multiple determinants, and it is important to consider the interactions of biological factors (such as medical complications and genetic endowment), environmental factors (such as demographic factors, quality of educational experience, socioeconomic, and psychosocial factors), and developmental factors (such as specific cognitive abilities and general development as measured by infant general development assessment) [11, 12]. Frequently there is an association between perinatal risk and poor social circumstances. Several studies have demonstrated that social factors, particularly low educational level of the parents and socioeconomic status, play an important role in the intellectual outcome of both healthy full-term and preterm infants and those who had perinatal medical complications [12-15].

The population of Very Low Birthweight (VLBW, birthweight between 1001-1500 grams) and Extremely Low Brithweight (ELBW, birthweight less than 1000 grams or 750 grams) infants is known to be at increased risk for a broad spectrum of health and developmental problems, and also an increased incidence of psychosocial disadvantages (e.g., poverty, single parenthood, youthful maternal age, and limited parental education), producing a "doubly vulnerable" population, which places their development in even greater jeopardy [16, 17]. The assessment of subtle developmental and behavioural delays in infants is complicated, and currently there are few sensitive measures available for the early identification of learning problems in infants. Conventional developmental assessment tools, such as the Bayley Scales of Infant Development, [18] only provide global indicators of development and fail to measure specific skills that may provide sensitive predictions of later learning.

The assessment of specific cognitive skills, in particular working memory, rather than a global development score in infancy, has been advocated by a number of investigators [19-21]. Working memory is defined as "the ability to maintain an appropriate problem solving set for the attainment of a future goal" [1, p. 201]. Working memory deficits have been linked to a range of developmental problems, including attentional deficit disorder (ADD), learning difficulties, and autism, all of which are more prevalent in children born preterm [22, 23]. Studying a group of infants at high-risk for learning difficulties should make it easier to identify factors that are predictive of later learning problems. This may lead to a greater understanding of the etiology of these problems in all children.

In Welsh and Pennington's model of working memory, certain information remains at the forefront of cognition, despite distraction, and hence is active for the purpose of guiding appropriate responses. An important characteristic of working memory is that it is prospective, that is, its purpose is to attain a goal. Fuster [24] suggested that this is achieved not only by holding information in mind, but also by guiding goal directed actions. Graham and Harris [25] stated that working memory is also necessary in tasks which require strategy selection, monitoring, and revision of actions. This implies that working memory not only enables information to be held in mind but also to be manipulated. It is generally agreed that these behaviours are governed by the prefrontal cortex of the brain [24, 26]. This part of the brain is late in developing and therefore may be particularly vulnerable to damage in preterm infants.

Evidence from Animal and Lesions Studies in Humans

Evidence for the link between working memory and prefrontal lobe has come from a wide range of sources including studies of the effects of brain lesions [27-30], neurophysiological, and neuroimaging investigations of animals, and both normal and clinical human populations [31-35]. Several researchers [i.e., 24, 36, 37] suggested that the frontal lobe may be divided into three regions: dorsolateral, orbital, and medial cortex. It has been shown that the dorsolateral region of the prefrontal cortex mediates the functioning of working memory [24].

Originally, most experimental studies examining working memory consequences of damage to the dosolateral region of the prefrontal lobe was conducted on animals [38-40]. These studies, which involved ablation or temporary inactivation of the dorsolateral part of the prefrontal lobe of the brain, provided vital information about the location of various cognitive functions within the brain. In ablation studies, large lesions of the prefrontal cortex produced decrements in performance on the Delayed Response (DR) task which was designed to measure working memory in the literature [41, 42]. In the DR task, an infant sits before two identical hiding locations (e.g., cloth covers, cups or wells) that are separated by a small distance. While the infant watches, a desired object is hidden in one location, location A. After a delay, the infant is allowed to reach and search for the object. Then while the infant watches, the object is hidden at the second location, location B. After a delay, the infant is allowed to reach and search for the object. The sequence of hiding locations in A and B in the DR task is random. Temporary, reversible depression or inactivation of the cortex by cooling [43], or the injection of drugs [44], induced a similar marked deterioration in performance on such tasks. The importance of these latter studies is that they showed that the effect was reversible and could be repeated on the same subject, clearly demonstrating that it was due to inactivity of the prefrontal cortex and not to some side effects of surgical intervention, and that it was consistent and repeatable. No deficits in DR task performance appeared on depressing or cooling other areas of the brain such as the parietal cortex. Although most of the above studies were conducted on adult primates, these studies provided vital information about a link between the prefrontal cortex and working memory.

Data on the effects of brain lesions on behaviour in humans are derived mainly from case reports of individuals who have sustained specific brain lesions [e.g., 27, 45, 46, 47], or from studies of clinical populations who have sustained somewhat diffuse brain injuries [e.g., 48, 49-51]. Many of the findings from these clinical observations have now been corroborated and extended in normal subjects using neuroimaging techniques, such as magnetic resonance imaging (MRI), positron emission tomography (PET), and single photon emission computed tomography [e.g., 31, 32, 33]. The evidence obtained suggests that damage to any part of the dorsolateral frontal lobe due to trauma, tumour, vascular accident or other disease processes produces deficits in working memory, leading to poor temporal integration of behaviour [51-56]. The subject fails to remember information or is not motivated to remember, and has a limited capacity to adapt to new situations because of difficulties in planning future actions that deviate from ordinary routines.

Impairment of Working Memory

Patients with frontal lobe damage have consistently been found to display deficits in working memory on a large variety of different assessment tools. For example, a number of studies using DR tasks with visual, auditory, and kinesthetic stimuli have clearly demonstrated the difficulties experienced by patients with frontal lobe damage [57-60]. For example, they could not do these tasks when time delays imposed by a research on a task.

These problems with working memory are not seen in normal subjects and patients with other cortical lesions, such as temporal-lobe damage and posterior cortical lesions [38, 57].

The Development of Frontal Lobe in Human Infants

The prefrontal cortex is one of the last regions of the central nervous system to undergo full myelination, and developmental changes originating from frontal lobe development are evident in several periods of life [61]. The most active periods of development of the prefrontal cortex appear to be in the first 2 years of life, then between 7 and 9 years, and finally in adolescence. The development of the frontal lobe in infants deserves particular mention because during this period remarkable and rapid changes occur in both the neural physiology and the behaviour of the human being. For the frontal cortex, the period of maximum synaptic excess appears to be in the second half of the first year [62], after which there occurs a protracted period of decline in synaptic density through selective elimination of little used pathways. Recent studies of human brain activity using positron emission tomography (PET) technique documented developmental changes in rates of glucose metabolism [63]. These changes are characterised by a rise in metabolism in the frontal region at approximately 6-8 months of age, followed by a prolonged period of decline in rates of metabolism which parallels the decline in synaptic density [63]. Thus, it seems that the significant and rapid changes related to anatomy and function of the fontal lobe occur in the second half of the first year after birth and continue more slowly after this early period.

There is ample evidence that working memory also develops dramatically during the second half of the first year of life. For example, infants can hold information in mind for increasing periods of time and use this information to direct and regulate their responses. Behaviours of this type have been shown in numerous studies to be related to the prefrontal cortex.

Bell and Fox [64] further demonstrated a relationship between working memory and prefrontal lobe functioning and showed individual differences in frontal-brain electrical activity, as shown in EEG recordings and performance on the AB task. Infants at eight months of age who succeeded on the AB task exhibited greater power values in the frontal EEG during baseline recordings than infants who were unable to do the task [64, 65].

Additional evidence for the importance of prefrontal cortex maturation for the development of working memory abilities has come from studies of children with phenylketonuria [66]. Even when treated, this genetically transmitted error of metabolism can have the specific consequence of reducing the levels of the neurotransmitter dopamine in the dorsolateral prefrontal cortex. This results in impaired performance on tasks thought to measure working memory, such as the AB task [41, 42]. The standard AB task was originally described by Piaget [67] to measure the changes in the concept of object permanence in human infants. In Piaget's AB task, an infant sits before two identical hiding places, often referred to as occluders (e.g., two identical cloth covers or two identical lids) that are separated by a small distance. While the infant watches, a desired object is hidden in one location (A). After a delay, the infant is allowed to reach and search for the object. This hiding and search at location A is repeated. Then while the infant watches, the object is hidden at the second location (B). After the delay, the infant is allowed to reach and search for the object. Infants frequently make the error of searching again at location A, committing what is known as the classic AB error. Thus both electrophysiological and behavioural data provide support for the relation between the development of the prefrontal cortex and the emergence of working memory in the first year of life.

During this important maturation process in the first year of life, any damage or disturbance to the development of the prefrontal cortex due to disease, trauma, or conditions associated with perinatal risk factors (i.e., medical complications, extremely low birthweight, shorter gestation age) may therefore lead to working memory dysfunctioning. Diamond and Goldman-Rakic [68] used animal models to examine whether lesions of the dorsolateral prefrontal cortex would have the same effect on infant monkeys as on adult monkeys. Two of the infant rhesus monkeys were tested longitudinally on the AB and the DR tasks. They received bilateral lesions of the dorsolateral prefrontal cortex at 5½ months. They were then tested on the AB task at 6 months. The findings showed that the infant monkeys that had the prefrontal lesions displayed poorer performance on the AB task than their age mates who did not have the prefrontal lesions. The lesions produced the same effect in infant monkeys as they did in adult monkeys with prefrontal lesions: they all reached incorrectly when the delay increased to 2-5 seconds s after the toy changed to the new hiding position.

Damage to the prefrontal lobe due to trauma and disease in infancy may have lifelong effects on working memory abilities, and may cause learning difficulties during school years [28, 69]. In comparison with adults, childhood frontal lobe lesions produce a more pervasive impairment, interfering with the acquisition of age-appropriate working memory skills. Most studies on the relationship between working memory development and frontal lobe damage in children are based on older children [49, 70]. However, a recent case study by Anderson, Damasio, Tranel, and Damasio [71] reported that an infant who had right frontal region damage at 3 months showed severe learning difficulties and behavioural problems at school, and failure in career development in adulthood despite average intelligence (as measured by traditional intelligence tests at school age and during adulthood). The study found that the impairments largely reflected a failure to develop working memory. These findings are consistent with the notion that early damage to prefrontal regions can lead to severe disruption of working memory, while not significantly affecting many aspects tapped by standard intelligence tests. They also suggest that the prefrontal cortex may have limited neuronal plasticity which contributes to poor working memory if the damage occurs early. This may be due to disruption to the laying down of the neural architectures which are viewed as the foundation of cognitive development. A detailed examination of the relationship between prefrontal cortex development and the development of working memory in a large sample of human infants has not been possible because of the relative lack of obvious prefrontal lesions in infants and the expense and lack of availability of neural imaging technology.

The prefrontal cortex of infants who are born preterm is even more immature and prone to damage from the multitude of adverse medical complications to which these frail infants may be exposed. Lesions or atypical development of the prefrontal cortex occurring as a consequence of these hazardous events may have a detrimental effect on the development of working memory which may have long-term consequences in terms of learning difficulties at school age. Indeed it has been found that children born preterm are at an increased risk for learning difficulties and attentional deficits when they reach school age and it has been suggested that this may be due to early abnormality in the development of the prefrontal cortex and consequently of working memory [23, 72].

Failure of working memory has been shown to underlie learning difficulties and attention deficits in children and these problems are particularly common in children born preterm. Historically, the assessment of working memory in infants was thought impossible. However, recent neuropsychological research has suggested that the A*B* task provide avenues for research on working memory.

This study was undertaken to compare the performance of preterm and full-term infants of the same corrected age (8 months) age and 10-11 month chronological age on tests related to working memory.

The following two hypotheses will be tested through the study:

Hypothesis 1: There will be significant difference between preterm and full-term infants of the same chronological age in the performance of working memory task (i.e., exposure to extrauterine environmental stimuli is the key factor influencing the development of working memory.

Hypothesis 2: There will be significant difference between preterm and full-term infants of the same corrected age in the performance of working memory task (i.e., maturation of the central nervous system from the time of conception is the key factors influencing the development of working memory).

METHODS

Study Design

This research involves the comparison of a cohort of ELBW infants ($n = 37$) and two comparison groups of full-term infants ($n = 37$ in each group) matched for gender and the age since expected date of delivery. The purpose of having two full-term comparison groups is to increase the statistical power. All infants were assessed on the working memory task. This measure formed the dependent variable.

Infants were also assessed on the confounding factors in the present study: perinatal variables which consist of medical complications, birthweight, and gestation age. All infants were assessed on the above variables at 8 months after the expected date of delivery (preterm infants were 10 to 11 months chronological age at this time). Term infants were reassessed at an age equivalent to the chronological age of the matched preterm infant at the time of the first assessment. This retest provided a comparison with the preterm infants on the basis of chronological age.

Participants

Participants consisted of two groups – preterm and fullterm infants.

1. Preterm infants: The mothers of 41 preterm infants, who attended the Growth and Development Unit at Mater Children's Hospital in Brisbane, Australia, responded to

an invitation to participate in this study. These preterm infants were all born at the Mater Mothers' Hospital, Brisbane, Australia, between May 1998 and July 1999. Inclusion criteria for preterm infants were:

< 1500 g birthweight,
< 32 weeks of gestation,
eight months of age after expected date of delivery,
no evidence of severe visual, auditory or neurological impairment, or severe congenital anomalies,
living in the Brisbane metropolitan area, and
mother was English-speaking.

Of the 41 preterm infants, 37 were included in the study group. Two infants were excluded from the study due to severe intellectual and neurological problems and two other infants were excluded from the data analysis due to errors in the administration of some of the test items. There were two sets of twins and one set of triplets.

2. Full-term Infants: Names and addresses of potential full-term comparison infants who were the same sex as the matched preterm infants, born at the Mater Mothers' Hospital on the same expected date of delivery, were obtained from medical records at the hospital. Parents were then contacted by a letter, and provided with an information sheet, and a follow-up telephone call. A total of 207 letters were sent, and of these 74 mothers of infants with birth weights of > 2500g were selected to match the corresponding preterm infants on a first-come basis. Inclusion criteria for full-term infants were:

> 2500 grams birthweight,
38-42 weeks of gestation,
same sex as matched preterm infant,
born on the same expected date of delivery as the matched preterm infant,
no evidence of perinatal complications or congenital abnormalities,
living in the Brisbane metropolitan area,
mother was English speaking, and
developmentally normal

In summary, all infants recruited into this study were born at the same hospital and tested at eight months (+ or - 2 weeks) after the expected date of delivery. Full term infants were reassessed when they were 10-11 month chronological age. All subjects lived within a 50-kilometre radius of the Mater Mothers' Hospital and did not have identifiable disabilities at the time of assessment.

Participation in the project was voluntary and informed consent was obtained from at least one parent of each child. Ethical approval for the project was obtained from the Mater Children's and Mater Mothers' Hospital Ethics Committees, and the Queensland University of Technology Research Ethics Committee.

Working Memory Task

The assessment of working memory was based on a task derived from the A*B* and DR tasks which have been described in the literature [41, 42]. In the A*B* task, an infant sits before two identical hiding locations (e.g., cloth covers, cups or wells) that are separated by a small distance. While the infant watches, a desired object is hidden in one location, location A. After a delay, the infant is allowed to reach and search for the object. This hiding and searching at location A is repeated. Then while the infant watches, the object is hidden at the second location, location B. After a delay, the infant is allowed to reach and search for the object. Infants frequently make the error of searching again at location A committing what is known as the classic A*B* error. The sequence of hiding locations in the DR task is random, whereas the hiding locations in the A*B* task are determined by the number of correct searches at location A.

Procedure

The administration procedure is described below.

1. *Materials.* The following materials were used for the Infant Working Memory task: one yellow cup (used to cover the toys), two red cups, three blue cups, and three small toys for hiding under the cups.
2. *Pre-test.* This involved the experimenter putting a toy on the table in front of the infant while the infant was watching. The infants were allowed to retrieve the toy immediately to test whether they could reach it. If it was unclear whether the infant had reached for the toy (e.g., if the infant showed an interest in the examiner or waited for several seconds before reaching to the toy), this procedure was repeated.

Ability to successfully retrieve the hidden objects is influenced by the infant's interest in and attention to the task [73]. To maintain infant's attention to the task, the colours of the occluders (the cups under which the goal objects were hidden), were changed at set points in the test administration.

Administration of the Infant Working Memory task

1-cup task. The Infant Working Memory task started with a 1-cup task. One yellow opaque cup and three small round toys were used. A toy was placed directly in front of the infant, at a distance of approximately 20 cm. While the child watched, the opaque yellow cup was placed by the examiner over the toy so that the toy was invisible. For this trial and all subsequent trials the mother was asked to prevent the infant from reaching by gently holding him/her whilst the object was being covered and also during the imposition of a delay between hiding and retrieving the object. She was instructed, prior to the task, to release her child when the examiner said "find the toy." The infant's ability to remove the occluder and reach for the object underneath was then noted. Three trials were given for each of the delay periods (0, 4 and 10 s).

2-cup task. For the 2-cup task, two red opaque cups and the same three toys were used. One cup was positioned 11 cm to the right of the infant's midline, at a distance of 20 cm from the infant. The other was positioned 11 cm to the left, also at a distance of 20 cm from the infant. Testing began by positioning the goal object in front of the cup on the infant's left hand side. The cup was then moved to cover the object. The infant was then permitted to retrieve the object and allowed a few seconds to play with it. The toy was hidden in the following positions: right, right, left, left, and right for the remaining 5 trials. Then the delay time between hiding the object and retrieving was increased to 2 seconds. For the 2 s delayed period trial, the order for hiding the toy was: right, left, left, right, right, and left. The hiding locations for the 4 s delay was the same as that of the 0 s delay and the hiding locations for the 10 s delay was the same as for the 2 s delayed time condition.

3-cup task. In the 3-cup task, three blue cups and the same toys were used. In this condition, the toy was always hidden to the left and the right side of the infant and never in the middle. The order for the hiding location was the same as for the 2-cup condition. For the 2- and 3-cup difficulty level, the toy was always hidden on the left side first, because perseverative reaching has been demonstrated to be more common on an infant's right side [74].

For the 1-cup task, three trials were presented at each time delay of the task. From the 2-cup to 3-cup Infant Working Memory task, six trials were presented at each time delay of the task. Three round toys with three colours (red, yellow, and blue) were used as objects for hiding under the cups. These three toys were used for each trial each for the first three trials at each time delay level based on the colour sequence of red, yellow, and blue. The procedure for the presentation of toys were the same for the second three trials at each time delay level. During the inter-trial (i.e., between infant's retrieval and the preparation of next trial) interval, the experimenter gave the hidden toy to the infant to play with for approximately 20 s while the next trial was prepared. The inter-trial interval was about 20 seconds. A summary of the tasks is presented in Table 2.

Criteria used for termination and continuation of the task

Each infant was tested on the 1-cup, 2-cup, and 3-cup tasks. In each of these conditions, the infant started from the easiest level of time delay, 0 seconds. If the infant failed to reach to the appropriate occluder on three consecutive trials at any delay level, the next trial was administered with one extra cup and 0 s delay, otherwise testing continued at the next level of delay with the same number of cups. The criteria used for terminating the task or moving to the next level are described in more detail below.

1. 1-cup task. Three presentations of this task could be given at each time delay (0, 4, 10 s). If the infant succeeded in removing the cup and obtaining the object underneath within the time limit on at least two of three presentations, then the task was administered at next level of time delay. If the infant failed to obtain the object on all three trials at a given time delay, following completion of three trials at 10 s delay the examiner moved on to the 2-cup task with a 0 s time delay.
2. 2-cup task. Six presentations of the 2-cup task were given at each delay time. There were four delay times (0, 2, 4, and 10 s), making a total of 24 trials. If the infant succeeded in reaching to the correct position on at least three consecutive trials on a given time delay, the next level of time delay was then presented. During the 2-cup task, if the infant failed to reach to the appropriate occluder on three consecutive

trials at any delay level, testing of the 2-cup task was terminated, and the 3-cup task was administered with 0 s time delay.
3. 3-cup task. The criterion to pass this task was the same as in the 2-cup task. In this condition, if the infant failed to retrieve the toy on three consecutive trials at any delay level, the tester stopped the testing.

Table 1. Infant working memory task

Tasks	Number of hiding places	Occluder (cup/s)	Delay time between hiding and reaching	Location of hidden object
1 cup	1	Yellow cup	Level 1: 0 s delay Level 2: 4 s delay Level 3: 10 s delay	
2 cups	2	Red Cups	Level 1: 0 s delay Level 2: 2 s delay Level 3: 4 s delay Level 4: 10 s delay	L R **R** L L **R** R L L **R** R **L** L R **R** L L **R** R L L **R** R **L**
3 cups	3	Blue cups	Level 1: 0 s delay Level 2: 2 s delay Level 3: 4 s delay Level 4: 10 s delay	L R **R** L L **R** R L L **R** R **L** L R **R** L L **R** R L L **R** R **L**

Note. R in the table refers to the right side, L refers to the left side of the infant. The bold type refers to the change to a new hiding position that provided a measure of inhibition to a prepotent response.

Scoring scheme for working memory

As shown in Table 2, finding a hidden object in the 1-cup task requires infants to remember the hidden object rather than a location, and to be able to reach the hidden object. These are the criteria for the infants to perform the Infant Working Memory task. Finding a hidden object in location A in the 2- and 3-cup tasks requires working memory for location. Increasing the delay time between hiding and retrieval increases the difficulty of the task for infants [75].

Therefore working memory was scored on the memory for location, and this was scored on the basis of the 2- and 3-cup tasks in location A. A score of one was awarded if the infant remembered the location of the toy on the first trial of both 2- and 3-cup tasks, and on subsequent trials when the hiding position was the same position as on the previous trial (i.e., all the A trials which are the ones not in bold type in Table 2). The task administration was organised so that this was always the 1st, 3rd and 5th trial at each time delay level. The total number of correct trials from all A trials attempted was then calculated. Possible scores ranged from 0-12 for both the 2- and 3-cup tasks (i.e., a possible overall total range of 0-24).

Data Analysis

All data were analysed using the SPSS package version 17.0. Each preterm infant had two comparison term infants matched for gender and age. The comparison between the study group and comparison groups on working memory tasks at eight months corrected age and

10-11 months chronological age was analysed by multivariate analysis of variance to test Hypothesis 1 and Hypothesis 2.

If there was a significant difference between preterm and full-term infants, the confounding variables which may explain this difference were examined. Perinatal variables which might confound the effects of prematurity, such as medical risks, birthweight, and gestation age, were also examined using ANOVA to compare the differences between the two preterm and one full-term infant groups.

RESULTS

The aim of this analysis was to compare the performance of preterm and full-term infants of the same chronological age (i.e., 10-11 months after expected date of delivery) and the same corrected age (i.e., eight months after expected date of delivery) on working memory task.

The univariate ANOVAs showed that each of the components of working memory contributed significantly to the differences between groups for working memory measure. There was a significant difference between the preterm group and full-term infants group on the working memory task.

There were significant differences between preterm and full-term infants at 10-11 months chronological age in the performance of working memory. Preterm infants showed significantly poorer performance than the full-term infant groups on working memory. These results supported Hypothesis 1, which stipulated that there will be significant difference between preterm and full-term infants of the same chronological age in the performance of working memory task (i.e., exposure to extrauterine environmental stimuli is the key factor influencing the development of working memory

It was also found that there were significant differences between preterm and full-term infant groups at eight months corrected age on working memory. Specifically, preterm infants as a group had significantly poorer performances on working memory compared with the full-term infant groups at eight months corrected age. These results supported Hypothesis 2, that postulated that the performance of preterm infants is different to full-term infants of the same corrected age on measure of working memory.

From this point, all of the analyses refer to the performance of infants at 8 months corrected age, and aim to identify those factors which might contribute to the differences in performance on working memory task between preterm and term infants.

It is possible that some factors associated with being preterm affected performance of working memory more than prematurity per se. These factors include medical complications, lower birthweight and shorter gestation age. Further analyses were conducted to assess the effect of perinatal variables which might have significantly affected preterm infants' performance on the working memory measures.

Preterm infants were firstly grouped on the basis of their severity of medical complication as follows. None of the full term infants had serious perinatal complications and they were combined to form one group.

Table 3. Comparison of Preterm and Full-term Infants on working memory Tasks at 10-11 Month Chronological Age and Eight Months Corrected Age

Executive function	Preterm	Full-term group	F	p
1. Working memory M (SD) Chronological age	5.75 (3.11) **1.67 (.57) A1**	13.42(4.01) **2.50 (.40) A2**	21.78	.00
2. Working memory M (SD) Corrected age	5.75 (3.11) **A1**	9.40 (4.45) **A2**	11.82	.00

1. high-risk preterm group ($n = 18$), group 1;
2. low-risk preterm group ($n = 19$), group 2; and,
3. no medical complications (term infants $n = 74$), group 3.

The results of high risk preterm infants, low-risk preterm infants and full term infants are shown in Table 4

The preterm infants who had a high medical risk in the perinatal period performed worse than those who did not have these medical risk factors on working memory, although the differences in performance were not statistically significant. The scores of both the preterm infant groups were lower than those of full-term infants on working memory measure. These differences reached statistical significance between both groups of preterm infants and full-term infants on working memory. The difference between preterm infants who had high medical risk and full-term infants was greater than that between low-risk infants and full-term infants on working memory, suggesting that medical risk influences the development of working memory.

Preterm infants were grouped on the basis of their birthweights as follows. None of the full-term infants was low birthweight and they were combined to form one group:

1. < 1000 g birthweight ($n = 21$), group 1;
2. 1000-1500 g birthweight group ($n = 16$), group 2; and,
3. normal birthweight group (term infants, $n = 74$), group 3.

The results of infants with less than 1000g birthweight, infants with 1001-1500g birthweight and normal birthweight infants are shown in Table 5

Table 4. The Comparison of Preterm Infants at High Medical Risk, Low Medical Risk, and Full-term Infants on Measures of Executive Function and Sustained Attention at Eight Months Corrected Age

Variables	High-risk preterm infants	Low-risk preterm infants	Full-term Infants	F	p	Tukey's HSD
Working memory M (SD)	4.61 (2.95)**A1**	6.84 (2.93) **A2**	9.36 (4.22) **A3**	12.34	.00	A1 vs.A3 (.00) A2 vs.A3 (.03)

Table 5. The Comparison of < 1000 g Birthweight Infants, 1000-1500 g Birthweight Infants and Full-term Infants on Working Memory Mmeasure at Eight Months Corrected Age.

Variables	< 1000 g birthweight	1000-1500 g birthweight	Full-term Infants	F	p	Tukey's HSD
Working memory M (SD)	5.23 (3.36)A1	6.43 (2.70) A2	9.36 (4.22)A3	11.01	.00	A1 vs.A3 (.00) A2 vs.A3 (.02)

Table 6. The Comparison of < 28 Weeks Gestation Infants, 28-32 Weeks Gestation Infants and Full-term Infants on Working Memory Measure at Eight Months Corrected Age

Variables	< 28 weeks M (SD)	28-32 weeks M (SD)	Full-term Infants M (SD)	F	p	Tukey's HSD
Working memory M (SD)	5.53 (2.66) A1	5.90 (3.43) A2	9.36 (4.22) A3	10.54	.00	A1 vs.A3 (.00) A2 vs.A3 (.00)

The preterm infants who had < 1000 g birthweight performed worse than those who had ≥ 1000 g birthweight on working memory although the differences in performance were not statistically significant. The scores of both groups of preterm infants were poorer than those of full-term infants on working memory. These differences were statistically significant between both groups of preterm infants and full-term infants on working memory. Thus the differences between the preterm infants who had < 1000 g birthweight and full-term infants appear greater than that between the infants with ≥ 1000 g birthweight and full-term infants on working memory, suggesting that ELBW may significantly influence the development of working memory.

Preterm infants were grouped on the basis of their gestation age. None of the full-term infants had low gestation age and they were combined to form one group.

1. 28 weeks gestation age ($n = 15$), group 1;
2. 28 to 32 weeks gestation age ($n = 22$), group 2; and
3. normal gestation age (full-term infants, $n = 74$), group 3.

Table 6 shows that scores were poorer for the infants < 28 weeks gestation than for the preterm infants with ≥ 28 weeks gestation on working memory, and the scores of both groups of preterm infants were poorer than those of full-term infants on working memory. These differences reached statistical significance between preterm infants and the group of full-term infants on working memory.

DISCUSSION

Preterm and full-term infants of the same chronological age and same corrected age were compared on measures of working memory in order to assess the differential effects of maturation (biological maturity) and length of exposure to extrauterine environmental stimuli on the development of these abilities. Although a number of studies suggest that global development seems to be largely the result of maturational influence [76-78], others have reported that "neural sculpting" occurs as the result of exposure to environmental influences [79, 80]. Currently little is known about the impact of the environment on the development of brain mechanisms that mediate specific cognitive abilities, such as working memory.

It was found that preterm infants were inferior to full-term infants on working memory tasks at both the same chronological age and the same corrected age, but the differences in performance were much less when the infants were compared at the same corrected age. This suggests that maturation had a greater impact than exposure to environmental stimuli on the development of working memory. However, as differences between the preterm and full term infants remained even when they were compared on corrected age, other factors must also have impact on the development of working memory in these infants. It was also found that high-risk perinatal complications, extremely low birthweight (<1000 g) and very low gestation age (< 28 weeks) were associated with poor performance on working memory task.

Preterm infants represent a heterogeneous population which varies with respect to gestation age, birthweight, adequacy of interuterine growth, and the diversity of medical complications to which they may have been exposed. All too often in the literature these differences have been ignored and data from preterm infants has been lumped together. It is however essential to consider the effect which these factors may have over and above the effects of prematurity per se.

The perinatal risk factors examined in the present study were high medical risk, extremely low birthweight, and shorter gestation age. A "high medical risk preterm infant" was defined as an infant who had one or more of the following perinatal medical complications, previously identified as associated with poor outcomes. [5, 13, 81-88]. These were: Home Oxygen Dependency, Cerebral Ventricular Hemorrhage, Ventricular Dilatation, and Periventricular Hemorrhage-Intraventricular Hemorrhage. VD did not occur in any of the infants in the present study so it was not used for the analysis. Eighteen infants fell into this "high medical risk" category, and the remaining 19 preterm infants were defined as "low medical risk."

ELBW was defined as birthweight < 1000 g. Preterm infants in the < 1000 g birthweight group did not differ from the preterm infants with ≥ 1000 g birthweight group with regards to medical risk status. Two gestation age groups comprised infants with gestation age < 28 weeks and preterm infants with ≥ 28 weeks gestation age. Infants with gestation age < 28 weeks were regarded as having shorter gestation age. Likewise, preterm infants born at < 28 weeks gestation were not significantly different to those with 28-32 weeks gestation in terms of medical risk status. There was therefore an opportunity to consider the effect of birthweight and gestation age independent of medical complications.

In each case, the high-risk group (i.e., the medical complications group, the <1000 g birthweight group, and the < 28 weeks gestation group) performed more poorly than their low risk counterparts (i.e., the low medical risk group, the > 1000 g birthweight group, and the >

28 weeks gestation group) on working memory measure although these differences did not reach statistical significance. The performance of both the high risk and low risk preterm groups on measure of working memory were also consistently poorer than that of the full-term group, and this reached levels of statistical significance more frequently for the high risk preterm groups than for the low risk groups. The results of the effects of perinatal factors on the performance of working memory are summarised in Table 7 below. These findings suggest that medical risk, lower birthweight, and lower gestation age adversely affect performance on working memory measure.

The findings of this study are consistent with those of other researchers, who have reported that perinatal risk factors influence cognitive development during the first year of life [89-91]. Similar deficits in working memory have also been reported in studies of school age children who were born preterm and who experienced high medical risk [23, 92]. For example, Luciana et al. [23] found that preterm born children at 7 to 9 years of age who had high medical risk differed from full-term infants on working memory tasks, and Taylor, Klein, et al. [93] also suggested that medical risk may influence the long term developmental outcomes of preterm infants.

The results are also consistent with previous studies of children with extremely low birthweight, whether defined as birthweight < 1000 g [72] or < 750 g [92], which have reported lower scores on the performance of working memory tasks. However the children in these studies were older than the children in the present study. The effect of SGA may also influence the performance of working memory in the preterm infants with < 1000 g birthweight group in the current study. For example, the poorer performance of the ELBW infants on working memory may have been due to the fact that there were eight SGA infants in the ELBW group. Several studies, such as that of McCarton et al. [94] have reported that SGA preterm infants tend to perform more poorly than their AGA counterparts on general developmental assessment measures. In the current study, SGA preterm infants tended to show poorer scores on the working memory measure than AGA preterm infants, but these differences did not reach statistically significant differences as the number of SGA infants in the present study was too small. Evidence for direct central nervous system effects of intrauterine undernutrition is primarily based on animal studies. Laboratory studies in rats and guinea pigs that have experienced intrauterine growth retardation have shown decreased brain weight, and reduced amount of brain DNA, protein, and myelin lipids [95]. While extrapolation from animal studies is questionable this does raise the possibility that SGA infants may experience cognitive impairments as the result of reduced brain growth.

This study appears to be the first to examine the effect of gestation age on the performance of working memory. The effects of gestation age on subsequent cognitive development has been the topic of considerable debate. Many studies have included a heterogeneous group of preterm infants with a wide range of gestation ages. The effects of gestation age on subsequent development have consequently often been confounded by a higher incidence of perinatal complications and poor psychomotor development in the infants of lower gestation age [96-100]. In this study, both preterm infants with < 28 weeks gestation and infants with 28-32 weeks gestation had lower scores than the full-term infants on working memory. The differences between both preterm groups and full-term infants reached statistical significance on measure of working memory. This suggests that a shorter gestation age is no more detrimental to performance in these areas than prematurity per se.

Table 7. Influence of Perinatal Risk Factors on Performance of Working Memory Measure When Compared to Full-term Infants

Variables	Medical risk		Birthweight		Gestation age	
	High risk	Low risk	< 1000 g	> 1000 g	< 28 weeks	> 28 weeks
	p	p	p	p	p	p
Working memory	.03*	.00***	.00***	.02*	.00***	.00***

Note. The figures in the table above are summarized from Table 4, 5 and 6.
Significant difference between preterm infant group and full-term infant group: *$p < .05$, ** $p < .01$, *** $p < .001$

There is considerable evidence that tasks which require the holding of information in memory involve the dorsolateral prefrontal cortex [101, 102]. The deficits in working memory observed in the high perinatal risk groups may be associated with the adverse effects of these perinatal risk factors on the prefrontal cortex which is very immature and sensitive in the preterm infants [17, 103, 104]. Mouradian, Als, and Coster [105] suggested that deficits in working memory might be due to late maturing cortical organization, particularly of the prefrontal regions. Myelination of the brain has been demonstrated to occur in a systematic fashion starting at the end of the first trimester and continuing at least until the end of the second year [106]. Between 23 and 32 weeks of gestation, structural differentiation of the central nervous system is at its most rapid (i.e., neuronal differentiation, glial cell growth, myelination, axonal and dendritic growth and synapse formation). The preterm infants in the present study were born between 24 to 32 weeks gestation just at this time of brain development. Most of these preterm infants were in the Neonatal Intensive-care Unit for up to three months after they were born. The environment in the Neonatal Intensive-care Unit may not be conductive to the development of the brain and the perinatal risk factors which occurred during this period may have further adversely affect brain development. The prefrontal cortex, which appears to play a central role in regulating working memory, is a late maturing area of the brain, and is consequently likely to be particularly vulnerable to damage in preterm infants [107]. Those preterm infants with these detrimental perinatal events are at particular risk for the abnormal prefrontal cortex functioning, hence the deficits in working memory.

The deficits of working memory observed in preterm infants may have long term consequences in terms of learning difficulties at school age. During school years, children born preterm who experienced high perinatal risks (i.e., high medical risks, extremely low birthweight, shorter gestation age) during the perinatal period have been found to have higher rates of deficits in cognitive and neuropsychological abilities, mathematics achievement, and adaptive behaviours, as well as higher rates of special education placements as compared with their full-term counterparts [2, 23, 93, 108]. It is possible that this is due to early abnormality in the development of the prefrontal cortex and consequent working memory impairment. Anderson et al. [71] suggested that this might possibly result in inability to ever acquire aspects of working memory.

In summary, there were significant differences between preterm and full-term infants' scores on working memory at both 10-11 month chorological age and eight month corrected age. Medical risk factors, extremely low birthweight, and shorter gestation age confounded the effects of prematurity for working memory.

Limitation of the Study

There are several limitations of this study. First, due to the restricted timeframe, long-term outcomes cannot be assessed. Hence a link cannot be made to the preterm infants between the deficits in working memory found in the present study and learning difficulties in school. Second, the examiner was not blind to the preterm/term status of the infants and this may have affected the administration and coding of the tests. Third, the relatively small sample of preterm infants who could be recruited within the time constraints for the present study restricted the range for statistical analyses that could be carried out and thus limited their power. Finally, the strict selection criteria chosen to yield a group of relatively healthy preterm infants may have biased the sample and made it unrepresentative of the general population of every preterm infant. For the above reasons the results should be interpreted with some caution.

CONCLUSION

Differences were found between preterm and full-term infants on measures of working memory at both the same corrected and same chronological age. Maturation was found to be an important factor influencing the development of working memory. However other factors associated with prematurity were also found to affect performance on working memory measure.

The present research examined the factors which may significantly affect the differences between preterm and full-term infants. In particular, high medical risk, lower birthweight, and shorter gestation age all affected the differences between preterm and full-term infants on of working memory measure.

REFERENCES

[1] Welsh, MC; Pennington, BF. Assessing frontal lobe functioning in children: View from *Developmental Psychology., Developmental Neuropsychology*. 1988, 4(3), 199-230.
[2] Hack M; Friedman H; Fanaroff AA. Outcomes of extremely low birth weight infants. *Pediatrics.,* 1996, 98(5), 931-7.
[3] O'Shea, TM; Klinepeter, L; Goldstein, DJ; Jackson, BW; Dillard, RG. Survival and developmental disability in infants with birth weights of 501 to 800 grams, born between 1979 and 1994. *Pediatrics.,* 1997, 100(6), 982-6.
[4] Rickards, AL; Kelly, EA; Doyle, LW; Callanan, C. Cognition, academic progress, behavior and self-concept at 14 years of very low birth weight children. Developmental and Behavioral *Pediatrics.,* 2001, 22(1), 11-8.

[5] Sostek, AM. Prematurity as well as intraventricular hemorrhage influence developmental outcome at 5 years. In: Friedman SL; Sigman MD; Sigel IE; eds. *The psychological development of low-birthweight children*. Norwood, NJ: Ablex, 1992, 259-74.

[6] Taylor, HG; Hack, M; Klein, N; Schatschneider, C. Achievement in children with birth weights less than 750 grams with normal cognitive abilities: Evidence for specific learning disabilities. *Journal of Pediatric Psychology.*, 1995, 20(6), 703-19.

[7] Klebanov, PK; Brooks-Gunn, J; McCormick, MC. Classroom behavior of very low birth weight elementary school children. *Pediatrics.*, 1994, 94(5), 700-8.

[8] Aylward, GP. Update on early developmental neuropsychological assessment: The early neuropsychological optimality rating scales. In: Tramontana MG; Hooper SR; eds. *Advances in child neuropsychology*. New York: Springer-Verlag, 1994, 172-200.

[9] Ross, G; Lipper, E; Auld, PAM. Cognitive abilities and early precursors of learning disabilities in very-low-birthweight children with normal intelligence and normal neurological status. *International Journal of Behavioral Development.*, 1996, 19(3), 563-80.

[10] Siegel, LS. A multivariate model for the early detection of learning disabilities. In: CW; Greenbaum, JG; Auerbath, eds. *Longitudinal studies of children at psychological risk: Cross-national perspectives*. Norwood, NJ: Ablex, 1992, 99-132.

[11] Koller, H; Lawson, K; Rose, SA; Wallace, I; McCarton, C. Patterns of cognitive development in very low birth weight children during the first six years of life. *Pediatrics.*, 1997, 99(3), 383-9.

[12] Laucht, M; Esser, G; Schmidt, MH. Developmental outcome of infants born with biological and psychosocial risks. *Journal of Child Psychology and Psychiatry and Allied Disciplines.*, 1997, 38(7), 843-53.

[13] Landry, SH; Denson, SE; Swank, PR. Effects of medical risk and socioeconomic status on the rate of change in cognitive and social development for low birth weight children. *Journal of Clinical and Experimental Neuropsychology.*, 1997, 19(2), 261-74.

[14] Roberts, E; Bornstein, MH; Slater, AM; Barrett, J. Early cognitive development and parental education. *Infant and Child Development.*, 1999, 8, 49-62.

[15] Thompson, RJ; Gustafson, KE; Oehler, JM; Catlett, AT; Brazy, JE; Coldstein, RF. Developmental outcome of very low birth weight infants at four years of age as a function of biological risk and psychosocial risk. *Journal of Developmental and Behavioral Pediatrics.*, 1997, 18(2), 91-6.

[16] Aylward, GP. *Infant and early childhood neuropsychology*. New York: Plenum Press, 1997.

[17] Aylward, GP. Perinatal asphyxia: Effects of biological and environmental risks. *Clinics in Perinatology.*, 1993, 20, 433-49.

[18] Bayley, N. Bayley scale of infant development: Manual. 2nd ed. San Antonio; TX: *The Psychological Corporation*, 1993.

[19] Aylward, GP; Pfeiffer, SI; Wright, A; Verhulst, SJ. Outcome studies of low birth weight infants published in the last decade: A meta-analysis. *Journal of Pediatrics.*, 1989, 115, 515-20.

[20] McCall, RB. What process mediates predictions of childhood IQ from infant habituation and recognition memory? Speculations on the roles of inhibition and rate of information processing. *Intelligence.*, 1994, 18, 107-25.

[21] Siegel, LS. The development of working memory in normally achieving and subtypes of learning disabled children. *Child Development.*, 1989, 60, 973-80.
[22] Gathercole, SE; Pickering, SJ. Working memory deficits in children with low achievements in the national curriculum at 7 years of age. *British Journal of Educational Psychology*. 2000, 70, 177-94.
[23] Luciana, M; Lindeke, L; Georgieff, M; Mills, M; Nelson, CA. Neurobehavioral evidence for working-memory deficits in school-aged children with histories of prematurity. *Developmental Medicine and Child Neurology.*, 1999, 41, 521-33.
[24] Fuster, JM. *The prefrontal cortex: Anatomy, physiology, and neuropsychology of the frontal lobe.* New York: s, 1997.
[25] Graham, S; Harris, KR. Addressing problems in attention, memory, and executive functioning. In: GR; Lyon, NA; Krasnegor, eds. *Attention, memory, and executive function*. Baltimore: Paul H. Brookes, 1996, 349-65.
[26] Goldman-Rakic, PS. Specification of higher cortical functions. In: Broman SH, Grafman J; eds. *Atypical cognitive deficits in developmental disorders: Implication for brain function*. Hillsdale, NJ: Lawrence Erlbaum, 1994, 3-17.
[27] Milner, B. Effects of different brain lesions on card sorting. *Archives of Neurology.*, 1963, 9, 90-100.
[28] Eslinger, PJ; Grattan, LM; Damasio, H; Damasio, AR. Developmental consequences of childhood frontal lobe damage. *Archives of Neurology.*, 1992, 49, 764-9.
[29] Hecaen, H. Mental symptoms associated with tumors of the frontal lobe. In: JM; Warren, K; Akert, eds. *The frontal granular cortex and behavior*. New York: McGraw-Hill 1964.
[30] Shallice, T; Burgess, PW. Deficits in strategy application following frontal lobe damage in man. *Brain.*, 1991, 114, 727-41.
[31] Grady, CL. Neuroimaging and activation of the frontal lobes. In: BL; Miller, JL; Cummings, eds. *The human frontal lobes: Functions and disorders*. New York: The Guilford Press, 1999, 196-230.
[32] Hoon, A; Melhem, ER. Neuroimaging: Applications in disorders of early brain development. *Developmental and Behavioral Pediatrics.*, 2000, 21(4), 291-302.
[33] Jagust, W. Neuroimaging and the frontal lobes: Insight from the study of neurodegenerative diseases. In: Miller BL; Cummings JL; eds. *The human frontal lobes: Functions and disorders*. New York: The Guilford Press, 1999, 107-22.
[34] Lepage, M; Beaudoin, G; Boulet, C; O'Brien, I; Marcantoni, W; Bourgouin, P; et al. Frontal cortex and the programming of repetitive tapping movements in man: Lesion effects and functional neuroimaging. *Cognitive Brain Research.*, 1999, 8, 17-25.
[35] Marenco, S; Coppola, R; Daniel, DG; Zigun, JR; Weinberger, DR. Regional cerebral blood flow during the Wisconsin Card Sorting Test in normal subjects studied by xenon-133 dynamic SPECT: Comparison of absolute values, percent distribution values, and covariance analysis. *Psychiatry Research: Neuroimaging.*, 1993, 50, 177-92.
[36] Barkley, RA. Behavioral inhibition, sustained attention, and executive functions: Constructing a unifying theory of ADHD. *Psychological Bulletin.*, 1997, 121(1), 65-94.
[37] Kaufer, DI; Lewis, DA. Frontal lobe anatomy and cortical connectivity. In: Miller BL; Cummings JL; eds. *The human frontal lobes: Functions and disorders*. New York: The Guilford Press 1999, 27-44.

[38] Petrides, M. Frontal lobe and working memory: Evidence from investigations of the effects of cortical excisions in nonhuman primates. In: Boller F; Spinnler H; Hendler JA; eds. *Handbook of neuropsychology*. Amsterdam: Elsevier Science, 1994, 59-82.

[39] Petrides, M. Learning impairments following excisions of the primate frontal cortex. In: Levin HS; Eisenberg HM; Benton AL; eds. *Frontal lobe function and dysfunction*. New York: Oxford University, Press 1996, 256-72.

[40] Goldman-Rakic, PS; Rosvold, HE. The effects of selective caudate lesions in infant and juvenile rhesus monkeys. *Brain Research.*, 1972, 42, 53-66.

[41] Diamond, A. Development of the ability to use recall to guide action; as indicated by infants' performance on A*B*. *Child Development.*, 1985, 56, 868-83.

[42] Diamond, A; Doar, B. The performance of human infants on a measure of frontal cortex function, the delayed response task. *Developmental Psychobiology.*, 1989, 22(3), 271-94.

[43] Fuster, JM. Role of prefrontal cortex in delay tasks: Evidence from reversible lesion and unit recording in the monkey. In: Levin HS; Eisenberg HM; eds. *Frontal function and dysfunction*. New York: Oxford University Press 1991, 59-71.

[44] Sawaguchi, T; Goldman-Rakic, PS. The role of D1-dopamine receptor in working memory: Local injections of dopamine antagonists into the prefrontal cortex of rhesus monkeys performing an oculomotor delayed-response task. *Journal of Neurophysiology.*, 1994, 71(2), 515-28.

[45] Guitton, D; Buchtel, HA; Douglas, RM. Frontal lobe lesions in man cause difficulties in suppressing reflexive glances and in generating goal-directed saccades. *Experimental Brain Research*, 1985, 58, 455-72.

[46] Levine, SC. Effects of early unilateral lesions: Changes over the course of development. In: Turkewitz G; Devenny DA; eds. *Developmental time and timing*. In: NJ: Hillsdale, Lawrence Erlbaum, 1993, 143-65.

[47] Teuber, HL; Rudel, RG. Behavior after cerebral lesions in children and adults. *Developmental Medicine and Child Neurology.*, 1962, 4, 3-20.

[48] Benton, A. Prefrontal injury and behavior in children. *Developmental Neuropsychology.*, 1991, 7(3), 275-81.

[49] Mateer, CA; Williams, D. Effects of frontal lobe injury in childhood. *Developmental Neuropsychology.*, 1991, 7(2), 359-76.

[50] McDowell, S; Whyte, J; D'Esposito, M. Working memory impairment in traumatic brain injury: Evidence from a dual-task paradigm. *Neuropsychologia*, 1997, 35(10), 1341-53.

[51] Levin, HS; Song, J; Ewing-Cobbs, L; Roberson, G. Porteus Maze performance following traumatic brain injury in children. *Neuropsychology*, 2001, 15(4), 557-67.

[52] Bohm, B; Katz-Salamon, M; Smedler, A; Lagercrantz, H; Forssberg, H. Developmental risks and protective factors for influencing cognitive outcome at 5 1/2 years of age in very-low-birthweight children. *Developmental Medicine and Child Neurology.*, 2002, 44, 508-16.

[53] Chui, H; Willis, L. Vascular diseases of the frontal lobes. In: Miller BL; Cummings JL; eds. *The human frontal lobes: Functions and disorders*. New York: The Guilford Press, 1999, 370-402.

[54] Nakawatase, TY. Frontal lobe tumors. In: Miller BL; Cummings JL; eds. *The human frontal lobes: Functions and disorders*. New York: The Guilford Press, 1999, 436-45.

[55] Rieger, M; Gauggel, S. Inhibition of ongoing responses in patients with traumatic brain injury. *Neuropsychologia.*, 2002, 40, 76-85.
[56] Vasterling, JJ; Duke, LM; Brailey, K; Constans, JI; Allain, AN; Sutker, PB. Attention, learning, and memory performances and intellectual resources in Vietnam veterans: PTSD and no disorder comparisons. *Neuropsychology.*, 2002, 16(1), 5-14.
[57] Lewinsohn, PM; Zieler, RE; Libet, J; Eyeberg, S; Nielson, G. Short-term memory: A comparison between frontal and nonfrontal right- and left-hemisphere brain damaged patients. *Journal of Comparitive Physiology and Psychology.*, 1972, 81, 248-55.
[58] Milner, B. Disorders of memory after brain lesions in man. *Neuropsychologia.*, 1968, 6, 175-9.
[59] Petrides, M. Deficits on conditional associative-learning tasks after frontal- and temporal-lobe lesions in man. *Neuropsychologia.*, 1985, 23, 601-14.
[60] Stuss, DT. Interference effects on memory functions in postleukotomy patients: An attentional perspective. In: Levin HS; Eisenberg HM; Benton AL; eds. *Frontal lobe function and dysfunction.* New York: Oxford University Press, 1991, 157-72.
[61] Thatcher, RW. Maturation of the human frontal lobes: Physiological evidence for staging. *Developmental Neuropsychology.*, 1991, 7(3), 397-419.
[62] Huttenlocher, PR. Synaptogenesis in human cerebral cortex. In: G; Dawson, KW; Fischer, eds. *Human behavior and the developing brain.* New York: The Guilford Press, 1994, 137-52.
[63] Chugani, HT; Phelps, ME. Imaging human brain development with positron emission tomography. *Journal of Nuclear Medicine.*, 1990, 32, 23-5.
[64] Bell, MA; Fox, NA. The relations between frontal brain electrical activity and cognitive development during infancy. *Child Development.*, 1992, 63, 1142-63.
[65] Bell, MA. Frontal lobe function during infancy: Implications for the development of cognition and attention. In: Richards JE; ed. *Cognitive neuroscience of attention: A developmental perspective.* Mahwah, NJ: Lawrence Erlbaum, 1998, 287-316.
[66] Diamond, A; Prevor, MB; Callender, G; Druin, DP. Prefrontal cortex cognitive deficits in children treated early and continuously for PKU. *Monographs of the Society for Research in Child Development.*, 1997, 62(4), 1-205.
[67] Piaget, J. The construction of reality in the child. New York: *Basic Books*, 1954.
[68] Diamond, A; Goldman-Rakic, PS. Comparative development of human infants and infant rhesus monkeys of cognitive functions that depend on the prefrontal cortex. *Neuropsychological Abstracts.*, 1986, 12, 274.
[69] Scheibel, RS; Levin, HS. Frontal lobe dysfunction following closed head injury in children: Findings from neuropsychology and brain imaging. In: Krasnegor NA; Lyon GR; Goldman-Rakic PS; eds. *Development of the prefrontal cortex: Evolution, neurobiology, and behavior.* Baltimore: Paul H. Brookes, 1997, 241-63.
[70] Eslinger, PJ; Biddle, K; Pennington, B; Page, RB. Cognitive and behavioral development up to 4 years after early right frontal lobe lesion. *Developmental Neuropsychology.*, 1999, 15(2), 157-91.
[71] Anderson, SW; Damasio, H; Tranel, D; Damasio, AR. Long-term sequelae of prefrontal cortex damage acquired in early childhood. *Developmental Neuropsychology.*, 2000, 18(3), 281-90.

[72] Harvey, JM; O'Callaghan, MJ; Mohay, H. Executive function of children with extremely low birthweight: A case control study. *Developmental Medicine and Child Neurology.*, 1999, 41, 292-7.

[73] Horobin, K; Acredolo, L. The role of attentiveness, mobility history, and separation of hiding sites on Stage IV search behavior. *Journal of Experimental Child Psychology*, 1986, 41, 114-27.

[74] Hofstadter, M; Reznick, JS. Response modality effects: Human infant delayed-response performance. *Child Development.*, 1996, 67, 646-58.

[75] Diamond, A. Neuropsychological insights into the meaning of object concept development. In: Johnson MH; ed. *Brain development and cognition: A reader.* Cambridge, MA: Blackwell, 1993, 208-47.

[76] Hunt, JV; Rhodes, L. Mental development of preterm infants during the first year. *Child Development.*, 1977, 48, 204-10.

[77] Rutter, M. Developing minds: Challenge and continuity across the life span. London, England: Penguin, 1992.

[78] Ungerer, JA; Sigman, M. Developmental lags in preterm infants from one to three years of age. *Child Development.*, 1983, 54, 1217-28.

[79] Campos, JJ; Kermoian, R; Witherington, D; Chen, H; Dong, Q. Activity, attention and developmental transitions in infancy. In: PJ; Lang, RF; Simons, eds. *Attention and orienting: Sensory and motivational processes.* Mahwah, NJ: Lawrence Erlbaum, 1997, 393-415.

[80] Dawson, G; Frey, K; Panagiotides, H; Yamada, E; Hessel, D; Osterling, J. Infants of depressed mothers exhibit atypical frontal electrical brain activity during interactions with mothers and with a familiar nondepressed adult. *Child Development.*, 1999, 70, 1058-66.

[81] Cohen, SE; Parmelee, AH; Beckwith, L; Sigman, M. Cognitive development in preterm infants: Birth to 8 years. *Developmental and Behavioral Pediatrics.*, 1986, 7(2), 102-9.

[82] Gregoire, MC; Lefebvre, F; Glorieux, J. Health and developmental outcomes at 18 months in very preterm infants with bronchopulmonary dysplasia. *Pediatrics.*, 1998, 101(5), 856-60.

[83] Hertzig, ME. Neurological 'soft' signs in low-birthweight children. *Developmental Medicine and Child Neurology.*, 1981, 23, 778-91.

[84] Msall, ME; Buck, GM; Rogers, BT; Mereke, D; Catanzaro, NL; Zorn, WA. Risk factors for major neurodevelopmental impairments and need for special education resources in extremely premature infants. *Journal of Pediatrics.*, 1991, 119, 606-14.

[85] Piecuch, RE; Leonard, CH; Cooper, B; Sehring, SA. Outcome of extremely low birth weight infants (500 to 999 grams) over a 12-year period. *Pediatrics.*, 1997, 100(4), 633-7.

[86] Pine, TRL; Jackson, JC; Bennett, FC. Outcome of infants weighing less than 800 grams at birth:15 years' experience. *Pediatrics.*, 1995, 96, 479-83.

[87] Smith, KE; Landry, SH; Swank, PR; Baldwin, CD; Denson, SE; Wildin, S. The relation of medical risk and maternal stimulation with preterm infants' development of cognitive, language and daily living skills. *Journal of Child Psychology and Psychiatry.*, 1996, 37(7), 855-64.

[88] van de Bor, M; den Ouden, L; Guit, GL. Value of cranial ultrasound and magnetic resonance imaging in predicting neurodevelopmental outcome in preterm infants. *Pediatrics.*, 1992, 90(2), 196-9.

[89] Molfese, V; Thomson, B. Optimality versus complications: Assessing predictive values of perinatal scales. *Child Development.*, 1985, 56, 810-23.

[90] Piper, MC; Kunos, I; Willis, DM; Mazer, B. Effect of gestational age on neurological functioning of the very low-birthweight infant at 40 weeks. *Developmental Medicine and Child Neurology.*, 1985, 27, 596-605.

[91] Ross, G; Tesman, J; Auld, PM; Nass, R. Effects of subependymal and mild intraventricular lesions on visual attention and memory in premature infants. *Developmental Psychology.*, 1992, 28(6), 1067-74.

[92] Taylor, HG; Klein, N; Minich, NM; Hack, M. Middle-school-age outcomes in children with very low birthweight. *Child Development.*, 2000, 71, 1495-511.

[93] Taylor, HG; Klein, N; Schatschneider, C; Hack, M. Predictors of early school age outcomes in very low birth weight children. *Developmental and Behavioral Pediatrics.*, 1998, 19(4), 235-43.

[94] McCarton, CM; Wallace, IF; Divon, M; Vaughan, HG. Cognitive and neurologic development of the premature, small for gestational age infant through age 6, Comparison by birth weight and gestational age. *Pediatrics.*, 1996, 98(6), 1167-78.

[95] Neville, HE; Chase, HP. Undernutrition and cerebella development. *Experimental Neurology.*, 1971, 33(3), 485-97.

[96] Duffy, FH; Als, H; McAnulty, GB. Behavioral and electrophysiological evidence for gestational age effects in healthy preterm and full-term infants studies two weeks after expected due date. *Child Development.*, 1990, 61, 1271-86.

[97] Emsley, HC; Wardle, SP; Sims, DG; Cheswick, ML; Souza, SW. Increased survival and deteriorating developmental outcome in 23 to 25 week old gestation infants, 1990-1994 compared to 1984-1990. *Archives of Disease in Childhood.*, 1998, 78, F99-F104.

[98] Eyal, FG. The small-for-gestational-age preterm infant. In: FR; Witter, LG; Keith, eds. *Textbook of prematurity: Antecedents, treatment, and outcome.* Boston, MA: Little, Brown, 1993, 361-9.

[99] Synnes, AR; Ling, EWY; Whitfield, MF; Mackinnon, M; Lopes, L; Wang, G; et al. Perinatal outcomes of a large cohort of extremely low gestational age infants (twenty-three to twenty-eight completed weeks of gestation). *The Journal of Pediatrics.*, 1994, 125(6), 952-60.

[100] The Victorian Infant Collaborative Study Group. Outcome at 2 years of children 23-27 weeks' gestation born in Victoria in 1991-1992. *Journal of Pediatrics.*, 1997, 33, 161-5.

[101] Diamond, A; Kirkham, N; Amso, D. Conditions under which young children can hold two rules in mind and inhibit a prepotent response. *Developmental Psychology.*, 2002, 38(3), 352-62.

[102] Roberts, JRJ; Pennington, BF. An interactive framework for examining prefrontal cognitive processes. *Developmental Neuropsychology.*, 1996, 12(1), 105-26.

[103] Diamond, A; Lee, E. Inability of five-month-old infants to retrieve a contiguous object: A failure of conceptual understanding or of control of action? *Child Development.*, 2000, 71(6), 1477-94.

[104] Fletcher, JM; Brookshire, BL; Landry, SH; Bohan, TP; Davidson, KC; Francis, DJ; et al. Attentional skills and executive functions in children with early hydrocephalus. *Developmental Neuropsychology.*, 1996, 12(1), 53-76.

[105] Mouradian, LE; Als, H; Coster, WJ. Neurobehavioral functioning of healthy preterm infants of varying gestational ages. *Developmental and Behavioral Pediatrics.*, 2000, 21(6), 408-16.

[106] Battin, MR; Maalouf, EF; Counsell, SJ; Herlihy, AH; Rutherford, MA; Azzopardi, D; et al. Magnetic resonance imaging of the brain in very preterm infants: Visualization of the germinal matrix, early myelination, and cortical folding. *Pediatrics.*, 1998, 101(6), 957-62.

[107] Gilles, FH; Shankle, W; Dooling, EC. Myelinated tracts: Growth pattern. In: FH; Gilles, AD; Leviton, EC; Dooking, eds. *The developing human brain: Growth and epidemiologic neuropathology.* Baltimore: Williams & Wilkins 1983.

[108] Taylor, HG; Anselmo, M; Foreman, AL; Schatschneider, C; Angelopoulos, J. Utility of kindergarten teacher judgments in identifying early learning problems. *Journal of Learning Disabilities.*, 2000, 33(2), 200-10.

In: Working Memory: Capacity, Developments and...
Editor: Eden S. Levin

ISBN: 978-1-61761-980-9
© 2011 Nova Science Publishers, Inc.-

Chapter 7

THE ASSESSMENT AND TRAINING OF WORKING MEMORY FOR PREVENTION AND EARLY INTERVENTION IN CASE OF READING, WRITING AND ARITHMETICAL DIFFICULTIES IN CHILDREN

Antonella D'Amico
Department of Psychology, University of Palermo, Palermo, Italy

ABSTRACT

The first part of the chapter reviews the recent literature regarding the involvement of working memory functions in scholastic learning and its role as an underlying factor of reading, writing and arithmetical difficulties. In the second part of the chapter we find an experience of assessment and training of working memory for the prevention of reading, writing and mathematical learning difficulties. On the basis of this study, an Italian working memory test battery and a training programme have been developed, including a series of activities involving both verbal and visual-spatial working memory with different degrees of central executive demand.

INTRODUCTION

Working memory (Baddeley, 1986) is considered as a measure of the capacity to manipulate and transform material while remembering information.

Recent literature reports different models which seek to explain how working memory functions. Some approaches consider WM as the activated portion of long-term memory and emphasize the role of attention resources and control processes (Cowan, 2005; Engle, 2002).

The other well known working memory model proposed by Baddeley and Hitch (1974), which will be focused on in this chapter, considers working memory as a system composed of three main components: the central executive, the phonological loop and the visual-spatial sketchpad. The *central executive* (CE) is responsible for performing a series of high order functions, such as the inhibition of irrelevant information, switching between retrieval plans or between different strategies and the temporary activation of long-term memory information (Baddeley, 1996; Lehto, Juujärvi, Kooistra, & Pulkkinen, 2003; Miyake, Friedman, Emerson, Witzki, Howerter, & Wager, 2000); the *phonological loop* (PL) and the *visual-spatial sketchpad* (VSSP) are assumed to be slave systems coordinated by the central executive and are devoted respectively to storing phonological (Vallar & Baddeley, 1984) and visual-spatial information (i.e. Della Sala, Gray, Baddeley, Allamano, & Wilson, 1999; Logie, 1991; Logie & Pearson, 1997; Quinn, 1988; Quinn & McConnell, 1996). Thus, while the central executive component is considered to work with both verbal-phonological and visual-spatial information, the slave mechanisms are highly specialized and domain dependent. More recently (Baddeley, 2000) a fourth component has been added to the model: the *episodic buffer*. This is a limited-capacity temporary storage system that is capable of integrating information from a variety of sources and is assumed to feed information into and retrieve information from episodic LTM.

In order to fully understand the nature of the three component structures of the Working Memory model, it is necessary to discuss the issue of its measurement. Indeed, many tasks have been developed in order to assess working memory in children and adults.

Only the tasks involving the CE component are defined as working memory tasks, and they generally require the simultaneous storage and manipulation of verbal-phonological or visual-spatial information. One of the best known and used working memory tasks is the *Listening span task* (Daneman & Carpenter, 1980), which is considered to involve both the CE and the PL; in particular, the processing component of verbal information is supported by the central executive, whereas storage is provided by the phonological loop (Baddeley & Logie, 1999). The task involves processing a series of sentences and expressing a true/false judgment on their content. At the end of the list of sentences, participants have to recall the last word of each sentence.

The PL is generally measured through tasks classically used to measure verbal and phonological short-term memory span. Individuals are required to recall increasing lists of verbal information in the given order (digit names, words or non-words), and the span measure of the subject corresponds to the maximum length of the list correctly recalled.

Many studies have widely demonstrated that the type of verbal material that is used in the span tasks may lead to significant differences in individuals' span. Indeed, people show generally higher spans in tasks involving short words than in tasks involving long words (*length effect,* Baddeley, Thomson & Buchanan, 1975); people show higher spans in tasks involving phonologically dissimilar words than in tasks involving phonologically similar words (*phonological similarity effect*); people show higher spans in tasks involving known words than in tasks involving foreign words or non-words (*lexicality effect,* Hulme, Maughan & Brown, 1991). Finally, people show lower verbal spans when they are required to performs a concurrent task, such as to say "bla, bla" while a verbal list is presented (*articulatory suppression condition*, Baddeley, Lewis & Vallar, 1984), or simply if they are exposed to an unattended discourse while they are learning lists of verbal items (*unattended speech condition*, Salame & Baddeley, 1982). All these experimental effects have demonstrated the nature of PL. Indeed, both phonological and unattended speech effects demonstrated the existence of a store specialized for phonological material and sensible to phonological interference, where phonological traces are stored for a very short period of time before decay; the length and suppression effects have demonstrated the existence and the importance of the rehearsal mechanism, which allows the traces in the phonological store to be refreshed and reactivated, contrasting their decay. Lexicality effect, finally, is the evidence for a long-term memory contribution to short-term memory span. All the above described effects highlight that phonological abilities, articulatory rate and long term knowledge may significantly influence individuals' performance. In order to control these influences, Gathercole and colleagues developed the non-words repetition test (Gathercole & Baddeley, 1996; Gathercole & Pickering, 2000), defined as a "pure" measure of phonological short term memory since it does not require the use of verbal rehearsal (the children have simply to repeat one non-word at a time) and, using low wordlike nonwords, makes little use of long term knowledge.

Similar to the PL, the VSSP is also generally measured through tasks classically used to measure visual spatial short-term memory span. The most famous task is certainly the Corsi block recall, used to measure memory for visual sequences. In this task, the experimenter taps from two up to nine blocks following a series of fixed sequences, and the subject is required to reproduce the tapping sequences in the same serial order. Other VSSP tasks require the recognition and/or the reproduction of visual patterns (Della Sala et al., 1999; McLean & Hitch, 1999; Wilson, Scott, & Power, 1987).

A complete assessment of the three component structures of the working memory was developed by Pickering and Gathercole (2001) and by Alloway (2007). Both test batteries are suitable for use with children age 5 and older and include measures of CE function, measures of PL function and measures of VSSP function.

1. INDIVIDUAL DIFFERENCES IN WORKING MEMORY AND THEIR RELATIONSHIPS WITH READING, WRITING AND ARITHMETIC LEARNING

Several studies have evidenced the role of working memory in explaining individual differences in reading, writing (see Gathercole & Baddeley, 1993a, or Pickering, 2006, for a review) and arithmetic learning (i.e. Geary, 1993, 2003; Jordan, Hanich, & Kaplan, 2003; Swanson & Sachse-Lee, 2001) as well as its causal role in learning disabilities, and they will be briefly examined below.

1.1. Working Memory and Reading

Reading development and specific reading disorders, such as dyslexia, have been studied in depth in the last 20 years, and many authors have focused on the individuation of the factor leading to normal development and learning disorders. Many authors place phonological abilities at the core of reading abilities and phonological deficit as principal causal factors of dyslexia (Snowling, 1995), whereas other focused on rapid perception of auditory and visual information (Tallal, 1980). Many other studies, described below, have focused on the role of working memory in reading development and reading disorders using different methodologies such as longitudinal studies, matching-groups studies and experimental studies.

Longitudinal studies evidenced that working memory abilities assessed in preschool children predict their reading level during primary school. Mann and Liberman (1984) evidenced that children showing a reduced letter span of phonological similar and dissimilar letters showed reading difficulties during primary school. Only these tasks involving PL, however, predict *reading* learning performance, while tasks involving VSSP, such as the Corsi span task, were not associated with later levels of reading. Gathercole and Baddeley (1993b), moreover, demonstrated that preschool performance in non-word repetition tests predicts later performance in reading tasks involving phonological processes. Both results have been replicated by D'Amico (2000a), and evidenced that digit and word span, as well as non-word repetition measured in preschool children, predict their reading levels during primary school.

Other demonstrations of the strong association between working memory and reading come from studies where working memory abilities of children with learning difficulties are matched to those of normal achievers. Indeed, many studies have demonstrated that children with specific reading disabilities have lower performance in tasks involving the PL (digit span, word span or non-word repetition), while they seem to have normal performance in VSSP tasks (Siegel, 1994). However, it should be noted that children with specific reading disabilities do display sensitivity to the phonological similarity effect, word length effect and unattended speech effects (Ackerman & Dykman, 1993; D'Amico, 2000b; Hall, Wilson, Humphreys, Tinzmann & Bowyer, 1983; Hansen & Bowey, 1994; Holligan & Johnston, 1988; Johnston, Rugg & Scott, 1987; Sechi, D'Amico, Longoni & Levi, 1997). These results, taken together, seem to demonstrate that children with reading difficulties use phonological codes in short term memory and make use of rehearsal strategies as well as children with normal abilities, although their performance is poorer than that of good readers.

Other interesting results regarding the involvement of working memory in reading processes come from studies involving normal readers performing different reading tasks. Arthur, Hitch, Halliday (1994), proposed reading tasks to 8-year old children respectively requiring the use of visual or phonological reading strategies under articulatory suppression condition. Only the reading task requiring the use of phonological route was significantly damaged by the suppression condition, while performance in the reading task requiring the use of visual route was unaltered by the experimental condition. This result, which has been replicated by Kimura and Bryant (1983) in children and by Besner, Davies and Daniels (1981) and Baddeley and Lewis (1981) in adults, demonstrates the importance of PL processes for phonological reading.

Other studies focussing on reading comprehension demonstrated that it basically relies on CE processes. Glanzer, Dorfman and Kaplan (1981), evidenced that concurrent tasks involving CE processes (backward enumeration) had a destructive effect on reading comprehension performances. Similarly, Daneman and Carpenter (1980) and Baddeley, Logie Nimmo-Smith and Brereton (1985) evidenced that reading comprehension of a group of university students was highly associated with the performance in the Listening Span Task. In a subsequent study, Daneman and Carpenter (1983) have also evidenced that subjects with high Listening Span performance were more skilled in ambiguous text comprehension.

Interesting results come also from a study by Yuill, Oakhill, and Parkin (1989) involving children with selective difficulties in reading comprehension and normal phonological reading, who found significant differences in a working memory task requiring reading aloud multi-digit numbers and recalling the last number of each group. A series of other studies produced converging evidence of an association between reading comprehension and working memory tasks that require the processing and storage of words (De Beni, Palladino, Pazzaglia, & Cornoldi, 1998), sentences (Seigneuric, Ehrlich, Oakhill, & Yuill, 2000), and numbers (Yuill et al., 1989), but not with tasks that require the manipulation of shapes and patterns (Nation, Adams, Bowyer-Crane, & Snowling, 1999; Seigneuric et al., 2000).

Cain, Oakhill, and Bryant (2004) however, have argued that the relationship between working memory and comprehension could have been overestimated since all the considered tasks are verbally mediated. Thus, in order to explore the extent to which the predictive power of the working memory tasks is mediated by verbal ability, they studied the relation between working memory and text comprehension taking into account the contribution of verbal ability as well. Results, however, demonstrated that working memory and component skills of comprehension (inference making, comprehension monitoring, story structure knowledge) predicted unique variance in reading comprehension after word reading ability and vocabulary and verbal ability were controlled for. Thus, working memory should be regarded as one, even if unique, of several factors that can influence comprehension ability and comprehension development.

1.2. Working Memory, Writing and Spelling

There are not many studies about the role of working memory in writing and spelling abilities. However, obtained results demonstrated that central executive processes are involved in writing composition, while phonological Loop processes are involved in spelling and orthography.

Swanson and Berninger (1996a) evidenced that performance in listening span tasks (Daneman & Carpenter, 1980) are associated to text generation. A second study by the same authors (Swanson & Berninger, 1996b) investigated the role of working memory tasks involving CE, PL and VSSP in writing. Results evidenced that VSSP tasks were not related to writing abilities, while performances in CE tasks were related to text generation and the ability in PL tasks was related to the use of orthography and punctuation. The relationships between performances in tasks involving PL and orthography were confirmed in a study by Kroese, Hynd, Knight, Hiemenz and Hall (2000).

1.3. Working Memory and Mathematical Learning

As regards the relationships between working memory abilities and mathematical achievement, different studies have reported a linear relationship between performances in digit span (Gathercole, Pickering, Knight, & Stegmann, 2004; Hoosain & Salili, 1987) or in central executive tasks (Bull & Scerif, 2001; Gathercole et al., 2004) and mathematical abilities as evaluated using standardized achievement batteries. Other studies have demonstrated that conditions that overload the working memory capacity, e.g. solving mental calculations rather than written calculations, result in poorer performances both in adults (Hitch, 1978) and children (Adams & Hitch, 1997). Finally, a series of experimental studies have shown that concurrent tasks involving the central executive component (Furst & Hitch,

2000; Lemaire, Abdi, & Fayol, 1996; Logie, Gilhooly, & Wynn, 1994; Seitz & Schumann-Hengsteler, 2000), the phonological loop (Furst & Hitch, 2000; Haughey, in Hitch, Cundick, Haughey, Pugh, & Wrigth, 1987; Lau & Hoosain, 1999; Lee & Kang, 2002; Lemaire, Abdi & Fayol, 1996; Logie et al., 1994; Seitz & Schumann-Hengsteler, 2000) or the visual-spatial sketchpad (Heathcote, 1994; Lee & Kang, 2002) have a deleterious effect on the execution of calculation processes.

The role played by the different components of working memory in arithmetical performance has been further explored in a series of studies involving children with Arithmetical Learning Difficulties (ALD) and controls (e.g. Bull & Johnston, 1997; Bull, Johnston, & Roy, 1999; McLean & Hitch, 1999; Passolunghi & Siegel, 2001). The literature examined is quite consistent in highlighting an impairment of the central executive process in children with ALD. Indeed, these subjects perform worse than controls in more general executive tasks such as the Wisconsin Sorting Card Tasks (Bull et al., 1999), in central executive tasks that require a switch between numerical/ linguistic retrieval strategies (McLean & Hitch, 1999) and in working memory tasks with a high executive demand (Siegel & Ryan, 1989) which involve both numerical or linguistic material (Gathercole, Pickering, Ambridge, & Wearing, 2004; Passolunghi & Siegel, 2001; Swanson & Sachse-Lee, 2001).

The results concerning the role of PL and VSSP in children with ALD seem more controversial. While converging evidence has demonstrated that these subjects perform normally in non-word repetition (McLean & Hitch, 1999) and word span (Bull & Johnston, 1997; Passolunghi & Siegel, 2001), their results in the short-term recall of digits are often inconsistent. In a number of studies, low arithmetical achievers performed normally in digit span tasks (Bull & Johnston, 1997; Geary, Hamson & Hoard, 2000; Geary, Hoard, & Hamson, 1999), whereas in other studies they performed at a significantly lower level than controls (Passolunghi & Siegel, 2001; Swanson & Sachse-Lee, 2001; see also McLean & Hitch, 1999, who found group differences very close to the statistical significance).

With regard to the functioning of the visual-spatial sketchpad, McLean and Hitch (1999), reported that children with ALD and normal reading abilities showed impairment in the Corsi Block task, even though they performed normally in the short-term recall of random visual-spatial patterns (Matrix task, adapted from Wilson, Scott, & Power, 1987), a result more recently replicated by Swanson and Sachse-Lee (2001), using a very similar task.

For these reasons, a study by D'Amico & Guarnera (2005) was aimed at drawing a complete and extensive picture of all the working memory functions of children with arithmetical difficulties but with normal reading abilities, focusing particularly on the differences between tasks that use linguistic and numerical material. A group of Italian children with low arithmetical achievement and normal reading skills (mean age: 9 years) and a group of age-matched controls with normal arithmetical and reading achievement were involved in the study. The two groups were presented with a series of working memory tasks, involving CE, PL and VSSP components.

Results of the study supported the view that the CE and the VSSP play an important role in arithmetical abilities, while the involvement of the PL seems to have been overestimated in the literature that based its observation only on the digit span performance of children with ALD. Indeed children with ALD underperformed in all CE tasks involving linguistic information (Listening Span task), and numerical information (Digit Span Backward) or both linguistic and numerical information (Making Verbal Trails) as compared to the control group. These results, consistent with the evidence from recent literature (Gathercole et al.,

2004; Passolunghi & Siegel, 2001; Swanson & Sachse-Lee, 2001) and with the results of a further study by D'Amico and Passolunghi (2009), confirmed the hypothesis of a domain independent central executive disorder in children with ALD. The CE impairment could be one of the causal factors of the difficulty of children with ALD in tasks such as the mental and written calculations that require pupils to simultaneously retain information (the amount carried, the loan, etc.) and to transform the new incoming items (i.e. the new addends) as well as to inhibit a pre-activated retrieval strategy (Barrouillet, Fayol, & Lathulière, 1997; Bull & Scerif, 2001; Passolunghi & Siegel, 2001; Swanson & Sachse-Lee, 2001).

Concerning the PL, D'Amico and Guarnera (2005) evidenced that children with ALD underachieved only in the digit span forward while, consistent with Bull and Johnston (1997) and Passolunghi and Siegel (2001), they showed normal word span abilities as well as normal non-word repetition abilities (McLean and Hitch's study, 1999). This selective impairment in the short-term recall of numerical material would have highlighted a difficulty in the access and retrieval of information from the numerical lexicon. However, D'Amico and Passolunghi (2009), investigating the rate of access to long term information in children with arithmetic difficulties compared to controls, revealed that children with ALD were slower than the controls in naming both digits and letters, and did not show a selective impairment in the long-term representation of numbers.

Finally, children with ALD underachieved both in the visual-spatial passive short-term memory task (Matrix Task) and in the visual-spatial sequential memory task (Corsi Block Task). Even if the literature regarding this issue is not really consistent (Bull et al., 1999; McLean & Hitch, 1999; Swanson & Sachse-Lee, 2001; Passolunghi & Cornoldi, 2008), many of the difficulties of children with ALD could be explained with reference to their visual-spatial difficulties: consider that one of the subtypes of learning disabilities in mathematics described by Geary (1993, 2004) is actually considered to be caused by difficulties in spatially representing numerical and other forms of mathematical information and relationships. Actually, visual spatial abilities are involved in a lot of arithmetical tasks such as alignment process in performing arithmetical operations (Rourke, 1993; see also Rourke and Conway, 1997), mental calculations requiring the manipulation of a number in a "mental blackboard" (compared to the visual sketchpad) where individuals store information while performing an operation (Heathcote, 1994), comparison between quantities that are based on an analogical magnitude code and require subjects to generate and use the mental representation of the number line (Campbell, 1994; Dehaene, 1997) or pay attention to the order of each digit in multi-digit numbers.

Controversial results of literature are explainable if we consider several methodological difficulties of studies involving children with arithmetical difficulties and controls. Indeed, these studies generally involve groups of children with arithmetic difficulties, who show non-homogeneous levels and typologies of arithmetical difficulties: some of them show calculation difficulties whereas others show particular troubles with number comprehension (McCloskey, Caramazza & Basili, 1985). It is also possible that different components of working memory underlie different subgroups of arithmetic disabilities as was found for reading disabilities (Swanson, Howard, Saetz, 2006).

2. ASSESSMENT AND TREATMENT OF WORKING MEMORY FOR PREVENTING READING AND MATHEMATICAL DIFFICULTIES: A STUDY REPORT

Working memory abilities improve significantly during the first years of life. Different studies involving children demonstrated that their memory span increases significantly from the age of 3 to the age of 8-9 (Orsini, Grossi, Capitani, Laiacona, Papagno & Vallar, 1987; Gathercole et al., 2004).

This improvement is basically explained referring to cerebral maturation but also to the development of other cognitive functions (i.e. language) or to the use of coding, maintaining and retrieving strategies (Schneider & Pressley, 1989; Coyle & Bjorklund, 1997; Coyle, Read, Gaultney & Bjorklund, 1999). For instance, the increase of PL is considered to be linked to the increased rate of rehearsal, which enables the child to maintain growing amounts of verbal material in the phonological store (Gathercole & Baddeley, 1993a).

Increasing performance is also due to changes in coding and recall strategies. Indeed, it has been demonstrated that children younger than 7 years old typically rely on the visual spatial sketchpad to support recall of pictures of familiar objects. Older children, however, tend to use the phonological loop to mediate immediate memory performance where possible, and so recode the visual inputs into a phonological form via rehearsal (e.g., Hitch & Halliday, 1983).

Despite the fact that the capacity of each component of working memory shows a steady increase from the preschool years through adolescence, the basic modular structure of the WM is present from 6 years of age (Gathercole et al., 2004). This is very important because it implies the possibility to assess working memory in young children and, when low performances are evidenced, to set up early intervention programmes.

Studies aimed at improving working memory in children are not numerous. Ho, Cheung and Chan (2003), in a study involving children and adolescents, reported the significant effect on verbal memory of a training based on listening to musical pieces. Hays e Pereira (1972) and Whisler (1974) demonstrated that visual spatial training produced significant improvements in reading abilities of primary school children. Klingberg, Forssberg and Westerberg (2002) demonstrated that visual spatial training produces significant effects on the ability to perform the same visual spatial memory tasks, as well as a generalization effect in other visual-spatial tasks.

Based on this and other subsequent studies by Klingberg and colleagues (Klingberg, et al., 2002; Thorell, Lindqvist, Bergman, Bohlin & Klingberg, 2008), CogMed developed a computerised training programme designed to enhance working memory through intensive practice in working memory activities. Work sessions of about 35 minutes a day for six weeks were shown to have a positive impact on working memory performance and inattentive behaviours in children with ADHD (Klingberg et al., 2005) and in enhancing childrens' working memory (Holmes, Gathercole & Dunning, 2009).

In particular, the study by Thorell, Lindqvist, Bergman, Bohlin e Klingberg (2008) demonstrated that the Cogmed program has a positive impact in improving working memory abilities in preschool children with normal abilities thus preventing difficulties in early academic achievement that may have otherwise occurred.

D'Amico (2006) also reported significant effects of a working memory training program on memory abilities and mathematical learning in children of the first class of primary school. This study will be reported on in more detail, describing the results concerning reading and writing abilities of children as well.

2.1. Method

A test-treatment-retest experimental design was adopted in order to study the efficacy of working memory treatment and its role in reading and mathematical achievement.

During the test phase, two classes of children attending the first year of primary school were administered a series of working memory tasks. Moreover, teachers were asked to rate scholastic abilities of children participating in the study. During the treatment phase, one of the two classes (where lower scholastic achievements were rated) followed the training program described below, while the control class carried out the normal scholastic activities. During the retest phase children were again administered the same working memory tests and teachers rated their scholastic achievement. Moreover, reading, writing and arithmetical levels of children in both classes were assessed through standardised tests.

Test-treatment-retest phases are described in more details below.

2.2. Participants

32 children, attending the first two classes of an Italian primary school, took part in the research (whole group: mean age= 75.3 months SD = 3.7, 18 males, 14 females; group assigned to the experimental condition: mean age= 74.8 months, 10 males, 5 females; group assigned to the control condition: mean age= 75.7 months, 8 males, 9 females).

Children in the two classes shared the same three teachers of Italian, Mathematics and Anthropology. This was retained to minimise the effect of different teaching styles and educational methods between the two groups.

2.3. Material and Procedures

2.3.1. Test phase
Scholastic achievement
Given that children were just at the beginning of the first year of primary school, it was not possible to assess their scholastic achievement using standardised tests, which are usually administered beginning in the middle of the first year of primary school. Thus, teachers were requested to rate the reading, writing and arithmetic baselines of children involved in the study assigning them a score form 0 to 4, basing their judgement in part on final profiles of the children at the end of pre-school. In particular they rated children's abilities in reading comprehension, reading aloud, writing under dictation, single digit calculations and logical-spatial knowledge (up-down, right-left knowledge).

The teachers' ratings were then examined and the class that was assigned to the experimental condition obtained lower scores than the other class in all the considered variables. Some of the differences between classes in teachers' ratings were statistically significant, and in particular for quantity judgements ($F(1,30) = 5.39$, $p<.05$) and logical-spatial knowledge, $F(1,30) = 5.85$ $p<.05$).

Working memory abilities

All children were administered a series of working memory tasks, listed and described below.

Listening span task. In the Italian version by D'Amico (2002a) of the Daneman and Carpenter (1980) listening span task, the experimenter reads a set of sentences aloud, asking the child to express a true/false judgment on the content of each sentence and to recall, at the end of the set, the last word of each sentence. Examples of true and false sentences are respectively "The child has a red umbrella" or "The ship floats in the sky". "Sky" and "umbrella" are, in these examples, the words to be recalled at the end of the set presentation. The test is composed of 12 sets of increasing length from 2 to 5 sentences (three sets for each length); following the Daneman and Carpenter (1980) procedure, the listening span score corresponds to the longest set of sentences of which the last words have been correctly recalled. For assigning the score, the true/false judgment is irrelevant. Listening span task is considered to involve both CE and PL.

Digit span backward. Recalling digits in the inverse order of presentation is generally considered to involve both the phonological loop and the central executive (Morra, 1994; Pickering & Gathercole, 2001), as the sequence spoken by the experimenter must be stored and reversed to produce the correct answer. The administration procedure of the digit span backward (drawn from the Wechsler Scale for Children—Revised, 1974) is as follows: the experimenter reads a series of digits aloud (starting from sets of 2 digits up to sets of 8 digits), asking children to recall the digit set in the reverse order (i.e.: 3, 4, 8 becomes 8, 4, 3). The score corresponds to the maximum length of the digit set recalled in the reverse order of presentation.

Non-word repetition task. The non-word repetition task used in this study was developed by D'Amico (2002b) and required children to repeat, one at a time, a series of non-words pronounced by the experimenter. The task consists of 18 non-words from 5 to 9 phonemes in length. The Non-word Repetition score corresponds to the total number of phonemes correctly repeated. This task is considered to measure phonological short term memory.

Bisyllabic word span task. In order to measure PL processes, a word span task was used. It was developed by D'Amico (2000b) and consisted of a series of frequently occurring Italian bisyllabic words like "sole" (sun) and "gatto" (cat). The task administration and the scoring method were similar to those used for the digit span tasks: the experimenter read a series of words aloud (starting from sets of 2 items up to sets of 8 items), asking children to recall the words in the same order as the presentation. The Bisyllabic Word Span score corresponds to the maximum length of the word set recalled in the same serial order.

Digit span forward task. A second task used to measure the PL was the Digit Span Forward Task, drawn from the WISC-R Scale (Wechsler, 1974). The administration procedure is as follows: the experimenter reads a series of digits aloud (starting from sets of 2 items up to sets of 8 items), asking children to recall the item set in the same order as the presentation. The Digit Span Forward score corresponds to the maximum length of the item set recalled in the correct order of presentation.

Short-term memory for patterns and positions. In order to assess VSSP processes, a new task was developed (D'Amico, 2006). Each child is presented with ten 5x5 matrixes where the experimenter places an increasing number of cards (from 2 to 5) reproducing circles printed with different patterns. After 10 seconds, each matrix is removed and the child is presented with a blank matrix where he has to replace the same cards in the same positions.

Two scores are assigned; the pattern score reflects the numbers of correct patterns recalled, the position score reflects the number of correct positions recalled.

Visual-spatial working memory. A second VSSP task was also developed for the aims of the study (D'Amico, 2006). Children are presented with sets of pairs of figures presenting the same geometrical pattern or different geometrical patterns. The sets may be from 2 to 5 pairs in length. Firstly, children are requested to judge if the figures in each couple are the same or different. At the end of the set of pairs, they have to recall the second figure of each couple by pointing it out from a series of distracters. The score corresponds to the longest set of couples of which the last figures have been correctly recalled. For assigning the score, the same/different judgment is irrelevant. Since this task requires the simultaneous elaboration of visual spatial information and its maintenance in short term memory, it is considered to involve both VSSP and CE processes.

2.3.2. Treatment phase

The treatment phase had a duration of 1 hour, twice a week, for 6 weeks. The training was performed during school hours, in a playful context and in group sessions. The specific activities are described below.

Random number/letter generation. The trainer asked children to say aloud, in random order, the number in the range between 1 and 20 or the letter of the alphabet. Each child had to say one item, in turn, without repeating the item that has already been said by his classmates and without following a fixed sequence (i.e. number sequence of alphabetical sequence).

This activity, inspired to the well known random generation tasks (Baddeley, 1998) was intended to involve CE functions of information updating and long-term information retrieving, as well as PL functions, required to maintain the item already pronounced by classmates.

Serial and free recall of verbal material. The trainer read aloud a list of 20 words. Then, he asked each child, in turn, to recall each word without repeating words already pronounced by his classmates. The activities were performed with different word lists, which were composed of: 20 high frequency 2-syllable words (3 lists of concrete words and 1 list of abstract words), 20 high frequency 3-4 syllable words (3 lists of concrete words and 1 list of abstract words), 20 low frequency 2-syllable words (3 lists of concrete words and 1 list of abstract words).

The same activities were performed both in free order recall conditions or in serial recall condition. Similar to the previous one, this activity was intended to involve the CE and the PL functions.

Serial and free recall of names in categories with concurrent task. The trainer read aloud a list of 20 words requiring children to tap a hand on the desk every time they heard an animal's name. At the end of the list, they were required to recall all the non-animal names and then all the animals' names that they were presented with. This activity was intended to stimulate the executive control, since it required children to perform a categorization task, and then an inhibition and updating task, which are necessary to recall all the non target items (the non-animal names) and the target items (the animals' names). PL loop was also implicated in this activity, to the extent to which the manipulation of verbal material was required.

Figure matching. The activity is inspired by the well known game "Memory". The trainer placed 36 covered cards with 18 pairs of identical objects printed on the back on a desk. Each child turned up 2 cards in order to find the pairs with identical objects; every time that a child found a pair, it remained turned face up on the desk, otherwise, both cards were turned down again and another child played the game. This activity was intended to improve the VSSP, and in particular memory for figures and positions.

Memory for positions. Children were presented with a series of 3x3 matrixes with some coloured squares. After 10 seconds, the target matrix was removed and children were presented with a blank matrix where they had to colour the squares identical to the target matrix. This activity was intended to improve the VSSP and in particular memory for positions.

Memory for "live" positions. A large cardboard matrix 5x5 (150x150 centimetres) was placed on the floor, and the experimenter placed some bonbons on three, four or five squares in the matrix. After 10 seconds the bonbons were removed and the children were required, in turn, to place themselves in the same squares where the bonbons had previously been placed. When children recalled all the correct positions, they got the bonbons as a reward. In another version of the game, a group of children displayed the target positions in the matrix and then their classmates had to reproduce the same positions. These activities were intended to improve the VSSP in a more lively context.

Memory for "smiles" and positions. Children were presented with a series of 3x3 matrixes, where some emoticons had been drawn. After 10 seconds, the target matrix was removed and children were presented with a blank matrix where they had to draw the same emoticons in the same positions as they had been presented. This activity was intended to improve VSSP, and in particular memory for figures and positions.

Memory for visual-spatial routes. The trainer showed a 3x3 matrix, indicating a square as the starting point. Then the matrix was removed and children were given some visual spatial instructions such as "go to the square on the right", "go one square up", "go two squares down" and so on. At the end, the children were asked to indicate the final position with an X, on a black matrix. This activity was inspired by the "active matrix task" by Cornoldi, Friso, Giordano, Molin, Poli, Rigoni, & Tressoldi (1997) and required children to generate and to move inside a sort of mental space. It was intended to improve visual-spatial memory, with an involvement of high level executive processes.

2.3.3. Retest phase

At the end of treatment, the class assigned to the experimental condition and the control class were submitted to a second phase of assessment of working memory, with the same tasks used in the test phase. Then, teachers were again required to rate (assigning a score from 0 to 4) reading, writing and arithmetic achievement of children at the end of the school year.

Since effect of treatment on scholastic achievement was evaluated based only on teachers' ratings, scores obtained by children in the standardised tests of reading, writing and arithmetic were used in order to verify the concurrent validity of teachers' ratings. In particular, reading has been assessed using the standardised MT battery (Cornoldi & Colpo, 1981). This test allows assessment of children's accuracy and speed in reading aloud, requiring them to read aloud a passage, while the experimenter scores the reading errors and the time taken to read it. Moreover, the test allows assessment of reading comprehension, requiring pupils to read a passage to themselves and to answer 10 questions about its content. The reading comprehension score corresponds to the total number of correct answers.

Writing under dictation was assessed using a passage drawn from Tressoldi and Cornoldi's test battery (1991). All children are collectively required to write under dictation and the total number of spelling errors are recorded.

The AC-MT standardised test was used for the assessment of number comprehension and calculation (Cornoldi, Lucangeli & Bellina, 2002). This test allows the calculation of four scores of Written Calculation, Number Knowledge, Accuracy and Speed using both collective and individual testing. Written Calculation tasks and Number Knowledge tasks are paper and pencil tasks in which the participant must solve four written multi-digit calculations (two additions and two subtractions) and to perform a series of number magnitude judgments, with an increasing and decreasing number arrangement and tasks of numerical syntax comprehension. Accuracy and Speed correspond respectively to the total accuracy and the total time taken to perform some individual tasks such as 6 mental simple calculations, 2 written simple calculations, 1-20 counting, 1-10 numbers dictation and retrieval of arithmetical facts.

2.4. Results

The descriptive statistics of participants and the summary of main effects and interactions are reported in Table 1.

A series of factorial analyses of variance (ANOVA) with repeated measures were performed to evaluate the differences between the experimental group and controls in all the considered tasks. Results do not reveal any significant effect of Group in the considered variables, while the effect of Time factor was significant for digit span forward task, Listening span task and STM for positions.

A significant interaction Group x Time in visual spatial working memory task, and an interaction close to statistical significance in STM for positions evidenced that children in the experimental group, after treatment, improved their working memory abilities in these tasks significantly more than children in the control group.

Table 1. Descriptive statistics of children in Experimental group and in the Control group and summary of main effects and interactions

	Experimental Group (N 15; 10 M, 5 F)		Control Group (N 17; 8 M, 9 F)		ANOVAs		
	Test M (*DS*)	Retest M (*DS*)	Test M (*DS*)	Retest M (*DS*)	Group $F(1, 30)$	Time $F(1, 30)$	Group x Time $F(1, 30)$
Working memory							
Non-word repetition task	118.3 (*3.5*)	118.1 (*4.5*)	117.5 (*5.7*)	117.3 (*5.8*)	.25	.21	.001
Bisyllabic word span task	3.7 (*1.1*)	4 (*.7*)	3.8 (*.6*)	3.8 (*.7*)	.003	2.23	1.23
Digit span forward task	4.4 (*.6*)	4.8 (*.9*)	4.2 (*.8*)	4.8 (*1.2*)	.13	8.89**	.49
Digit span backward	2.4 (*.9*)	2.5 (*.7*)	2.5 (*.8*)	2.5 (*.6*)	.08	.14	.001
Listening span task	1.3 (*.9*)	1.5 (*1.3*)	1.1 (*.9*)	2 (*.9*)	.47	6.07*	2.41
Visual-spatial working memory	.8 (*.6*)	1.7 (*1.1*)	1.6 (*.8*)	1 (*.6*)	.17	.76	12.95***
STM for patterns	9.6 (*2.7*)	9.5 (*2*)	9.6 (*2.2*)	9.6 (*2.1*)	.001	.06	.06
STM for positions	8.4 (*2.6*)	11.5 (*3.3*)	9.2 (*3.1*)	10.1 (*1.5*)	.15	10.97**	3.45 [a]
Scholastic achievement (teachers' ratings)							
Reading and writing							
Reading Comprehension	1.8 (*1.08*)	2.6 (*1.18*)	2.17 (*1.01*)	2.94 (*.89*)	.99	78.47***	.40
Reading aloud	1.66 (*1.17*)	2.6 (*1.12*)	1.88 (*1.05*)	2.76 (*.90*)	.27	73.6***	.58
Writing under dictation	1.73 (*1.16*)	2.46 (*1.12*)	1.94 (*1.02*)	2.53 (*1.12*)	.13	46.13***	.56
Arithmetic							
Quantity knowledge	2.07 (*1.10*)	2.67 (*.81*)	2.82 (*.73*)	3 (*.71*)	3.77 [a]	14.31 ***	4.26*
Calculations	2.00 (*1.00*)	2.6 (*.9*)	2.12 (*.99*)	2.53 (*.62*)	.006	25.2***	.87
Spatial relationships	2.07 (*1.03*)	2.6 (*1.05*)	2.82 (*.72*)	2.7 (*.77*)	1.9	7.5*	18.43***

*$p < .05$, **$p < .01$, ***$p < .001$, [a]$p = .07$

Similarly, a series of ANOVAs were performed using teachers' ratings as dependent variables. Results (reported in Table 1) did not reveal any Group effect. Significant Time effects for all the considered variables, on the contrary, demonstrated that all the children improved their scholastic achievement from the beginning of the school year to the end.

Significant Group x Time interactions in Quantity Knowledge and Spatial Relationship teachers' ratings demonstrated that children in the experimental group improved their scholastic achievement in these arithmetical areas significantly more than children in the control group.

The validity of the retest teachers' ratings was confirmed through a series of correlation analyses that revealed many significant associations between teachers' rating and standardised test scores, and in particular between teachers' ratings in Reading aloud and MT Correctness and Speed ($r=-.60$ $p<.001$ and $r=-.66$ $p<.001$), between teachers' ratings in Reading comprehension and MT Reading comprehension ($r=.32$ $p=.07$, close to significance), and between teachers' ratings in Writing under dictation and Tressoldi and Cornoldi's Writing under dictation ($r=.70$ $p<.001$). Teachers' ratings in Quantity knowledge were associated to AC-MT Number knowledge ($r=.40$ $p<.05$) and AC-MT Accuracy ($r=-.36$ $p<.05$). Teachers' ratings in Calculation were associated to AC-MT Number knowledge ($r=.37$ $p<.05$) and Speed ($r=-.39$ $p<.05$). Teachers' ratings in Spatial relationships were associated to AC-MT Number knowledge ($r=.54$ $p<.005$), Accuracy ($r=-.36$ $p<.05$) and Speed ($r=-.38$ $p<.05$).

2.5. Discussion

This study demonstrates that methodologies coming from experimental research may be efficiently applied in an educational context. Indeed, all the treatment activities were performed during school hours, in the school context and with the class-group. This gave an entertaining and playful aspect to the entire treatment, motivating interest and participation of the children.

As reported in the results section, the working memory treatment had a significant effect on improving visual spatial working memory abilities of children belonging to the experimental group. In fact, the activities intended to improve the VSSP were particularly suitable to be performed in group sessions. Children enjoyed playing, and engaged more in these activities than in the verbal ones. Last but not least, in the Memory for "live" positions, children also received a reward for their performances.

A second result of the study was that children in the experimental group showed a significantly higher improvement than children in the control group in quantity knowledge and spatial relationships teachers' ratings. As reported in the test section, children in the experimental group had shown lower performance than the children in the control group in these aspects of arithmetic achievement; if we consider that both groups shared the same teachers and the same scholastic programme, it is quite plausible to infer that the strengthening of these abilities in the experimental group was also due to the working memory treatment. This interpretation is also supported by the interconnected evidence that children in the experimental group improved their performance in visual spatial memory tasks but not in verbal memory tasks and, at the same time, they obtained improved scholastic ratings in some aspects of arithmetic but not in reading. As reported in the first part of this chapter, psychological literature has revealed that VSSP is an important underlying factor of arithmetic processes, while it does not seem implicated in reading processes. All things considered, it is possible to claim that an improvement of VSSP processes in children of experimental groups might have lead to a subsequent improvement of their arithmetical abilities, and to overcoming the difficulties that had been recorded by teachers at the beginning of the school year.

CONCLUSION

In conclusion, all the studies described in this chapter denote the growing interest of researchers regarding working memory and its role in explaining individual learning differences. The interest in working memory, moreover, is not specific to psychologists interested in cognitive processes research, as it is shared also by clinical psychologists working with children with learning or cognitive disabilities, and by educators and teachers.

Assessment of working memory, indeed, may give important insights to school and clinical psychologists in order to cope with the sometimes puzzling problem of diagnosis of learning disabilities. Indeed, many children, during the first years of primary school, show difficulties in reading, writing or arithmetic, and it is even more frequent when socio-cultural disadvantages or educational dysfunctional conditions are present.

Under these circumstances, it is very hard to say whether the learning failure symptoms shown by children reflect a learning disability or rather they simply reflect learning difficulties, which may be overcome by more intense teaching sessions and practice. One of the approaches that could be used in order to distinguish between children with false positive and true positive learning disability, thus, could be an in-depth assessment of their working memory processes. If children show good functions in all working memory processes, their diagnosis might plausibly be formulated as learning difficulty, and the relative prognosis might be more optimistic. Otherwise, if the working memory functions of children appear to be compromised, it is more probable that the observed learning failure symptoms reflect a learning disability.

Assessment of working memory, moreover, may help school psychologists and teachers to formulate prediction of risk for specific learning difficulties, and to indicate some children for additional attention starting in pre-school.

It should be noted, however, that working memory individual profiles may also be improved by specific intervention programmes, as the research's findings previously described have evidenced.

These results stress the potentialities of working memory treatment programmes for the early intervention in children at risk for learning disabilities and for cognitive rehabilitation of declared cases of learning disabilities or ADHA. Indeed, working memory improvements, in turn, often lead to better reading, writing and arithmetic performances, as well as to a reduction of ADHD's symptoms.

Given the importance of the assessment and training of working memory, one of our recent efforts has been to develop an Italian working memory test followed by a treatment program (D'Amico & Lipari, *in press*), aimed at measuring and improving working memory functions in **5 to 15 year olds**.

The test, actually under standardisation on a sample of about 500 primary school children, has a two-level structure. The first level, following Baddeley and Hitch's working memory model (1974; Baddeley, 1986) is composed of three measures of phonological loop (non-word repetition, word span and digit span), three measures of visual-spatial sketchpad (visual pattern span, visual-spatial pattern span, visual-spatial sequences span), and three tasks involving central executive functions (listening span, counting span, visual-spatial span).

The second level is composed of 5 tasks aimed at examining different cognitive processes which are considered to be involved in working memory functions (Baddeley, 2000; Barrouillet, Bernardin & Camos 2004; Cowan, 1995; Miyake et al., 2000). In particular, three tasks (number-letter shifting, random number generation and Navon task) measure respectively the executive functions of shifting, updating and inhibition. The remaining two tasks measure rate of access to long term memory and speed of processing (letter, number and picture naming, and visual target search).

The treatment programme includes many of the activities already used in the study previously described, along with other new activities aimed at improving the use of memo-techniques, as well as at improving attentional processes involved in working memory and speed of processing.

REFERENCES

[1] Ackerman, P. T. & Dykman, R. A. (1993). Phonological processes, confrontational naming, and immediate memory in dyslexia. *Journal of learning disabilities*, *26(9)*, 597-609.

[2] Adams, J. W. & Hitch, G. J. (1997). Working memory and children's mental addition. Journal of Experimental Child Psychology, 67, 21-38.

[3] Alloway, T. P. (2007). The Automated Working Memory Assessment. London: Psychological Corporation

[4] Arthur, T. A. A., Hitch G. J. & Halliday, M. S. (1994). Articulatory loop and children's reading. British Journal of Psychology, 85, 283-300.

[5] Baddeley, A. D. (1986). Working Memory. Oxford: Oxford University Press.

[6] Baddeley, A. D. (1996). Exploring the central executive. Quarterly Journal of Experimental Psychology, 49A, 5-28.

[7] Baddeley, A. D. (1998). Random generation and the executive control of working memory. Quarterly Journal of Experimental Psychology. 51A, 819–852.

[8] Baddeley, A. D. (2000). The episodic buffer: A new component of working memory? Trends in Cognitive Science, 4, 417-423.

[9] Baddeley, A. D. & Hitch, G.J. (1974). Working Memory. In G. Bower (Ed.), The Psychology of Learning and Motivation, 8, 47-90

[10] Baddeley, A. D. & Lewis, V. J. (1981). Inner active processes and reading: The inner voice, the inner ear, and the inner eye. In A. M. Lesgold & C. A. Perfetti (Eds), Interactive Processes in Reading, pp. 107-129. Hillsdale, NJ: Lawrence Erlbaum Associates Inc.

[11] Baddeley, A. D. & Logie R.H.. (1999). Working memory: The multiple component model. In: Miyake A, Shah P, editors. Models of Working Memory, pp. 28–61. New York: Cambridge University Press.

[12] Baddeley, A. D., Lewis, V. J. & Vallar, G. (1984). Exploring the articulatory loop.

Quarterly Journal of Experimental Psychology, 36, 233-252.
[13] Baddeley, A. D., Logie, R. H., Nimmo-Smith, I. & Brereton, N. (1985). Components of fluid reading. Journal of Memory and Language, 24,119-131.
[14] Baddeley, A. D., Thomson, N. & Buchanan, M. (1975). Word length and the structure of short term memory. Journal of Verbal Learning and Verbal Behavior, 14, 575-589.
[15] Barrouillet, P., Bernardin, S. & Camos, V. (2004). Time constraints and resource sharing in adults' working memory spans. Journal of Experimental Psychology. General, 133(1), 83–100.
[16] Barrouillet, P., Fayol, M. & Lathulière, E. (1997). Selecting between competitors in multiplication tasks: an explanation of the errors produced by adolescents with learning disabilities. International Journal of Behavioural Development, 21, 253-275.
[17] Besner, D., Davies, J. & Daniels, S. (1981). Reading for meaning: The effects of concurrent articulation. Quarterly Journal of Experimental Psychology, 33a, 415-437.
[18] Bull, R. & Johnston, R. S. (1997). Children's arithmetical difficulties: contributions from processing speed, item identification, and short-term memory. Journal of Experimental Child Psychology, 65, 1-24.
[19] Bull, R., Johnston, R. S. & Roy, J. A. (1999). Exploring the roles of the visual-spatial sketch pad and central executive in children's arithmetical skills: Views from cognition and developmental neuropsychology. Developmental Neuropsychology, 15, 421-442.
[20] Bull, R. & Scerif, G. (2001). Executive Functioning as a predictor of children's mathematics ability: inhibition, switching, and working memory. Developmental Neuropsychology, 19(3), 273-293.
[21] Cain, K., Oakhill, J. & Bryant, P. E. (2004). Children's reading comprehension ability: Concurrent prediction by working memory, verbal ability, and component skills. Journal of Educational Psychology, 96, 31-42.
[22] Campbell, J. I. D. (1994). Architectures for numerical cognition. Cognition, 53, 1-44.
[23] Cornoldi, C. & Colpo, G. (1981). La verifica dell'apprendimento della lettura. O.S., Firenze.
[24] Cornoldi, C., Friso, G., Giordano, L., Molin, A., Poli, S., Rigoni, F. & Tressoldi, P. E. (1997). Abilità visuo-spaziali. Intervento sulle difficoltà non verbali di apprendimento. Trento: Erickson.
[25] Cornoldi, C. & Lucangeli, D. Bellina (2002). AC-MT. Test di valutazione delle abilità di calcolo. Trento, Erickson.
[26] Cowan, N. (1995). Attention and memory: An integrated framework. New York: Oxford University Press.
[27] Cowan, N. (2005). Working memory capacity. New York, NY: Psychology Press.
[28] Coyle, T. R. & Bjorklund, D. F. (1997). Age differences in, and consequently of, multiple- and variable strategy use on a multitrial sort recall task. Developmental Psychology, 33, 372-380.
[29] Coyle, T. R., Read, L.E., Gaultney, J. F. & Bjorklund, D. F. (1999). Giftedness and variability in strategic processing on a multitrial memory task: evidence for stability in gifted cognition. Learning and Individual Differences, 10, 273-290.
[30] D'Amico A. (2000a). Il ruolo della memoria fonologica e della consapevolezza fonemica nell'apprendimento della lettura. Ricerca longitudinale. Psicologia Clinica dello Sviluppo. Anno IV, 1, 125-143.
[31] D'Amico, A. (2000b). Lo span di memoria verbale e la ripetizione di parole e non

parole. Confronto tra buoni e cattivi lettori. Rassegna di Psicologia. Vol. XVII.1, 51-72.
[32] D'Amico, A. (2002a). Lettura, Scrittura, Calcolo. Processi cognitivi e disturbi dell'apprendimento. Edizioni Carlo Amore, Roma.
[33] D'Amico, A. (2002b). Processi implicati nella ripetizione di non parole verosimili ed inverosimili. Ricerche di Psicologia, XXV(3), 7-22.
[34] D'Amico A. (2006). Potenziare la memoria di lavoro per prevenire l'insuccesso in matematica. Età Evolutiva, vol. 83, 90-99.
[35] D'Amico A. & Guarnera, M. (2005). Exploring Working Memory in Children with low Arithmetical Achievement. Learning and Individual Differences, 15, 189-202.
[36] D'Amico A. e Lipari C. (in press). Batteria per la Valutazione ed il Trattamento della Memoria di Lavoro. Firera & Liuzzo Publishing, Roma.
[37] D'Amico A. & Passolunghi M. C. (2009). Naming speed and Effortful and Automatic Inhibition in Children with Arithmetic Learning Disabilities. Learning and Individual Differences , 19, 170-180.
[38] Daneman, M. & Carpenter, P. A. (1980). Individual differences in working memory and reading. Journal of Verbal Learning and Verbal Behavior, 19, 450-466.
[39] Daneman, M. & Carpenter, P. A. (1983). Individual differences in integrating information between and within sentences. Journal of Experimental Psychology: Learning Memory and Cognition, 9, 561-584.
[40] De Beni, R., Palladino, P., Pazzaglia, F. & Cornoldi, C. (1998). Increases in intrusions errors and working memory deficit of poor comprehenders. Quarterly Journal of Experimental Psychology, 51A, 305-320.
[41] Dehaene, S. (1997). The number sense. New York: Oxford University Press.
[42] Della Sala, S., Gray, C., Baddeley, A. D., Allamano, N. & Wilson, L. (1999). Pattern span: A tool for unwelding visuo-spatial memory. Neuropsychologia, 37, 1189-1199.
[43] Engle, R. W. (2002). Working memory capacity as executive attention. Current Directions in Psychological Science, 11, 19-23.
[44] Furst, A. J. & Hitch, G. J. (2000). Separate roles for executive and phonological components of working memory in mental arithmetic. Memory and Cognition, 28(5), 774-782.
[45] Gathercole, S. E. & Baddeley, A. D. (1993a). Working Memory and Language. Lawrence Erlbaum Association. London.
[46] Gathercole, S. E. & Baddeley, A. D. (1993b). Phonological working memory: a critical building block for reading development and vocabulary acquisition? European Journal of Psychology and Education, Vol. VIII (3), 259,272.
[47] Gathercole, S. E. & Baddeley, A. D. (1996). The Children's Test of Nonword Repetition. New York: Psychological Corporation.
[48] Gathercole, S. E. & Pickering, S. J. (2000). Assessment of working memory in six and seven year-old children. Journal of Educational Psychology, 92, 377-390.
[49] Gathercole, S. E., Pickering, S. J., Ambridge, B. &Wearing, H. (2004). The Structure of Working Memory From 4 to 15 Years of Age. Developmental Psychology, 40(2), 177–190.
[50] Gathercole, S. E., Pickering, S. J., Knight, C. & Stegmann, Z. (2004). Working memory skills and educational attainment: evidence from national curriculum assessments at 7 and 14 years of age. Applied Cognitive Psychology, 18,1-16.
[51] Geary, D. C. (1993). Mathematical disabilities: Cognitive, neuropsychological, and

genetic components. Psychological Bulletin, 114, 345–362.
[52] Geary, D. C. (2003). Learning disabilities in arithmetic: problem solving differences and cognitive deficits. In H. L. Swanson, K. R. Harris & S. Graham (Eds.), Handbook of Learning Disabilities, pp. 199-212. The Guilford Press, New York.
[53] Geary, D. C. (2004). Mathematics and Learning Disabilities. Journal of Learning Disabilities 37(1), 4-15.
[54] Geary, D. C., Hamson, C. O. & Hoard, M. K. (2000). Numerical and arithmetical cognition: A longitudinal study of process and concept deficits in children with learning disability. Journal of Experimental Child Psychology, 77, 236-263.
[55] Geary, D. C., Hoard, M. K. & Hamson, C. O. (1999). Numerical and arithmetical cognition: Patterns of function and deficits in children at risk for a mathematical disability. Journal of Experimental Child Psychology, 74, 213-219.
[56] Glanzer, M., Dorfman, D. & Kaplan, B. (1981). Short-term storage in the processing of text. Journal of Verbal Learning and Verbal Behavior, 20, 656-670.
[57] Hall, J. W., Wilson, K. P., Humphreys M. S., Tinzmann, M. B. & Bowyer, P. M. (1983). Phonemic-similarity effects in good vs. poor readers. Memory and Cognition, 11(5), 520-527.
[58] Hansen, J. & Bowey, J. (1994). Phonological analysis skills, verbal working memory and reading ability in second-grade children. Child Development, 65, 938-950.
[59] Hays, B. M. & Pereira, E. R. (1972). Effect of visual memory training on reading ability of kindergarten and first grade children. Journal of Experimental Education, 41(1), 33-38.
[60] Heathcote, D. (1994). The role of visuo-spatial working memory in the mental addition of multi-digit addends. Current Psychology of Cognition, 13, 207-245.
[61] Hitch, G. J., Cundick, J., Haughey, M., Pugh, R. & Wright, H. (1987). Aspects of counting in children's arithmetic. In: J. E. Sloboda, & D. Rogers, (eds.), Cognitive processes in mathematics, Oxford: Oxford University Press.
[62] Hitch, G. J. (1978). The role of short-term working memory in mental arithmetic. Cognitive Psychology, 10(3), 302-323.
[63] Hitch, G. J. & Halliday, M. S. (1983). Working memory in children. Philosophical Transactions of the Royal Society, Series B, 302, 324-340.
[64] Ho, Y., Cheung, M. & Chan, A. S. (2003). Music Training Improves Verbal but Not Visual Memory: Cross-Sectional and Longitudinal Explorations in Children. Neuropsychology, 17(3), July, 439–450.
[65] Holligan, C. & Johnston, R. (1988). The use of phonological information by good and poor readers in memory and reading tasks. Memory and Cognition, 16(6), 522-532.
[66] Holmes J., Gathercole S. E. & Dunning D. L. (2009). Adaptive training leads to sustained enhancement of poor working memory in children. Developmental Science, 12(4), 9-15.
[67] Hoosain, R. & Salili, F. (1987). Language differences in pronunciation speed for numbers, digit span and mathematical ability. Psychologia, 30, 34-38.
[68] Hulme, C., Maughan, S. & Brown, G. D. A. (1991). Memory for familiar and unfamiliar words: evidence for a long-term memory contribution to short-term memory span. Journal of Memory and Language, **30**, 685-701.
[69] Johnston, R. S., Rugg, M. D. & Scott, T. (1987). Phonological similarity effects, memory span and developmental reading disorders: the nature of relationship. British

Journal of Psychology, 78, 205-211.

[70] Jordan, N. C., Hanich, L. B. & Kaplan, D. (2003). Arithmetic fact mastery in young children: A longitudinal investigation. Journal of Experimental Child Psychology, 85,103-119.

[71] Kimura, Y. & Bryant, P. (1983). Reading and writing in English and Japanese: A cross cultural study of young children. British Journal of Developmental Psychology, 1, 143-154.

[72] Klingberg, T., Fernell, E., Olesen, P., Johnson, M., Gustafsson, P., Dahlström, K., Gillberg, C. G., Forssberg, H. & Westerberg, H. (2005). Computerized training of working memory in children with ADHD – a randomized, controlled trial. J American Academy of Child and Adolescent Psychiatry, 44(2), 177-186.

[73] Klingberg, T., Forssberg, H. & Westerberg, H. (2002). Training of Working Memory in Children With ADHD. Journal of Clinical and Experimental Neuropsychology, 24(6), 781-791.

[74] Kroese, J. M., Hynd, G. W., Knight, D. F., Hiemenz, J. R. & Hall, J. (2000). Clinical appraisal of spelling ability and its relationship to phonemic awareness (blending, segmenting, elision, and reversal), phonological memory, and reading in reading disabled, ADHD, and normal children. Reading and Writing: An Interdisciplinary Journal, 13, 105-131.

[75] Lau, C. W. & Hoosain, R. (1999). Working memory and language difference in sound duration: A comparison of mental arithmetic in Chinese, Japanese, and English. Psychologia: An International Journal of Psychology in the Orient, 42(3), 139-144.

[76] Lee, K. M. & Kang, S. Y. (2002).Arithmetic operation and working memory: differential suppression in dual tasks. Cognition, 83, B63–B68

[77] Lehto, J. E., Juujärvi, P., Kooistra, L. & Pulkkinen, L. (2003). Dimensions of executive functioning: Evidence from children. British Journal of Developmental Psychology, vol. 21, 59-80.

[78] Lemaire, P., Abdi, H. & Fayol, M. (1996). The role of working memory resources in simple cognitive arithmetic. European Journal of Cognitive Psychology, 8(1), 73-103.

[79] Logie, R. H. (1991). Visuo-spatial working memory: Visual working memory or Visual buffer? In C. Cornoldi & M. McDaniel (Eds.), Imagery and Cognition, pp. 77-102. Berlin: Springer-Verlag.

[80] Logie, R. H., Gilhooly, K. J. & Wynn, V. (1994). Counting on working memory in arithmetic problem solving. Memory and Cognition, 22(4), 395-410.

[81] Logie, R. H. & Pearson, D. G. (1997). The inner eye and the inner scribe of visuo-spatial working memory: Evidence from developmental fractionation. European Journal of Cognitive Psychology, 9, 241-257.

[82] Mann, V. A. & Liberman, I. Y. (1984). Phonological awareness and verbal short term memory. Journal of learning disabilities., 17, 592-598.

[83] McCloskey, M., Caramazza, A. & Basili, A. (1985). Cognitive mechanisms in number processing and calculation: evidence from dyscalculia. Brain Cognition, 4, 171-196.

[84] McLean, J. F. & Hitch, G. J. (1999). Working memory impairments in children with specific arithmetic learning difficulties. Journal of Experimental Child Psychology, 74(3), 240-260.

[85] Miyake, A., Friedman, N. P., Emerson, M. J., Witzki, A. H., Howerter, A. & Wager, T. D. (2000). The unity and diversity of executive functions and their contributions to

complex frontal lobe tasks: A latent variable analysis. Cognitive Psychology, 41, 49-100.

[86] Morra, S. (1994). Issues in working memory measurement: Testing for M capacity. International Journal of Behavioural Development, 17, 143-159.

[87] Nation, K., Adams, J. W., Bowyer-Crane, C. A. & Snowling, M. J. (1999). Working memory deficits in poor comprehenders reflect underlying language impairments. Journal of Experimental Child Psychology, 73, 139-158.

[88] Orsini, A., Grossi, D., Capitani, E., Laiacona, M., Papagno, C. & Vallar, G. (1987). Verbal and spatial immediate memory span: normative data from 1355 adults and 1112 children. Italian Journal of Neurological Sciences, 8, 539-548.

[89] Passolunghi, M. C. & Cornoldi, C. (2008). Working memory failures in children with arithmetical difficulties. Child Neuropsychology, 14, 387-400.

[90] Passolunghi, M. C. & Siegel, L. S. (2001). Short-term memory, working memory and inhibitory control in children with difficulties in arithmetic problem solving. Journal of Experimental Child Psychology, 80, 44-57.

[91] Pickering, S. J. (2006). Working memory in dyslexia. In T. P. Alloway & S. E. Gathercole (Eds.), Working memory and neurodevelopmental disorders (7-40). Hove, UK: Psychological press.

[92] Pickering, S. J. & Gathercole, S. E. (2001). Working Memory Test Battery for Children. London: Psychological Corporation.

[93] Quinn, J. G. (1988). Interference effects in the visuo-spatial sketchpad. In: M., Denis, J. EngleKamp, & J. T. E. Richardson, (Eds.), Cognitive and neuropsychological approaches to mental imagery (181-189). Amsterdam: Martinus Nijhoff.

[94] Quinn, J. G. & McConnell, J. (1996). Irrelevant pictures in visual working memory. Quarterly Journal of Experimental Psychology, 40A, 200-215.

[95] Rourke, B. P. (1993). Arithmetic disabilities, specific and otherwise: A neuropsychological perspective. Journal of Learning Disabilities, 26(4), 214-226.

[96] Rourke, B. P. & Conway, J. A. (1997). Disabilities of arithmetic and mathematical reasoning: Perspectives from neurology and neuropsychology. Journal of Learning Disabilities, 30, 34-46.

[97] Salame, P. & Baddeley, A. D. (1982). Distruption of memory by unattended speech: implication for the structure of working memory. Journal of Verbal Learning and Verbal Behavior., 21, 150-164.

[98] Schneider, W. & Pressley, M. (1989). Memory development between 2 and 20. Springer Verlag, Berlin.

[99] Sechi, E., D'Amico, A., Longoni, A. M. & Levi, G. (1997). Le componenti della memoria verbale a breve termine nei bambini con disturbo specifico di lettura. Psichiatria dell'Infanzia e dell'Adolescenza, Vol.64(6).

[100] Seigneuric, A., Ehrlich, M. F., Oakhill, J. & Yuill, N. (2000). Working memory resources and children's reading comprehension. Reading and Writing, 13, 81-103.

[101] Seitz, K. & Schumann-Hengsteler, R. (2000). Mental multiplication and working memory. European Journal of Cognitive Psychology, 12(4), 552-570.

[102] Siegel, L. S. (1994). Working memory and reading: a life span perspective. International Journal of Behavioral Development, 17(1), 109-124.

[103] Siegel, L. S. & Ryan (1989). The developmental Working memory in normally achieving and subtypes of learning disabled children. Child Development, 60, 973-980

[104] Snowling, M. J. (1995). Phonological processing and developmental dyslexia. Journal of Research in Reading, 18, 132-138.
[105] Swanson, H. L. & Berninger, V. W. (1996a). Individual differences in children's writing: A function of working memory or reading or both processes? Reading and Writing, Aug; Vol 8(4), 357-383
[106] Swanson, H. L. & Berninger, V. W. (1996b). Individual differences in children's working memory and writing skill. Journal of Experimental Child Psychology. Nov; Vol 63(2), 358-385.
[107] Swanson, H. L., Howard, C. B. & Sáez, L. (2006). Do different components of working memory underlie different subgroups of reading disabilities? Journal of Learning Disabilities, 39(3), 252-69.
[108] Swanson, H. L. & Sachse-Lee, C. (2001). Mathematical problem solving and working memory in children with learning disabilities: both executive and phonological processes are important. Journal of Experimental Child Psychology, 79, 294-321.
[109] Tallal, P. (1980). Auditory temporal perception, phonics, and reading disabilities in children, Brain and Language, 9, 182–198.
[110] Thorell, L. B., Lindqvist, S., Bergman, S., Bohlin, G. & Klingberg, T. (2009). Training and transfer effects of executive functions in preschool children. Developmental Science, 12(1), 106-113.
[111] Tressoldi, P. & Cornoldi, C. (1991). Batteria per la valutazione della scrittura e della competenza ortografica. O.S., Firenze.
[112] Vallar, G. & Baddeley, A. D. (1984). Fractionating of working memory: neuropsychological evidence for a short-term memory store. Journal of Verbal Memory and Verbal Behavior, 23, 151-161.
[113] Wechsler, D. (1974). Manual for the Wechsler Intelligence Scale for Children-Revised. New York: Psychological Corporation.
[114] Whisler, N. G. (1974). Visual-memory training in first grade: Effects on visual discrimination and reading ability. Elementary School Journal, 75(1), 50-54.
[115] Wilson, J. T. L., Scott J. H. & Power, K. G. (1987). Developmental differences in the span of visual memory for pattern. British Journal of Developmental Psychology, 5, 249-255.
[116] Yuill, N., Oakhill, J. & Parkin, A. (1989). Working memory, comprehension ability and the resolution of text anomaly. British Journal of Psychology, 80, 351-361.

In: Working Memory: Capacity, Developments and…
Editor: Eden S. Levin

ISBN: 978-1-61761-980-9
© 2011 Nova Science Publishers, Inc.-

Chapter 8

WORKING MEMORY IN SENTENCE COMPREHENSION AND PRODUCTION

Matthew J. Traxler[*,1], *David Caplan*[2], *Debra L. Long*[1] *and Gloria S. Waters*[3]

[1]University of California, Davis, CA, USA
[2]Massachusetts General Hospital, Harvard University
[3]Boston University, Boston, MA, USA

ABSTRACT

Sentence comprehension and production both involve temporary activation, storage, and manipulation of partially structured representations. Comprehenders sometimes buffer individual words and phrases as they register and process new input and relate new to previously presented input. Speakers must activate conceptual representations, search for corresponding lexicalized concepts, place them in the appropriate order, and apply the proper inflections before they can begin articulation. All of this activity requires some ability retain information in an active state and manipulate this information. Considerable research on both healthy and neurologically impaired individuals has focused on describing the working memory system or systems that support this temporary activation and manipulation of information. This paper provides an overview of the theoretical and methodological issues that characterize research in this area, with a particular emphasis on sentence processing. We will make a number of suggestions for improving the methods used to research working memory in sentence comprehension and production.

---

* Address Correspondence to:Matt Traxler, Department of Psychology, UC Davis, 1 Shields Avenue, Davis, CA 95616, 530 752 2087 (fax) 530 902 8526 (o), mjtraxler@ucdavis.edu

I. MODELS OF WORKING MEMORY AND SENTENCE COMPREHENSION

Cognitive psychologists have long recognized that limitations on attention influence human cognition. While individuals possess vast quantities of stored information and are exposed to an equally vast and changing set of sensory stimuli, they can access and manipulate only a tiny fraction of that information at any given time. Tasks such as language comprehension, that require accessing and using stored and incoming information, must also be carried out using mechanisms and processes that do not overtax human information processing limitations. Cognitive psychologists use the term *working memory* to describe mechanisms that allow individuals to maintain and manipulate information in the service of cognitive tasks, such as language comprehension and production, logical reasoning, decision making, arithmetic, and so on.

Alan Baddeley's model of working memory (Baddeley, 1974; 2000; Baddeley & Hitch, 1974; see also Cowan, 2010; Engle, 2010; Jonides et al., 2008) provides the most prominent general model of the human working memory system. On this account, verbal, visual, and episodic buffers are used to maintain information in an active state as computations are being performed. The capacity of the individual buffers, sometimes called *slave systems*, is limited, and decisions need to be made about how activated information is to be organized (i.e., chunking). The operations of the buffers are directed by a *central executive*, which keeps track of the contents of the slave systems and makes decisions about task scheduling. The Baddeley working memory model has successfully accounted for a variety of empirical phenomena related to chunking, including effects of similarity between newly encountered stimuli and pre-existing knowledge (Baddeley et al., 2009). Cognitive psychologists working on language have borrowed many of Baddeley's ideas to explain how comprehenders process language. For instance, at the level of discourse, Ericsson & Kintsch (1995) have developed the concept of a long term working memory system that can take advantage of pre-existing knowledge structures in long-term memory to help make decisions about how information should be chunked.

This review focuses on the sentence level. Comprehending any sentence involves determining how the words in the sentence are related to one another, a process that is called *dependency formation*. For example, in sentence (1), there is a relationship between the words *guy* and *wrote*, and *know* and *guy*:

(1) This is the *guy* that some of us *know* who *wrote* about working memory.

In sentence (1), the word *guy* appears in an unusual position (compare to: *some of us know this guy* and *this guy wrote about working memory*). The consensus view in linguistics and psychology is that the initial noun *guy* must be held in an incompletely interpreted state as other parts of the sentence are being processed, because it is not immediately apparent what syntactic and semantic role that noun plays. In fact, the word *guy* plays two different syntactic and semantic roles, those of object and theme of the verb *know* and subject and agent of the verb *wrote*. Those syntactic and semantic roles become clear only after the comprehender has reached the verbs *know* and *wrote*. Thus, comprehenders must exploit working memory resources to hold the initial noun *guy* in an active state until the appropriate dependencies can be formed.

Psycholinguists have appealed to working memory capacity limits to explain why some sentences are harder to process than others (e.g., Gibson, 1998; Just & Carpenter, 1992; King & Just, 1991; Wanner & Maratsos, 1978). These accounts differ in detail, but they all argue that processing speed, accuracy, or both will suffer when the demands imposed by sentence-structuring processes exceed the working memory system's tolerances. Recent studies have identified characteristics of language that can increase demands on working memory. Some accounts have focused on the putative computational demands imposed by dependency forming processes themselves (Andrews et al., 2006; Traxler et al., 2002; Waters & Caplan, 2005). Other accounts have appealed to general encoding and retrieval processes that can be complicated by some aspects of linguistic material. In particular, similarity-based interference between activated elements has been shown to impair sentence interpretation (Gordon et al., 2001; van Dyke & McElree, 2006). These two perspectives need not be in conflict, as both complexity and interference appear to influence dependency formation and interpretation. However, syntactic complexity can slow comprehenders down even when there is minimal opportunity for similarity-based interference to have an effect (Betancourt et al., 2009; Mak et al., 2002, 2006; Traxler et al., 2002, 2005).

The application of the working memory concept to sentence processing can be naturally extended to account for individual differences in sentence processing proficiency. Within the normal population, some individuals interpret sentences quickly and accurately, while others have more difficulty. If working memory capacity imposes limitations on processing and interpretation, lower working memory capacity measures would be expected to correlate with less efficient sentence processing, which would be more evident at points of greater working memory load in sentences that make more working memory demands. Patients who have suffered brain damage following strokes, tumors, or accidents can also have difficulty processing sentences (Caplan & Hildebrandt, 1988; Martin, 2003), as can patients with dementing disorders. Psycholinguists and neurologists have appealed to individual differences in working memory capacity to explain variability in the normal population as well as sentence-processing and comprehension deficits in patient populations (Just & Carpenter, 1992; Caplan & Waters, 1999; Waters & Caplan, 1996).

Despite its utility in providing an explanation for variation in sentence processing efficiency, the working memory theory of sentence comprehension has been criticized on theoretical and empirical grounds. One line of criticism maintains that there is no working memory system separate from language processing mechanisms; i.e., that people's language processing system(s) are used to perform working memory tasks, and there is no separate short-term store or Central Executive devoted to working memory as in Baddeley's account (MacDonald and Christiansen, 2002; Acheson & MacDonald, 2009; Misyak, Christiansen & Tomblin, 2009; see also McElree, 2001, Verhaeghen et al., 2004; Cowan, 1995, for different views of working memory capacity). MacDonald and Christiansen argued for a large role for comprehension processes in working memory tasks, and Acheson and MacDonald argued that production processes, particularly phonological encoding, also have a large role in working memory tasks. In a similar vein, Martin and Ayala (2004) reported that aphasic patients' performance on verbal and pointing digit and word span was predicted by their lexical-semantic and phonological processing abilities, with higher correlations between span and lexical tasks that shared processing. However, these results do not establish that processing of phonological, lexical and lexical semantic representations totally accounts for performance on short-term/working memory tasks. In Martin and Ayala's study, for instance, correlations between lexical and span tasks were in the .5 range (the highest was .77), accounting for less than 50% of the shared variance between lexical processing and span. Models of short-term/working memory include mechanisms such as decay and interference parameters that either have no direct counterparts or are not subject to the same processes as similar mechanisms in models of lexical processing, (Page and Norris, 1996; Nairne et al., 1997) and, conversely, models of sentence processing utilize mechanisms that correspond to short-term/working memory (within the terms of the model), such as the "context units" in simple recurrent network models of comprehension (MacDonald & Christiansen, 2002; Weckerly and Elman, 1992). Thus, there is no getting away from dealing with memory in either short-term/working memory or sentence comprehension.

The application of the concept of working memory to sentence processing has led researchers to consider two related questions. The first is what component of working memory is involved in sentence comprehension. Baddeley's model provides two mechanisms whereby verbal information can be stored – the verbal slave system (the Phonological Buffer and the Articulatory Loop), in which information is maintained in a phonological and articulatory form, and the Central Executive, in which information is maintained in more abstract form (not fully specified in Baddeley's model), either of which might support maintenance of information in sentence comprehension. R. Martin and her colleagues have suggested that another component of the working memory system maintains lexical semantic representations. The second question is whether the working memory capacity underlying sentence processing is shared with other cognitive tasks (the *shared resources* hypothesis), or whether sentence processing has its own distinct working memory system (the *dedicated resource hypothesis*). Baddeley's model includes separate verbal and spatial slave systems, and subsequent research has provided evidence for similar verbal and spatial specializations within the Central Executive component of his model (e.g., Miyake et al., 2001). Advocates of the dedicated resources hypothesis carry this fractionation one step further to separate the memory system utilized in language processing from that used in other verbally mediated tasks. We review these topics in turn.

II. WORKING MEMORY COMPONENTS AND SENTENCE COMPREHENSION

Initial data suggesting that phonological representations were maintained in memory during sentence processing came from studies of patients with deficits in the Phonological Store and Articulatory Loop ("short term memory" patients), whose comprehension of various types of sentences was shown to be abnormal. However, in an exhaustive review of all published cases, Caplan and Waters (1990) argued that these data were inconclusive. Experimental evidence against the phonological representation maintenance model came from cross modal lexical priming results (Love and Swinney, 1996) that showed priming of both contextually supported and unsupported meanings of homophones immediately after their occurrence, no priming further into the sentence, and priming of only contextually supported meaning at an even later point when the homophone was related to a verb. This pattern suggests that the stored representation, whose activation level increases at the point when it is needed, is lexical semantic or conceptual in nature. Waters et al.(1992) reached a similar result for written sentences on the basis of a cost of phonological plausibility of unacceptable sentences containing homophone antecedents and either surface (verb-gap) anaphors or pronouns in plausibility judgment with whole sentence but not with rapid serial visual presentation (RSVP); i.e., participants found it harder to reject "The children sleighed in the park and the murderer in cold blood" as implausible than "The children skied in the park and the murderer in cold blood" only in whole sentence, not RSVP. Evidence that a short duration semantic memory system plays a role in sentence processing also comes from patients who have shown no sensitivity to semantic variables in short term memory tests and who have a characteristic problem in sentence comprehension consisting of difficulty understanding sentences in which multiple pieces of information must be maintained in memory before they are integrated into a concept (e.g., *The boy liked the large, black, expensive, handmade briefcase*; vs. *The boy liked the briefcase that was large, black, expensive, and handmade*). However, the abnormalities in sentence comprehension seen in the semantic short term memory patients are not those predicted by the working memory model of sentence comprehension (see above). If the verbal memory slave systems are not used in memory during sentence comprehension and lesions of the semantic short-term memory system do not lead to working-memory-related comprehension deficits, then some other component of the system must support sentence interpretation processes. The only possible remaining component is the Central Executive, and many researchers have concluded that the Central Executive is the working memory component that is critical for comprehension.

III. FRACTIONATION OF THE CENTRAL EXECUTIVE AND SENTENCE COMPREHENSION

The second question researchers have addressed is whether the Central Executive is fractionated into a component that supports aspects of sentence processing and one that supports other verbally mediated functions (the *dedicated resource theory*) or not (the *shared resource* model; Just & Carpenter, 1992; King & Just, 1991; Just, Carpenter, & Keller, 1996). There have been two approaches to this question – the study of individual differences, and the study of dual task effects. The logic is as follows: If individuals differ in their working memory capacity, and if those working memory differences underlie both linguistic and non-linguistic verbal processing, then individual differences in working memory capacity should correlate with the individual differences in the magnitude of the effects of variables that affect working memory demands in sentences. Similarly, if a single working memory system underlies both linguistic and non-linguistic verbal processing, increasing the working memory demands of each type of process should lead to superadditive interactions in dual task performance when linguistic and non-linguistic verbal tasks are performed together.

III. A. Individual Differences Studies

Support from individual differences research for the shared resources hypothesis can be found in individual differences in sentence processing efficiency. One well known study classified participants as being "high" or "low" in working memory capacity based on the sentence span test (King & Just, 1991). In this study, participants read syntactically simpler sentences, such as (2), and syntactically complex sentences, such as (3),

(2) The reporter that attacked the senator apologized after the meeting.
(3) The reporter that the senator attacked apologized after the meeting.

Sentences such as (3) typically take longer to process than sentences such as (2) (see Traxler et al., 2002, for a review of several accounts that explain why). In this study, the difference between processing times for the two sentences was claimed to be greater for individuals who had low working memory scores than for individuals who had high working memory scores. While lower span participants appeared to have greater difficulty with more complex sentences than higher span participants, there are some complications. First, the critical interactions between working memory, sentence complexity, and sentence segment were not reported in ANOVAs (see Waters & Caplan, 1996). Second, as explained below, ANOVA is not an appropriate method to investigate individual differences where the underlying characteristic varies continuously. Studies using more appropriate analyses have not found effects of working memory on on-line processing of more complex sentences (Traxler et al., 2005; Traxler, 2007, 2009).

Other studies have also found effects of working memory on aspects of sentence processing. Pearlmutter and MacDonald (1995), for example, found that high-span readers, but not low-span readers, were influenced by semantic characteristics in a form of mild garden-path sentence, represented by (4):

(4) The soup cooked in the pot but was not ready to eat.

High span readers, but not low span readers, showed a processing cost at and following the word "but," which disambiguates the sentence, when reading times for sentences such as (4) were compared to unambiguous controls (...*soup was cooked in the pot but*...). Traxler and colleagues (2005) found evidence that high-span readers were more sensitive to semantic information, animacy specifically, which helped speed their reading of sentences containing object-relative clauses. However, these studies do not vary complexity along the lines discussed above, but they do provide evidence that some aspects of sentence processing, perhaps ones related to semantics, differ as a function of working memory.

In contrast with the shared resources account, the dedicated resources account proposes that certain sentence interpretation processes are supported by a pool of working memory resources that does not serve any other purpose and is not tapped by non-linguistic cognitive processes (Caplan & Waters, 1999; Waters & Caplan, 1996). The fact that the Daneman and Carpenter (1990) sentence-span test correlates with performance on a variety of language tasks (Daneman & Carpenter, 1983; Daneman & Merikle, 1996) indicates that this is likely to be the case only for a selected number of language operations. Caplan and Waters' account draws a distinction between cognitive processes that are responsible for lexical access, parsing, and the assignment of a standard semantic interpretation -- *interpretive processes* -- and cognitive processes that operate on the outcome of interpretive processes -- *post-interpretive processes* – and claims that a specialized working memory system supports interpretive processes. Studies of clinical populations provide support for the dedicated resources hypothesis (Waters et al, 1995; Waters & Caplan, 1996; Caplan, Waters and DeDe, 2007). In these studies, patients with Alzheimer's Disease completed working memory tests, such as sentence span. They also completed sentence-processing tasks involving self-paced listening or self-paced reading. The results indicated that patients could parse and interpret sentences, even if the sentences had complex syntax with non-canonical ordering of constituents, despite having measured working memory capacities of zero. If the reading span test tapped the same working memory system that underlies parsing and interpretation, these patients should have been incapable of understanding sentences.[1]

The view of working memory and sentence processing that calls into question the concept of working memory resources altogether (MacDonald & Christiansen, 1992) objects to this model on theoretical grounds. According to this viewpoint, cognitive processes are undertaken by connectionist networks where knowledge is stored as connection weights between individual representational units. In such a system, some stimuli may produce faster and more accurate responses than others because of the way they drive activation in the network, but, as noted above, there is nothing in the system that corresponds to working memory capacity. Theorists who advocate this approach are especially dubious about the distinction between automatic and non-automatic processes. Under traditional views of working memory, tasks that are "automatic" are carried out rapidly, outside conscious awareness, without conscious volition, and do not impose measurable load on working memory resources. To determine whether a given task is difficult because it occupies working memory resources, one needs an independent assessment of whether a given process is automatic. If not, the shared resources theory cannot be falsified. If a task leads to slowed processing or decreased accuracy, the shared resources account would attribute that result to overtaxing working memory capacity. However, if a task does not lead to slowed processing or decreased accuracy, that result could be explained away simply by classifying the task as "automatic."

In fact, there is a close relationship between practice and response time for a variety of cognitive tasks, including sentence processing and interpretation (Wells et al., 2009; Long & Prat, 2008; Tooley, 2009). Sentences that have simpler syntactic structures (e.g., subject-verb-object) tend to be more frequent than sentences that have more complex structures (e.g., sentences involving object extraction), so contrasts of simple and complex syntax usually also involve contrasts of frequent and less-frequent structure. Hence, differences in the way comprehenders respond to different kinds of sentences could be attributed to practice effects. Studies in which participants have been repeatedly exposed to sentences with rare and

---

[1] A recent study suggested that these findings could have been an artifact of the segmentation technique used in the self-paced listening task (Kemper & Liu, 2007). However, this study suffers from some of the methodological flaws identified in the "Individual Differences Approach" section of this article, including testing small numbers of participants, using an extreme-groups design, and applying the inappropriate statistical methods. Further, the stimuli used in the study maximize opportunities for similarity-based confusion (i.e., the nouns were generics such as doctor and banker). Finally, the study did not explore variables that are known to correlate with working memory and that have been shown to mediate working-memory's effects on sentence processing tasks, such as processing speed.

complex structures show that, over time, their processing speed for those sentence types increases. Standard working memory accounts suggest that working memory capacity is a fixed individual characteristic, so such changes in sentence processing efficiency would have to be the results of improvements in automaticity, rather than capacity. By contrast, accounts such as MacDonald and Christiansen's would suggest that improvements in efficiency result from changes in connectivity within the relevant pool of processing units.

III. B. Dual-Task Studies

In dual-task studies of sentence comprehension, participants undertake a language processing task at the same time they are undertaking an unrelated secondary task. One of the first such studies contrasted processing of sentences such as (2) and (3) (repeated here; Wanner & Maratsos, 1978):

(2) The reporter that attacked the senator apologized after the meeting.
(3) The reporter that the senator attacked apologized after the meeting.

In this experiment, participants read the sentences one word at a time. The secondary task involved reading and remembering lists of unrelated words. The secondary task was imposed either at the beginning of the sentence, when participants reached the relative clause (*that attacked the senator/that the senator attacked*), or towards the end of the sentence. Participants' sentence processing performance was indexed using a composite measure of reading speed and recall accuracy. The results indicated that composite scores were lower when the external load was imposed during processing of the relative clause, but not if the load was imposed before or after that point. Wanner and Maratsos interpreted the results as showing that sentence interpretation processes used the same working memory resources as memory processes related to the external load.

More recently, dual-task experiments have contrasted the effects of different kinds of external loads on speed and accuracy of sentence processing (Fedorenko et al., 2006, 2007; Gordon et al., 2002). These studies used phrase-by-phrase self-paced reading to assess processing speed. In some of the experiments, the external load was imposed prior to the sentence. In other cases, the external load was imposed incrementally, simultaneous with the display of each sentence fragment. In Fedorenko and colleagues' (2006) study, the external load was either one (easy condition) or three (hard condition) unrelated words. In addition, the nouns were either drawn from the same category as the nouns in the sentence (generic nouns such as *doctor* and *accountant*; match condition) or from a different category (proper names, non-match condition). In the easy (one memory noun) conditions, object relatives such as (3) produced longer reading times than subject relatives (2), regardless of the type of noun that was used. When participants had to remember three memory nouns, the object-relative penalty in the non-match condition (names) was much less than the object relative penalty in the match condition (generic nouns). Fedorenko and colleagues interpreted this result as showing that retaining the nouns, whether generic or names, tapped the same resource as the sentence processing operations. However, there are some aspects of their results that do not fit neatly within this conclusion. In particular, the results indicated that in the non-match conditions, the object relative penalty was less than half as large (~200 msec) when the external load consisted of three nouns compared to when the external load consisted of one noun (~450 msec). The shared resources position would predict either no difference in load, if maintaining up to three names is automatic or does not tie up many working memory resources in the context of processing a sentence with generic nouns, or a difference in the opposite direction, if maintaining names occupies resources that are shared with the sentence processing task. Also, the finding that secondary tasks produce interactions with sentence complexity when the content of the secondary load is confusable with the content of the sentence itself could be due to the comprehender being forced recall both item and source information about lexical items that are hard to distinguish from one another. The demands of this aspect of the task on attention could be the source of the interactions that have been reported (cf. Engle's concept of working memory capacity as being determined by attentional flexibility).

A second study in this line (Fedorenko et al., 2007) assessed sentence processing performance using different kinds of secondary tasks that arguably tap different representational modalities. One type of secondary task was arithmetic, which arguably taps verbal working memory because digits can be treated essentially as names. Another type of secondary task involved the estimation of angles that would result if two geometric figures were combined or the shape that would result when blocks were added to a base figure. This geometric task arguably taps a non-linguistic visual-spatial processing system. The prediction, then, was that the arithmetic task would have a greater influence on sentence processing performance than the visual task, because the math task occupies the same resource as sentence processing (verbal working memory), while the visual task does not. When participants simultaneously read sentences and performed mental arithmetic, the difficulty of the secondary task interacted with sentence structure. The relative clause of object relatives (3) generally produced longer reading times than subject relatives (2), and the magnitude of this difference was greater when the math task was more difficult. By contrast, the size of the object relative penalty was the same no matter how difficult the visual secondary task was. To explain this pattern of results, Fedorenko and colleagues suggested that "linguistic processing and other verbal working memory tasks that involve similar integration processes rely on a shared pool of working memory resources."

Fedorenko and colleagues' (2006, 2007) results did not replicate in two subsequent studies (Evans et al, 2010. The first was an exact replication of Fedorenko and colleagues (2007, Experiment 1); there were effects of both mathematical and syntactic complexity at the expected regions (found by Fedorenko et al) but not the theoretically crucial interaction of these factors. The second was a replication of Fedorenko and colleagues' (2007, Experiment 2) to which eye tracking was added. Again, the behavioral reaction times showed effects of mathematical and syntactic complexity at the expected regions but no interaction. The eye-tracking study produced an interaction between the complexity of an arithmetic and a syntactic task in second pass fixations on complex segments of complex sentences, suggesting that the interaction that Fedorenko and colleagues found occurs during later sentence processing, consistent with Caplan and Waters view of a shared working memory resource for "post interpretive" processing.

IV. METHODOLOGICAL ISSUES

Many studies of working memory and language suffer from serious methodological flaws, which severely restrict their usefulness. These methodological problems include using inappropriate individual-differences measures, treating continuous variables as dichotomous, the use of median splits or extreme-group designs, using inappropriate statistical modeling techniques to evaluate hypotheses, and failing to address the "third variable" problem. Let us examine each of these in turn.

It is common practice for researchers to measure working-memory capacity using a version of the sentence span task (Daneman & Carpenter, 1980). One major variant of this produces a number of correct responses that can range from 0 to 60. Researchers assume that the underlying trait, working-memory capacity, varies continuously, but commonly-used scoring methods for the sentence span test categorize individuals as belonging to one of 7 categories (spans of "0" through "6"). Treating the data in this way has the potential to artificially reduce variability in the working-memory scores, which may inflate the estimates of actual correlations between working-memory capacity and sentence-processing performance.

A second problem related to measurement of working memory capacity concerns the tests themselves. The most commonly used version, sentence span, has sub-standard reliability (Waters & Caplan, 2003). This is true when the most common scoring method, category scores, is used, but it persists even when a continuous measure of working-memory capacity is extracted from the raw responses. When sentence span is combined with other measures of working-memory capacity, such as operation span (Turner & Engle, 1989), alphabet span, and minus span, split-half reliability rises to acceptable levels. Still, it is common practice in the sentence-comprehension literature for only a single working-memory test to be applied (e.g., Clifton, Traxler, et al., 2003; Di Domenico & Di Matteo, 2009). Since reliability places an upper limit on validity, studies that use unreliable working-memory measures should be interpreted with extreme caution.

Having obtained working memory estimates, researchers commonly create artificial groups by lumping together participants using arbitrary cutoff points. This is done mainly so that the data set can be analyzed using common statistical methods, such as ANOVA. To shoe-horn data into a format appropriate for ANOVA, researchers often create two equal sized groups using a median split. Participants who score below the median are assigned to one group, the rest are assigned to the other group. Depending on the true nature of the relation between working memory and task performance in the population, this technique can either over-estimate or under-estimate the magnitude of the correlation. Consider a situation in which reaction time and working-memory capacity are modestly correlated. If two working-memory groups are created based on a median split, the means that are calculated for each group will collapse across important variation within groups. That is, the within-group variation that contributes to the reliable correlation is eliminated when the means are calculated, likely leading to a deflation of the relation between working memory and reaction time. This problem is exacerbated by small sample sizes (e.g., Di Domenico & Di Matteo, 2009; Prat et al., 2007).

In the extreme-groups variant of the ANOVA design, working-memory measures are taken, and participants who score in the middle of the scale are excluded from the analyses (sometimes, working-memory tests are used to screen out individuals from participating in sentence-processing tasks). This methodology carries its own risks (Preacher et al., 2005). Like the median split, extreme-groups analyses can mischaracterize the relation between the individual-difference variable and the criterion variable (e.g., sentence reading times; comprehension scores) by artificially reducing or inflating variability in the individual-difference measure. Inflation of the relation results when collapsing across the criterion measure at the extremes of the individual-difference variable yields mean differences that are larger than the correlation between the two variables. In addition, the extreme group design presupposes a linear relation between the individual-difference and criterion variables. This need not be the case. Thus, extreme-group designs defeat the primary purpose of engaging in individual differences research, describing the true relation between different variables. Fortunately, the problem can be remedied by including participants who score in the middle of the individual differences scale and by using the appropriate statistical methods to handle continuous variables.

ANOVA is commonly used to identify interactions between working memory capacity and text characteristics, such as syntactic complexity, based on the experimental logic described above. But ANOVA may not provide accurate estimates of the true relation between working memory and sentence processing performance. Emerging statistical tools solve many of the problems associated with ANOVA. Multi-level modeling (also known as Hierarchical Linear Modeling), for example, avoids the problems associated with the dichotomization of continuous variables and has been successfully applied to investigate individual differences in sentence processing and comprehension (Raudenbusch & Bryk, 2001; Blozis & Traxler, 2007; Traxler et al., 2005; Traxler, 2007). Multilevel models simultaneously estimate 1) the effects of text characteristics on performance, and 2) the way individual characteristics such as working memory influence how text characteristics affect performance. Unlike standard ANOVA, multi-level modeling allows multiple individual difference characteristics to be evaluated simultaneously in a fairly straightforward fashion.

Even if we ignore all of the complications that arise from using ANOVA to evaluate individual-difference hypotheses, and accept the modeling results as being 100% veridical, we still can not take the outcome of these analyses at face value. This is because working-memory scores correlate with a variety of other individual-difference measures. Thus, if we conduct a study that finds an interaction of working-memory capacity with some sentence property, we still can not be certain that working memory is the underlying individual characteristic that is actually driving the interaction. Working memory could serve as a proxy for one or more un-measured variables. This is more than just a hypothetical objection since recent studies that directly compare working memory and other individual difference variables have shown that working memory gets "pushed out" of the model when other individual characteristics are taken into account. To date, at least three different individual-difference variables have been shown to negate working memory as a mediator of performance: processing speed, vocabulary knowledge, and relational processing (Andrews et al., 2006; Traxler et al., in press; Traxler & Tooley, 2007).

Previous studies have sometimes found that working-memory capacity correlates with reading time, in particular, sentence-processing time. As noted above, Pearlmutter and MacDonald (1995), for example, found that high-span readers, but not low-span readers, were influenced by semantic characteristics of sentences. Traxler and colleagues (2005) also found evidence that high-span readers were more sensitive to semantic information, animacy specifically, which helped speed their reading of sentences containing object-relative clauses. However, in both of these studies, working-memory capacity was the only individual-difference variable that was examined. More recently, processing speed (as measured by reading times for filler sentences, as well as simple- and choice-reaction time) has been included in models alongside working-memory capacity. In each instance (Caplan et al., in press; Traxler et al., in press), working memory capacity ceased to mediate sentence processing performance, when processing speed was evaluated simultaneously.

Vocabulary knowledge is another variable that needs to be accounted for when sentence processing performance is assessed. In a study that evaluated working memory and vocabulary knowledge (as indicated by the Nelson-Denny vocabulary test), readers processed *object-complement* ambiguities, such as (5) (Traxler & Tooley, 2007):

(5) Susan knew her sister would arrive late.

Sentence (5) is ambiguous, because the noun phrase *her sister* is taken to be the object of the preceding verb *knew*, but it is actually the subject of an embedded sentence, *her sister would arrive late*. Eye-movement studies usually detect mild processing cost at the matrix verb *would arrive* (Trueswell et al., 1993), when sentences such as (5) are compared to unambiguous controls, such as (6):

(6) Susan knew that her sister would arrive late.

When working memory capacity was entered by itself in a multi-level model, it predicted the difficulty that readers had at, and following, the point of syntactic disambiguation. However, when vocabulary knowledge was evaluated simultaneously with working memory capacity, working memory no longer accounted for significant variance in readers' sentence-processing performance.

Tests of relational processing ability have also been contrasted with working-memory capacity as a predictor of sentence-processing performance (Andrews et al., 2006). Relational (also referred to as *computational*) processing maps onto the "processing" component of the "storage and processing" conceptualization of working-memory capacity. Andrews and colleagues (p. 1328) define complexity as "the number of arguments or entities related in a single decision. Each argument corresponds to a dimension, and the number of dimensions corresponds to the number of interacting variables that constrain responses or decisions." Sentence processing involves relating elements at multiple levels simultaneously, and sentences can differ in terms of the number of arguments or propositions that must be related, as well as in the number of constituents that must be buffered before being related. Thus, individual differences in the ability to engage in relational processing has the potential to mediate sentence-processing performance, independent of the "storage" component of working memory capacity. As with processing speed and vocabulary knowledge, tests of relational processing ability push working memory capacity out of the picture when both are used to predict the magnitude of syntactic complexity effects.

Finally, there may be third variable problems associated with the sentence stimuli themselves. When researchers manipulate complexity, they are usually manipulating frequency, but they may also be manipulating the implicit prosodic contour that participants generate while reading silently. One study of relative clause attachment ambiguity found that working memory predicted the degree of preference for one attachment versus another (Traxler, 2007). In sentences such as (7), the relative clause *who hurt herself* can attach to either of the preceding nouns, *daughter* or *queen*:

(7) The daughter of the queen who hurt herself arrived late.

In (8), gender cues drive attachment to the first noun, daughter:

(8) The daughter of the king who hurt herself arrived late.
In (9), the relative clause must attach to the second noun:

(9) The daughter of the king who hurt himself arrived late.

In this study, there were no effects associated with the relative clause itself, but readers with higher sentence-span scores had less difficulty processing the latter part of the sentence when the relative clause attached to the first noun than when it attached to the second. Readers with lower sentence-span scores showed no preference either way. In a follow-up study (Traxler, 2009), implicit prosody was manipulated by inserting a line break between the second noun (*queen/king*), and the relative clause. This line break changes the timing of the input processes, which gives readers more time to process and consolidate the noun-phrase complex into a unified whole before they begin to process the relative clause. Under these conditions, both off-line judgment and on-line preference assessment show that readers have less difficulty when the relative clause attaches to the first noun (Swets et al., 2007). This degree of preference did not correlate with working-memory capacity, suggesting that both higher and lower capacity readers were structuring the sentence in the same way. The shared resources hypothesis would predict greater preference for the more recent (second) noun with decreases in working-memory capacity, but this was not observed (see also Felser et al., 2003). Thus, rather than being an effect of syntactic complexity or recency, sentence-processing outcomes can reflect the influence of other text effects. Syntactic complexity effects and interactions can plausibly be attributed to resource limitations, but the effects of other text characteristics may not be straightforwardly blamed on restricted working memory.

V. MODELS OF WORKING MEMORY CAPACITY AND SENTENCE PRODUCTION

When generating an utterance, speakers must construct phrases and sentences so that information about how the meanings of words are related to one another (e.g., *John slapped Bill* vs. *Bill slapped John*) is properly conveyed. This includes choosing the appropriate words, placing them in the correct order according to grammatically-specified constraints, and inflecting them according to language-specific morphological and syntactic requirements. Models of language production agree to a large extent on the major stages of the sentence production process (e.g., Bock, 1995; Bock & Levelt, 1994; Dell, 1986; Eberhard, Cutting, & Bock, 2005; Fromkin, 1973; Garrett, 1975, 1982; Kempen & Hoenkamp, 1987; Vigliocco & Hartsuiker, 2002): 1) formulation of a message, which represents the speaker's intended meaning; 2) grammatical encoding, which translates the non-linguistic message into an ordered sequence of inflected words; and 3) phonological encoding, which translates the sequence of words into a sequence of sounds to be uttered. Bock and Levelt (1994) organized grammatical encoding into two sets: functional encoding and positional processing.

Functional encoding associates concepts activated at the message level with linguistic semantic values such as thematic roles, creating the "Functional Level" in which hierarchical relations between syntactic nodes encode these semantic values. For instance, the functional level translates the concept [DOG BITES MAN] into the linguistic semantic values of {dog = Agent; man = Patient; bite = Action} and assigns these linguistic semantic values a hierarchical structure [$_S$[$_{NP}$dog] [$_{VP}$[$_V$ bite] [$_{NP}$man]]]. Language-specific semantic features, such as whether the manner of an action is encoded in a verb (e.g., *trot*) or a prepositional phrase (e.g., *walked with caution*) and verb argument structure (e.g., the fact that *considered* can be followed by an object – *the proposal* – or a sentential complement – *the proposal was terrific*), are utilized in this process.

Positional processing creates linearly-organized sequences of words and associated morphological markers (the "Positional Level") on the basis of the representations constructed during functional encoding. Positional processing itself consists of two processes. The first -- Constituent Assembly -- creates linear orders of words and phrases. The order of phrases and the order of words within phrases are determined largely by hierarchical relationships from functional encoding and by grammatical properties of the language (e.g., Subject-Verb-Object (English) *vs.* Subject-Object-Verb (Japanese); Adjective-Noun (English) *vs.* Noun-Adjective (French)). A variety of studies have identified other factors involved in word order choice (e.g., Arnold et al., 2000; Bock, 1986, 1987a, 1987b; Bock & Warren, 1985; F. Ferreira, 1994; F. Ferreira & Henderson, 1998; Gibson et al., 1996; Hawkins, 1994; Kelly et al., 1986; Stallings et al., 1998).

The second positional-level process -- Inflection -- relates features of words to one another, resulting in inflectional markers that specify relations between words (e.g., subject-verb agreement; Bock & Miller, 1991; Eberhard et al., 2005; Franck et al., 2002; Hartsuiker et al., 2001; Vigliocco & Nicol, 1998). The mechanism implementing inflection is argued to be feature-passing, in which feature values are passed along a hierarchical syntactic structure from a source (the subject noun) to a target (the verb) under constraints provided by the grammar. Franck et al. (2002) provided evidence for feature-passing in a sentence-initial fragment completion task using stimuli like (1).

(1) a. The helicopter for the flights over the canyon...
    b. The helicopter for the flight over the canyons...

Participants produced more incorrect plural completions (*were* rather than *was*) in (1a) than in (1b) -- an "agreement mismatch error effect." On a feature-passing account, these errors arise because features of nouns incorrectly percolate up a syntactic tree; as shown above, the larger number of errors in (1a) than in (1b) is due to the fact that the hierarchical distance up the tree from the interfering plural noun to the subject noun is shorter in (1a) (*flights*) than in (1b) (*canyons*). This contrasts with a simple linear memory recall account of errors, which predicts more errors in (1b) than in (1a) because the interfering plural noun is linearly closer to the verb in (1b) (*canyons*) than in (1a) (*flights*).

There are potential links between the operations described above and WM. Memory limitations limit how far downstream in the utterance phrasal structure can be planned and words inserted into syntactic positions. Inflection is also affected by memory limitations. When confronted with long-distance dependencies, information must be kept active or must be reactivated when needed. Evidence for a limit on the ability to retain or retrieve information relevant to morphological features comes from the fact that the size of the agreement mismatch error effect increases as the intervening material is lengthened (Bock & Cutting, 1992). Though most theories postulate a large role for WM in sentence production (see Bock, 1982, and Levelt, 1989, for classic models, and Badecker & Kuminiak, 2007, for a recent view), as in comprehension, whether the WM system that supports sentence production also is used in other tasks is unclear.

There are a few studies of the effects of WM on aspects of Grammatical Encoding. Using an individual differences approach to this question, Bock and Cutting (1992) reported a significant correlation of speaking span (adapted from Daneman & Green, 1986) with agreement error rate. Using an interference approach, Fayol et al. (1994) found effects of concurrent tasks on written agreement errors. Combining both, Hartsuiker and Berkhuysen (2006) reported increased agreement errors only in low-span participants under concurrent load conditions. These results are broadly consistent with the view that WM capacity affects agreement, but they are few and weak. Bock and Cutting found a reliable effect in only one of their three studies, and Bock and Miller (1991) found no correlation between speaking span and agreement error rates in the one experiment in which they reported such an analysis. Fayol et al. themselves considered that error rates might have mainly reflected controlled checking processes found in written but not spoken production. A critical message property (distributivity) did not interact as was predicted with span or load in Hartsuiker and Berkhuysen's study. To our knowledge, there are no experimental studies of the effects of WM on constituent assembly.

Aging provides another opportunity to examine the effect of WM on sentence production. WM capacities decline with age, and many declines in performance in specific cognitive domains have been shown to be at least partially mediated by age-related declines in WM. This has suggested to many researchers that aspects of sentence production that decline with age are likely to do so because of changes in these capacities (e.g., Altmann & Kemper, 2006; Wingfield & Stine-Morrow, 2000).

Evidence for this hypothesis comes from several sources. In corpus analyses, the syntactic complexity of spoken and written language, measured by counts of different types of embedded clauses and of clauses per utterance, has been found to decline in old age in samples of writing from diaries (Kemper, 1987) and essays (Kemper et al., 2001a) and in spontaneous speech (Kemper & Mitzner, 2001) and spoken responses to questions (Kemper & Sumner, 2001; Kemper et al., 2001b). These declines were related to WM measures (Kemper et al., 1989, 2001a, b; Kemper & Sumner, 2001) but not to level of education. These studies suggest WM-mediated age-related changes in syntactic planning.

Experimental studies of language production have helped to identify the specific processes that are affected by age, and researchers have related some of these declines to working memory. Using a constrained production task in which participants constructed a sentence using a visually-presented subject and verb followed by two to four cue words (nouns), Kemper, Herman, and Lian (2003a) reported that an increased number of cue words led to larger increases in latency to produce a sentence, and smaller increases in grammatical complexity and idea density, in old compared to young adults. Similarly, increased complexity of a cue verb (complement-taking verbs (*wished*), vs. transitive verbs (*called*) and intransitive verbs (*smiled*)) led to greater increases in production latency and smaller increases in grammatical complexity and idea density for older than for young adults. Kemper, Herman, and Lian argued that increasing the number of cue words or the complexity of a cue verb increased WM load by increasing the number of responses from which a selection must be made, and that older individuals are less able to meet the demands of this increase in load. In a third study (Kemper, Herman, & Liu, 2004), sentences were generated from presented stems that cued simpler right-branching or more complex left-branching completions. Young adults' sentences, but not older adults' sentences, were longer, more grammatically complex and more dense in propositions for right-branching than left-branching stems. The authors argued that older adults' reduced WM capacity creates a "ceiling" on sentence complexity that is reached by the simplest right-branching structures. However, some studies do not show age differences in sentence production. Altmann and Kemper (2006) found minimal differences between sentences produced by older and young adults in a task that required forming a sentence from two nouns and a verb, where noun animacy and verb type were varied. Davidson, Zacks, and Ferreira (2003) used a cued production task and varied the number of options for sentence construction associated with a verb (verb argument structure). They found equal increases in onset latencies and number of dysfluencies in completions as a function of the number of possible argument structures of the verb in young and old participants. The difference between these results and those of Kemper, Herman, and Lian may lie in the features of the verbs that were varied, the features of sentence production that were measured, the use of different strategies by old and young participants in different tasks, and other factors.

Kemper et al.'s hypothesis that age-related changes in sentence production are related to age-related changes in WM was based on correlation analyses of WM capacity and general features of sentences (propositional density; overall grammatical complexity) in unconstrained tasks. This hypothesis has also been approached experimentally using the logic of dual task interference. If the hypothesis is correct, production should be disproportionately affected in older adults under a concurrent load. Kemper, Herman, and Lian (2003b) found that language production of both young and older adults was affected by performance of a concurrent walking or finger-tapping task, with different effects in the two groups. Young adults showed greater dual task costs on grammatical complexity and length of utterance, and older adults showed greater costs on speech rate. These results are not consistent with the WM account of age differences in sentence production, since grammatical complexity and length of utterance are features of sentences that had been thought to be mediated by WM. The study was also rendered hard to interpret because the groups were not matched at baseline: Older adults' baseline language was less fluent and complex than young adults'.

Overall, there is good evidence that sentence planning becomes more difficult with age, and some evidence that this is related to reduced WM, though the details of the processes that decline with age, and the relation of age-related changes in sentence production to WM remain unclear. There are, however, several gaps are related to the methods and analyses that have been used in the study of sentence production in aging to this point; many of these are the same as those discussed above regarding sentence comprehension. One that applies only to studies of production is that only "input side" WM has been assessed in most studies. Daneman and Green (1986) suggested that verbal WM should be divided into "input" and "output" systems, and Daneman (1991) has shown that "speaking span" is better correlated with verbal output tasks such as fluency than is "listening span." That said, it may be that sentence production differs from sentence comprehension in the specialization of the working memory system that supports it. If so, the reasons for the difference would be of interest to understand (e.g., the difference may be in the extent to which perceptual vs. motor planning skills rely on general functional abilities; see Burke et al., 2000, for discussion).

IV. SUMMARY AND CONCLUSIONS

Our chief goals in this review were to describe the working memory system that supports language interpretation and production processes and to evaluate studies that purport to show that working memory limitations play a causal role in comprehension and production performance. On the comprehension side, individual differences studies have produced evidence that working memory capacity correlates with sentence processing efficiency. Unfortunately, many of the individual differences studies suffer from methodological limitations that cast doubt on their conclusions. These doubts are further enhanced by more recent studies in which working memory measures were pitted directly against other individual difference variables. In those studies, working memory fails to predict sentence processing performance when other variables were assessed simultaneously. Dual task studies also support a connection between working memory capacity and sentence comprehension performance, but the observed effects may occur at a post-interpretive stage of processing. On the production side, processes involved in constituent assembly and inflection may be affected by working memory limitations. However, only a few studies have addressed whether limitations in working memory capacity correlate with increased morphological coding errors. Further, while increases in production errors are associated with normal and abnormal aging, which is broadly compatible with reductions in working memory capacity with aging, other individual characteristics, including processing speed, also decline with age. Hence, there is great need for studies that simultaneously assess multiple individual characteristics and their relationship to production processes. Such studies have begun to appear on the comprehension side and we expect to see similar advances in the near future in research on production.

ACKNOWLEDGMENT

This project was supported by awards from the National Science Foundation (#1024003) and the National Institutes of Health (#1R01HD048914-01A2).

REFERENCES

Acheson, D.J., & MacDonald, M.C. (2009). Twisting tongues and memories: Explorations of the relationship between language production and verbal working memory. *Journal of Memory and Language*, 60, 329-350.

Altmann, L.J.P., & Kemper, S. (2006). Effects of age, animacy, and activation order on sentence production. *Language and Cognitive Processes, Special Issue: Language Production Across the Life Span*, 21, 322-354.

Andrews, G., Birney, D., & Halford, G.S. (2006). Relational processing and working memory capacity in comprehension of relative clause sentences. *Memory & Cognition*, 34, 1325-1340.

Arnold, J.E., Eisenband, J.G., Brown-Schmidt, S., & Trueswell, J.C. (2000). The rapid use of gender information: Evidence of the time course for pronoun resolution from eyetracking. *Cognition*, 76, B13-B26.

Baddeley, A. (1986). *Working Memory*. Oxford, England: Oxford University Press.

Baddeley, A.D., & Hitch, G.J.L. (1974). Working Memory. In G.A. Bower (Ed.), *The Psychology of Learning and Motivation: Advances in Research and Theory*, 8, 47-89.

Baddeley, A.D., Hitch, G.J., & Allen, R.J. (2009). Working memory and binding in sentence recall. *Journal of Memory and Language*, 61, 438-456.

Badecker, W., & Kuminiak, F. (2007). Morphology, agreement, and working memory retrieval in sentence production: Evidence from gender and case in Slovak. *Journal of Memory and Language*, 56, 65-85.

Betancourt, M., Carreiras, M., & Sturt, P. (2009). The processing of subject and object relative clauses in Spanish: An eye-tracking study. *The Quarterly Journal of Experimental Psychology*, 62, 1915-1929.

Blozis, S.A., & Traxler, M.J. (2007). Analyzing individual differences in sentence processing performance using multilevel models. *Behavior Research Methods*, 39, 31-38.

Bock, J.K. (1982). Toward a cognitive psychology of syntax: Information processing contributions to sentence formulation. *Psychological Review*, 89, 1-47.

Bock, J.K. (1986). Syntactic persistence in sentence production. *Cognitive Psychology*, 18, 355-387.

Bock, J.K. (1987a). An effect of the accessibility of word forms on sentence structures. *Journal of Memory and Language*, 26, 119-137.

Bock, J.K. (1987b). Co-ordinating words and syntax in speech plans. In A.W. Ellis (Ed.), *Progress in the Psychology of Language*, 3, 337-390. Hillsdale, NJ: Erlbaum.

Bock, K. (1995). Producing agreement. *Current Directions in Psychological Science*, 4, 56-61.

Bock, K., & Cutting, J.C. (1992). Regulating mental energy: Performance units in language production. *Journal of Memory and Language*, 31, 99-127.

Bock, K., Levelt, W. (1994). Language production: Grammatical encoding. In M.A. Gernsbacher, *The Handbook of Psycholinguistics* (pp. 945-984). San Diego, CA: Academic Press.

Bock, K., & Miller, C.A. (1991). Broken agreement. *Cognitive Psychology*, 23, 45-93.

Bock, J.K., & Warren, R.K. (1985). Conceptual accessibility and syntactic structure in sentence formulation. *Cognition*, 21, 47-67.

Burke, D.M., MacKay, D.G., & James, L.E. (2000). Theoretical approaches to language and aging. In T.J. Perfect & E.A. Maylor (Eds.), *Models of Cognitive Aging: Debates in Psychology* (pp. 204-237). New York, NY: Oxford University Press.

Caplan, D., DeDe, G., Waters, G., Michaud, J., & Tripodis, Y. (in press). Effects of age, speed of processing, and working memory on comprehension of sentences with relative clauses. *Psychology and Aging*.

Caplan, D., & Hildebrandt, N. (1988). *Disorders of Syntactic Comprehension*. Cambridge, MA: MIT Press.

Caplan, D., & Waters, G.S. (1990). Short-term memory and language comprehension: A critical review of the neuropsychological literature. In G. Vallar & T. Shallice (Eds.), *Neuropsychological Impairments of Short-Term Memory* (pp. 337-389). New York, NY: Cambridge University Press.

Caplan, D., & Waters, G.S. (1999). Verbal working memory and sentence comprehension. *Behavioral and Brain Sciences*, 22, 77-126.

Caplan, D., Waters, G., & DeDe, G. (2007). Specialized verbal working memory for language comprehension. In A.R.A. Conway, C. Jarrold, M.J. Kane, A. Miyake, & J.N. Towse (Eds.), *Variation in Working Memory* (pp. 272-302). New York, NY: Oxford University Press.

Clifton, C., Jr., Traxler, M.J., Mohamed, M.T., Williams, R.S., Morris, R.K., & Rayner, K. (2003). The use of thematic role information in parsing: Syntactic processing autonomy revisited. *Journal of Memory and Language*, 49, 317-334.

Cowan, N. (1995). *Attention and memory*. Oxford Psychology Series (No. 26). New York: Oxford University Press.

Cowan, N. (2010). The magical mystery four: How is working memory capacity limited, and why? *Current Directions in Psychological Science*, 19, 51-57.

Daneman, M. (1991). Working memory as a predictor of verbal fluency. *Journal of Psycholinguistic Research*, 20, 445-464.

Daneman, M., & Carpenter, P.A. (1980). Individual differences in working memory and reading. *Journal of Verbal Learning & Verbal Behavior*, 19, 450-466.

Daneman, M., & Carpenter, P.A. (1983). Individual differences in integrating information between and within sentences. *Journal of Experimental Psychology: Learning, Memory, & Cognition*, 9, 561-584.

Daneman, M., & Green, I. (1986). Individual differences in comprehending and producing words in context. *Journal of Memory and Language*, 25, 1-18.

Daneman, M., & Merikle, P.M. (1996). Working memory and language comprehension: A meta-analysis. *Psychonomic Bulleting & Review*, 3, 422-433.

Davidson, D.J., Zacks, R.T., & Ferreira, F. (2003). Age preservation of the syntactic processor in production. *Journal of Psycholinguistic Research*, 32, 541-566.

Dell, G.S. (1986). A spreading activation theory of retrieval in sentence production. *Psychological Review*, 93, 283-321.

Di Domenico, A., & Di Mattteo, R. (2009). Processing Italian relative clauses: Working memory span and word order effects on RTs. *The Journal of General Psychology*, 136, 387-406.

Eberhard, K.M., Cutting, J.C., & Bock, K. (2005). Making syntax of sense: Number agreement in sentence production. *Psychological Review*, 112, 531-559.

Engle, R.W. (2010). Role of working memory capacity in cognitive control. *Current Anthropology*, 51, S17-S26.

Ericsson, K.A., & Kintsch, W. (1995). Long-term working memory. *Psychological Review*, 102, 211-245.

Evans, W.S., Caplan, D., Waters, G. (under review) Effects on arithmetical and syntactic complexity on gaze fixations under dual task conditions

Fayol, M., Largy, P., & Lemaire, P. (1994). Cognitive overload and orthographic errors: When cognitive overload enhances subject-verb agreement errors: A study in French written language. *The Quarterly Journal of Experimental Psychology A: Human Experimental Psychology*, 47, 437-464.

Fedorenko, E., Gibson, E., & Rohde, D. (2006). The nature of working memory capacity in sentence comprehension: Evidence against domain-specific working memory resources. *Journal of Memory and Language*, 54, 541-553.

Fedorenko, E., Gibson, E., & Rohde, D. (2007). The nature of working memory in linguistic, arithmetic and spatial integration processes. *Journal of Memory and Language*, 56, 246-269.

Felser, C., Marinis, T., & Clahsen, H. (2003). Children's processing of ambiguous sentences: A study of relative clause attachment. *Language Acquisition: A Journal of Developmental Linguistics*, 11, 127-163.

Ferreira, F. (1994). Choice of passive voice is affected by verb type and animacy. *Journal of Memory and Language*, 33, 715-736.

Ferreira, F., & Henderson, J.M. (1998). Linearization strategies during language production. *Memory & Cognition*, 26, 88-96.

Franck, J., Vigliocco, G., Nicol, J. (2002). Subject-verb agreement errors in French and English: The role of syntactic hierarchy. *Language and Cognitive Processes*, 17, 371-404.

Fromkin, V.A. (1973). *Speech Errors as Linguistic Evidence.* Oxford, England: Mouton.

Garrett, M.F. (1975). The analysis of sentence production. In G.H. Bower (Ed.), *The Psychology of Learning and Motivation*, 9 (pp. 133-177). New York, NY: Academic Press.

Garrett, M.F. (1982). Production of speech: Observations from normal and pathological language use. In A. Ellis (Ed.), *Normality and Pathology in Cognitive Functions* (pp. 19-76). London, England: Academic Press.

Gibson, E. (1998). Linguistic complexity: Locality of syntactic dependencies. *Cognition*, 68, 1-76.

Gibson, E., Schutze, C.T., & Salomon, A. (1996). The relationship between the frequency and the processing complexity of linguistic structure. *Journal of Psycholinguistic Research*, 25, 59-92.

Gordon, P.C., Hendrick, R., & Johnson, M. (2001). Memory interference during language processing. *Journal of Experimental Psychology: Learning, Memory, and Cognition*, 27, 1411-1423.

Gordon, P.C., Hendrick, R., & Levine, W.H. (2002). Memory-load interference in syntactic processing. *Psychological Science*, 13, 425-430.

Hartsuiker, R. J. & Berkhuysen, P. N. (2006) Language production and working memory: The case of subject-verb agreement. *Language and Cognitive Processes*, 21, 181-204.

Hartsuiker, R.J., Anton-Mendez, I., & van Zee, M. (2001). Object attraction in subject-verb agreement construction. *Journal of Memory and Language*, 45, 546-572.

Hawkins, J.A. (1994). A performance theory of order and constituency. *Cambridge Studies in Linguistics*, 73. Cambridge, England: Cambridge University Press.

Jonides, J., Lewis, R.L., Nee, D.E., Lustig, C.A., Berman, M.G., & Moore, K.S. (2008). The mind and brain of short-term memory. *Annual Review of Psychology*, 59, 193-224.

Just, M.A., & Carpenter, P.A. (1992). A capacity theory of comprehension: Individual differences in working memory capacity. *Psychological Review*, 99, 122-149.

Just, M.A., Carpenter, P.A., & Keller, T.A. (1996). The capacity theory of comprehension: New frontiers of evidence and arguments. *Psychological Review*, 103, 773-780.

Kelly, M. H., Bock, J. K., & Keil, F. C. (1986). Prototypicality in a linguistic context: Effects on sentence structure. *Journal of Memory and Language*, 25, 59-74.

Kempen, G., & Hoenkamp, E. (1987). An incremental procedural grammar for sentence formulation. *Cognitive Science*, 11, 201-258.

Kemper, S. (1987). Constraints on psychological processes in discourse production. In H.W. Dechert & M. Raupach (Eds.), *Psycholinguistic Models of Production* (pp. 185-188). Westport, CT: Ablex.

Kemper, S., Greiner, L.H., Marquis, J.G., Prenovost, K., & Mitzner, T.L. (2001). Language decline across the life span: Findings from the nun study. *Psychology and Aging*, 16, 227-239.

Kemper, S., Herman, R., & Lian, C. (2003a). Age differences in sentence production. *The Journals of Gerontology: Series B: Psychological Sciences and Social Sciences*, 58B, S260-P268.

Kemper, S., Herman, R.E., & Lian, C.H.T. (2003b). The costs of doing two things at once for young and older adults: Talking while walking, finger tapping, and ignoring speech of noise. *Psychology and Aging*, 18, 181-192.

Kemper, S., Herman, R.E., & Liu, C.J. (2004). Sentence production by young and older adults in controlled contexts. *The Journals of Gerontology: Series B: Psychological Sciences and Social Sciences*, 59, P220-P224.

Kemper, S., Kynette, D., Rash, S., O'Brien, K. (1989). Life span changes to adults' language: Effects of memory and genre. *Applied Psycholinguistics*, 10, 49-66.

Kemper, S., & Liu, C.J. (2007). Eye movements of young and older adults during reading. *Psychology and Aging*, 22, 84-93.

Kemper, S., & Mitzner, T.L. (2001). Language production and comprehension. In J.E. Birren & K. Warner (Eds.), *Handbook of the Psychology of Aging, 5th Edition* (pp. 378-398). San Diego, CA: Academic Press.

Kemper, S., & Sumner, A. (2001). The structure of verbal abilities in young and older adults. *Psychology and Aging*, 16, 312-322.

Kemper, S., Thompson, M., & Marquis, J. (2001). Longitudinal change in language production: Effects of aging and dementia on grammatical complexity and propositional content. *Psychology and Aging*, 64, 600-614.

King, J., & Just, M.A. (1991). Individual differences in syntactic parsing: The role of working memory. *Journal of Memory and Language*, 30, 580-602.

Levelt, W.J.M. *Speaking: From Intention to Articulation*. Cambridge, MA: MIT Press.

Long, D.L., & Prat, C.S. (2008). Individual differences in syntactic ambiguity resolution: Readers vary in their use of plausibility information. *Memory and Cognition*, 36, 375-391.

Love, T., & Swinney, D. (1996). Coreference processing and levels of analysis in object-relative constructions: Demonstration of antecedent reactivation with the cross-modal priming paradigm. *Journal of Psycholinguistic Research*, 25, 5-24.

MacDonald, M.C., & Christiansen, M.H. (1992). Reassessing working memory *Psychological Review*, 109, 35-54.

MacDonald, M.C., & Christiansen, M.H. (2002). Reassessing working memory: Comment on Just and Carpenter (1992) and Waters and Caplan (1996). *Psychological Review*, 109, 35-54.

Mak, W.M., Vonk, W., & Schriefers, H. (2002). The influence of animacy on relative clause processing. *Journal of Memory and Language*, 47, 50-68.

Mak, W., Vonk, W., & Schriefers, H. (2006). Animacy in processing relative clauses: The hikers that rocks crush. *Journal of Memory and Language*, 54, 466-490.

Martin, N. & Ayala, J. (2004). Measurement of auditory-verbal STM span in aphasia: Effects of item, task, and lexical impairment. *Brain and Language*, 89, 464-483.

Martin, R.C. (2003). Language processing: Functional organization and neuroanatomical basis. *Annual Review of Psychology*, 54, 55-89.

McElree, B.D. (2001). Working memory and focal attention. *Journal of Experimental Psychology: Learning, Memory, and Cognition*, 27, 817-835.

Misyak, J.B., Christiansen, M.H. & Tomblin, J.B. (2009). Statistical learning of nonadjacencies predicts on-line processing of long-distance dependencies in natural language. In N. Taatgen, H. van Rijn, J. Nerbonne & L. Schomaker (Eds.), Proceedings of the 31st Annual Cognitive Science Society Conference (pp. 177-182). Austin, TX: Cognitive Science Society.

Miyake, A., Friedman, N.P., Rettinger, D.A., Shah, P., & Hegarty, M. (2001). How are visuospatial working memory, executive functioning, and spatial abilities related? A latent-variable analysis. *Journal of Experimental Psychology: General*, 130, 621-640.

Nairne, J. S., Neath, I., Serra, M., & Byun, E. (1997). Positional distinctiveness and the ratio rule in free recall. *Journal of Memory and Language, 37,* 155-166.

Page, M.P.A. and Norris, D.G. (1998) The Primacy Model: a New Model of Immediate Serial Recall, *Psychological Review, 104,* 761-781.

Pearlmutter, N.J. & MacDonald, M.C. (1995). Individual differences and probabilistic constraints in syntactic ambiguity resolution. *Journal of Memory and Language.* 34, 521-542.

Prat, C.S., Keller, T.A., & Just, M.A. (2007). Individual differences in sentence comprehension: A functional magnetic resonance imaging investigation of syntactic and lexical processing demands. *Journal of Cognitive Neuroscience*, 19, 1950–1963.

Preacher, K.J., Rucker, D.D., MacCallum, R.C., Nicewander, W.A. (2005). Use of the extreme groups approach: A critical reexamination and new recommendations. *Psychological Methods*, 10, 178-192.

Raudenbush, S.W. & Bryk, A.S. (2001). Hierarchical Linear Models: Applications and Data Analysis Methods (2E). Thousand Oaks, CA: Sage Publications, Inc.

Stallings, L.M., MacDonald, M.C., & O'Seaghdha, P.G. (1998). Phrasal ordering constraints in sentence production: Phrase length and verb disposition in heavy-NP shift. *Journal of Memory and Language*, 39, 392-417.

Swets, B., Desmet, T., Hambrick, D.Z., & Ferreira, F. (2007). The role of working memory in syntactic ambiguity resolution: A psychometric approach. *Journal of Experimental Psychology: General*, 136, 64-81.

Tooley, K.M. (2009, March). *Is syntactic priming in sentence comprehension really just implicit learning?* Paper presented to the 22nd annual CUNY Conference on Human Sentence Processing. Davis, CA.

Traxler, M.J. (2007). Working Memory Contributions to Relative Clause Attachment Processing: A Hierarchical Linear Modeling Analysis. *Memory and Cognition*, 35, 1107-1121.

Traxler, M.J. (2009). A hierarchical linear modeling analysis of working memory and implicit prosody in the resolution of adjunct attachment ambiguity. *Journal of Psycholinguistic Research*, 38, 491-509.

Traxler, M.J., Long, D.L., Johns, C.L., Tooley, K.M., Zirnstein, M., & Jonathan, E. (in press). Modeling individual differences in eye-movements during reading: Working memory and speed-of-processing effects. *Journal of Eye-Movement Research*.

Traxler, M.J., Morris, R.K., & Seely, R.E. (2002). Processing of subject and object relative clauses: Evidence from eye movements. *Journal of Memory and Language*, 47, 69-90.

Traxler, M.J., & Tooley, K.M. (2007). Lexical mediation and context effects in sentence processing. *Brain Research*, 1146, 59-74.

Traxler, M.J., Williams, R.S., Blozis, S.A., & Morris, R.K. (2005). Working Memory, Animacy, and Verb Class in the Processing of Relative Clauses. *Journal of Memory & Language*, 53, 204-224.

Trueswell, J.C., Tanenhaus, M.K., & Kello, C. (1993). Verb-specific constraints in sentence processing: Separating effects of lexical preference from garden-paths. *Journal of Experimental Psychology: Learning, Memory, and Cognition*, 19, 528-553.

Turner, M.L., & Engle, R.W. (1989). Is working memory capacity task dependent? *Journal of Memory and Language*, 28, 127-154.

van Dyke, J.A., & McElree, B. (2006). Retrieval interference in sentence comprehension. *Journal of Memory and Language*, 55, 157-166.

Verhaeghen, P., Cerella, J, & Basak, C. (2004). A working memory workout: How to change to size of the focus of attention from one to four in ten hours or less. Journal of Experimental Psychology: Learning, Memory, and Cognition, 30, 1322-1337.

Vigliocco, G., & Hartsuiker, R.J. (2002). The interplay of meaning, sound, and syntax in sentence production. *Psychological Bulletin*, 128, 442-472.

Vigliocco, G., & Nicol, J. (1998). Separating hierarchical relations and word order in language production: Is proximity concord syntactic or linear. *Cognition*, 68, B13-B29.

Wanner, E., & Maratsos, M. (1978). An ATN approach to comprehension. In M. Halle J. Bresnan, & G.A. Miller (Eds.). *Linguistic Theory and Psychological Reality*. Cambridge, MA: MIT Press.

Waters, G., & Caplan, D. (2005). The relationship between age, processing speed, working memory capacity, and language comprehension. *Memory*, 13, 403-413.

Waters, G.S., & Caplan, D. (1996a). Processing resource capacity and the comprehension of garden path sentences. *Memory and Cognition*, 24, 342-355.

Waters, G.S., & Caplan, D. (1996b). The capacity theory of sentence comprehension: Critique of Just and Carpenter (1992). *Psychological Review*, 103, 761-772.

Waters, G.S., & Caplan, D. (2003). The reliability and stability of verbal working memory measures. *Behavior Research Methods, Instruments, & Computers*, 35, 550-564.

Waters, G.S., Caplan, D., & Leonard, C. (1992). The role of phonology in reading comprehension: Implications of the effects of homophones on processing sentences with referentially dependent categories. *The Quarterly Journal of Experimental Psychology A: Human Experimental Psychology*, 44, 343-372.

Waters, G.S., Caplan, D., & Rochon, E. (1995). Processing capacity and sentence comprehension in patients with Alzheimer's disease. *Cognitive Neuropsychology*, 12, 1-308.

Weckerly J, Elman J. A PDP approach to processing center-embedded sentences. Proceedings of the Fourteenth Annual Meeting of the Cognitive Science Society; Hillsdale, NJ: Lawrence Erlbaum Associates; 1992. pp. 414–419.

Wells, J.B., Christiansen, M.H., Race, D.S., Acheson, D.J., & MacDonald, M.C. (2009). Experience and sentence processing: Statistical learning and relative clause processing. *Cognitive Psychology*, 58, 250-271.

Wingfield, A., & Stine-Morrow, E.A.L. (2000). Language and speech. In F.I.M. Craik, & T.A. Salthouse (Eds.), *The Handbook of Aging and Cognition* (pp. 359-416). Mahwah, NJ: Erlbaum.

In: Working Memory: Capacity, Developments and… ISBN: 978-1-61761-980-9
Editor: Eden S. Levin © 2011 Nova Science Publishers, Inc.-

Chapter 9

WORKING MEMORY COMPONENTS AND VIRTUAL REORIENTATION: A DUAL-TASK STUDY

Alessandro O. Caffò, Luciana Picucci, Manuela N. Di Masi and Andrea Bosco
University of Bari, Bari, Italy

ABSTRACT

In the history of cognitive psychology, one of the most studied, analyzed, cited, revised and criticized theoretical model was the Baddeley & Hitch's (1974) Working Memory Model. A binding attribute of working memory is its limited capacity, as evidenced by the studies on span measures. The methodology most often used to investigate such limited capacity is dual-task paradigm. In the present experiment a dual task procedure was employed to evaluate the requirements of working memory resources in a virtual spatial memory task (reorientation paradigm, Cheng, 1986; Hermer & Spelke, 1994, 1996). In previous studies (Hermer-Vazquez et al., 1999; Ratliff & Newcombe, 2005; Ratliff & Newcombe, 2008), a dual task procedure was employed to shed light on the hypothesis that spatial language would be an essential for the integration of geometric and non-geometric (feature) information (for a review, see Cheng and Newcombe, 2005; Cheng, 2008). Nowadays, contrasting results do not permit to accomplish with this hypothesis and integration of different classes of information remains at level of open debate. The present experiment was aimed at providing new evidence for the aforementioned topic employing the virtual version of the reorientation task (Bosco et al., 2008; Picucci et al., 2009; Bosco et al, 2010; Picucci et al, 2010) and two well-known concurrent tasks: articulatory suppression for verbal and spatial tapping tasks for visuo-spatial working memory components, respectively. These tasks were already employed in navigation-based experiments (e. g. Garden et al, 2002; Coluccia et al, 2007). If visuo-spatial working memory is substantially involved in reorientation, then it might expect that spatial tapping would impair the encoding relationships among target, landmark and geometric characteristics of the environment largely than articulatory suppression. On the other hand, a large decrease in performance following articulatory suppression will lead to conclude that the language hypothesis might be correct. Sixty participants were randomly assigned to one of three different dual task experimental conditions:

Articulatory Suppression Task, Spatial Tapping Task and No Concurrent Task. The articulatory suppression task involved a sequence of monosyllabic syllables when pronounced by Italian speakers i. e. Ba/Be/Bi/Bo/Bu/Da/De/Di/Do/Du. The spatial tapping task involved the participant in tapping repeatedly on wooden keys of a custom-made keypad.

Data showed a main effect of the dual task interference, with a significant decrease in performance as effect of visuo-spatial as well as verbal dual task. Moreover, the difference between the two dual tasks was also significant demonstrating that visuo-spatial interference worsened the performance significantly more than verbal one. These results seem to shed new light on current debate, since they lead to conclude that reorientation task engages critically visuo-spatial, and with a minor extent, verbal component of working memory.

INTRODUCTION

According to the human information processing approach proposed by Atkinson & Shiffrin (1968), an immediate memory system is used for the reproduction of information immediately after presentation, but it is even more important as a support system capable of maintaining the information needed for a large range of human activities. Some years later, Baddeley and Hitch (1974) introduced and made popular the multi-component model of working memory. The model of working memory proposed by Alan Baddeley and Graham Hitch in 1974 is one of the longest lived and most widely used models in cognitive psychology. It holds a central place in experimental psychology and continues to be extremely successful in guiding and stimulating research in applied and theoretical domains. This model proposes that two "slave systems" are responsible for short-term maintenance of information, and a "central executive" is responsible for the supervision of information integration and for coordinating the slave systems. One slave system, the phonological loop, stores phonological information (i. e., the sound of language) and prevents its decay by continuously articulating its contents, thereby refreshing the information in a rehearsal loop. It can, for example, maintain a seven-digit telephone number for as long as one repeats the number to oneself again and again. The other slave system, the visuo-spatial sketch pad, stores visual and spatial information. It can be used, for example, for constructing and manipulating visual images, and for the representation of mental maps. The sketch pad can be further broken down into a visual subsystem (dealing with, for instance, shape, color, and texture), and a spatial subsystem (dealing with location) (Logie, 1986; Logie and Marchetti, 1991). The central executive is responsible for directing attention to relevant information, suppressing irrelevant information and inappropriate actions, and for coordinating cognitive processes when more than one task must be done at the same time. Baddeley (2000) extended the model by adding a fourth component, the "episodic buffer", which holds representations that integrate phonological, visual, and spatial information, and possibly information not covered by the slave systems (e. g., semantic information, musical information). The component is episodic because it is assumed to bind information into a unitary episodic representation. The episodic buffer resembles Tulving's concept of episodic memory (Tulving, 1972, 1983), but it differs in that the episodic buffer is a temporary store. One attribute of working memory about which there would at the time have been very little dispute is its apparently limited capacity, as evidenced in the limited span of immediate memory. Baddeley and Hitch (1974) investigated the effects of a concurrent serial recall task on performance in reasoning, comprehension, and free recall. They argued: "Such a concurrent memory load might reasonably be expected to absorb some of the storage capacity of a limited capacity working memory system" (p. 50). It would therefore disrupt performance in any criterion task that relied on such a system. They found, for example, that a concurrent memory load of six items impaired performance in all three sorts of task. They also showed that phonemic similarity among the stimulus items impaired both reasoning and comprehension, and that suppressing any relevant articulatory activity by requiring subjects to produce irrelevant vocalizations ("articulatory suppression") impaired performance in free recall (Richardson, Longoni, & Di Masi, 1996) and, to a lesser extent, in reasoning. These results were taken to support the notion of working memory as a short-term store that had access to phonemic coding.

In keeping with this view, Baddeley and co-authors (Baddeley, 1986) proposed a model of working memory in which the main assumption is to consider short-term memory as a system for the temporary storage and processing of information. In an impressive series of studies, Baddeley and colleagues tested the basic hypothesis and main implications of their model. In particular, in the first study in this series, Baddeley and Hitch (1974) used a dual-task technique requiring their subjects to hold a certain quantity of material (a series of two to eight digits) in short-term memory, absorbing most of their immediate memory capacity. At the same time they were asked to perform another task (learning, reasoning, or comprehending). Results showed that increases in WM load reduced performance correspondingly, confirming the WM hypothesis. However, the participant was able to execute the required concurrent cognitive task even when the entire WM capacity was absorbed by the digit memory task.

On the basis of these and other data, Baddeley (1986) abandoned the assumption of a unitary short-term memory system, hypothesizing that the limits of digit span may involve a WM subsystem, leaving other components of WM relatively unimpaired. In these terms, it is important to consider the type of information that accesses the system and, of course, the nature of the task to be carried out. More recently, Baddeley (2000) has taken his position further, suggesting the existence of a new WM subsystem—the episodic buffer—responsible for connections of WM with episodic LTM. The episodic buffer is seen as a separate limited capacity system within working memory that uses a multimodal code. The function of the episodic buffer can be described in terms of both processing and storage. As regards processing, the buffer serves as a workbench for assembling unitary multidimensional representations in different codes (visual, phonological, semantic, etc.) from different perceptual (visual, auditory, tactile, etc.) and mnemonic (episodic, semantic, etc.) sources (Baddeley, 2000, 2003; Repovs and Baddeley, 2006). As regards storage, the episodic buffer temporarily accommodates unitary multidimensional representations (Repovs and Baddeley, 2006; Baddeley and Wilson, 2002). Evidence of the maintenance of unitary multidimensional representations in working memory was provided by a set of studies, showing interference between phonological and visuo-spatial representations in working memory (Logie et al., 2000).

In conclusions four separate components have been suggested for the architecture of the WM system: (1) an articulatory loop dealing with verbal material (e. g., in the immediate memory of digits); (2) a visuo-spatial sketch (scratch) pad for maintaining/manipulating visuo-spatial information; and (3) a central executive with control and supervising functions and (4) an episodic buffer. They are involved in a wide series of complex cognitive tasks from reasoning to spatial updating during navigation.

Spatial Updating: The Case of Reorientation

In the previous paragraph we concluded that WM components are crucial for complex functions like spatial updating. Indeed, when we move in the environment, we continuously look around searching for clues. Equally, animals who are trapped and successively freed, or who emerge from their lairs, search for information about their position in the environment. Since the seminal work of Cheng (1986) we know that, after being disoriented, animals reorient using the metric information given by the lengths and angles that form the shape of the surrounding environment. Specifically, he trained rats to find food hidden in one of two corners of a rectangular cage with no distinctive features, the long wall being to the left of a short wall. If the rats remained oriented, they distinguished well between the two corners which had the same geometric characteristics, but, if they were disoriented blindfolding them, removing them from the cage and then reinserting after a few seconds, the rats searched for the food equally often at the geometrically identical corners. Cheng also noticed that the animals did not simply use geometric information, but they also relied on it exclusively, despite the presence of non geometric information. In fact, when the rectangular environment was characterized with non-geometric features, such as wall markings or particular smells, that removed the ambiguity between the two geometrically congruent corners, the rats ignored the landmark information. Rather, they continued to search equally between the correct and reverse corners. Thanks to this simple experimental procedure, Cheng showed that the rats encoded the geometric properties of the space (i. e., the length of the walls and their relation at the corners, being the short wall to the left of the long wall, and vice versa), but were not able to incorporate the non-geometric features in their representation of the environment to guide their reorientation. The paradigm of reorientation has been employed successfully not only with animals (i. e. rats, pigeon, chickens, rhesus monkey, fishes; see: Chiandetti, Regolin, Sovrano, & Vallortigara, 2007; Sovrano & Vallortigara, 2006; Vallortigara, Zanforlin, & Pasti, 1990 for chickens; Kelly, Spetch, & Heth, 1998 for pigeons; Gouteux, Thinus-Blanc, & Vauclair, 2001 for monkeys; Sovrano, Bisazza, & Vallortigara, 2002, 2003, 2005, 2006, for fish), but also with humans, either children and adults, providing interesting results highlighting the concurrent development of language and spatial skills.

The Role of Language in the Integration of Geometric and Feature Cues

Children at 18-24 months of age have shown search patterns similar to those Cheng found with rats, for a hidden toy within a symmetric rectangular environment (Hermer and Spelke, 1994, 1996). In a rectangular room with all white walls, young children employed geometric information to reorient, dividing their searches for the hidden toy evenly between the correct and reverse corners. When the research assistant added a colored wall, although children had enough information to distinguish the correct corner and to successfully solve the task, children perseverated in searching at the two geometrically correct corners; in other words, their search rates remained identical to those in the all-white room.

Hermer and Spelke claimed that children fail to conjoin geometric and non-geometric information because they use an encapsulated and task-specific mechanism: the geometric module, based on the conceptualization of "module" proposed by Jerry Fodor (2000).

While adult rats and human children until 24 months of age both show evidence of dominance of the geometric information that guides reorientation and of a neglect of non-geometric information, human adults are able to combine geometric and non-geometric spatial information to reorient in a symmetric rectangular environment. Hermer-Vazquez et al. (1999) found that, coherently with the last assumption, human adults can successfully reorient and find the correct corner in a rectangular room with three white walls and one blue wall. However, when adults were concurrently engaged in a verbal shadowing task that consisted in repeating words to produce continuous speech, they were no longer able to flexibly combine the two kinds of spatial information and rely only on to the geometric information to reorient. Otherwise, adults who performed a nonverbal control task (i. e. a rhythmic shadowing task) were easily able to combine geometric and non-geometric information to reorient. These results seems to suggest that the joint use of geometric and featural information requires linguistic support, in particular knowledge and ability to use the spatial language (i. e. terms such as "left" and "right"), which specify spatial relationship between environmental information. Hermer-Vazquez et al. (1999), on the basis on these data, concluded that adults are able to bypass the encapsulation found among young children by acquiring spatial language and employ linguistic processing to make use of non-geometric features in conjunction with geometric information. In particular, they claimed that a language skill, which is a system of representation, connects to other systems of representation, so allowing the conjoining between information derived from distinct sources. Another interesting fact is that children develop the skill to appropriately use spatial language, and the spatial terms "left" and "right", around the age of six. At this age, they can successfully complete the reorientation task with the employment of both geometric and feature cues. Hermer-Vazquez et al. (2001) investigated this coincidence of ages further. They administered a variety of cognitive tests, including nonverbal intelligence, digit span, visuo-spatial span, production and comprehension of spatial terms (above–below, in front–behind, left–right), to a group of 6 years old children and tested them in the reorientation task. The only predictor of children's ability to reorient using features as well as geometry was their production of the terms "left" and "right". Based on these data, Hermer-Vazquez et al. (2001) argued that acquisition and control of such linguistic terms was essential in allowing for rapid and flexible use of features in reorientation.

Reorientation: Beyond Spatial Language

Following Newcombe and Ratliff (2007) there is an alternative explanation of Hermer-Vasquez et al. (1999) data. Indeed, in the Hermer-Vazquez et al. (1999) study, adults were only told, prior to the disorientation procedure, that "you will see something happening that you should try to notice" and that would be required later. After these instructions, which seem rather vague, and with no practice trials, participants began the searching task performing the concurrent shadowing task in a rectangular room with a blue wall, followed by search without shadowing. The same procedure was used also in an all-white rectangular room. It is possible that, if the participants would have been clearly informed on the demands of the task, they would have searched the correct corner at the same rate both in the verbal shadowing condition and in the no shadowing condition. Secondly, the concurrent task employed by Hermer-Vazquez et al. (1999) might disrupt the ability to use featural landmarks for other reasons than interference with a linguistic encoding process. It is possible that a concurrent task per se reduces the ability to integrate different types of spatial information. Hermer-Vazquez et al. (1999) used a nonverbal rhythm-clapping task to exclude this possibility, but this control concurrent task could be inadequate because it might engage different processing mechanisms than those involved in conjoining different sources of spatial information (Newcombe, 2005).

Other Authors have led several studies using Hermer-Vazquez et al.'s dual-task paradigm. Ratliff and Newcombe (2005, 2008) have replicated the Experiment 1 proposed in Hermer-Vazquez, Spelke, and Katsnelson (1999), adopting an upgrading: they gave participants additional, explicit, instructions about the nature of the searching task and participants underwent a practice trial prior to performing the reorientation task. Participants in the explicit instructions condition successfully used the blue wall as a landmark significantly more than the participants in the replication condition. This greater success in using the blue wall led to a higher rate of correct corner searches for participants who received the explicit instructions than for the replications condition participants. It appears that giving participants additional instructions and some practice trials removes the effect that verbal shadowing has on conjoining geometric and featural information. These findings cast some doubts on the assumption that the verbal shadowing task can hinder adult spatial skills in conjoining both geometric and featural information. Another issue addressed by Ratliff and Newcombe (2005) concerns about the non verbal rhythm-shadowing condition used by Hermer-Vazquez et al. (1999). The rhythm-clapping task is thought to involve cerebellar regions of the brain, and it would not be expected to be basically involved with integration of spatial information (Woodruf-Pak, Papka, & Ivry, 1996). Experiment 2 by Ratliff and Newcombe (2005, 2008) investigate how a nonverbal spatial task (i. e. a visual-imagery task based on Brooks, 1968) can interfere with the integration of geometric and featural information during the reorientation task. The most interesting result is that participants engaged in the spatial secondary task ignored the landmark as if they were in the all white wall room. Participants that were not engaged in the concurrent spatial task successfully employed the blue wall to solve correctly the searching task. The concurrent spatial task seems to reduce participants' skill to conjoin the geometric and featural information during reorientation. Nonetheless, the participants in the verbal shadowing condition used the blue wall as a landmark for reorienting significantly more than in the spatial visualizing condition. The overall result is that the spatial secondary task of Ratliff & Newcombe (2005) seemed to interfere more than the verbal shadowing task to flexibly conjoin geometric and featural information. These findings contrast with the proposed theory of Hermer-Vazquez et al. (1999) that the acquisition of spatial language is responsible for integration of geometric and featural information.

The Experiment

The present experiment was aimed at providing new evidences for the aforementioned open debate utilizing the virtual version of the reorientation task (Bosco et al., 2008; Picucci et al., 2009) and two very well known concurrent tasks: articulatory suppression for verbal and spatial tapping task for visuo-spatial working memory components, both already employed in navigation-based tasks (e. g. Garden, Cornoldi, & Logie, 2002). If visuo-spatial working memory is substantially involved, we might expect that spatial tapping would impair the learning of spatial relationships among target, landmark and geometrical characteristics in a larger manner than articulatory suppression. On the other hand, a decrease in performance following articulatory suppression will lead to conclude that the language hypothesis is correct.

In the present experiment, a dual task procedure was carried out to evaluate the requirements of general working memory resources in a reorientation task. In two studies carried out previously (Hermer-Vazquez et al., 1999; Ratliff et al., 2005), a dual task procedure was employed to assess the hypothesis on spatial language as the most important factor in the integration of geometrical and featural information. Hermer-Vazquez, et al. (1999) found that a verbal shadowing task (immediately repeating an irrelevant discourse heard through headphones, syllable by syllable or word by word) impaired performance of the canonical reorientation task. On the other hand, a rhythm-shadowing task had minimal effect on reorientation. In particular, adults who performed verbal shadowing seemed to be able to encode geometrical cues, neglecting the coloured wall. This finding accounted for the hypothesis that verbal shadowing overrides the possibility to handle spatial language (as "on the right/left of...") and consequently to conjoin geometrical and featural information during the encoding. In contrast with these results, Ratliff & Newcombe (2005, 2008) found that a spatial concurrent task seemed to be more interfering with adults' ability to combine geometrical and featural information than the verbal shadowing task such as that used in Hermer-Vazquez, et al. (1999). This finding suggested that spatial language is not an essential precursor for the integration of geometrical and featural information. Moreover, a large body of data supported this hypothesis. They converged in demonstrating that nonhuman species (see Cheng & Newcombe, 2005, for a review) resolve accurately the reorientation task making use of both geometric and featural properties of the environment in absence of linguistic skills.

METHOD

Participants

Participants were 60 right-handed, university students (30 women and 30 men) ranging in age 19-29 years (age, mean: 23. 7, sd: 3. 2). Their vision was normal or corrected to normal. They received a course credit for the participation and took part at the experiment after they have given their written consent.

Apparatus and Material

Freeware software, the C-G Arena was used (Jacobs et al. 1997, 1998). A computer monitor (19" wide) displayed a colored view of an environment from the perspective of one positioned on the floor of the environment. The environment had an internal structure composed by a circular, invisible arena, in which the participants could move and explore freely the environment in a first-person perspective, controlling their movements with a joystick. Since we are talking of first-person perspective, the monitor did not display any image of the participant.

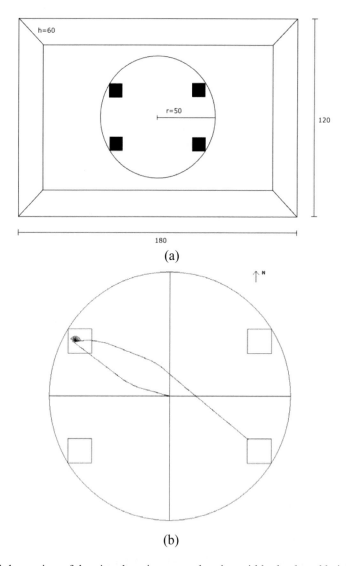

Figure 1. (a) A bird-eye view of the virtual environment showing width, depth and height of the rectangular environment, the circular arena and its radius, and the four black response patches. (b.) A Screenshot of the output file showing the route travelled by the participant in the testing environment. The path began in the centre of the environment and finished when the participant reached the correct response patch, then the participant was trapped and teleported to the next environment.

The virtual space. The computer screen showed a perspective as if the participants were 15 units above the arena floor. This allowed the participants to feel completely comfortable with the searching task described in detail below. The arena was 50 units in radius and had a height of zero units. Consequently, participants were unable to see it; nonetheless, their movements were restricted in the arena circle. The arena held four quadrants: northeast (NE), northwest (NW), southeast (SE), and southwest (SW). The quadrants were invisible components of the computer-generated display (see Figure 1b.). A rectangular environment with proportion of 2:3 was created, as proposed in the original experiment of Hermer and Spelke (1996), measuring 180 x 120 x 60 units and housing an invisible arena (see Figure 1a). As it is usual in VR experiments, a correspondence between physical and a virtual space was introduced. For instance, Jacobs et al. (1998) took a length of a stride to be the equivalent of 1 m. Hartley et al. (2004) used the virtual subject's height as scale. In this study, a standard walking speed was employed. Equating the speed of the participant's view (25 units/s) to a standard walking speed (4. 5 km/h) we estimated the rectangular environment to be approximately 9 x 6 x 3 mt. With this regard, it may be noted, however, that any strategies adopted is partially arbitrary. Three types of environments were generated. They differed both in terms of layout information and in terms of featural information: rectangular environments with four white walls, rectangular environments with three white walls and a blue wall on one of the short sides. Ceiling was light grey and floor was medium grey. Experimental session counted in fifteen trials. Each trial was composed of a learning phase and a testing phase (see description below). Trials were presented in three counterbalanced blocks, each block containing five trials.

The C-G learning environment. The learning environment consisted of a rectangular environment that could have all white walls, or a blue short wall, depending on the experimental conditions. A yellow sphere, 7 units in radius, was placed in one corner (see Figure 2). Four 10 x 10 units square response patches were located on the floor, inside the perimeter of the invisible arena, in relation to each corner. The response patches were leveled with the arena floor and their color was black. The use of a series of response patches was inspired by Kelly and Bishof (2005, 2008). They used the response patches in a reorientation study that employed static images depicting three-dimensional environments.

The C-G testing environment. The testing environment had the same shape and walls of the learning environment. Instead of the sphere, there were four blue identical boxes (7 x 7 x 7 units), one for each corner (see Figure 2). The four response patches were maintained. The target corresponded to one of the patches.

Joystick and keyboard. Participants used a joystick to explore the C–G Arena. Holding the joystick forward moved the participant's view forward about 25 units/s. Holding the joystick to the left or to the right turned the participant's view about 30–40°/s to the left or to the right, respectively. Holding the joystick backward did not produce any movement, because human being did not walk backwards in real life, so the joystick was modified in order to disable the backward walking. Pressing the space bar on the computer keyboard allowed teleport from learning environment to the testing environment.

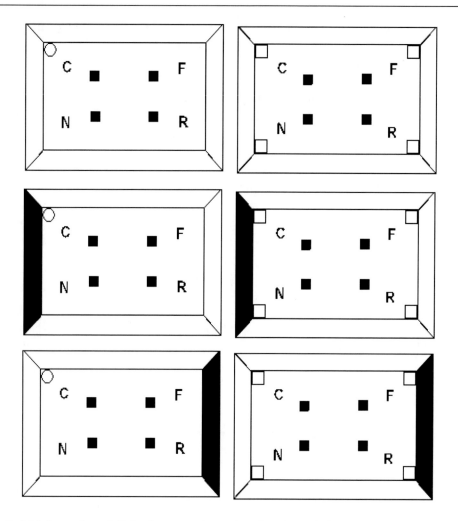

Figure 2. A bird-eye view of all the three experimental environments, in learning (on the left) and testing phases (on the right), respectively. A rectangular environment with all white walls, a rectangular environment with three white walls and one coloured wall near to the target, a rectangular environment with three white walls and one coloured wall far from the target.

Design and Procedures

Prior to the start of the experiment, each participant was randomly assigned to one of three different dual task conditions: *Articulatory Suppression Task*, *Spatial Tapping Task* and *No Concurrent Task*. The material and the procedure of dual task paradigm employed here match those reported in Coluccia, Bosco and Brandimonte (2007), Garden, et al. (2002), and Law et al. (2006). The articulatory suppression task involved a sequence of monosyllabic syllables when pronounced by Italian speakers i. e. Ba/Be/Bi/Bo/Bu/Da/De/Di/Do/Du. The spatial tapping task involved a custom-made keypad consisting of a matrix of 3 x 3 square, black, wooden keys. Each key measured 3 x 3 cm. with 1 cm. intervening gaps between squares. The number of trials for each of the three rooms (all white walls, blue wall near to / far from the target) was five.

Articulatory suppression task: the participants were instructed to repeat aloud the sequence of syllables presented above at a rate of one syllable per second, and were given practice in doing so. Suppression commenced immediately prior to entering the learning environment and continued throughout the exploration of the features of the environment itself. Suppression ceased when the subjects entered the testing environment, during the search for the target, and then was performed again in the next learning environment, and so on for all the experimental trials.

Spatial tapping task: the participants were instructed to tap each of the nine keys at a rate of one tap per second in a specified pattern: a forward movement form the top–left square to the bottom–right square, followed by the reversed sequence of movements. As in articulatory suppression condition, the movement was repeated during the exploration in the learning environment, and ceased when the participants entered the testing environment. Moreover, they were asked to tap with their left hand, while with the right hand they moved the joystick in order to navigate the environment. Participants were instructed that they should perform the concurrent task throughout the time they visited the learning environment and to stop when entering the testing environment. The research assistant monitored the participants closely to ensure that these instructions were followed.

Each participant entered into the laboratory and sat on a chair in front of a computer screen and a joystick. The eyes of the participants were approximately 50 cm from the centre of the screen. The physical FOV (Field of View) has been calculated to be 42° on the horizontal axis and 34° on vertical axis. They read and signed a consent form, then read the following written instructions:

> Instruction A - What you need to do. You will start out in a learning environment, where you will see a yellow sphere in one of the four corners. Please, explore the environment using the joystick and pay attention to all the features of the environment. Walk and look until you feel comfortable, then nod your head to the research assistant: you will be teleported to the testing environment. You will find yourself in an environment identical to the previous one, but with one blue box at each corner. Your initial orientation will be randomly settled during the transitions between learning and testing environments. The yellow sphere will not change place, it will stay in the same place, but it will be hidden by one blue box. Your goal is to walk around the environment and locate the corner where the sphere is placed. You should reach the black response patch on the floor, associated to the corner, only when you are reasonably convinced of your choice. You will know you have found the correct position when you hear a beep; otherwise, you should look for another corner, until you hear the sound.

> Instruction B - How to move and look about. Pushing the cloche of the joystick, you can move forward. Pushing it to the left or to the right you can turn on to the left or to the right, respectively. You can withdraw from the experiment at any time with no penalty. If you have any questions about the experiment, ask the research assistant now. Once you are done with it, we will give you more details about the study.

After this reading, all participants were requested to practice with the desktop virtual environment apparatus. Prior to the start of the experiment, a training phase provided the participants the opportunity to reach an adequate level of practice with: (a) joystick, (b) procedure of the experimental session, including the two concurrent tasks, (c) goal of the task.

The training phase was carried out in order to avoid or to minimize distortions due to different level of experience when facing a virtual reality apparatus, especially in children and elderly people (Moffat & Resnick, 2002; Newhouse et al. 2007). Another technique adopted to control for this kind of bias is to ask participants how much they are confident with computer technologies. Participants answered to a short questionnaire, in order to assess their ability in the use of personal computers and videogames and console games. The use of personal computer and widespread software, such as word processing, electronic sheets etc., give us information related to the familiarity with a computer monitor and to the degree of interaction participants have with it. The use of videogames and console games gave us information related to familiarity with virtual environments, and with the tools for navigating in these environments. A low or high attendance in the employment of joystick, cloche, game pads, can determine relevant differences in performance in virtual navigation tasks (e. g. Gagnon, 1985).

Learning phase. After completing the training, participants entered the learning environment, facing randomly one of the four walls. In this phase, participants were explicitly requested to visit the environment looking for the yellow sphere, in order to subsequently find it in the testing environment (where the yellow sphere was hidden). When they felt comfortable with the task, they gave a signal to the research assistant, who promptly pressed the space bar and teleported the participants into the testing environment.

Virtual disorientation. During the interval between learning and testing phase, lasting 2 seconds, the computer screen was switched-off. The C–G Arena application allowed changing randomly the participants' point of view with respect to the one they had in the learning environment. This procedure induced interference in the egocentric mental representation of the relative position of the target with respect to participants' view. In other terms, in the testing environment participants had to refer to their allocentric mental representation of space: that is, the relationship between layout and featural cues (geometric and non-geometric characteristics) of the environment and the sphere's position. This kind of interference due to changing initial orientation in testing environment will be referred to as virtual disorientation in the rest of the paper.

Testing phase. Participants' initial facing position in the testing environment was randomly settled (see above). They were requested to explore the environment to find the yellow sphere hidden in one of the four boxes. Participants knew that the yellow sphere was hidden but not moved from the original location. Thereafter, they were requested to discover the box housing the sphere by reaching the response patch corresponding to that box. If the chosen response patch was correct, participants heard a sound, and a trap captured her/him and another trial began. If the response patch was wrong, participants had to search for another corner until they had found the right one, as in typical searching tasks. Each participant was involved in three experimental conditions, each condition was composed of five trials, and for a total of fifteen trials (order of conditions was counterbalanced across participants): rectangular environment with all white walls, rectangular environment with one blue-wall near to the target, rectangular environment with one blue-wall far from the target. Location of the target was balanced across trials.

Response coding. The output files, generated by the program, showed the layout of the invisible, circular arena, and the route traveled by the participants both to explore the environment in the learning phase and to reach the response patches in the testing phase. In rectangular environment with four white walls the responses were recorded as appropriate if the participants searched either at the correct corner "C" or at its rotationally equivalent "R" corner. In the rectangular blue-wall environment the responses were recorded as appropriate if the participants searched at the correct corner "C". If the participant searched in "R" corner, s/he made an error related to the shape of the room. This error was coded as "geometric appropriate error." The errors in "N" corner were due to the ineffectiveness of both (a) the distinction between left and right (sense information) and (b) the assessment of geometrical information. This error was coded as "landmark appropriate error" since "C" and "N" shared the landmark. "F" did not possess specificity in terms of error type.

The analysis presented here focused on the participants' first search in each trial (see Figure 1b). The first search within each trial was coded twice, (a) on-line, during the experimental session by a research assistant (blind to the experimental hypotheses) specifically trained in evaluating if a response patch was intentionally reached, and (b) off-line by means of visual inspection of an output showing the route traveled by the participants in the testing environments (see Figure 1b). A third rater assessed the disagreements (less than 2% on more than 900 outputs examined).

RESULTS

Firstly, a one-way between-subject ANOVA with C and R pooled proportion of first searches as dependent variable and type of concurrent task as a three level factor (articulatory suppression, spatial tapping, no concurrent task) was performed on the performance showed in the all white wall condition. The analysis did not show the main effect of the independent variable with $F(2, 57) = 1.25$, $p > 0.1$. Performance on the blue wall rooms was evaluated through a mixed factors ANOVA, with proportion of errors as dependent variable, type of concurrent task (as in previous analysis), proximity of landmark to the target (near to vs. far from) and kind of error (R, F, and N angles) as independent variables. Results showed a main effect of the type of concurrent task with $F(2, 57) = 4.14$, $p < 0.05$; (MSe= 0.01; partial eta-square=0.13; control: 0.02, spatial: 0.07, verbal: 0.04); a main effect of proximity $F(1, 57) = 9.47$, $p < 0.01$; (MSe= 0.01; partial eta-square=0.14; near to the target: 0.02, far from the target: 0.05) and a main effect of the kind of error $F(2, 114) = 9.65$, $p < 0.001$; (MSe= 0.01; partial eta-square=0.14; R: 0.03, F: 0.03, N: 0.07). No significant interaction emerged. Post – hoc comparison (Scheffé) for the type of concurrent task indicated that the proportion of errors in the spatial tapping condition was significantly higher than that both the control ($p < 0.01$), and the articulatory suppression condition ($p < 0.05$). A statistically significant difference emerged between articulatory suppression and control ($p < 0.05$). Proximity showed the expected advantage of the landmark near to with respect to far from the target. Finally, post – hoc comparisons for errors showed that the rate of searching in the "N" corner (sense error) was significantly higher than the rate of searching in the "R" angle ($p < 0.01$), and "F" angle ($p < 0.01$). No difference between "R" and "F" emerged.

DISCUSSION

The principal aim of this experiment was to assess the role of different subsystems of working memory in reorientation paradigm and in this way to appraise the role of language in the integration of geometric and featural characteristics of the environment. This aim was fostered by the fact that previous studies on this topic were not completely comparable in terms of materials employed and generating divergent results. For example, the verbal shadowing task used in Hermer-Vazquez, et al. (1999) - immediately repeating an irrelevant discourse heard through headphone - appears higher demanding than the rhythm concurrent task. Indeed, repeating words could activate a lexical-based long-term memory trace, with a possible drawback in terms of general loads of the cognitive system. This suggestion could explain to some extent the fact that the interference effect of verbal concurrent task was higher than that of the rhythm concurrent task employed in that research. Likewise, the spatial concurrent task used in Ratliff and Newcombe (2005, 2008) - visualizing a series of four line diagrams and categorizing each intersecting point in the diagram according to one of two spatial categories - entails visual imagery and only partially verbal abilities (especially in the categorization phases). On these grounds, it cannot be considered simply as a visuo-spatial working memory task. It is worthwhile to note that the selection of the concurrent tasks in previous studies was constrained by procedural problems met by the researchers in the real environment experimental setting. On the contrary, the VR technologies provide a broader autonomy in selecting the appropriate concurrent task. Consequently, spatial tapping tasks and articulatory suppressions, both employed in our experiment, perfectly fitted experimental needs. They are comparable in terms of general cognitive load and are known to affect visuo-spatial and verbal components of working memory, respectively (Cornoldi & Vecchi, 2003). As expected, both the concurrent tasks produced a decrease in performance, although spatial tapping seems to interfere in a greater extent than articulatory suppression. These results seem to partially harmonize previous findings, since they lead to conclude that the reorientation task engages critically visuo-spatial and, with a minor extent, verbal components of working memory. Recently, Landau and Lakusta (2009) suggest that, within simple environments, navigation is primarily supported by cues that are easy to verbalize like typical landmarks (i.e. "a blu wall"). The reorientation task involved such kind of environment leading the participants to adopt a verbal coding disturbed by verbal interference.

Spatial interference in Ratliff and Newcombe (2005, 2008) revealed a decrease in performance due to an additional amount of first searches in R angle. In contrast, in the present experiment the spatial interference caused a large amount of first search in N angle. An explanation is referred to the notion of *size of the enclosure*. Indeed, previous findings demonstrated that in large environments, human (children: Learmonth, et al., 2001; 2002) and non-human (e.g. chicks: Sovrano et al., 2006) animals tended to solve the task using essentially featural (landmark) information, whereas in small environments the shape of the enclosure seemed to have the primacy in guiding spatial navigation.

In light of this consideration, we might conclude that spatial has a larger effect than verbal interference on reorientation, but produces increase of geometric errors in small-scale environment, as in the study of Ratliff and Newcombe (2005, 2008), or an increase of featural errors in large-scale environment, as in the present study.

REFERENCES

[1] Atkinson, R. C. & Shiffrin, R. M. (1968). Human memory: A proposed system and its control processes. In: K. W. Spence, & J. T. Spence, (Eds.), *The psychology of learning and motivation: Advances in research and theory. (Vol. 2)*. New York: Academic Press.

[2] Baddeley, A. D. & Hitch, G. (1974). *Working memory*. In: G. H. Bower (Ed.), *The psychology of learning and motivation: Advances in research and theory*. New York: Academic Press.

[3] Baddeley, A. (1986). *Working memory*. Oxford: Clarendon Press

[4] Baddeley, A. D. (2000). The episodic buffer: A new component of working memory? *Trends in Cognitive Science, 4,* 417-423.

[5] Baddeley, A. & Wilson, B. A. (2002). Prose recall and amnesia: Implications for the structure of working memory. *Neuropsychologia, 40*(10), 1737-1743.

[6] Baddeley, A. (2003). Working memory: looking back and looking forward. *Nature Reviews Neuroscience, 4(10),* 829–839.

[7] Bosco, A., Picucci, L., Caffo', A., Lancioni, G. E. & Gyselinck, V. (2008). Assessing human reorientation inside virtual reality environments: the role of working memory components and task characteristics. *Cognitive Processing, 9,* 299–309.

[8] Bosco, A., Picucci, L., Caffò. A. O. & Lancioni, G. E. (2010). Current Debate on Human Spatial Reorientation: How Geometric and Non-Geometric Cues Interact. In J. Valentín & L. Gamez (Eds), *Environmental Psychology: New Developments*. New York: Nova Science Publishers.

[9] Brooks, L. (1968). Spatial and verbal components of the act of recall. *Canadian Journal of Psychology, 22,* 349–368.

[10] Cheng, K. (1986). A purely geometric module in rat's spatial representation. *Cognition, 23,* 149-178.

[11] Cheng, K. & Newcombe, N. S. (2005). Is there a geometric module for spatial orientation? Squaring theory and evidence. *Psychonomic Bulletin & Review, 12,* 1-23.

[12] Cheng, K. (2008). Whither geometry? Troubles of the geometric module. *Trends in Cognitive Sciences. 12(9),* 355-361.

[13] Chiandetti, C., Regolin, L., Sovrano, V. A. & Vallortigara, G. (2007). Spatial reorientation: the effects of space size on the encoding of landmark and geometry information. *Animal Cognition, 10(2),* 159-168.

[14] Coluccia, E., Bosco, A. & Brandimonte, M. A. (2007). The role of visuo-spatial working memory in map learning: New findings from a map drawing paradigm. *Psychological Research, 71,* 359-372.

[15] Cornoldi, C. & Vecchi, T. (2003). *Visuo-spatial working memory and individual differences*. Psychology Press: Hove and New York, UK/USA.

[16] Fodor, J. (2000). *The mind doesn't work that way*. MIT Press, Cambridge.

[17] Gagnon, D. (1985). Videogames and spatial skills: An exploratory study. *Educational Communication and Technology Journal, 33(4),* 263-275.

[18] Garden, S., Cornoldi, C., Logie, R. H. (2002). Visuo-spatial working memory in navigation. *Applied Cognitive Psychology, 16,* 35-50.

[19] Gouteux, S., Thinus-Blanc, C. & Vauclair, J. (2001). Rhesus monkeys use geometric and nongeometric information during a reorientation task. *Journal of Experimental Psychology: General, 130,* 505-519.

[20] Hartley, T., Trinkler, I. & Burgess, N. (2004). Geometric Determinants of Human Spatial Memory. *Cognition, 94(1),* 39-75.

[21] Hermer, L. & Spelke, E. (1994). A geometric process for spatial reorientation in young children. *Nature, 370,* 57-59.

[22] Hermer, L. & Spelke, E. (1996). Modularity and development: The case of spatial reorientation. *Cognition, 61,* 195-232.

[23] Hermer-Vasquez, L., Spelke, E. S. & Katsnelson, A. S. (1999). Sources of flexibility inhuman cognition: Dual-Task studies of space and language. *Cognitive Psychology, 39,* 3-36.

[24] Hermer-Vazquez, L., Moffet, A. & Munkholm, P. (2001). Language, space, and the development of cognitive flexibility in humans: The case of two spatial memory tasks. *Cognition, 79(3),* 263-299.

[25] Jacobs, W. J., Laurance, H. E. & Thomas, K. G. F. (1997). Place learning in virtual space I: Acquisition, overshadowing, and transfer. *Learning and Motivation, 28,* 521–541.

[26] Jacobs, W. J., Thomas, K. G. F., Laurance, H. E. & Nadel, L. (1998). Place learning in virtual space II. Topographical relations as one dimension of stimulus control. *Learning and Motivation, 29,* 288-308.

[27] Kelly, D. M., Spetch, M. L. & Heth, C. D. (1998). Pigeons' (Columba livia) encoding of geometric and featural properties of a spatial environment. *Journal of Comparative Psychology, 112,* 259-269.

[28] Kelly, D. M. & Bischof, W. F. (2005). Orienting in images of a 3-D environment. *Experimental of Psychological Human Perception and Performance, 31,* 1391–1403.

[29] Kelly, D. M. & Bischof, W. F. (2008). Orienting in virtual environments: How are surface features and environmental geometry weighted in an orientation task? *Cognition, 109,* 89-104.

[30] Landau, B. & Lakusta, L. (2009). Spatial representations across species: geometry, language, and maps. *Current Opinion in Neurobiology, 19,* 1-8.

[31] Law, A. S., Logie, R. H. & Pearson, D. G. (2006). The impact of secondary tasks on multitasking in a virtual environment. *Acta Psychologica, 122(1),* 27-44.

[32] Learmonth, A. E., Newcombe, N. S. & Huttenlocher, J. (2001). Toddlers' use of metric information and landmarks to reorient. *Journal of Experimental Child Psychology, 80,* 225-244.

[33] Learmonth, A. E., Nadel, L. & Newcombe, N. S. (2002). Children's use of landmarks: Implications for modularity theory. *Psychological Science, 13,* 337-341.

[34] Logie, R. H. (1986). Visuo-spatial processing in working memory. *Quarterly Journal of Experimental Psychology, 38A,* 229-247.

[35] Logie, R. H. & Marchetti, C. (1991). Visuo-spatial working memory: Visual, spatial or central executive?. In: R. H. Logie, M. Denis, (Eds), *Mental images in human cognition.* Amsterdam: Elsevier.

[36] Logie, R. H., Della Sala, S., Wynn, V. & Baddeley, A. D. (2000). Visual similarity effects in immediate verbal serial recall. *Quarterly Journal of Experimental Psychology Section A: Human Experimental Psychology, 53(3),* 626-646.

[37] Moffat, S. D. & Resnick, S. M. (2002). Effects of age on virtual environment place navigation and allocentric cognitive mapping. *Behavioral Neuroscience, 116(5),* 851-859.

[38] Newcombe, N. S. (2005). Evidence for and against a geometric module: The roles of language and action. In J. Rieser, J. Lockman, & C. Nelson (Eds.), *Minnesota symposium on child psychology. Action as an organizer of learning and development, 33,* 221–241. Mahwah, NJ: Lawrence Erlbaum.

[39] Newcombe, N. S. & Ratliff, K. R. (2007). Explaining the development of spatial reorientation: modularity-plus-language versus the emergence of adaptive combination. In J. M. Plumert & J. P. Spencer (Eds), *The emerging spatial mind.* Oxford University Press.

[40] Newhouse, P. A., Newhouse, C. D. & Astur, R. (2007). Gender differences in visual-spatial learning using a virtual water maze in pre-pubertal children. *Behavioral Brain Research, 7,* 183–187.

[41] Picucci, L., Caffò, A. O. & Bosco, A. (2009). Age and sex differences in a virtual version of the reorientation task. *Cognitive Processing, 10(2),* 272-275.

[42] Picucci, L., Bosco, A., Caffò, A. O., D'Angelo, G., Soleti, E., Lancioni, G. E. & Di Masi, M. N. (2010). A New Methodology to Assess Individual Differences in Spatial Memory: The Computer-Generated Version of the Reorientation Paradigm. In: G. Salvati, & V. Rabuano, (Eds), *Cognitive Psychology Perspectives.* New York: Nova Science Publishers.

[43] Ratliff, K. R. & Newcombe, N. S. (2005). Human spatial reorientation using dual task paradigms. *Proceedings of Annual Cognitive Science Society, 27,* 1809-1814.

[44] Ratliff, K. R. & Newcombe, N. S. (2008). Is language necessary for human spatial reorientation? Reconsidering evidence from dual task paradigm. *Cognitive Psychology, 56,* 142-163.

[45] RepovŠ, G. & Baddeley, A. (2006). The multi-component model of working memory: Explorations in experimental cognitive psychology. *Neuroscience, 139(1),* 5-21.

[46] Richardson, J. T. E., Longoni, A. M. & Di Masi, N. (1996). Persistence of the phonological trace in working memory. *Cahiers de Psychologie Cognitive – Current Psychology of Cognition, 15,* 557–81.

[47] Sovrano, V. A., Bisazza, A. & Vallortigara, G. (2002). Modularity and spatial orientation in a simple mind: Encoding of geometric and non geometric properties of a spatial environment by fish. *Cognition, 85,* 51-59.

[48] Sovrano, V. A., Bisazza, A. & Vallortigara, G. (2003). Modularity as a fish (Xenotoca eiseni) views it: Conjoining geometric and non-geometric information for spatial reorientation. *Journal of Experimental Psychology: Animal Behavior Processes, 29,* 199-210.

[49] Sovrano, V. A., Bisazza, A. & Vallortigara, G. (2005). Animals' use of landmarks and metric information to reorient: Effects of the size of the experimental space. *Cognition, 97(2),* 121-133.

[50] Sovrano, V. A., Bisazza, A. & Vallortigara, G. (2006). How fish do geometry in large and in small spaces. *Animal Cognition, 10(1),* 47-54.

[51] Sovrano, V. A. & Vallortigara, G. (2006). Dissecting the geometric module: a sense linkage for metric and landmark information in animals' spatial reorientation. *Psychological Science, 17,* 616–621.

[52] Tulving, E. (1972). Episodic and semantic memory. In E. Tulving & W. Donaldson (Eds.), *Organization of Memory*. New York: Academic Press.
[53] Tulving, E. (1983). *Elements of Episodic Memory*. Oxford: Clarendon Press.
[54] Vallortigara, G., Zanforlin, M. & Pasti, G. (1990). Geometric modules in animals' spatial representations: A test with chicks (Gallus Gallus Domesticus). *Journal of Camparative Psychology, 104,* 248-254.
[55] Woodruff-Pak, D. S., Papka, M. & Ivry, R. B. (1996). Cerebellar involvement in eyeblink classical conditioning in humans. *Neuropsychology, 10(4),* 443-458.

In: Working Memory: Capacity, Developments and... ISBN: 978-1-61761-980-9
Editor: Eden S. Levin © 2011 Nova Science Publishers, Inc.-

Chapter 10

USING fMRI TO EXAMINE THE BRAIN – BASES OF WORKING MEMORY

Michael A. Motes[1,2,], Ehsan Shokri Kojori[1], Neena K. Rao[1], Ilana J. Bennett[1] and Bart Rypma[1,2]*

[1]Center for BrainHealth & School of Behavioral and Brain Sciences,
University of Texas at Dallas, TX, USA
[2]Department of Psychiatry, University of Texas Southwestern Medical Center, TX, USA

ABSTRACT

Considerable knowledge has been gained about the brain bases of working memory through research with functional magnetic resonance imaging (fMRI). However, using fMRI to explore the component processes that support working memory is difficult due to the timing of component processes and the lag of the hemodynamic response underlying the blood oxygen level dependent (BOLD) response in fMRI. Resolving controversies regarding the role of various brain regions in encoding, maintaining, retrieving, searching, and comparing information held in working memory requires isolating BOLD signal changes in response to the engagement of each of these component processes. A variety of fMRI experimental design and analysis techniques have been used for this purpose. These have included regression analyses with models based on canonical or subject-derived hemodynamic response functions, varying the duration of component process intervals, using component process intervals that exceed the ideal time needed for the hemodynamic response to return to baseline, regression modeling of parts of component process intervals, and including partial-trials in which only a subset of the component processes are engaged. The present chapter provides an overview of the technical challenges in using fMRI to examine the brain bases of working memory component processes, briefly reviews study designs and analysis methods that have been used to explore the brain bases of working memory, and offers suggestions for future research directions.

---

[*] Corresponding author: Center for BrainHealth, University of Texas at Dallas, 2200 W. Mockingbird Lane, Dallas, TX 75235, Phone: 972-883-3254, Fax: 972-883-3231, Email: Michael.Motes@utd.edu

INTRODUCTION

Working memory (WM) has a key role in higher-level cognitive processes including reasoning (Goel & Grafman, 1995), problem-solving (Prabhakaran, Rypma, & Gabrieli, 2001; Seyler, Kirk, & Ashcraft, 2003), and comprehension (Ehrlich, Brebion, & Tardieu, 1994), and it is also considered fundamental to general intelligence (Engle, Tuholski, Laughlin, & Conway, 1999; Wechsler, 1997). Given its entrenched role in the cognitive system, it is not surprising that considerable research effort has been invested in examining the brain bases of working memory. To date, a plethora of studies on humans and other animals have shown the involvement of prefrontal cortex (PFC) in working memory tasks, and given the evidence, it seems rather uncontroversial to say that PFC mediates working memory function (see Curtis & D'Esposito, 2003; Levy & Goldman-Rakic, 2000; Rypma, 2006). However, controversy does exist regarding the specific working memory functions mediated by PFC (see Feredoes & Postle, 2007; Rypma, 2006; Wickelgren, 1997), and within the fMRI literature, this controversy is further complicated by issues surrounding optimal fMRI designs and analysis techniques (Cairo, Liddle, Woodward, & Ngan, 2004; Motes & Rypma, 2010; Rypma, 2006). In the present chapter, we summarize design and analysis challenges in using fMRI to examine the brain bases of WM component processes, review our recent work on the use of a *partial-trial* method for examining the brain bases of WM component processes, and provide suggestions for future research.

Component Processes Supporting WM

Although many definitions of WM exist (see Miyake & Shah, 1999), research has provided a relatively consistent pattern of data suggesting that WM is not a unified construct. WM consists of multiple component processes that subserve the overall goal of holding information in a temporarily accessible state, often reorganizing or recoding the information, and making the information available for other operations. At a minimum, research has shown that WM is supported by encoding, maintenance, and search or retrieval processes (see Baddeley, 1986; Miyake & Shah, 1999; Repovs & Baddeley, 2006; cf. Just & Carpenter, 1992).

WM is further supported by executive processes that can be brought online when a goal requires the manipulation of information (e.g., when ordering information [D'Esposito, Postle, Ballard, & Lease, 1999; Eldreth et al., 2006; Postle, Berger, & D'Esposito, 1999] or performing computations [Seyler et al., 2003]). WM is known to be capacity limited (e.g., Glanzer & Razel, 1974; Luck & Vogel, 1997; Miller, 1956; but see Repovs & Baddeley, 2006). For example, one estimate puts WM capacity as low as four (+/- 1) items (see Cowan, 2001; 2005). However, when the amount of information to be remembered exceeds the capacity limit, WM executive processes can be brought online to reorganize memory codes in an attempt to fit them within the capacity limit (e.g., a 10-digit phone number regrouped or "chunked" into two sets of three numbers and a set of four numbers; see Baddeley, 1986; Miller, 1956) and thus produce substantial increases in capacity (Ericcson, Chase, & Falloon, 1980).

fMRI Studies Have Shown PFC Involvement in WM Depends on Demand

Across a variety of tasks, fMRI studies have shown that PFC is involved in WM and that PFC activity increases when processing demands placed on WM increase, such as, when the information to be remembered exceeds basic WM capacity (e.g., D'Esposito et al., 1995; D'Esposito, Postle, Ballard, & Lease, 1999; Rypma et al., 1999; see Rypma, 2006). Three general classes of tasks have been used in fMRI research to explore the role of PFC in WM for supra-capacity information. These classes of tasks are item recognition tasks (IRT), IRTs with explicit memory reorganization requirements, and n-back tasks.

IRT trials consist of separate sample, delay, and probe periods designed to isolate the engagement of different cognitive processes. On each trial, a participant is presented a sample memory-set that they are instructed to *encode*; then, they are to *maintain* a mental representation of the memory-set over a delay; and finally, they are to *decide* whether a probe item appeared within the memory-set. Thus, IRT designs ideally, and at a minimum, allow for the separate assessment of the brain-bases of WM encoding, maintenance, and decision-making component processes engaged during the different task periods.

Some fMRI IRT studies have included manipulations of the memory set-size, or the amount of material to be remembered, in efforts to examine the brain-bases of demand placed on WM (Cairo, Liddle, Woodward, & Ngan, 2004; Habeck et al., 2005; Jha & McCarthy, 2000; Narayanan et al., 2005; Rypma & D'Esposito, 1999; Rypma et al., 2002; Veltman et al., 2003; Zarahn, Rakitin, Abela, Flynn, & Stern, 2005). IRT studies have tried to isolate memory set-size effects to encoding, maintenance, and decision task periods to determine when PFC resources are differentially utilized, possibly in the service of spontaneously re-encoding memory-sets that exceed WM capacity. However, this research has produced mixed results. Some fMRI studies have reported set-size effects within PFC for both the encoding and maintenance periods (Cairo et al., 2004; Narayanan et al., 2005; but see Feredoes & Postle, 2007, for group versus individual difference accounts), with larger set-sizes producing greater activity. Some studies have revealed set-size effects within PFC only during encoding (Postle et al., 1999; Rypma & D'Esposito, 1999; but see Rypma et al., 2002, for an individual differences account). Finally, some studies have exclusively focused on set-size effects during maintenance and have found mixed evidence, with one study finding that larger set-sizes produced greater PFC activity (Leung, Gore, & Goldman-Rakic, 2002) but another not finding a relationship between set-size and the degree of PFC activity (Jha & McCarthy, 2000).

A second class of tasks used in fMRI research to explore the role of PFC and other brain regions in WM component processes has involved WM demand manipulations through explicit requirements to mentally reorganize information being remembered (Bor, Cumming, Scott, & Owen, 2004; Bor, Duncan, Wiseman, & Owen, 2003; D'Esposito, Postle, Ballard, & Lease, 1999; Eldreth et al., 2006; Feredoes & Postle, 2007; Postle, Berger, & D'Esposito, 1999; Wagner, Maril, Bjork, & Schacter, 2001). In such studies, participants have been asked to study a randomly arranged memory-set, reorder the set over a delay (e.g., alphabetize or semantically order), and then judge the ordinal position of a probe in the reordered memory-set. Similar to the IRTs with implicit instructions described earlier, studies have revealed that explicit manipulation instructions have led to increased PFC activity during the maintenance period (D'Esposito et al., 1999; Postle et al., 1999; Wagner et al., 2001), suggesting that the information is first encoded and then PFC executive resources are elicited to re-encode the material during the maintenance period (but see Eldreth et al., 2006, and Feredoes & Postle, 2007, for individual differences accounts).

N-back tasks compose the third class of tasks used in fMRI research to explore the role of PFC WM component processes by including WM demand manipulations. For n-back tasks, trial items are presented sequentially, one at a time, and participants are to judge whether an item is the same as an item appearing some number of items, n, earlier. WM demand is manipulated by increasing n. Meta-analyses of n-back fMRI data have identified cortical regions that have tended to show activation across variations of n-back tasks: bilateral dorsolateral PFC, bilateral premotor and medial supplemental motor regions, frontal pole, bilateral ventrolateral PFC, and bilateral medial and lateral parietal regions (Owen, McMillan, Laird, & Bullmore, 2005). Of these regions, frontal pole, dorsolateral PFC, ventrolateral PFC, medial supplementary motor, and superior and inferior parietal regions also have been shown to be sensitive to n-back set-size (e.g., Veltman, Rombouts, & Dolan, 2003). However, n-back tasks require memory updating, because the to-be-remembered set is consistently updated by the addition of the probe to the memory set and the deletion of the target after the response, and it has been argued that updating places additional demand on WM and reduces capacity estimates from n-back tasks compared to other WM tasks (Cowan, 2000; Rypma et al., 1999). Thus, studies dissociating set-size and updating effects need to be conducted.

In general, these fMRI studies have shown that PFC involvement in WM varies with the amount of material to be remembered. Greater PFC involvement has been shown to occur when the memory-set exceeds basic capacity limits. However, mixed findings reported across fMRI studies limit certainty regarding the component processes being mediated by PFC, particularly whether PFC set-size effects are related to encoding, maintenance, or decision-making component processes (see Rypma, 2006).

Complications due to Hemodynamic Lag in fMRI

One challenge with isolating PFC involvement in trial-periods designed to capture the engagement of WM component processes is the nature of the fMRI signal. The fMRI signal is dependent on a hemodynamic response that lags in time behind the neural response of interest (see Heeger & Ress, 2002). FMRI measures a blood oxygen-level dependent (BOLD) response, where an increase in oxygenated blood within a brain region produces an increase in the intensity of the fMRI signal measured from that region.

Fundamental research on the fMRI BOLD response has shown it to be sensitive to the characteristics of stimuli being processed. The BOLD response within visual cortex, for example, varies largely proportionally with characteristics like the degree of visual contrast in visual stimuli and the duration and frequency of visual presentations (Boynton, Engel, Glover, & Heeger, 1996; Glover, 1999). Thus, the prevailing logic is that BOLD signal-change within a region is an index of regional neural activity and proportional to the degree of neural activity.

Event-related IRT fMRI designs might seem ideal for investigating the brain bases of WM component processes because the trial periods allow for some restriction or isolation of the component processes, but because of the hemodynamic lag, the measured BOLD signal-change for a given trial-period is not independent of hemodynamic influences from other adjacent trial-periods. This colinearity is depicted in Figure 1. Independent idealized BOLD signal-change functions for sample, delay, and probe periods from two IRT trials are depicted. The BOLD signal-change estimates in Figure 1 were generated by convolving canonical hemodynamic response functions (HRF; two-gamma functions; generated with AFNI Waver, Cox, 1996), commonly used for regression modeling of the BOLD response in fMRI analysis (Friston, Ashburner, Kiebel, Nichols, & Penny, 2006), with boxcar models of the trial-periods. The delay period in the example is longer than the sample and probe periods, and therefore, the idealized BOLD signal-change is greater due to the summing of BOLD responses over the longer period. Thus, the idealized responses are based on the assumption of steady neural activity over the three periods. The idealized *full-trial* BOLD response depicted in Figure 1 (seen as the dashed line) was created by summing over the sample, delay, and probe period responses at corresponding time-points (i.e., full-trial(t) = sample(t) + delay(t) + probe(t), where t=time-point), as would be expected for temporally adjacent events (Dale & Buckner, 1997). The summed contributions of the BOLD response for each trial-period at each time-point to overall BOLD signal-change over the full trial are depicted in the formulas in Figure 1. The invariant temporal spacing of adjacent IRT trial periods leads to the depicted colinearity in the BOLD responses to each period. This colinearity limits the possibility of estimating the unique portions of the BOLD response attributable to each period (Cairo et al., 2004; Manoach, Greve, Lingren, & Dale, 2003; Ollinger, Shulman et al., 2001), because there are not enough unique samples of the BOLD response necessary to obtain estimates of the signal-change for each component trial period in the full-trial.

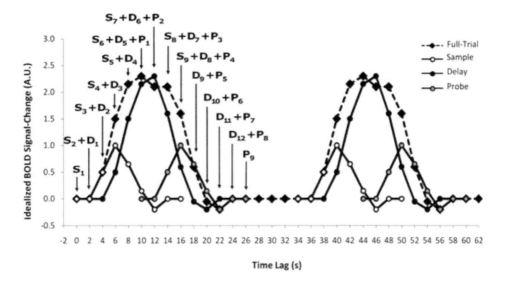

Figure 1. Idealized BOLD signal-change functions for sample, delay, and probe periods from an item response task and the resulting idealized BOLD signal-change function for a full trial from the task. Open circles depict sample period BOLD signal-change functions, filled black circles depict delay period BOLD signal-change functions, and filled gray circles depict probe period BOLD signal-change functions. Filled black diamonds depict idealized BOLD signal-change functions for a full-trial, summing over the individual BOLD responses to each period. A.U. = arbitrary units.

Methods Used to Estimate IRT Trial-Period BOLD Signal-Change

PFC BOLD responses over IRT trial-periods have been explored using a variety of methods. Regression analyses with models based on canonical and subject-derived HRFs have been used (e.g., Sakai, Rowe, & Passingham, 2002). Modeling responses based on canonical or subject-derived HRFs, however, has been shown to misestimate the magnitude of signal-change (Handwerker, Ollinger, & D'Esposito, 2004), is biased toward producing stronger effects for participants and brain regions having task-related HRFs that match the chosen shape, and does not allow for estimating particular characteristics of the response, such as rise time and latency to the peak. Varying the duration of the delay interval also has been used (e.g., Cairo et al., 2004; Rowe, Toni, Josephs, Frackowiak, & Passingham, 2000). Varying the duration of the interval increases the signal-change variability attributable to this interval, improving the validity of a detected maintenance effect; however, this method does not eliminate the colinearity problem. Using long maintenance intervals that exceed the ideal time needed for the encoding HRF to return to baseline (Jha & McCarthy, 2000) and modeling only the middle or later parts of the maintenance response (e.g., Feredoes & Postle, 2007; Rypma & D'Esposito, 1999) also have been used. These methods reduce the influence of the sample period BOLD responses on detection of delay period effects; however, they also do not entirely eliminate the colinearity problem and do not allow for the estimation of early and late delay period effects.

We used an arguably more refined partial-trial method to explore the brain-bases of WM component processes (Motes & Rypma, 2010).[1] In our study, participants (N=11, age $M = 26$, range = 19-41; 6 females) worked through full-trials consisting sample, delay, and probe periods. Participants were instructed to encode a sample set of letters, maintain a representation of the letter-set over a delay, and then decide whether a probe letter was in the memory-set or not. They also worked through *partial-trials* in which they were exposed to only the sample period of a full trial, the sample and delay periods of a full trial, or the sample and probe periods of a full trial.

The advantage of this method was that the combination of full- and partial-trials provided unique samples of the BOLD response necessary to account for the unknown signal-change parameter estimates for each component trial period in the full-trial (see Figure 2). Therefore, this partial-trial paradigm, with the sample, delay, and probe periods, allowed for the examination of brain regions mediating WM IRT encoding, maintenance, and decision-making processes, and the manipulation of memory set-size across full- and partial-trials allowed for the examination of the engagement of PFC during the trial-periods in response to supra- and sub-capacity memory-sets. The memory capacity estimates, based on Cowan's K (Cowan, 2001) and accuracy in the 6-item condition, that we obtained in the study supported the classification of six items as being above WM capacity and two items as being below capacity ($M = 4.45$ items).

---

[1] The imaging data were collected on a Philips Achieva 3T scanner equipped with an 8-element, SENSE, receive-only head coil (MPRAGE sequence: 1 mm isovoxel; sagittal; TE = 3.7 ms; flip angle = 12°; and seven functional EPI sequences: voxel = 3.5 x 3.5 x 4 mm; 36 slices/volume; 180 volumes/run; TR = 2000 ms, TE = 30 ms; flip angle = 70°; matrix = 64x64; axial; inferior to superior interleaved, with 6 "dummy" scans at the beginning of each functional run to remove T1 saturation effects).

The partial-trial paradigm was proposed to isolate BOLD responses to distinct but adjacent processing periods within a trial by having participants engage those component

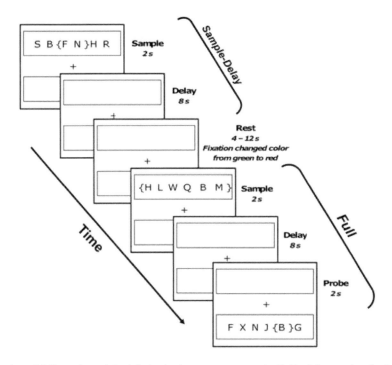

Figure 2. Examples of full- and partial-trials in the item response task. Full-trials consisted of a 2 s sample period in which participants would encode either two or six sample letters appearing within (yellow) brackets, an 8 s delay period in which they were to mentally maintain the encoded letters, and a 2 s probe period in which they were to decide whether a probe letter appearing within (blue) brackets was in the memory-set or not. Partial-trials consisted of sample only, sample and delay, and sample and probe parts of full trials. For the depicted sample and delay partial-trial, participants would encode the letters appearing within the (yellow) brackets, mentally maintain the letters over the 8 s delay, but then "rest" when the fixation changed from green to red. Adapted from Motes & Rypma, 2010.

processes in isolation or in combinations such that unique estimates of the BOLD responses for each processing period can be obtained. Ollinger and colleagues, for example, demonstrated that unique BOLD response estimates (within the calcarine sulcus) to a low-contrast visual stimulus immediately followed by a high-contrast visual stimulus could be obtained for each stimulus event if intermittent presentations of the low-contrast stimulus alone (i.e., not followed by the high-contrast stimulus) occurred during data acquisition (Ollinger, Corbetta, & Shulman, 2001; Ollinger, Shulman, et al., 2001). In fact, the obtained estimates were relatively equal in magnitude and in shape to obtained estimates from separate runs in which the low- or high-contrast stimulus was presented alone. We deconvolved the voxel-wise time-series data for individual participants using a basis function expansion approach, as opposed to a traditional fixed-shape regression approach. This approach allowed for the examination of WM component-related BOLD signal-changes without assumptions regarding the exact shape of the signal-change curves. We used a piecewise linear B-spline regression analysis (Graybill & Iyer, 2004: Saad et al., 2006; Ward, 1998/2006; for details, see Motes & Rypma, 2010), and this linear regression analysis yielded nine response amplitude parameter estimates (*B*) for the 2- and 6-letter sample conditions and for the 2- and 6-letter probe conditions, and 12 *B*s for the 2- and 6-letter delay conditions. Thus, for each voxel, the predicted BOLD response was equal to the sum of the three sets of scaled B-spline basis functions for each of the trial-periods for each of the set-size conditions, that is,

$$\hat{y}(t) = \sum_{i=0}^{8} B_{6E_i} T_{6E_i}(t) + \sum_{i=0}^{11} B_{6M_i} T_{6M_i}(t) + \sum_{i=0}^{8} B_{6D_i} T_{6D_i}(t) +$$

$$\sum_{i=0}^{8} B_{2E_i} T_{2E_i}(t) + \sum_{i=0}^{11} B_{2M_i} T_{2M_i}(t) + \sum_{i=0}^{8} B_{2D_i} T_{2D_i}(t)$$

where the subscripted 6 and 2 indicate the number of items in the memory set; the subscripted *E*, *M*, and *D* indicate sample, delay, and probe trial periods, respectively; $T_i(t)$ = *i*th tent basis function for the condition; and B_i = scaling parameter for the *i*th tent basis function for the condition.[2]

We then used a random-effects, 2 (Set-Size) X 3 (Trial-Period), repeated-measures ANOVA to identify regions where the set-size effects significantly differed over the trial-periods. The derived BOLD signal-change estimates for each condition were used for the group analysis. For each participant, the area under the curve (AUC) for the BOLD response estimates obtained from the linear B-spline regression analysis was calculated for each condition at each voxel, AUC = .5(B_1) + B_2 + B_3 + ... + .5(B_n), and the resulting AUC matrices were spatially normalized to Talairach space (Talairach & Tornoux, 1988). We then used these AUC estimates as the dependent measures for the ANOVA modeling.

Through these analyses, we discovered three clusters[3] of voxels where the effects of set-size significantly differed over the three trial periods (Figure 3), and all were within PFC. One cluster was in left lateral PFC, extending from lateral superior frontal gyrus ventrally to middle frontal gyrus, inferior frontal gyrus, and superior insula regions. One cluster was in right lateral PFC, extending ventrally across middle frontal gyrus to inferior frontal gyrus. Finally, one cluster was in medial PFC, extending bilaterally into superior frontal regions and cingulate gyri.

For each trial-period by set-size condition, we extracted and further examined the BOLD signal-change parameter estimates (i.e., the Bs from the subject-level B-spline regression analyses) from each of the clusters for each participant. The patterns were similar across the three clusters, except that the effects were stronger for the left and medial clusters than for the right cluster. The data showed greater involvement of the three PFC regions during both the sample and delay periods when processing the 6-letter sets compared to the 2-letter sets (data for left PFC illustrated in Figure 4, full data appear in Motes & Rypma, 2010). For all three regions, positive signal-change occurred for both the 6-letter and the 2-letter conditions during the sample period, but the 6-letter condition showed greater signal-change than the 2-letter condition. For all three regions, positive signal-change occurred for both the 6-letter and the 2-letter conditions during the delay period, but only for the latter lags in this period in the 2-letter condition. The 6-letter condition also was associated with greater signal-change than

---

[2] Prior to the regression analysis, the fMRI data for each participant were corrected for slice-timing offset, corrected for motion, and spatially filtered with a Gaussian kernel (FWHM = 8 mm). For each run, the data for each voxel were then scaled so that the deconvolution parameter estimates were expressed in terms of percent signal-change (i.e., for each voxel, rescaled y_t = 100 * y_t/M_y).

[3] The cluster-threshold was based on Monte Carlo simulations using AlphaSim software (Ward, 2000). With the cluster-level α = .05, voxel-level α = .005 and significant clusters = 1225 μL at 2 mm isovoxel or ~153 voxels.

the 2-letter condition. Finally, for all three regions, positive signal-change occurred for both the 6-letter and the 2-letter conditions during the probe period. However, the 2-letter condition was associated with greater signal-change than the 6-letter condition, particularly within right PFC.

Thus, the results from our partial-trial study revealed differential involvement of PFC across the three trial periods for the two set-sizes, that is, differential involvement of PFC in the WM component processes. When the memory-set exceeded the WM capacity of 4 items, PFC was more active during the sample and delay periods, suggesting greater involvement in encoding and maintenance processes. However, the finding that these PFC regions exhibited sustained activity over the delay period for the supra-capacity (6-letter) memory-sets but not for the sub-capacity (2-letter) sets suggests that these regions mediate processes qualitatively different from pure WM maintenance. The sub-capacity sets should have been associated with sustained activity over the delay period if these regions were mediating pure maintenance. Sustained activity for supra-capacity sets over the delay, but not for the sub-capacity sets, suggests that the delay interval might have been exploited for the engagement of WM executive processes in an attempt to organize the supra-capacity information to fit WM capacity constraints (Rypma, Berger, & D'Esposito, 2002; Rypma & Prabhakaran, 2009).

For the partial-trial study, we further analyzed the data to determine whether full-trial effects could be accounted for by the summing of the BOLD responses found for the separate trial periods. We obtained full-trial signal-change estimates using piecewise linear B-spline regression analysis, but we used models for full-trial and sample-only, sample and delay, and sample and probe partial-trials for each set-size condition in the subject-level regression analyses. Then, from the clusters identified in the above trial-period analysis, we obtained mean percent signal-change estimates for the 6-letter set and 2-letter set full-trials (e.g., Figure 5, solid lines with filleddiamonds and squares, respectively). As seen in Figure 5, peaks occurred toward the beginning and end of the full-trial functions, similar to findings from other IRT studies (e.g., Curtis, Rao, & D'Esposito, 2004; D'Esposito, Postle, Ballard, & Lease, 1999; D'Esposito, Postle, & Rypma, 2000; Feredoes & Postle, 2007; Jha & McCarthy, 2000; Leung et al., 2002; Narayanan et al., 2005; Rypma & D'Esposito, 1999). These peaks

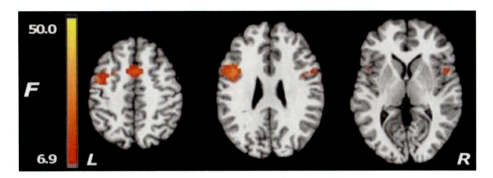

Figure 3. Statistical parameter maps showing PFC regions where BOLD signal-change estimates differed as a function of trial-period and set-size. Results from the random-effects, group ANOVA of the area under the BOLD signal-change curve. Clusters were significant with the cluster-level $\alpha = .05$ and voxel-level $\alpha = .005$ for the F-statistics for the interaction effect. Data are color-scaled based on the F-statistics per voxel. Adapted from Motes & Rympa, 2010.

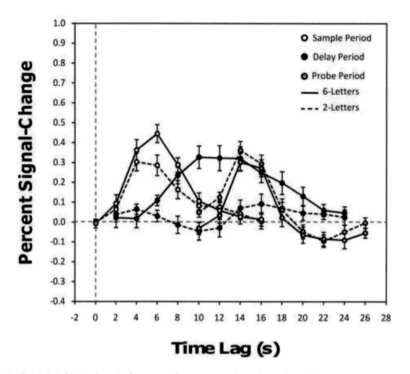

Figure 4. Left PFC BOLD signal-change estimates as a function of working memory trial-period and set-size. Solid black lines depict 6-item trial effects and dashed lines depict 2-item trial effects. Open circles depict sample period effects, black circles depict delay period effects, and gray circles depict probe period effects. Bars represent standard errors. Adapted from Motes & Rympa, 2010.

might appear to suggest greater encoding (sample period) and decision-making (probe period) effects relative to the maintenance (delay period) effect, as has been proposed in the research literature (see Curtis & D'Esposito, 2003). However, functions created by summing over corresponding time-points in the sample, delay, and probe BOLD signal-change estimates from the examination of the trial-period effects (i.e., full(t) = sample(t) + delay(t) + probe(t)) from Figure 4 are also depicted in Figure 5. The mean of the summed percent signal-change estimates for the 6-letter set (dashed line and open diamonds) and 2-letter set (dashed line and open squares) were correlated with their corresponding full-trial functions, as would be expected for temporally proximal events (Dale & Buckner, 1997), and the linear correlations between these data revealed that the summed functions fit the full-trial response functions well, with all rs (n=14) > .99, ps < .001.

Thus, the relative contributions of brain activity or cognitive functions during trial-periods just based on full-trial BOLD response data should be interpreted with considerable caution. Visual inspection of the full-trial effects might lead one to conclude that encoding and decision-making effects are greater than maintenance effects, and in fact, the analyses in which the partial-trial data were included suggest that this interpretation generally might be true. The data from the 2 letter-set delay condition compared to the sample and probe conditions clearly support this interpretation. However, the data from the 6 letter-set delay condition also supports this interpretation if the assumption of the summing of the hemodynamic response over sustained neural activity is met. With the assumption that the

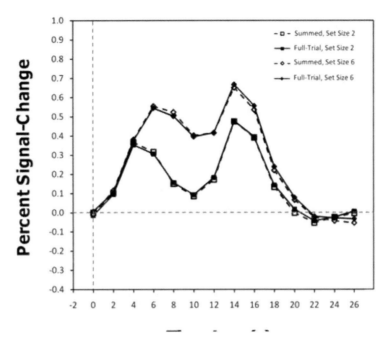

Figure 5. Left PFC BOLD signal-change estimates as a function of time from the onset of a full trial and set-size. Solid black lines depict full trial estimates, and dashed lines depict the summed parameters of the sample, delay, and probe period effects from Figure 4. Filled and open diamonds depict 6-letter set effects, and filled and open squares depict 2-letter set effects.

BOLD response sums over sustained neural events, the peak BOLD response over the delay period should be greater than the peak response for either the sample or probe periods if the same rate and magnitude of neural activity occurs over the three periods, as in Figure 1. The peak for the delay period for the 6 letter-set condition, however, was roughly equal to (or slightly less than) the peaks from the sample and probe periods. Thus, with the additivity assumption, it appears that the maintenance-related activity, even for the supra-capacity memory-sets, was lower than the encoding and decision-making activity, suggesting more intermittent maintenance-related neural activity within these PFC regions.

Finally, for the present chapter, we reanalyzed these partial-trial data, examining only the data from the first three runs, and the reanalysis revealed a need to consider dynamics over a session in the identification of the brain bases of WM component processes. The majority of studies using fMRI to investigate the brain bases of WM, including the partial-trial study described above, have relied on steady-state analysis methods designed to identify mean signal changes over a run or set of runs. When we reanalyzed only the first three runs of the original seven-run data, however, we found interaction effects within the left and medial PFC regions, similar to what we found using all seven runs, but we also found interaction effects within other brain regions (see Table 1 and Figure 6A). For the three runs, interaction effects also occurred bilaterally within superior and middle temporal regions, left superior parietal cortex, left parahippocampus and hippocampus, parts of the cerebellum, and parts of the left basal ganglia and thalamus. For the sample period, the only significant difference was within cerebellum, with 6-items producing greater signal-change than 2-items (Figure 6B and means in Table 1). For the delay period, significant differences were observed within left lateral and

Table 1. For RAI, Right, Anterior, and Inferior coordinates are negative, and Left, Posterior, and Superior are positive

| Region | Number of voxels | Talairach Coordinates (RAI) for Voxel with Peak F Value ||| Mean Percent Signal-Change ||||||
| | | x | y | z | Encoding || Maintenance || Judgment ||
					6-items	2-items	6-items	2-items	6-items	2-items
L. Inferior Frontal	1123	43	-5	26	1.19	0.76	2.09	0.43	-0.06	0.82
Cerebellum	737	9	59	-26	0.75	0.17	0.6	0.13	0.37	0.87
Medial Frontal	536	-3	1	54	1.47	0.74	2.34	0.59	-0.4	0.47
L. Fusiform	510	49	53	-16	0.38	0.31	0.5	-0.27	-0.14	0.56
R. Superior/Middle Temporal	434	-53	33	6	0.22	-0.29	-0.32	-0.29	-0.65	0.41
L. Superior Parietal	332	29	67	40	1.13	1.1	1.64	0.33	0.28	0.79
L. Superior/Middle Temporal	221	45	7	-8	-0.04	-0.31	0.1	-0.05	-0.31	0.49
R. Cerebellum	216	-25	53	-26	0.7	0.22	0.85	0.22	0.29	0.76
L. Parahippocampus/Hippocampus	205	33	13	-18	-0.16	-0.42	0.07	-0.37	-0.46	0.48
L. Cerebellum	204	23	45	-20	0.86	0.2	0.58	0.17	0.1	0.72
R. Cerebellum	196	-27	61	-50	0.89	0.46	1.33	-0.11	-0.002	0.71
L. Basal Ganglia/Thalamus	181	7	15	-8	0.6	0.064	0.41	0.18	0.04	0.56

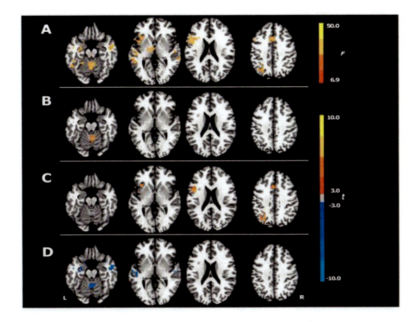

Figure 6. Statistical parametric maps showing regional differences in BOLD signal-change estimates as a function of trial-period and set-size for 3 fMRI runs. Figure A depicts significant trial-period by set-size interaction effects (illustrated in red to yellow). Results from the random-effects, group ANOVA of the area under the BOLD signal-change curve. Clusters were significant with the cluster-level $\alpha = .05$ and voxel-level $\alpha = .005$ for the F-statistics for the interaction effect. Data are color-scaled based on the F-statistics per voxel. Figure B depicts significant differences between 6-letter sets and 2-letter sets for the sample period. Figure C depicts significant differences between 6-letter sets and 2-letter sets for the delay period. Figure D depicts significant differences between 6-letter sets and 2-letter sets for the probe period. For B, C, and D, red to yellow illustrates greater effects for 6-letter sets compared to 2-letter set, and blue to cyan illustrates greater effects for 2-letter sets compared to 6 letter sets. Clusters were significant with the voxel-level $\alpha = .005$ for the t-statistics for the 6-letter set versus 2-letter set comparison.

medial PFC (as in the analysis of the full seven runs), left inferior frontal cortex, and left parietal cortex, with 6-items producing greater signal-change than 2-items in all regions (Figure 6C & means in Table 1). Finally, for the probe period, significant differences were observed in cerebellum, bilateral superior/middle temporal cortex, and left parahippocampus/hippocampus, with greater signal-change occurring in the 2-item condition than in the 6-item condition (Figure 6D and means in Table 1).

Together, these data suggest that the nature of the brain activity supporting WM component processes changed over the course of the study. The PFC activation patterns remained relatively consistent across the analyses of the three and seven runs, with the exception of the right lateral PFC effects being observed only after analyzing data from all seven runs. Yet, the data analysis from the first three runs suggests that other regions or processes recruited early in the study were not used across the duration of the study. The processing strategies being used over the study, particularly the encoding and decision-making components, appear to have changed from the earlier to the later runs.

CONCLUSION

The research reviewed in the present chapter has emphasized the role of PFC in WM component processes. The data show that developing an understanding of the role of PFC in WM component processes and understanding the brain bases of WM component processes, in general, requires examining the nature of processing changes both within trials and over a session. Furthermore, the data suggest that more refined fMRI designs and analysis methods will be required to resolve issues regarding the role of PFC in WM component processes given the nature of the BOLD response as an index of neural activity.

The partial-trial study presented in this chapter demonstrates the efficacy of using fMRI partial-trial methods for further disambiguating the role of PFC (and other regions) in WM component processes and also shows the potential value of using the partial-trial method for examining other hypotheses regarding the role of PFC in WM. The partial-trial method allowed for the isolation of unique BOLD responses to the temporally adjacent trial-periods and revealed the differential involvement of PFC in periods designed to isolate component processes supporting WM for supra- and sub-capacity memory sets. With modifications, the partial-trial method should be useful for disambiguating the role of PFC in executive mediation when given explicit material manipulation instructions (D'Esposito, Postle, Ballard, & Lease, 1999; Eldreth et al., 2006; Postle, Berger, & D'Esposito, 1999), when performing mental computations (Seyler et al., 2003), and when remembering information over a long delay (Jha & McCarthy, 2000). Additionally, the partial-trial method also could be useful for evaluating PFC process-specific (D'Esposito et al., 2000; Curtis & D'Esposito, 2003; Petrides, 1996; Rypma, 2006) versus modality-specific hypotheses (Goldman-Rakic, 1987; Levy & Goldman-Rakic, 2000). Indeed, although the partial-trial study suggests the differential involvement of PFC in encoding, maintaining, and making decisions about sub- and supra-capacity memory-sets, more refined designs will more precisely specify the WM component processes PFC is mediating (e.g., evaluating search and comparison processes during the probe period).

Finally, with respect to dynamics, it is well known that the brain functions via interactions between connected regions, with white matter connecting brain regions making up a large proportion of brain tissue. Thus, understanding the brain bases of WM component processes will require employing approaches that consider functional brain regions within a network of interacting nodes. In fact, one study that used a correlational connectivity approach revealed that visual, parietal, and prefrontal regions became highly correlated during load-dependent sample periods but that left lateralized inferior parietal, premotor and supplementary motor, and inferior prefrontal regions became highly correlated during load-dependent maintenance periods (Woodward et al. 2006), differentiating brain networks mediating encoding and maintenance processes supporting WM. The data suggest that functional connectivity between attention regions mediates load-dependent encoding processes but that functional connectivity between subvocal and phonological rehearsal regions mediates maintenance processes. Additionally, another study that used coherence as a measure of connectivity revealed that frontal eye fields showed greater functional connectivity with oculomotor areas during delay periods when a motor representation (i.e., a directional saccade) was the optimal memory code but that frontal eye fields showed greater functional connectivity with PFC, in particular, and other heteromodal brain regions when a sensory visuospatial representation was the optimal memory code (Curtis, Sun, Miller, & D'Esposito, 2005), thus showing variations in frontal eye field connectivity patterns for different memory representations. An additional promising avenue of research in brain dynamics is in the development and use of causal connectivity techniques. Causal connectivity techniques, such as Granger causality, can establish directional causal influences among functional brain regions wherein the past activity of brain regions is used to explore possible causal influences on the future activity of other brain regions of interest (Goebel, Roebroeck, Kim, & Formisano, 2003). Even though, the slow hemodynamic response, noise issues, and reduced sampling rate have put some practical restrictions on the application of this connectivity analyses to fMRI data, causal connectivity techniques have proven to be very informative for identifying the directionality of interactions between brain regions mediating cognitive processes (e.g., Biswal, Eldreth, Motes, Rypma, in press; Rypma et al., 2006). With the development of appropriate fMRI research designs, they hold the promise of allowing for the further characterization of network interactions supporting WM component processes.

REFERENCES

[1] Baddeley, A. D. (1986). *Working Memory.* New York: Oxford University Press.
[2] Biswal, B. B., Eldreth, D. A., Motes, M. A. & Rypma, B. (in press). Task-dependent individual differences in prefrontal connectivity. *Cerebral Cortex.*
[3] Bor, D., Cumming, N., Scott, C. E. M. & Owen, A. M. (2004). Prefrontal cortical involvement in encoding strategies, independent of stimulus modality. *European Journal of Neuroscience., 19,* 3365-3370.
[4] Bor, D., Duncan, J., Wiseman, R. J. & Owen, A. M. (2003). Encoding strategies dissociate prefrontal activity from working memory demand. *Neuron, 37,* 361-367.
[5] Boynton, G. M., Engel, S. A., Glover, G. H. & Heeger, D. J. (1996). Linear systems analysis of functional magnetic resonance imaging in human V1. *The Journal of Neuroscience, 16,* 4207-4221.
[6] Cairo, T. A., Liddle, P. F., Woodward, T. S. & Ngan, E. T. C. (2004). The influence of working memory load on phase specific patterns of cortical activity. *Cognitive Brain Research, 21,* 377–387.
[7] Curtis, C. E. & D'Esposito, M. (2003). Persistent activity in the prefrontal cortex during working memory. TRENDS in *Cognitive Sciences, 9,* 415-423.
[8] Curtis, C. E., Rao, V. Y. & D'Esposito, M. (2004). Maintenance of spatial and motor codes during oculomotor delayed response tasks. *Journal of Neuroscience, 24,* 3944-3952.
[9] Curtis, C. E., Sun, F. T., Miller, L. M. & D'Esposito, M. (2005). Coherence between fMRI time-series distinguishes two spatial working memory networks. *NeuroImage, 26,* 177-183.
[10] Cowan, N. (2001). The magical number 4 in short-term memory: A reconsideration of mental storage capacity. *Behavioral and Brain Science, 24,* 87-185.
[11] Cowan, N. (2005). *Working Memory Capacity.* New York: Psychology Press.

[12] Cox, R. W. (1996). AFNI: Software for analysis and visualization of functional magnetic resonance neuroimages. *Computers and Biomedical Research, 29,* 162-173.
[13] Dale, A. & Buckner, R. L. (1997). Selective averaging of rapidly presented individual trials using fMRI. *Human Brain Mapping, 5,* 329-340.
[14] D'Esposito, M., Detre, J. A., Alsop, D. C., Shin, R. K., Atlas, S. & Grossman, M. (1995). The neural basis of the central executive system of working memory. *Nature, 378,* 279-281.
[15] D'Esposito, M., Postle, B. R., Ballard, D. & Lease, J. (1999). Maintenance versus manipulation of information held in working memory: An event-related fMRI study. *Brain Cognition, 41,* 66–86.
[16] D'Esposito, M., Postle, B. R. & Rypma, B. (2000). Prefrontal cortical contributions to working memory: evidence from event-related fMRI studies. *Experimental Brain Research, 133,* 3-11.
[17] Ehrlich, M. F., Brebion, J. & Tardieu, H. (1994). Working-memory capacity and reading comprehension in young and older adults. *Journal of Psychological Research, 56,* 110-115.
[18] Eldreth, D. A., Patterson, M. D., Porcelli, A. J., Biswal, B. B., Rebbechi, D. & Rypma, B. (2006). Evidence for multiple manipulation processes in prefrontal cortex. *Brain Research, 1123,* 145-156.
[19] Engle, R. W., Tuholski, S. W., Laughlin, E. & Conway, A. R. A. (1999). Working memory, short-term memory and general fluid intelligence: A latent variable approach. *Journal of Experimental Psychology*: General, *128,* 309-331.
[20] Ericcson, K. A., Chase, W. G. & Falloon, S. (1980). Acquisition of a memory skill. *Science,* 1181-1182.
[21] Feredoes, E. & Postle, B. (2007). Localization of load sensitivity of working memory storage: Quantitatively and qualitatively discrepant results yielded by single-subject and group-averaged approaches to fMRI group analysis. *NeuroImage, 35,* 881-903.
[22] Friston, K. J., Ashburner, J. T., Kiebel, S. J., Nichols, T. E. & Penny, W. D. (2006). *Statistical Parametric Mapping: The Analysis of Functional Brain Images.* London: Academic Press.
[23] Goebel, R., Roebroeck, A., Kim, D. S. & Formisano, E. (2003). Investigating directed cortical interactions in time-resolved fMRI data using vector autoregressive modeling and Granger causality mapping. *Magnetic Resonance Imaging, 21,* 1251-1261.
[24] Glanzer, M. & Razel, M. (1974). The size of the unit in short-term storage. *Journal of Verbal Learning and Verbal Behavior, 13,* 114-131.
[25] Glover, G. H. (1999). Deconvolution of impulse response in event-related BOLD fMRI. *NeuroImage, 9,* 416-429.
[26] Goel, V. & Grafman, J. (1995). Are the frontal lobes implicated in "planning" functions? Interpreting data from the Tower of Hanoi. *Neuropsychologia, 33,* 623–642.
[27] Goldman-Rakic, P. S. (1987). Circuitry of primate prefrontal cortex and regulation of behavior by representational memory. In: Plum, F., Mountcastle, F. (Eds.), Handbook of Physiology (vol. 5). Washington DC: The American Physiological Society, 373-517.
[28] Graybill, F. A. & Iyer, H. K. (1994). Regression Analysis: Concepts and Applications. Belmont, CA: Duxbury Press.
[29] Habeck, C., Rakitin, B. C., Moeller, J., Scarmeas, N., Zarahn, E. & Brown, T. et al., (2005). An event-related fMRI study of the neural networks underlying the encoding,

maintenance, and retrieval phase in a delayed-match-to-sample task. Brain Research *Cognitive Brain Research, 23,* 207–220.

[30] Handwerker, D. A., Ollinger, J. M. & D'Esposito, M. (2004). Variation of BOLD hemodynamic responses across subjects and brain regions and their effects on statistical analyses. *NeuroImage, 21,* 1639-1651.

[31] Heeger, D. J. & Ress, D. (2002). What does fMRI tell us about neuronal activity. *Nature Reviews Neuroscience, 3,* 142-151.

[32] Jha, A. P. & McCarthy, G. (2000). The influence of memory load upon delay-interval activity in a working-memory task: An event-related functional MRI study. *Journal of Cognitive Neuroscience, 12,* 90-105.

[33] Just, M. A. & Carpenter, P. A. (1992). A capacity theory of comprehension: Individual differences in working memory. *Psychological Review, 98,* 122-149.

[34] Leung, H. C., Gore, J. C. & Goldman-Rakic, P. S. (2002). Sustained mnemonic response in the human middle frontal gyrus during on-line storage of spatial memoranda. *Journal of Cognitive Neuroscience, 14,* 659–671.

[35] Levy, R. & Goldman-Rakic, P. S. (2000). Segregation of working memory functions within the dorsolateral prefrontal cortex. *Experimental Brain Research, 133,* 23-32.

[36] Luck, S. J. & Vogel, E. K. (1997). The capacity of visual working memory for features and conjunctions. *Nature, 390,* 279-281.

[37] Manoach, D. S., Greve, D. N., Lindgren, K. A. & Dale, A. M. (2003). Identifying regional activity associated with temporally separated components of working memory using event-related functional MRI. *NeuroImage, 20,* 1670–1684.

[38] Miller, G. A. (1956). The magical number seven, plus or minus two: Some limits on our capacity for processing information. *Psychological Review, 63,* 81-97.

[39] Miyake, A. & Shah, P (1999). Models of working memory: Mechanisms of active maintenance and executive control. NY: Cambridge University Press.

[40] Motes, M. A. & Rypma, B. (2010). Working memory component processes: Isolating BOLD signal-changes. *NeuroImage, 49,* 1933-1941.

[41] Murdock, B. B., Jr., (1962). The serial position effect of free recall. *Journal of Experimental Psychology, 64,* 482-488.

[42] Narayanan, N. S., Prabhakaran, V., Bunge, S. A., Christoff, K., Fine, E. M. & Gabrieli, J. D. E. (2005). The role of prefrontal cortex in the maintenance of verbal working memory: An event-related fMRI analysis. *Neuropsychology, 19,* 223-232.

[43] Ollinger, J. M., Corbetta, M. & Shulman, G. L. (2001). Separating processes within a trial in event-related functional MRI II. Analysis. *NeuroImage, 13,* 218–229.

[44] Ollinger, J. M., Shulman, G. L. & Corbetta, M. (2001). Separating processes within a trial in event-related functional MRI I. The method. *NeuroImage, 13,* 210-217.

[45] Owen, A. M., McMillan, K. M., Laird, A. R. & Bullmore, E. (2005). N-back working memory paradigm: A meta-analysis of normative functional neuroimaging studies. *Human Brain Mapping, 25,* 46-59.

[46] Postle, B. R., Berger, J. S. & D'Esposito, M. (1999). Functional neuroanatomical double dissociation of mnemonic and executive control processes contributing to working memory performance. *Proceedings of the National Academy of Sciences* U. S. A., *96,* 12959-12964.

[47] Prabhakaran, V., Narayanan, K., Zhao, Z. & Gabrieli, J. D. E. (2000). Integration of diverse information in working memory with the frontal lobe. *Nature Neuroscience, 3,* 85-90.

[48] Repovs, G. & Baddeley, A. (2006). The multi-component model of working memory: explorations in experimental cognitive psychology. *Neuroscience, 139,* 5–21.

[49] Rosen, B. R., Buckner, R. L. & Dale, A. M. (1998). Event-related functional MRI: Past, present, and future. *Proceedings of the National Academy of Sciences,* USA, *95,* 773-780.

[50] Rowe, J. B., Toni, I., Josephs, O., Frackowiak, R. S. & Passingham R. E. (2000). The prefrontal cortex: response selection or maintenance within working memory? *Science, 288,* 1656-1660.

[51] Rypma, B. (2006). Factors controlling neural activity during delayed-response task performance: Testing a memory organization hypothesis of prefrontal function. *Neuroscience, 139,* 223-235.

[52] Rypma, B., Berger, J. S. & D'Esposito, M. (2002). The influence of working-memory demand and subject performance on prefrontal cortical activity. *Journal of Cognitive Neuroscience, 14,* 721-731.

[53] Rypma, B., Berger, J. S., Prabhakaran, V., Martin-Bly, B., Kimberg, D. Y., Biswal, B. B. & D'Esposito (2006). Neural correlates of cognitive efficiency. *NeuroImage, 33,* 969-979.

[54] Rypma, B. & D'Esposito, M. (1999). The roles of prefrontal brain regions in components of working memory: Effects of memory load and individual differences. *Proceedings of the National Academy of Sciences,* USA, *96,* 6558-6563.

[55] Rypma, B. & Prabhakaran, V. (2009). When less is more and when more is more: The mediating roles of capacity and speed in brain-behavior efficiency. *Intelligence, 37,* 207-222.

[56] Rypma, B., Prabhakaran, V., Desmond, J. E., Glover, G. H. & Gabrieli, J. D. E. (1999). Load-dependent roles of frontal brain regions in the maintenance of working memory. *NeuroImage, 9,* 216-226.

[57] Rypma, B., Prabhakaran, V., Desmond, J. E. & Gabrieli, J. D. E. (2001). Age differences in prefrontal cortical activity in working memory. *Psychology and Aging, 16,* 371-384.

[58] Saad, Z. S., Chen, G., Reynolds, R. C., Chistidis, P. P., Hammett, K. R., et al., (2006). Functional imaging analysis context (FIAC) analysis according to AFNI and SUMA. *Human Brain Mapping, 27,* 417-424.

[59] Sakai, K., Rowe, J. B. & Passingham, R. E. (2002). Active maintenance in prefrontal area 46 creates distractor-resistant memory. *Nature Neuroscience, 5,* 479-484.

[60] Seyler, D. J., Kirk, E. P. & Ashcraft, M. H. (2003). Elementary subtraction. Journal of Experimental Psychology: Learning, *Memory, and Cognition, 29,* 1339–1352.

[61] Talairach, J. & Tornoux, P. (1988). Co-planar stereotaxic atlas of the human brain. NY: Thieme Medical Publishers.

[62] Veltman, D. J., Rombouts, S. A. & Dolan, R. J. (2003). Maintenance versus manipulation in verbal working memory revisited: an fMRI study. *NeuroImage, 18,* 247-256.

[63] Wagner, A. D., Maril, A., Bjork, R. A. & Schacter, D. L. (2001). Prefrontal contributions to executive control: fMRI evidence for functional distinctions within lateral prefrontal cortex. *NeuroImage, 14,* 1337-1347.

[64] Ward, B. D. (2000). Simultaneous inference for FMRI data [Computer software manual]. Retrieved from http://afni. nimh. nih. gov/afni/doc/manual/AlphaSim.

[65] Ward, B. D. (1998/2006). Deconvolution analysis of FMRI time series data [Computer software manual]. Retrieved from http://afni. nimh. nih. gov/afni/doc/manual/3dDeconvolve.

[66] Wechsler, D. (1997). The Wechsler Adult Intelligence Scale—Third Edition. San Antonio, TX: The Psychological Corporation.

[67] Wickelgren, I. (1997). Getting a grasp on working memory. *Science, 275,* 1580-1582.

[68] Woodward, T. S., Cairo, T. A., Ruff, C. C., Takane, Y., Hunter, M. A. & Ngan, T. C. (2006). Functional connectivity reveals load dependent neural systems underlying encoding and maintenance in verbal working memory. *Neuroscience, 139,* 317-325.

[69] Zarahn, E., Rakitin, B., Abela, D., Flynn, J. & Stern, Y. (2005). Positive evidence against human hippocampal involvement in working memory maintenance of familiar stimuli. *Cerebral Cortex, 15,* 303-316.

In: Working Memory: Capacity, Developments and…
Editor: Eden S. Levin

ISBN: 978-1-61761-980-9
© 2011 Nova Science Publishers, Inc.

Chapter 11

AGING AND SHORT-TERM MEMORY FOR FACE IDENTITY OF EMOTIONAL FACES

Sandra J. E. Langeslag and Jan W. van Strien*
Erasmus Affective Neuroscience Lab, Institute of Psychology,
Erasmus University Rotterdam, The Netherlands

ABSTRACT

Age differences have been observed in emotional modulation of long-term memory (LTM) but have not yet been investigated in short-term memory (STM) in a comparable manner. In this study, age differences in the effect of stimulus emotionality on STM for stimulus content were examined. Younger (18-29 years) and older (61-77 years) adults completed a STM task with angry, happy, and neutral faces. Memory for face identity was increased for angry and neutral compared to happy faces. The response bias was most conservative for angry, and most liberal for happy faces. No age differences were observed in this emotional modulation of STM. It is argued that this is not due to lack of statistical power or to participant characteristics, but rather to the constraint nature of the task (probe-guided retrieval and short retention interval). The current findings do not suggest that emotional modulation of STM changes across the lifespan.

Keywords: working memory; emotion; faces; expressions; aging

INTRODUCTION

Many studies have examined age differences in emotional long-term memory (LTM), and age differences have been observed in several of these studies (see Mather & Carstensen, 2005, for a review). To our knowledge, only one study has investigated age differences in

---

* Corresponding author S. Langeslag is now at: Erasmus MC – Sophia Children's Hospital, Department of Child and Adolescent Psychiatry, P.O. Box 2060, NL-3000 CB Rotterdam, The Netherlands, Email address: s.langeslag@erasmusmc.nl, Tel: +31 (0)10 703 7071, Fax: +31 (0)10 703 2111

emotional short-term memory (STM). In that study, younger and older adults viewed unpleasant and pleasant pictures and were instructed to memorize the intensity of the feeling that a picture elicited. Older adults showed superior memory for pleasant versus unpleasant feelings, while younger adults showed the opposite pattern (Mikels, Larkin, Reuter-Lorenz, & Carstensen, 2005). Findings in the LTM domain, however, typically concern memory for the emotional stimuli themselves, instead of memory for the elicited feelings. We performed the present study to examine age differences in STM for the content of emotional stimuli.

Both STM and LTM decline with aging, starting already in young adulthood (Park & Reuter-Lorenz, 2009). Recall memory, which is dependent on the process of recollection, declines more with age than recognition memory, for which the process of familiarity suffices (Light, Prull, La Voie, & Healy, 2000). Age may also influence the emotional modulation of memory (Mather & Carstensen, 2005). In general, it is assumed that people remember salient emotional information better than non-emotional information (Kensinger, 2004). Age differences in emotional processing would arise in the form of a so-called positivity effect, which is "a trend for adults to increasingly process positive information and/or decreasingly process negative information compared with other information with advancing age" (Langeslag & Van Strien, 2009, p. 376; Mather & Carstensen, 2005; but see Uttl & Graf, 2006). This positivity effect has been observed not only when comparing younger (approx. 18-30 yrs) with older adults (approx. 60-80 yrs), but also when comparing younger with middle-aged adults (approx. 40-55 yrs) (Charles, Mather, & Carstensen, 2003).

The goal of the present study was to examine age differences in STM for emotional stimulus content. In studies involving STM for face identity of emotional faces, younger adults had better memory for angry compared to happy and neutral faces (Jackson, Wolf, Johnston, Raymond, & Linden, 2008; Jackson, Wu, Linden, & Raymond, 2009). Memory for the identity of faces is important in both younger and older adults' daily life. It is called upon in social interactions in which it is relevant to remember the identity of those individuals that reveal their judgement, mood, or intentions through their facial expressions. Here we used the emotional face STM paradigm of Jackson et al. (2008; 2009) to test age differences in STM for the content of the emotional stimuli (i.e. face identity), and not for the emotion conveyed (e.g. facial expression or feeling/emotion elicited).

For LTM, a previous study has demonstrated a positivity effect in memory for emotional faces. Younger adults recognized positive and negative faces equally well and older adults recognized positive faces better than negative faces (Mather & Carstensen, 2003). In another LTM study, however, such positivity effect was not observed. Younger adults recognized negative faces best, neutral faces intermediately and positive faces least, whereas older adults recognized neutral faces better than positive faces (Grady, Hongwanishkul, Keightley, Lee, & Hasher, 2007). In three more LTM studies, age differences in the effect of facial expression on recognition memory were absent all together (D'Argembeau & Van der Linden, 2004; Leigland, Schulz, & Janowsky, 2004; Spaniol, Voss, & Grady, 2008). It is unclear why the findings of these LTM studies differ, but it may have to do with differences in the length of the delay between the study and test phases (which varied between 5 and 30 minutes), the specific facial expressions used, and the different recognition measures that were computed (discrimination indices or proportional scores (see also Uttl & Graf, 2006)).

The above mentioned findings concern the ability to distinguish faces that were or were not previously encountered, which is called discrimination. To fully consider recognition memory, a measure of response bias needs to be considered as well (Snodgrass & Corwin,

1988). The response bias reflects the tendency to classify a certain stimulus as previously encountered, irrespective of its actual old or new status. Generally, people adopt a more liberal response bias for emotional than neutral stimuli (Ochsner, 2000; Windmann & Kutas, 2001), yielding higher hit and false alarm rates for emotional than neutral stimuli. This more liberal response bias for emotional stimuli would ensure that information that is relevant for survival and/or reproduction is not missed or forgotten, and is thought to be mediated by the prefrontal cortex (Windmann & Kutas, 2001). In some LTM studies, age differences in emotional modulation of response bias were absent (Charles et al., 2003; Comblain, D'Argembeau, Van der Linden, & Aldenhoff, 2004; Spaniol et al., 2008), whereas in other studies age differences in emotional modulation of false alarm rate or response bias were observed that are consistent with the positivity effect (Fernandes, Ross, Wiegand, & Schryer, 2008; Kapucu, Rotello, Ready, & Seidl, 2008; Thapar & Rouder, 2009).

Based on previous studies regarding STM for the identity of emotional faces (Jackson et al., 2008; Jackson et al., 2009), we expected to find increased discrimination for angry faces in younger adults. With respect to the response bias, previous LTM studies (Ochsner, 2000; Windmann & Kutas, 2001) led to the hypothesis that the response bias would be more liberal for emotional than neutral faces. With respect to age differences in emotional STM, the hypotheses that positivity effects would occur in discrimination and/or response bias were put to the test. Such positivity effects would imply that older adults would have relatively better memory and/or a more liberal response bias for happy than angry faces compared to younger adults. However, because of previous conflicting results of LTM studies we were not sure whether to expect age differences in emotional modulation of discrimination and response bias in STM.

METHOD

Participants

Participants were 20 younger (mean age 20.7 years; age range 18-29 years; 10 men) and 20 older (mean age 68.9 years; age range 61-77 years; 10 men) adults who volunteered to take part. Participants were not depressed[1], reported to be in good neurological and psychiatric health and did not use centrally-active drugs. The older adults were not demented, as they had a Mini Mental State Exam (MMSE) score of at least 27 (Derix et al., 2003; Folstein, Folstein, & McHugh, 1975). Participants' education was scored on a scale ranging from 1 (primary education) to 8 (master degree) (De Bie, 1987). The younger participants ($M = 7.0$, $SD = 0.2$) tended to have completed more formal education than the older participants ($M = 6.2$, $SD = 1.7$), $F(1,38) = 3.8$, $p = .058$. Visual acuity, if necessary corrected with glasses or contact lenses, was assessed using a Landolt-C card. Although the younger participants ($M = 2.0$, $SD = 0.5$) had higher visual acuity than the older participants ($M = 1.3$, $SD = 0.4$), $F(1,38) = 27.5$, $p < .001$, all participants had a visual acuity of at least 0.8 and asserted

---

[1] Younger participants were considered non-depressed if they scored less than 13 on the Beck Depression Inventory (BDI) (Beck, Ward, Mendelson, Mock, & Erbaugh, 1961; Lasa, Ayusi-Mateos, Vázquez-Barquero, Díez-Manrique, & Dowrick, 2000) and older adults if they scored less than 11 on the Geriatric Depression Scale (GDS) (Yesavage et al., 1983).

sufficient capability to view the faces. Participants were rewarded with course credit or money (at a rate of €7.50 per hour). The study was approved by the local ethics committee and the participants gave written informed consent prior to testing.

Stimuli and Memory Task

The stimuli for the STM task were 18 gray-scaled faces from the Ekman and Friesen (1976) series: six men each displaying angry, happy and neutral facial expressions (cf. Jackson et al., 2008; Jackson et al., 2009; Langeslag, Morgan, Jackson, Linden, & Van Strien, 2009). The faces subtended a visual angle of 2.7° vertically and 2.4° horizontally and were presented against a white background. A trial consisted of the following displays, see Figure 1. First, a black fixation cross that increased and decreased in size indicated the start of a trial. During the encoding phase, an array of four stimuli was presented for two seconds. These stimuli were one to four faces, resulting in a memory load of one to four, with scrambled faces occupying the locations not filled by faces. The stimuli were arranged in a two by two grid around a black fixation cross (0.4°) in the centre of the screen with the centre of each stimulus 1.8° away from the fixation cross. During the retention phase, a fixation cross was presented for one second. During the retrieval phase, a probe face occurred in the centre of the screen. The participants had to decide whether or not the probe face matched one of the faces in the preceding encoding array (50% match trials). The response terminated the retrieval phase, and initiated the next trial.

It is important to note that this STM task (Jackson et al., 2008; Jackson et al., 2009) was an identity matching task, and not an emotion matching task. Because faces of only six individuals (each displaying all three expressions) were used, each face was repeated multiple times during the experiment. This actually ensured that the task tapped into STM and not into LTM, because participants had to decide whether a probe face, even though it may have been present in LTM storage because of its appearance on previous trials, matched any of the encoding faces in the current trial only. Furthermore, all of the faces within one trial displayed the same facial expression. This made facial expression uninformative for the task and prevented the occurrence of attentional biases towards or away from faces with certain expressions during encoding. This design allowed the investigation of age differences in the influence of expression on STM without the potentially confounding influence of age differences in attentional biases (Isaacowitz, Wadlinger, Goren, & Wilson, 2006a; Isaacowitz, Wadlinger, Goren, & Wilson, 2006b; Mather & Carstensen, 2003) during encoding.

Procedure

Upon arrival in the lab, the participants completed the above mentioned screening procedures. Following, the participants were introduced to the memory task and were told that the scrambled faces and the facial expressions could be ignored because those would not be useful for the task at hand. Participants were instructed to respond to the probe face by pressing the 'A' (match) or the 'L' (mismatch) keys on a keyboard, with their left and right index fingers respectively, as accurately as possible. Participants were asked to try to maintain fixation at the fixation crosses at all times.

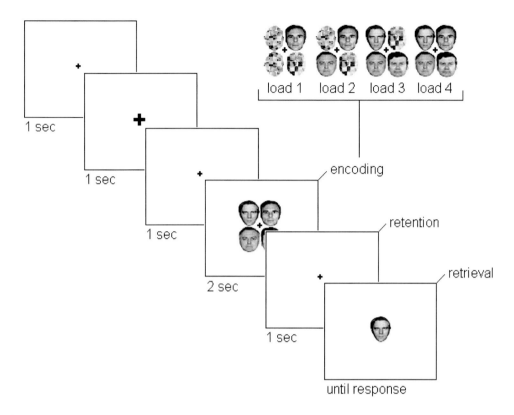

Figure 1. Trial overview.

After some practice trials, the participants completed a total of 192 experimental trials: 3 facial expressions x 4 loads x 2 match/mismatch x 8 trials per condition. The order of the trials was random with respect to memory load, facial expression, face identity, location occupied, and match/mismatch. The task was divided into four blocks interleaved with short breaks. After the final block, the participants rated the valence and arousal they experienced when viewing each face with a computerized version of the Self-Assessment Manikin (SAM) (Lang, 1980).

Analyses

The hit rates (H, i.e. proportion correct 'match' responses) and false alarms rates (FA, i.e. proportion incorrect 'match' responses) were computed using the correction recommended by Snodgrass and Corwin (1988). Memory performance was represented by the discrimination index $Pr = H - FA$, where $Pr = 1$ reflects perfect performance and $Pr = 0$ reflects chance performance, and by the response bias index $Br = FA / (1 - Pr)$. The response bias index describes the tendency of participants to respond 'match' irrespective of the true match or mismatch status of the probe stimulus, where $Br > 0.5$ indicates a liberal response bias and $Br < 0.5$ indicates a conservative response bias (Snodgrass & Corwin, 1988)[2].

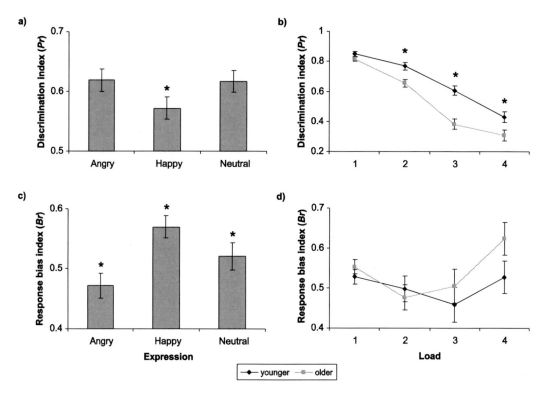

Figure 2. a) The discrimination index was lowest for happy faces, * both $ps < .014$ b) Older adults had a lower discrimination index than younger adults in loads 2 to 4, * all $ps < .020$ c) The response bias was most liberal for happy faces, intermediately liberal for neutral faces and least liberal for angry faces, * all $ps < .023$ d) No age differences occurred with respect to the response bias index.

The data were analyzed with repeated measures analysis of variance (rmANOVA). Valence and arousal ratings were analyzed with the factors Expression (angry, happy, neutral), and Age group (younger, older). Memory performance measures Pr and Br were analyzed with factors Expression, Load (1, 2, 3, 4), and Age group. When applicable, degrees of freedom were corrected with the Greenhouse-Geisser correction. The F values, the uncorrected dfs, the epsilon (ε) values and corrected probability levels are reported. A two-sided significance level of 5% was selected. Significant effects were followed-up by independent samples t-tests when testing age group effects and by paired samples t-tests when testing expression or load effects. In the case of load effects, consecutive loads were compared.

---

[2] When analyzing d' and C, as discrimination and bias indices respectively, the same pattern of results was obtained.

RESULTS

Valence and Arousal Ratings

Valence. There were a significant effect of Expression, $F(2,76) = 189.1$, $\varepsilon = .74$, $p < .001$, and a significant Expression x Age group interaction, $F(2,76) = 4.3$, $\varepsilon = .74$, $p = .028$. Both the younger and older participants associated angry faces with lowest valence (younger: $M = 3.1$, $SD = 0.8$, older: $M = 3.5$, $SD = 1.3$), neutral faces with intermediate valence (younger: $M = 4.7$, $SD = 0.5$, older: $M = 4.7$, $SD = 0.9$), and happy faces with highest valence (younger: $M = 7.4$, $SD = 0.8$, older: $M = 6.7$, $SD = 1.0$), all $ps < .001$. Yet, the older participants rated happy faces as less pleasant than the younger participants did, $p = .015$. There was no significant main effect of Age group, $F < 1$, ns.

Arousal. A significant effect of Expression, $F(2,76) = 19.3$, $\varepsilon = .98$, $p < .001$, and a significant Expression x Age group interaction, $F(2,76) = 7.9$, $\varepsilon = .98$, $p = .001$, were observed. The younger participants rated angry ($M = 5.4$, $SD = 1.3$) and happy faces ($M = 5.8$, $SD = 1.4$) as more arousing than the neutral faces ($M = 3.8$, $SD = 1.3$), both $ps < .001$. The arousal ratings for angry and happy faces were not significantly different, $p = .29$. The older participants rated happy faces as most arousing ($M = 5.3$, $SD = 0.8$), both $ps < .003$, and angry ($M = 4.1$, $SD = 1.1$) and neutral faces ($M = 4.4$, $SD = 1.2$) as equally arousing, $p = .50$. This age difference occurred because the older participants rated angry faces as less arousing than the younger participants did, $p = .002$. The main effect of Age group was not significant, $F(1,38) = 2.4$, $p = .13$.

Memory Performance

Discrimination index. There was an effect of Expression, $F(2,76) = 4.1$, $\varepsilon = .99$, $p = .016$, showing that discrimination was inferior for happy faces, both $ps < .014$, whereas discrimination was similar for angry and neutral faces, $p = .88$, see Figure 2a. This effect of Expression was not modulated by Age group or Load, all $Fs < 1.1$, all $ps > .40$. The effect of Load, $F(3,114) = 200.2$, $\varepsilon = .92$, $p < .001$, showed that discrimination decreased with increasing load, all $ps < .001$. The effect of Age group, $F(1,38) = 16.6$, $p < .001$, showed that older participants had a lower discrimination index than younger participants. Moreover, the significant Load x Age group interaction, $F(3,114) = 6.9$, $\varepsilon = .92$, $p < .001$, indicated that significant age differences were present in loads 2 to 4, all $ps < .020$, but not in load 1, $p = .095$, see Figure 2b.

To control for the potentially confounding effect of the observed age differences in valence and arousal ratings, separate ANCOVAs for each expression were conducted with the covariates Valence rating and Arousal rating, and the factor Age group. Valence rating and Arousal rating had no significant effect on the discrimination index for each expression, all $Fs < 2.1$, all $ps > .15$. Moreover, the main effects of Age group, signifying decreased performance in the older compared to the younger adults, remained significant after controlling for age differences in valence and arousal ratings for all expressions, all $Fs > 5.6$, all $ps < .03$.

Response bias index. There was a main effect of Expression, $F(2,76) = 12.8$, $\varepsilon = .96$, $p < .001$. The response bias was different for each of the three expressions; it was most conservative for angry faces, slightly liberal for neutral faces, and most liberal for happy faces, all $ps < .023$, see Figure 2c. This effect of Expression was not modulated by Age group or Load, all $Fs < 1.1$, all $ps > .33$. Further, there was a significant effect of Load, $F(3,114) = 5.3$, $\varepsilon = .81$, $p = .004$. The response bias decreased from load 1 to 2, $p = .033$, was similar between loads 2 and 3, $p = .83$, and increased again between load 3 and 4, $p < .001$, see Figure 2d. Neither the main effect of Age group, nor the Load x Age group interaction was significant, both $Fs < 1.6$, both $ps > .21$.

To control for the potentially confounding effect of the observed age differences in valence and arousal ratings, additional ANCOVAs were conducted for each expression separately. For all expressions, the covariates Valence rating and Arousal rating, and the factor Age group together did not have a significant effect on the response bias index, all $Fs < 1.1$, all $ps > .37$.

Sex Differences

To examine the influence of sex of the participant, ANOVAs with the additional factor Sex (male, female) were performed. For the valence ratings, the arousal ratings, and the discrimination index, none of the effects including Sex were significant, all $Fs < 2.0$, all $ps > .15$. For the response bias index, the Expression x Sex interaction was significant, $F(2,72) = 4.4$, $\varepsilon = .90$, $p = .019$. Independent samples t-tests showed that female participants had a more liberal response than male participants for neutral faces, $p = .003$, but that no sex differences occurred for angry and happy faces, both $ps > .27$. None of the other effects including the factor Sex reached significance, all $Fs < 4.1$, all $ps > .05$.

DISCUSSION

The goal of the current study was to investigate the occurrence of age differences in emotional modulation of STM performance. The expression of the to-be-remembered faces influenced memory for face identity in two ways. First, discrimination between faces that were or were not presented previously was increased for angry and neutral compared to happy faces. Second, the response bias was most conservative for angry faces and most liberal for happy faces. Most important for the current research question, no interactions between facial expression and age group were observed on the discrimination and response bias indices. We found no positivity effect or any other age differences in the emotional modulation of STM, even when we controlled for the observed age differences in valence and arousal ratings. The absence of age differences in emotional modulation of STM can be explained in various ways, namely as a consequence of task characteristics, lack of statistical power, or insufficient cognitive control in the older participants, each of which will be discussed in turn below.

The socio-emotional selectivity theory states that the older adults' limited remaining life time urges them to focus on emotion-related goals, while younger adults would focus more on knowledge-related goals (Carstensen, Isaacowitz, & Charles, 1999). But, the more externally constraint a task is, the less influence these emotion goals may have on task performance (Mather, 2006). Indeed, age differences in emotional memory are typically less pronounced in LTM recognition and cued recall tests than in free recall tests (e.g. Langeslag & Van Strien, 2008; Langeslag & Van Strien, 2009). The current STM task resembles LTM recognition tests in the sense that retrieval is guided by the presentation of a probe that requires a forced-choice decision. In addition, assuming that emotion-related goals influence only late stages of processing (Mather & Carstensen, 2005), the influence of these emotion-related goals may have been further reduced by the short time interval between encoding and retrieval phases of the STM task. The valence and arousal ratings tasks, in contrast, were less externally constraint as participants could complete them at their own pace. Indeed, emotion-related goals appeared to have an impact on these rating tasks as age differences in valence and arousal ratings were observed.

The absence of an age effect on the emotional modulation of STM could further have been due to a relative lack of power with 20 participants per age group, even though we did observe effects of age on discrimination in general. With 20 participants per group, power is 80% to detect large effects at a significance level of 10% (Cohen, 1992). Nevertheless, age differences in emotional modulation were absent, even when increasing power by adopting a more lenient significance level (Stevens, 2002) of 20%, or even 30%. Age-independent effects of facial expression, in contrast, were observed with the stringent significance level of 5%. Any modulating effects of age would probably be much smaller than the general effect of facial expression on STM.

It has been suggested that age differences in emotional processing occur only when older adults have sufficient cognitive control (Mather & Carstensen, 2005; Mather, 2006). The current absence of age differences could therefore also have been the result of testing a sample of older adults with inadequate cognitive control or limited resource availability. Although our older adults had completed less formal education than the younger adults, which is a nearly inevitable consequence of generational differences in educational possibilities, they were relatively well-educated and had intact cognitive functioning as assessed by the MMSE. It can therefore be assumed that our older participants' cognitive control was (above) average, thereby satisfying the prerequisite for the occurrence of age differences in emotional processing. Furthermore, although the condition with a memory load of one face was undemanding (as evident from the high and equivalent memory performance of younger and older adults), age differences in the effect of facial expression did not even occur in the low memory load condition. Also the findings of age differences in the valence and arousal ratings of the faces suggests that the absence of age differences in emotional modulation of STM was not due to participant characteristics such as a deficiency in cognitive control. They also dispute the notion that our older participants might not have been old enough for age differences to be detected. Indeed, a positivity effect in LTM has previously been observed with both older and middle-aged adults (Charles et al., 2003). In conclusion, we think that task characteristics rather than a lack of power or participant characteristics are responsible for the absence of age differences in emotional modulation of STM.

In this study, both younger and older adults showed better memory for angry and neutral over happy faces. In previous studies, younger adults remembered angry faces better than happy and neutral faces (Jackson et al., 2008; Jackson et al., 2009) or remembered angry and happy faces better than neutral faces (Langeslag et al., 2009). It is unclear why the present finding of increased discrimination of neutral over happy faces occurred. It could have been due to methodological differences between this and previous studies. In one of the previous studies, participants were required to rehearse a pair of letters subvocally to prevent recruitment of verbal STM processes (Jackson et al., 2009), and in another study participants were instructed to make speeded responses (Langeslag et al., 2009). In a combined genetics and fMRI study, genetic variations have been shown to influence STM for happy faces in particular (Wolf, Jackson, Kissling, Thome, & Linden, 2009). Other individual differences such as affective disposition and personality (see e.g. Feldman Barrett, Tugade, & Engle, 2004; Hamann & Canli, 2004) may have contributed to the discrepancy between this and previous studies as well.

The response bias was most conservative for angry faces and most liberal for happy faces. Compared to neutral faces there was a decreased tendency to indicate that an angry probe face matched the content of memory storage, whereas there was an increased tendency to indicate that a happy probe face matched the content of memory storage. The more liberal response bias for happy compared to neutral faces was in line with our hypothesis, and this liberal way of responding to happy faces appears to have substantially reduced discrimination of these faces. The conservative bias for angry faces was an unexpected finding because previous LTM studies have demonstrated more liberal response biases for both negative and positive stimuli (Grider & Malmberg, 2008; Ochsner, 2000; Windmann & Kutas, 2001). However, in one previous experiment the response bias tended to be more conservative for negative compared to neutral stimuli too (Ochsner, 2000). Notably, in both that previous and the current study, participants were instructed to focus on a non-emotional aspect of the stimulus, namely picture brightness and face identity respectively. More research is needed to examine how response bias for negative and positive information is perhaps differentially affected by the instruction to focus on emotional or non-emotional aspects of a stimulus.

Our investigation of age differences in emotional STM used only three different facial expressions. Although there appears to be a general age-related decline in the ability to label facial expressions, this decline does not appear to be similar for all expressions (Ruffman, Henry, Livingstone, & Phillips, 2008). It would therefore be interesting to examine age differences in emotional STM for faces using faces with other expressions, such as fear, disgust, sadness or surprise, as age differences may be observed in STM for these expressions. In addition, the stimuli used in this study were all male faces, whereas the participants were both men and women. In the analysis of sex differences, it was observed that women had a more liberal response for neutral faces than men. Although this could have been caused by some opposite sex effect, it is unclear why this more liberal response bias would have occurred only for the neutral and not for the emotional faces. Because no effects of participant sex were observed on the discrimination index, the valence ratings and the arousal ratings, we believe that the absence of age differences in emotional modulation of STM is not attributable to the use of male facial stimuli. Still, it might be better to use pictures of both male and female faces in future studies.

To summarize, we report here the first study in which age differences in emotional modulation of STM were investigated in a way that matched previous LTM studies. That is, age differences in the effect of stimulus emotionality on memory for stimulus content were examined. No age differences were observed in the effect of facial expression on STM for face identity. We argue that the current absence of age differences in the emotional modulation of STM is not due to insufficient statistical power or inadequate cognitive control in the older adults. Instead, it might be due to the restricted nature of the STM task. With the mean population age rising, research on the lifespan development of emotional processing, which includes emotional STM, becomes more and more important. Future research could further explore whether, and under what circumstances, age differences in emotional STM occur.

REFERENCES

[1] Beck, A. T., Ward, C. H., Mendelson, M., Mock, J. & Erbaugh, J. (1961). An inventory for measuring depression. *Archives of General Psychiatry, 4*, 561-571.

[2] Carstensen, L. L., Isaacowitz, D. M. & Charles, S. T. (1999). Taking time seriously: A theory of socioemotional selectivity. *American Psychologist, 54*, 165-181.

[3] Charles, S. T., Mather, M. & Carstensen, L. L. (2003). Aging and emotional memory: The forgettable nature of negative images for older adults. *Journal of Experimental Psychology: General, 132*, 310-324.

[4] Cohen, J. (1992). A power primer. *Psychological Bulletin, 112*, 155-159.

[5] Comblain, C., D'Argembeau, A., Van der Linden, M. & Aldenhoff, L. (2004). The effect of ageing on the recollection of emotional and neutral pictures. *Memory, 12*, 673-684.

[6] D'Argembeau, A. & Van der Linden, M. (2004). Identity but not expression memory for unfamiliar faces is affected by aging. *Memory, 12*, 644-654.

[7] De Bie, S. E. (1987). *Standaardvragen 1987-voorstellen voor uniformering van vraagstellingen naar achtergrondkenmerken en interviews [standard questions 1987-proposals for unification of inquiries after background characteristics and interviews]* (2nd ed.). Leiden: Leiden University Press.

[8] Derix, M. M. A., Korten, E., Teunisse, S., Jelicic, M., Lindeboom, J., Walstra, G. J. M. & Van Gool, W. A. (2003). *Nederlandse versie van de cambridge examination for mental disorders of the elderly-revised*. Lisse: Swets & Zeitlinger BV.

[9] Ekman, P. & Friesen, W. (1976). *Pictures of facial affect*. Palo Alto, CA: Consulting Psychological Press.

[10] Feldman Barrett, L., Tugade, M. M. & Engle, R. W. (2004). Individual differences in working memory capacity and dual-process theories of the mind. *Psychological Bulletin, 130*, 553-573.

[11] Fernandes, M., Ross, M., Wiegand, M. & Schryer, E. (2008). Are memories of older adults positively biased? *Psychology and Aging, 23*, 297-306.

[12] Folstein, M. F., Folstein, S. E. & McHugh, P. R. (1975). "Mini-mental state". A practical method for grading the cognitive state of patients for the clinician. *Journal of Psychiatric Research, 12*, 189-198.

[13] Grady, C. L., Hongwanishkul, D., Keightley, M., Lee, W. & Hasher, L. (2007). The effect of age on memory for emotional faces. *Neuropsychology, 21*, 371-380.

[14] Grider, R. C. & Malmberg, K. J. (2008). Discriminating between changes in bias and changes in accuracy for recognition of emotional stimuli. *Memory & Cognition, 36*, 933-946.

[15] Hamann, S. & Canli, T. (2004). Individual differences in emotion processing. *Current Opinion in Neurobiology, 14*, 233-238.

[16] Isaacowitz, D. M., Wadlinger, H. A., Goren, D. & Wilson, H. R. (2006a). Is there an age-related positivity effect in visual attention? A comparison of two methodologies. *Emotion, 6*, 511-516.

[17] Isaacowitz, D. M., Wadlinger, H. A., Goren, D. & Wilson, H. R. (2006b). Selective preference in visual fixation away from negative images in old age? an eye-tracking study. *Psychology and Aging, 21*, 40-48.

[18] Jackson, M. C., Wolf, C., Johnston, S. J., Raymond, J. E. & Linden, D. E. J. (2008). Neural correlates of enhanced visual short-term memory for angry faces: An fMRI study. *PLoS ONE, 3*, e3536.

[19] Jackson, M. C., Wu, C. -., Linden, D. E. J. & Raymond, J. E. (2009). Enhanced visual short-term memory for angry faces. *Journal of Experimental Psychology: Human Perception and Performance, 35*, 363-374.

[20] Kapucu, A., Rotello, C. M., Ready, R. E. & Seidl, K. N. (2008). Response bias in "remembering" emotional stimuli: A new perspective on age differences. *Journal of Experimental Psychology: Learning, Memory, and Cognition, 34*, 703-711.

[21] Kensinger, E. A. (2004). Remembering emotional experiences: The contribution of valence and arousal. *Reviews in the Neurosciences, 15*, 241-251.

[22] Langeslag, S. J. E., Morgan, H. M., Jackson, M. C., Linden, D. E. J. & Van Strien, J. W. (2009). Electrophysiological correlates of improved short-term memory for emotional faces. *Neuropsychologia, 47*, 887-896.

[23] Langeslag, S. J. E. & Van Strien, J. W. (2008). Age differences in the emotional modulation of ERP old/new effects. *International Journal of Psychophysiology, 70*, 105-114.

[24] Langeslag, S. J. E. & Van Strien, J. W. (2009). Aging and emotional memory: The co-occurrence of neurophysiological and behavioral positivity effects. *Emotion, 9*, 369-377.

[25] Lasa, L., Ayusi-Mateos, J. L., Vázquez-Barquero, J. L., Díez-Manrique, F. J. & Dowrick, C. F. (2000). The use of the beck depression inventory to screen for depression in the general population: A preliminary analysis. *Journal of Affective Disorders, 57*, 261-265.

[26] Leigland, L. A., Schulz, L. E. & Janowsky, J. S. (2004). Age related changes in emotional memory. *Neurobiology of Aging, 25*, 1117-1124.

[27] Light, L. L., Prull, M. W., La Voie, D. J. & Healy, M. R. (2000). Dual-process theories of memory in old age. In T. J. Perfect, & E. A. Maylor (Eds.), *Models of cognitive aging* (pp. 238-300) Oxford University Press.

[28] Mather, M. (2006). Why memories may become more positive as people age. In B. Uttl, N. Ohta & A. L. Siegenthaler (Eds.), *Memory and emotion: Interdisciplinary perspectives* (pp. 135-158) Blackwell Publishing.

[29] Mather, M. & Carstensen, L. L. (2003). Aging and attentional biases for emotional faces. *Psychological Science, 14*, 409-415.

[30] Mather, M. & Carstensen, L. L. (2005). Aging and motivated cognition: The positivity effect in attention and memory. *Trends in Cognitive Sciences, 9*, 496-502.

[31] Mikels, J. A., Larkin, G. R., Reuter-Lorenz, P. A. & Carstensen, L. L. (2005). Divergent trajectories in the aging mind: Changes in working memory for affective versus visual information with age. *Psychology and Aging, 20*, 542-553.

[32] Ochsner, K. N. (2000). Are affective events richly recollected or simply familiar? the experience and process of recognizing feelings past. *Journal of Experimental Psychology: General, 129*, 242-261.

[33] Park, D. C. & Reuter-Lorenz, P. (2009). The adaptive brain: Aging and neurocognitive scaffolding. *Annual Review of Psychology, 60*(1), 173-196.

[34] Ruffman, T., Henry, J. D., Livingstone, V. & Phillips, L. H. (2008). A meta-analytic review of emotion recognition and aging: Implications for neuropsychological models of aging. *Neuroscience and Biobehavioral Reviews, 32*, 863-881.

[35] Snodgrass, J. G. & Corwin, J. (1988). Pragmatics of measuring recognition memory: Applications to dementia and amnesia. *Journal of Experimental Psychology: General, 117*, 34-50.

[36] Spaniol, J., Voss, A. & Grady, C. L. (2008). Aging and emotional memory: Cognitive mechanisms underlying the positivity effect. *Psychology and Aging, 23*, 859-872.

[37] Stevens, J. P. (2002). *Applied multivariate statistics for the social sciences* (4th ed.). Philadelphia: Lawrence Erlbaum Associates.

[38] Thapar, A. & Rouder, J. N. (2009). Aging and recognition memory for emotional words: A bias account. *Psychonomic Bulletin & Review, 16*, 699-704.

[39] Uttl, B. & Graf, P. (2006). Age-related changes in the encoding and retrieval of emotional and non-emotional information. In B. Uttl, N. Ohta & A. L. Siegenthaler (Eds.), *Memory and emotion: Interdisciplinary perspectives* (pp. 159-187) Blackwell Publishing.

[40] Windmann, S. & Kutas, M. (2001). Electrophysiological correlates of emotion-induced recognition bias. *Journal of Cognitive Neuroscience, 13*, 577-592.

[41] Wolf, C., Jackson, M. C., Kissling, C., Thome, J. & Linden, D. E. J. (2009). Dysbindin-1 genotype effects on emotional working memory. *Molecular Psychiatry,*

[42] Yesavage, J. A., Brink, T. L., Rose, T. L., Lum, O., Huang, V., Adey, M. & Leirer, V. O. (1983). Development and validation of a geriatric depression screening scale: A preliminary report. *Journal of Psychiatric Research, 17*, 37-49.

Chapter 12

VARYING BACKGROUND COLOURS REVEALS THAT ENHANCED SHORT-TERM MEMORY FOR ANGRY FACES IS A VALENCE AND NOT AN AROUSAL EFFECT

Sandra J. E. Langeslag[1]*, Margaret C. Jackson[2], Jan W. van Strien[1] and David E. J. Linden[2]

[1]Erasmus Affective Neuroscience Lab, Institute of Psychology, Erasmus University Rotterdam, The Netherlands
[2]Wolfson Centre for Clinical and Cognitive Neurosciences, School of Psychology, Bangor University, UK

ABSTRACT

There is debate on whether the effect of stimulus emotionality on memory is a valence or an arousal effect. In a previous study, short-term memory (STM) was enhanced for angry compared to happy and neutral faces, and music-induced contextual arousal did not modulate this effect. The absence of such a contextual arousal effect could, however, have been due to the cross-modal nature of the study, as the contextual arousal was induced auditorily while the to-be-remembered stimuli were presented visually. In this study, we investigated the influence of visually-induced contextual arousal on the same STM task to determine whether the angry face benefit in STM is a valence or an arousal effect. Contextual arousal was successfully manipulated by presenting the background colours red, pink, and light pink. STM discrimination was enhanced for angry faces, and was not modulated by contextual arousal. High contextual arousal elicited by the red or pink backgrounds was accompanied by a more liberal response bias, regardless of facial expression. Because of this dissociation and because the effects of facial expression and background colour did not interact, it is concluded that the angry face benefit in STM is a valence and not an arousal effect. It is suggested

---

* Corresponding author S. Langeslag is now at: Erasmus MC – Sophia Children's Hospital, Department of Child & Adolescent Psychiatry, P.O. Box 2060, NL-3000 CB Rotterdam, The Netherlands, E-mail address: s.langeslag@erasmusmc.nl, Tel: +31 (0)10 703 7071, Fax: +31 (0)10 703 2111

that these stimulus valence and contextual arousal effects have different underlying mechanisms.

Keywords: short-term memory; working memory; emotion; faces; facial expressions; colours; valence; arousal

INTRODUCTION

Emotions can be classified along the two independent dimensions of valence and arousal. The valence of an emotion describes whether the emotion is unpleasant or pleasant, whereas arousal reflects the intensity of an emotion (Bradley & Lang, 1994). Emotional pictures, words, and faces are typically better remembered than equivalent neutral stimuli in long-term memory (Kensinger, 2004). In the last couple of years, also the effect of stimulus emotionality on short-term memory (STM) has become a topic of research (e.g. Perlstein, Elbert, & Stenger, 2002).

There is some debate on whether the effect of stimulus emotionality on memory is a valence or an arousal effect. Because emotional information (whether negative or positive) is typically more arousing than neutral information, the often observed memory benefit for emotional compared to neutral information suggests that the emotion enhancement effect is an arousal effect. It has, however, been observed that also low-arousing negative and positive stimuli are remembered better than equally low-arousing neutral information (Kensinger & Corkin, 2003; Ochsner, 2000), in which case the emotion enhancement effect appears to be a valence effect. Moreover, an emotion enhancement effect sometimes also occurred for negative but not for positive over neutral stimuli, even when the negative and positive stimuli were matched in arousal (e.g. Ochsner, 2000), again implying a valence effect, albeit of negative valence only. It has therefore been suggested that both valence and arousal of emotional stimuli are capable of influencing memory for those stimuli (see Kensinger, 2004, for a review).

In a couple of previous studies, STM has been found to be superior for angry compared to happy and neutral faces (Jackson, Wolf, Johnston, Raymond, & Linden, 2008; Jackson, Wu, Linden, & Raymond, 2009). In order to examine whether the effect of facial expression on STM was a valence or an arousal effect, the emotionality of the context was varied by playing calming or arousing background music, which did not modulate the memory benefit for angry faces (Jackson et al., 2009). The absence of such a contextual arousal effect could, however, have been due to the cross-modal nature of the study, as the contextual arousal was induced auditorily while the to-be-remembered stimuli were presented visually. Additionally, in the Jackson et al. (2009) study the general effect of playing background music was not directly investigated as there was no within-subject control condition without background music. Erk, Kleczar and Walter (2007) have shown the importance of including a no context condition as a control condition. In a STM test for letters they presented a neutral picture, an emotional picture or no picture during the retention interval. STM performance was equivalent in the emotional and no pictures conditions, and was inferior to those conditions in the neutral pictures condition. The presence of a neutral context may have decreased performance by increasing cognitive load or by distracting attention, for example. As the presence of emotional context did not impair performance compared to the no context condition, the emotionality of context appeared to counteract the impairing effect of the presence of context per se, for example by increasing general arousal levels.

The goal of the current study was to examine the effect of contextual arousal on STM for emotional faces in a way that takes into account the above-mentioned issues. First, we wanted to elicit the contextual arousal in the same modality as the emotionality of the faces, i.e. in the visual modality. Interestingly, background colours have been found to influence emotional processing, as questionnaires regarding murder or rape scenarios that were printed on pink paper elicited less angry reactions than did questionnaires printed on blue or white paper (Weller & Livingston, 1988). Variations in colour have further been associated with differences in (electro)physiological responses such as blood pressure, heart rate and brain waves (Cajochen, 2007; Yoto, Katsuura, Iwanaga, & Shimomura, 2007), suggesting that colour may influence arousal levels. Indeed, it has been shown that colour brightness is negatively related to arousal ratings, and that colour saturation is positively related to arousal ratings (Valdez & Mehrabian, 1994), and we therefore decided to use background colours to manipulate contextual arousal. The colours that we used were, in order of increasing brightness, decreasing saturation, and thus decreasing arousal: red, pink and light pink. Each of these background colours was presented throughout one entire block of the STM memory task. Because we wanted the background colours to confiscate processing resources as little as possible, the colours did not have a task attached. Second, we included a within-subjects control condition in which no other background colour was presented than the white background that was used in previous studies (Jackson et al., 2008; Jackson et al., 2009; Langeslag, Morgan, Jackson, Linden, & Van Strien, 2009).

Further, besides a measure of discrimination we also obtained a measure of response bias. The above mentioned findings concern the ability to distinguish faces that were or were not previously encountered, which is called discrimination. But to fully consider recognition memory, a measure of response bias needs to be considered as well (Snodgrass & Corwin, 1988). The response bias reflects the tendency to classify a certain stimulus as previously encountered, irrespective of its actual old or new status. Generally, people adopt a more liberal response bias for emotional than neutral stimuli (Ochsner, 2000; Windmann & Kutas, 2001), yielding higher hit and false alarm rates for emotional than neutral stimuli. This more liberal response bias for emotional stimuli would ensure that information that is relevant for survival and/or reproduction is not forgotten or missed (Windmann & Kutas, 2001).

We expected to replicate the increased STM performance for angry faces (Jackson et al., 2008; Jackson et al., 2009). Assuming that the background colours would not use processing resources needed for the STM task, we also expected that contextual arousal would not decrease performance. Crucially, any interaction between the effects of facial expression and contextual arousal would imply that the angry face benefit on STM has to do with arousal. The absence of such interaction, in contrast, would imply that the angry face benefit on STM is a valence effect.

METHOD

Participants

Twenty-four students (3 men, mean age 19.3 years, range 18-24) of the University of Wales Bangor, School of Psychology with normal (colour) vision volunteered to participate in return for course credit. The study was approved by the School's ethics committee in Bangor and all participants provided written informed consent before participation.

Stimuli

The stimuli for the STM task were 18 gray-scaled male faces (approximate visual angle of 2.9° vertically and 2.5° horizontally) from the Ekman and Friesen (1976) series: six individuals each displaying angry, happy and neutral facial expressions. The stimuli were presented within a white rectangle (approximate visual angle of 7.7° vertically and 6.9° horizontally) surrounded by a red, pink, light pink or white background, see Figure 1. The RGB values of these colours were: 255, 0, 0 (red), 255, 121, 121 (pink), 255, 207, 207 (light pink) and 255, 255, 255 (white). Note that because in the previous studies (Jackson et al., 2008; Jackson et al., 2009; Langeslag et al., 2009) the faces were always presented on a white background, the white background condition served as a control condition (see also Mehta & Zhu, 2009). Stimuli were displayed on a 15-inch Toshiba SA60-352 notebook (16-bit colour; resolution 1068 x 768 pixels), generated by E-Prime version 1.1.

Procedure

Participants were seated in front of a computer in a room without any windows. After completion of informed consent, the participants were introduced to the STM task. A background colour was present throughout the entire trial, which consisted of the following displays, see Figure 1. First, a fixation cross that grew and shrunk indicated that the trial was about to start. During the encoding phase an array of faces was presented for 2,000 ms. This encoding array consisted of either two different to-be-remembered faces and two different scrambled faces or of four different to-be-remembered faces, resulting in a STM load of two or four respectively. The faces were arranged in a two by two grid around a black fixation cross (0.5°) in the centre of the screen. A 1,000 ms retention display followed, consisting of a black fixation cross. During the retrieval phase a probe face appeared in the centre of the screen. The participants had to decide whether or not the probe face matched one of the faces in the preceding encoding array (50% match trials). Participants were instructed to respond to the probe faces by pressing the left ('match') or the right ('mismatch') mouse buttons with their right index and middle fingers respectively. The response terminated the retrieval phase and participants hit the spacebar to initiate the next trial. Participants were asked to maintain fixation at the fixation crosses at all times. After the practice trials, the lights were turned off and the participants completed the five blocks of the STM task, interleaved with breaks.

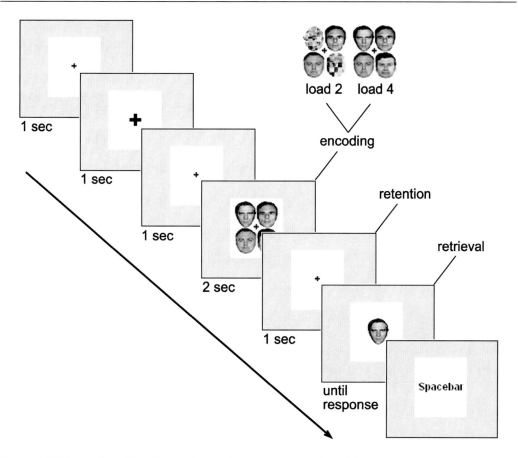

Figure 1 Trial overview. Note that the images here are not to scale and that the gray background was actually red, pink, light pink or white.

Trials with different facial expressions and STM loads were presented pseudo randomly within blocks. The induction of contextual arousal (i.e. background colour), in contrast, was blocked to ensure a lasting arousal state (Shackman et al., 2006) and to avoid between-trial carry-over effects. The order of the blocks with red, pink and light pink backgrounds (60 trials each) was counterbalanced across participants. Two blocks with a white background (30 trials each, 60 trials in total) interspersed the blocks with red, pink and light pink backgrounds to minimize between-block carry-over effects. It is important to note that the STM task was an identity, and not an emotion, matching task. Moreover, all of the faces within one trial displayed the same facial expression, making facial expression uninformative for the task.

After the final block of the STM task, the participants rated the valence and arousal of the faces and the red, pink and light pink colours with a computerized version of the Self-Assessment Manikin (SAM) (Lang, 1980).

Analyses

Hit rates (H, i.e. proportion correct 'match' responses) and false alarms rates (FA, i.e. proportion incorrect 'match' responses) were computed using the correction recommended by

Snodgrass and Corwin (1988). These hits and false alarm rates were used to compute the discrimination index $Pr = H - FA$, where $Pr = 1$ reflects perfect performance and $Pr = 0$ reflects chance performance, and the response bias index $Br = FA / (1 - Pr)$. The response bias index describes the tendency of participants to respond 'match' irrespective of the true match or mismatch status of the probe stimulus, where $Br > 0.5$ indicates a liberal response bias and $Br < 0.5$ indicates a conservative response bias (Snodgrass & Corwin, 1988).

Valence and arousal ratings of the faces and colours were analyzed with planned comparisons between angry, happy and neutral faces and between the red, pink and light pink colours. The discrimination and response bias indices Pr and Br^1 were tested using repeated measures ANOVAs with the factors Colour (red, pink, light pink, white), Expression (angry, happy, neutral) and Load (2, 4). When applicable, degrees of freedom were corrected with the Greenhouse-Geisser correction. The F values, the uncorrected dfs, the epsilon (ε) values and corrected probability levels are reported. A significance level of 5% (two-sided) was selected. Only effects involving the factors Colour and/or Expression are mentioned and significant effects were followed up by paired samples t-tests.

RESULTS

Valence and Arousal Ratings

See Table 1 for the valence and arousal ratings of the colours and faces.

Faces. Valence ratings were lowest for angry faces, intermediate for neutral faces and highest for happy faces, all $ts(23) > |6.1|$, all $ps < .001$. Arousal ratings were higher for angry and happy than for neutral faces, both $ts(23) > |4.2|$, both $ps < .001$, while arousal ratings for angry and happy faces did not differ, $t(23) = |0.3|, p = .75$.

Colours. Valence ratings were higher for pink than for red, $t(23) = |4.1|, p < .001$, with light pink non-significantly different in-between. Arousal ratings were highest for red, medium for pink and lowest for light pink, all $ts(23) > |3.6|$, all $ps < .002$. Thus, arousal was successfully manipulated using the colours red, pink, and light pink.

Table 1. Mean valence and arousal ratings (standard deviation in brackets) of the colours and faces

	Colours			Faces		
	Red	Pink	Light pink	Angry	Happy	Neutral
Valence	5.6 (2.2)	7.5 (1.2)	6.6 (1.9)	3.1 (0.9)	7.6 (1.0)	4.3 (0.6)
Arousal	7.3 (1.4)	5.9 (2.1)	3.8 (1.9)	5.1 (1.5)	5.0 (1.8)	3.4 (1.0)

Note. Valence and arousal ratings ranged from 1 (extremely unpleasant or calming) to 9 (extremely pleasant or arousing) (Lang, 1980).

---

[1] When analyzing d' and C, as discrimination and bias indices respectively, the same pattern of results was obtained.

Recognition Performance

See Table 2 for the discrimination and response bias indices in all conditions.

Discrimination index. A main effect of Expression was found, $F(2,46) = 4.6$, $\varepsilon = .75$, $p = .026$. Overall, discrimination was significantly better for angry than for happy faces, $p < .001$, nearly significantly better for angry than for neutral faces, $p = .074$, and not significantly different between happy and neutral faces, $p = .55$. This main effect was modulated by a significant Expression by Load interaction, $F(2,46) = 5.7$, $\varepsilon = .77$, $p = .011$. In load 4, discrimination was significantly better for the angry vs. happy and neutral faces, both $ps < .024$, see Figure 2a.

All main and interaction effects involving Colour were non-significant, all Fs < 1.3, all ps > .28. This absence of Colour effects shows that STM performance for emotional faces was not increased or decreased by the coloured backgrounds compared to the white background.

Response bias index. A significant main effect of Expression occurred, $F(2,46) = 7.8$, $\varepsilon = .96$, $p = .001$. Angry faces were associated with a more conservative bias than happy and neutral faces, both $ps < .022$. A significant Expression by Load interaction, $F(2,46) = 4.3$, $\varepsilon = .99$, $p = .019$, signified that only in load 4, the response bias was more conservative for the angry vs. happy and neutral faces, both $ps = .001$, see Figure 2b. This implies that under high memory load conditions, the participants were less inclined to respond 'match' to an angry probe face than to probe faces with happy or neutral expressions.

Table 2. Mean discrimination (*Pr*) and response bias (*Br*) indices in all conditions

		Pr Load 2	Pr Load 4	Br Load 2	Br Load 4
Angry	Red	.69	.51	.47	.46
	Pink	.72	.44	.48	.47
	Light pink	.71	.41	.41	.40
	White	.69	.46	.39	.40
Happy	Red	.71	.42	.47	.55
	Pink	.67	.28	.48	.60
	Light pink	.68	.35	.47	.56
	White	.70	.33	.46	.50
Neutral	Red	.70	.35	.48	.56
	Pink	.69	.41	.39	.58
	Light pink	.69	.31	.40	.51
	White	.76	.32	.44	.51

Note. A greater discrimination index indicates better recognition accuracy. A response bias larger than 0.5 indicates a liberal response bias, whereas a response bias smaller than 0.5 indicates a conservative response bias (Snodgras & Corwin, 1988).

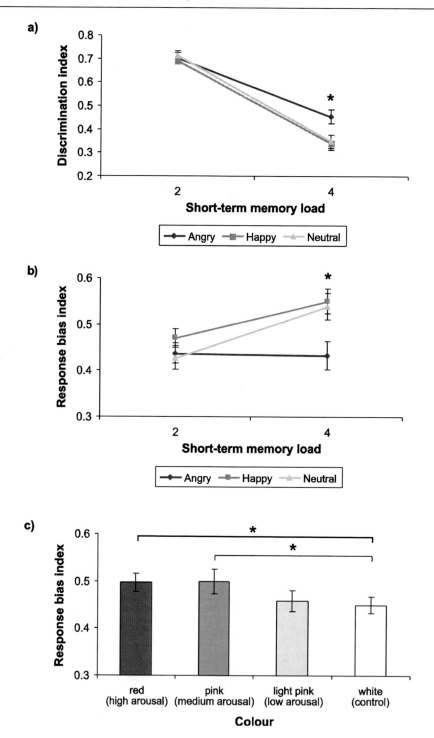

Figure 2. a) Discrimination index per facial expression and memory load. In load 4, discrimination was significantly better for angry faces, than for happy or neutral faces, * $ps < .024$ b) Response bias index per facial expression and memory load. In load 4, the response bias was more conservative for angry than for happy or neutral faces, * $ps = .001$ c) Response bias index per colour. Stimuli presented on a red (high arousal) or a pink (medium arousal) background were associated with more liberal response biases than stimuli presented on a white background (control), * $ps < .044$.

There was a trend towards a significant main effect of Colour, $F(3,69) = 2.7$, $\varepsilon = .83$, $p = .065$. Stimuli presented on a red (high arousal) or a pink (medium arousal) background were associated with more liberal response biases than stimuli presented on a white background (control), both $ps < .044$, with light pink (low arousal) non-significantly different in-between, see Figure 2c. This means that the participants were more inclined to respond 'match' to a probe face presented under high contextual arousal compared to control conditions. All interaction effects involving Colour were non-significant, all $Fs < 1.0$, *ns*.

CONCLUSION

The goal of the present study was to examine how STM for face identity of emotional faces would be influenced by visually-induced contextual arousal to clarify whether the effect of facial expression on STM is a valence or an arousal effect. Our manipulation of contextual arousal through colours was successful, given that the subjective ratings showed that red was associated with highest arousal, pink with medium, and light pink with lowest arousal.

As expected, we replicated previous findings of an increased discrimination index and thus enhanced STM for angry compared to happy and neutral faces (Jackson et al., 2008; Jackson et al., 2009), under high STM load (Langeslag et al., 2009). Moreover, participants were less inclined to incorrectly respond 'match' to angry compared to happy and neutral faces given that angry faces were associated a more conservative response bias when STM load was high. It is this conservative bias that appears to be the base of the angry face benefit in STM.

Contextual arousal did not affect discrimination between match and mismatch probe faces, which is in line with the study by Dougal (2003) as well as with the study using calming and arousing background music (Jackson et al., 2009). It does, however, stand in contrast to the results of the study by Erk et al. (2007), in which the context was formed by pictures that were presented during the retention interval. The context in that study appeared to be resource demanding, because performance was decreased when a neutral compared to no picture was presented. Our study suggests that background colours are not resource demanding, as they did not impair performance compared to the control condition with a white background. This makes manipulating background colours a promising approach for studying the effect of contextual arousal on cognitive processes.

As expected, the contextual arousal that the colours elicited influenced the response bias in the STM for faces. The response bias was more liberal in the high and medium arousal conditions compared to the control condition. This finding concurs with the finding of Dougal (2003) that neutral words studied in the presence of another emotional word (i.e. arousing context) were associated with a more liberal response bias at retrieval compared to neutral words studied in a the presence of another neutral word (i.e. non-arousing context). The arousing context in the current study may have increased the participant's tendency to respond 'match', may have increased the perceptual fluency with which the faces were processed at retrieval and/or may have increased the familiarity of the faces.

Despite the fact that contextual arousal and stimulus emotionality were manipulated in the same modality, the effects of background colour and facial expression did not interact. Although the colour pink was rated as more pleasant than the colour red, the response bias reflected the pattern of colour arousal rather than valence, suggesting that the effect of context on response bias is an arousal effect (cf. Dougal, 2003). Because the angry and happy faces were matched with respect to arousal, the influence of facial expression on STM performance on the other hand appears to be a valence effect, which is in line with previous findings (Jackson et al., 2009; Kensinger, 2007). The non-interacting and distinct effects of contextual arousal and facial expression on STM suggest that these arousal and valence effects have different underlying mechanisms. It has been suggested that the amygdala increases memory for arousing stimuli, whereas the prefrontal cortex increases memory for non-arousing valenced stimuli (Kensinger, 2004; Van Strien, Langeslag, Strekalova, Gootjes, & Franken, 2009), and a similar distinction may exist for the effects of emotional stimuli and contexts on memory.

To conclude, we report here the first study of the influence of visually-induced contextual arousal on visual STM for emotional faces. Whereas high contextual arousal was associated with a more liberal response bias regardless of expression, negative valence of facial expression was associated with an increased discrimination and more conservative bias regardless of background colour. Thus, the present results suggest that the effects of colour-induced contextual arousal and facial expression on STM are different. Because colour-induced arousal did not interact with the effect of facial expression on STM, this latter effect appears to be a valence and not an arousal effect. More research is needed to determine what cognitive and neural mechanisms underlie the effects of contextual arousal and facial expression on STM. In the mean time, the use of background colours to induce and manipulate contextual arousal appears a promising method that could be used in future research studying the effects of emotional context on cognitive tasks requiring visual presentation of stimuli.

ACKNOWLEDGMENT

MCJ and DEJL were supported by Wellcome Trust grant number 077185/Z/05/Z.

REFERENCES

[1] Bradley, M. M. & Lang, P. J. (1994). Measuring emotion: The self-assessment manikin and the semantic differential. *Journal of Behavior Therapy and Experimental Psychiatry, 25*, 49-59.
[2] Cajochen, C. (2007). Alerting effects of light. *Sleep Medicine Reviews, 11*, 453–464.
[3] Dougal, S. (2003). A dual process approach to emotional memory: Effects of emotion on familiarity and retrieval processes in recognition. University of Pittsburgh.
[4] Ekman, P. & Friesen, W. (1976). *Pictures of facial affect*. Palo Alto, CA: Consulting Psychological Press.
[5] Erk, S., Kleczar, A. & Walter, H. (2007). Valence-specific regulation effects in a working memory task with emotional context. *Neuroimage, 37*, 623-632.

[6] Jackson, M. C., Wolf, C., Johnston, S. J., Raymond, J. E. & Linden, D. E. J. (2008). Neural correlates of enhanced visual short-term memory for angry faces: An fMRI study. *PLoS ONE, 3*, e3536.

[7] Jackson, M. C., Wu, C. -., Linden, D. E. J. & Raymond, J. E. (2009). Enhanced visual short-term memory for angry faces. *Journal of Experimental Psychology: Human Perception and Performance, 35*, 363-374.

[8] Kensinger, E. A. (2004). Remembering emotional experiences: The contribution of valence and arousal. *Reviews in the Neurosciences, 15*, 241-251.

[9] Kensinger, E. A. (2007). Negative emotion enhances memory accuracy: Behavioural and neuroimaging evidence. *Current Directions in Psychological Science, 16*, 213-218.

[10] Kensinger, E. A. & Corkin, S. (2003). Memory enhancement for emotional words: Are emotional words more vividly remembered than neutral words? *Memory & Cognition, 31*, 1169-1180.

[11] Lang, P. J. (1980). Behavioral treatment and bio-behavioral assessment: Computer applications. In J. B. Sidowski, J. H. Johnson & T. A. Williams (Eds.), *Technology in mental health care delivery systems* (pp. 119-137) Ablex.

[12] Langeslag, S. J. E., Morgan, H. M., Jackson, M. C., Linden, D. E. J. & Van Strien, J. W. (2009). Electrophysiological correlates of improved short-term memory for emotional faces. *Neuropsychologia, 47*, 887-896.

[13] Mehta, R. & Zhu, R. J. (2009). Blue or red? Exploring the effect of color on cognitive task performances. *Science, 323*, 1226-1229.

[14] Ochsner, K. N. (2000). Are affective events richly recollected or simply familiar? the experience and process of recognizing feelings past. *Journal of Experimental Psychology: General, 129*, 242-261.

[15] Perlstein, W. M., Elbert, T. & Stenger, A. (2002). Dissociations in human prefrontal cortex of affective influences on working memory-related activity. *Proceedings of the National Academy of Sciences of the United States of America, 99*, 1736-1741.

[16] Shackman, A. J., Sarinopolous, I., Maxwell, J. S., Pizzagalli, D. A., Lavric, A. & Davidson, R. J. (2006). Anxiety selectively disrupts visuospatial working memory. *Emotion, 6*, 40-61.

[17] Snodgrass, J. G. & Corwin, J. (1988). Pragmatics of measuring recognition memory: Applications to dementia and amnesia. *Journal of Experimental Psychology: General, 117*, 34-50.

[18] Valdez, P. & Mehrabian, A. (1994). Effects of color on emotions. *Journal of Experimental Psychology: General, 123*, 394-409.

[19] Van Strien, J. W., Langeslag, S. J. E., Strekalova, N. J., Gootjes, L. & Franken, I. H. A. (2009). Valence interacts with the early ERP old/new effect and arousal with the sustained ERP old/new effect for affective pictures. *Brain Research, 1251*, 223-235.

[20] Weller, L. & Livingston, R. (1988). Effect of color of questionnaire on emotional responses. *The Journal of General Psychology, 115*, 433-440.

[21] Windmann, S. & Kutas, M. (2001). Electrophysiological correlates of emotion-induced recognition bias. *Journal of Cognitive Neuroscience, 13*, 577-592.

[22] Yoto, A., Katsuura, T., Iwanaga, K. & Shimomura, Y. (2007). Effects of object color stimuli on human brain activities in perception and attention referred to EEG alpha band response. *Journal of Physiological Anthropology, 26*, 373-379.

In: Working Memory: Capacity, Developments and…
Editor: Eden S. Levin

ISBN: 978-1-61761-980-9
© 2011 Nova Science Publishers, Inc.

Chapter 13

WORKING MEMORY DEFICITS IN SCHIZOPHRENIA: NEUROBIOLOGICAL CORRELATES AND TREATMENT

Haiyun Xu [1,2], Hong-Ju Yang[1] and Gregory M. Rose [1,2]

[1]Department of Anatomy,
[2] Center for Integrated Research in Cognitive and Neural Sciences, School of Medicine, Southern Illinois University Carbondale, Carbondale, IL USA

ABSTRACT

Working memory is a cognitive process dedicated to the transitory maintenance and online manipulation of information. Patients with schizophrenia, a heterogeneous brain disease, show several types of working memory deficits, including in visuospatial working memory, phonological working memory, and executive functioning. These deficits may underlie other schizophrenia symptoms and predict patient outcomes. Furthermore, there is increasing evidence suggesting that working memory deficits may provide a behavioral marker of genetic liability for schizophrenia. While the dominant role of the prefrontal dysfunction in working memory deficits of patients with schizophrenia has been appreciated, there is increasing evidence suggesting the existence of disturbed functional connectivity within brain networks subserving domain-specific components of working memory in schizophrenia. This functional deficit may result from dysfunctional neurotransmitter systems, of which the dopaminergic system has been best characterized, and/or white matter abnormalities which have been shown to be a consistent pathological finding in brains of schizophrenia patients. Working memory deficits in schizophrenia can be somewhat relieved by antipsychotics and various cognitive rehabilitation approaches. Atypical, but not typical, antipsychotics have shown some promise for relieving working memory deficits in patients with schizophrenia. Cognitive rehabilitation, an alternative to pharmacological treatment of cognitive deficits in patients with schizophrenia, also shows promise, but further work needs to be done to optimize this approach. Developing effective treatments for working memory impairments in schizophrenia patients remains an important therapeutic goal.

INTRODUCTION

Schizophrenia is a heterogeneous brain disease with disturbances in a range of mental processes including thought, perception, emotion, drive and behavior. Of the cognitive impairments in schizophrenia, working memory deficits are among the most prominent (Silver et al., 2003). Working memory is a low-capacity form of resettable memory that is usually short-term (seconds to minutes in duration; Baddeley, 1986). This working memory deficit has been suggested to contribute to other schizophrenia symptoms (Menon et al., 2001; Nestor et al., 1998) and to be a predictor for the outcome of schizophrenia patients (Green et al., 2000). Unaffected siblings of schizophrenics also have working memory deficits, suggesting that working memory dysfunction may be linked to the genetic susceptibility for schizophrenia (Cannon et al., 2000).

In addition to reviewing evidence of working memory deficits in schizophrenia and relating working memory deficits with other schizophrenia symptoms, this chapter will discuss the neurobiological correlates of working memory deficits in schizophrenia by focusing on aspects of prefrontal dysfunction, disturbed functional connectivity, dysregulation of the dopaminergic system, and white matter alterations in the schizophrenic brain. The closing sections describe recent efforts to treat working memory deficits in schizophrenia.

SCHIZOPHRENIA PATIENTS SHOW WORKING MEMORY DEFICITS

According to Baddeley's (1986) model, working memory involves three different component processes: a short-term storage buffer for visual information, termed the visuospatial scratch pad; a short-term storage buffer for verbal information, referred to as the phonological loop; and a central executive component that guides the manipulation and transformation of the information transiently held in these two storage buffers. A growing number of studies in patients with schizophrenia have shown deficits on tasks designed to measure the above elements of working memory.

Schizophrenics Show Visuospatial Working Memory Deficits

The seminal study by Park and Holzman (1992) first reported that patients with schizophrenia had deficits in oculomotor and haptic delayed-response tasks. (Schizophrenic subjects were also impaired in a test of verbal working memory; see next section.) However, the authors found that performance accuracy of schizophrenics did not differ from that of the normal controls in a sensory control task. Therefore, the authors concluded that the deficits observed in schizophrenics were likely to be due to a visuospatial working memory deficit rather than to a simple motor problem.

Since then, many other behavioral studies have confirmed that schizophrenia patients are impaired on visuospatial working memory tasks. For example, Fleming et al. (1997) reported that patients with schizophrenia were as adept as normal control subjects in judging the slope of a line (the judgment of line orientation task), but performed significantly worse than control subjects on delayed conditions and on both the visual span forward and visual span backward conditions. This pattern of results is highly suggestive of an impairment of visuospatial working memory. In a study by Tek et al. (2002), subjects with schizophrenia exhibited impaired performance relative to controls for spatial working memory measured by a task involving perceptual discrimination of spatial and object visual stimuli. This result is consistent with the outcome of another independent study (Chey et al., 2002) which observed significantly reduced spatial working memory span in the schizophrenia group compared to control subjects. Visuospatial working memory deficits, as defined by poor 'between search error' performance, are also evident in adolescent-onset schizophrenia (Vance et al., 2006). Moreover, spatial working memory deficits appear to be a stable marker for schizophrenia, as indicated by significant differences between normal controls and patients, both on a first test and a 4-month follow-up session (Park et al., 1999) and by the delayed-matching-to-sample tasks for novel shapes (Park et al., 2002).

Using functional magnetic resonance imaging (fMRI), altered brain activation during visuospatial working memory was revealed in patients with schizophrenia (McCarthy et al., 1994): responses were diminished in the left supramarginal gyrus (BA 40), left superior temporal lobe, left anterior cingulate, and within multiple sites of the left basal ganglia, as well as in the right precuneus region (BA 7). That most areas of diminished spatial working memory activation occurred in the left hemisphere suggests that verbal processes were activated less in schizophrenics compared to healthy volunteers. In addition, patients displayed activation in several brain regions where controls showed a reverse pattern. For example, patients showed activation in the culmen of the cerebellum, whereas healthy volunteers showed the opposite response (Kindermann et al., 2004). During the maintenance of visuospatial information, brain activation was significantly reduced in patients bilaterally in the superior parietal lobule, in the right middle occipital gyrus and in the right inferior temporal gyrus. Additionally, patients showed significantly increased activation of the right frontal eye field and the right inferior parital lobule (Henseler et al., 2009).

In another fMRI study, group differences in spatial working memory activation were revealed only in the region of dorsal lateral prefrontal cortex (DLPFC), with patients showing significantly less activation in this region when explicit manipulation requirements were present and at larger memory set sizes (Cannon et al., 2005). More interestingly, in a parametric fMRI study with four levels of a spatial N-back task, schizophrenic's activity initially increased in DLPFC and inferior parietal cortex bilaterally and in anterior cingulate with increasing load. However, at 3-back, activity dropped in DLPFC in comparison with controls. The results indicate that peak activation of the working memory system was reached at a lower processing load in schizophrenic patients than in healthy controls, while DLPFC activity declined at high processing loads (Jansma et al., 2004). These seemingly discrepant results suggest that the performance of visuospatial working memory tasks involves widespread networks in which prefrontal areas are major components. Consistent with this view, when performing a 2-back working memory task, patients with schizophrenia showed a pattern of reduced connectivity within the prefrontal-cerebellar and the cerebellar-thalamic limbs, but enhanced connectivity in the thalamo-cortical limb of the cortical-cerebellar circuit, relative to normal controls (Schlosser et al., 2003).

Schizophrenics Show Phonological Working Memory Deficits

Impaired verbal memory is well documented in patients with schizophrenia. A recent meta-analysis by Forbes et al. (2009) reviewed twenty-one tests or subtests with at least three contributing studies. For all of these tests, scores were significantly worse in schizophrenia than control groups, with absolute effect sizes ranging from 0.55 to 1.41. Although fourteen of these tests were associated with significant heterogeneity between studies, seven showed significant differences between schizophrenia and control groups that were not potentially attributable to heterogeneity or publication bias. These tests included: the long Digit Span Distraction Test (DSDT) (both non-distraction and distraction conditions), the short DSDT (non-distraction condition), digit span backwards, verbal learning tests, and verbal span tasks.

The evidence concerning deficits in phonological working memory in schizophrenia continues to grow, reinforced by recent fMRI studies mapping and comparing the brain activation patterns of schizophrenics and normal subjects when they perform the same tasks. Patients with schizophrenia showed greater activation than normal subjects in the left DLPFC, but did not differ in the right DLPFC, during the performance of a modified version of the Sternberg Item Recognition Paradigm (SIRP; Manoach et al., 1999). However, in another study in which participants performed two verbal working memory tasks while undergoing fMRI, patients showed less bilateral DLPFC activation and greater ventrolateral prefrontal cortex (VLPFC) activation relative to the comparison subjects (Tan et al., 2005). Moreover, patients with schizophrenia showed reduced activation of the right frontal operculum, the left intraparietal cortex and the right anterior cingulate cortex during the non-articulatory maintenance of phonological information, as well as attenuated deactivation of the hippocampus (Henseler et al., 2009). In addition, patients with schizophrenia exhibited bilateral deficits in dorsal frontal and parietal activation during both verbal and nonverbal working memory tasks (Barch and Csernansky, 2007). Although the results of all these fMRI studies are not entirely consistent, it is clear that phonological working memory deficits in schizophrenia patients are accompanied by alterations in regional brain activation.

Schizophrenics Show Executive Functioning Deficits

Executive functioning can be defined as the complex process of coordinating multiple sub-processes to achieve a particular goal (Elliott, 2003). Among the most used tasks that require executive function are: the Wisconsin Card Sorting Test (WCST); the Category Test; puzzle tests such as the Tower of Hanoi (TOH) and Tower of London (TOL); the Auditory Consonant Trigram Test, which requires sustained attention and simultaneous information processing; the *N*-back task; the self-ordered pointing task; and the letter-number sequencing (LNS) task.

Individuals with schizophrenia consistently show deficits on the above mentioned, and other, cognitive tasks designed to measure executive functioning. For example, in an early study of 60 schizophrenia patients and 34 nonpatient controls, 67 percent of the patients showed significant cognitive inflexibility as measured by perseverative error scores on the WCST (Morice, 1990). Similar deficits in WCST were reported in schizophrenia patients in other investigations (Kumra et al., 2000; Oie and Rund, 1999). Schizophrenia patients also demonstrated significant impairments in performance on TOL and Sentence Span (Morice and Delahunty, 1996). In the TOL test, patients showed deficits in planning accuracy and reduced subsequent planning time, a measure of time spent planning and thinking about the next problem solving mode (Fagerlund et al., 2006). Gold and colleagues (1997) demonstrated that schizophrenia patients have performance deficits in the LNS task, and that this impaired performance was correlated with WCST perseverative responses ($r = -0.52$). More impressively, Mahurin et al. (1998) demonstrated that schizophrenia patients have significant impairment across all of the executive-frontal tests, although these deficits are not uniform across symptom subtypes (Mahurin et al., 1998). Similarly, in a study by Perry et al. (2001) assessing schizophrenia patients and normal control subjects on a group of tests of executive function, schizophrenia patients were slower and committed more errors of commission on the Numerical Attention Test, required more moves to completion on the TOH test, achieved fewer correct responses on the LNS task, and committed significantly more perseverative responses and completed fewer categories on the WCST, compared to healthy subjects.

Despite consistent evidence showing executive function deficits in schizophrenics, there is still ongoing debate about the course of altered cognitive functioning in these patients. Several previous studies suggested a relative stability of cognitive functioning in patients with schizophrenia (Cervellione et al., 2007; Frangou et al., 2008; Oie et al., 2010). For example, executive function impairments seen in adolescent schizophrenics remained unchanged over a 2-year follow-up period (Cervellione et al., 2007), planning accuracy in early onset schizophrenia patients maintained at the same level of performance over a 4-year follow-up period (Frangou et al., 2008), and the performance of early onset schizophrenia patients on abstraction and perseveration (measured using the WCST) did not change over a 13-year follow-up period (Oie et al, 2010). On the other hand, other studies suggested a process of cognitive deterioration mainly within the first 5-10 years after the onset of schizophrenia (Albus et al., 1996; Braw et al., 2008; Lieberman et al., 2001; Saykin et al., 1994). For example, Braw et al. (2008) reported that multi-episode schizophrenia patients were significantly more impaired than the first-episode ones, with deficits mainly related to psychomotor speed, pattern memory, and executive functioning. As such, the authors proposed that the first years after onset may represent a therapeutic window for rehabilitation efforts focusing on the specific needs of schizophrenia patients. Without prompt and proper interventions, growing cognitive impairments may complicate rehabilitation efforts and will inevitably impact the patients' daily lives (Braw et al., 2008).

WORKING MEMORY DEFICITS IN SCHIZOPHRENICS ARE UNLIKELY ARTIFACTUAL

Although the above subsections reviewed a great body of evidence for working memory deficits in patients with schizophrenia, a potential caveat exists. Are the working memory deficits seen in schizophrenia the results of the disease *per se*, or secondary consequences of taking antipsychotic medications? In the following, we will summarize evidence ruling out the possibility that the working memory deficits in schizophrenia are merely side effects of antipsychotic treatment.

First of all, working memory deficits are present in unmedicated schizophrenia patients. Neuropsychological deficits, including deficits in verbal memory and learning, semantic memory, and visuomotor processing and attention have been seen in antipsychotic-naïve patients with first-episode schizophrenia (Albus et al., 2006; Hill et al., 2004; Saykin et al., 1994). Further, schizophrenic patients who had been free from antipsychotic drugs and all other medications at the time of testing (the medication-free period ranged from 2 weeks to 10 years) showed generalized impairment relative to controls and a selective deficit in memory and learning compared with other functions (Saykin et al., 1991). Similarly, patients who had been withdrawn from oral antipsychotic medications for at least 10 days prior to testing showed spatial working memory deficits (Carter et al., 1996). Conversely, bipolar patients taking antipsychotics showed intact spatial working memory (Park and Holzman 1992, 1993). These results suggest that the deficits in working memory performance seen in schizophrenics are not merely the result of antipsychotic treatment.

Second, clinically unaffected relatives of schizophrenia patients also show working memory deficits. For example, Park et al. (1995) found that the first-degree relatives of schizophrenic patients showed significant deficits in working memory on both oculomotor and visual-manual delayed response tasks. In a study by Conklin et al. (2000) the nonpsychotic relatives of patients with schizophrenia showed impairment on the backward digit span task, a measure of verbal working memory, but not on the forward digit span task, a measure of general attention. The results were replicated by the same group in a subsequent study (Conklin et al., 2005). In addition, the authors found that more relatives (20%) of patients with schizophrenia failed to reach a solution prior to task termination (in a self-ordered pointing task) compared to controls (2%), suggesting a deficit in object working memory. These results indicate that working memory deficit is associated with the diathesis for schizophrenia and may be a valuable indicator of susceptibility for this disorder.

WORKING MEMORY DEFICIT MAY PROVIDE A BEHAVIORAL MARKER OF GENETIC LIABILITY FOR SCHIZOPHRENIA

In support of the claim that memory deficits may indicate genetic predisposition toward schizophrenia, Cannon and colleagues (2000) reported that healthy monozygotic co-twins of affected individuals performed worse than did the healthy dizygotic co-twins of affected individuals, who in turn performed worse than did healthy control twins without a positive family history for schizophrenia, on the spatial span task of the Wechsler Memory Scale-Revised. In a subsequent study (Glahn et al., 2003) the group developed a spatial delayed-response task to measure spatial working memory. In this task the number of memoranda (locations) was parametrically varied, whereas the encoding time was held constant across trials. Individuals with limited storage capacity would be expected to perform increasingly worse on trials with higher memory sets sizes compared to individuals with more extensive stores. They found that impaired performance on the spatial delayed-response task increased in a dose-dependent fashion with increasing genetic predisposition toward schizophrenia.

Further evidence comes from studies of individuals with schizotypal personality disorder (SPD). Schizotypic individuals share genetic and psychological commonalities with schizophrenia, yet they are free of the possible confounds of antipsychotic medications, chronic hospitalization, and lifestyle changes. Individuals with SPD showed impairment as great as schizophrenics themselves on tests measuring working memory (Farmer et al., 2000; Heinrichs and Zakzanis, 1998; Mitropoulou et al., 2002, 2005). Verbal memory and learning are also impaired with SPD (Mitropoulou et al., 2005; Siever et al., 2002; Voglmaier et al., 1997). In addition, individuals with SPD show executive functioning deficits as assessed with the WCST (Diforio et al., 2000; Voglmaier et al., 1997).

Finally, neuroiamging studies have also supported a relationship between working memory deficits and genetic risk for schizophrenia. For example, Callicott et al. (2003) found increased activation in the right DLPFC of unaffected siblings of patients with schizophrenia compared to healthy controls during encoding and manipulation of information. Thermenos et al. (2004) showed that unaffected relatives of schizophrenics exhibited greater task-related activation in PFC and portions of thalamus. Brahmbhatt et al. (2006) showed that high-risk siblings abnormally activated their PFC, indicated by hyperactivation compared to controls during response selection to verbal stimuli. However, in a study by Meda et al. (2008), first-degree unaffected relatives of schizophrenia patients displayed reduced activation, most markedly in bilateral DLPFC/VLPFC and posterior parietal cortex, when encoding stimuli and in bilateral DLPFC and parietal areas during response selection. These different fMRI results, as discussed by others (Johnson et al., 2006; Manoach et al., 2003; Meda et al., 2008), are likely dynamic and dependent both on relative task difficulty and a particular individual's baseline efficiency on a particular task. As was discussed earlier, it has been proposed that at low memory loads schizophrenia patients are inefficient and over-activate, but at high loads exceeding their working memory capacity, their PFC is underactivated (Meda et al., 2008).

WORKING MEMORY DEFICITS UNDERLIE OTHER SCHIZOPHRENIA SYMPTOMS AND PREDICT PATIENT OUTCOMES

The ability to actively hold information 'online' and to manipulate information in the service of guiding behavior permits individuals to respond in a flexible manner, to formulate and modify plans, and to base behavior on internally held ideas and thoughts rather than being driven by external stimuli (Plum and Mountcastle, 1987). A defect in this ability can explain a variety of symptoms of schizophrenia, as proposed by Goldman-Rakic (1994). Theoretically, the inability to hold a discourse plan in mind and monitor speech output should lead to disorganized speech and thought disorder; the inability to maintain a plan for behavioral activities could lead to negative symptoms such as avolition or alogia; and the inability to reference a specific external or internal experience against associative memories could lead to an altered consciousness of sensory experience that might be expressed as delusions or hallucinations (Andreasen, 1997). Therefore, impaired working memory could underlie diverse impairments in schizophrenia. Indeed, impairments in verbal or spatial working memory have been correlated with deficits in a range of neuropsychological functions in patients with schizophrenia, including visual orientation, visual retention, memory for objects, memory for faces, executive function, and simple motor and complex sensorimotor function (Silver et al., 2003). Thus, schizophrenia patients' lower working memory capacity could be 'rate limiting' for the performance of other cognitive operations (Silver et al., 2003).

As might be expected, working memory deficits have been correlated with negative symptoms in patients with schizophrenia. For example, the findings of Carter et al. (1996) suggested that behavioral deficits during the 2-back visuospatial working memory were related to negative symptoms. Negative symptoms, indexed by the withdrawal-retardation subscale of the Brief Psychiatric Rating Scale (BPRS), were associated with poor performance in a 2-back auditory working memory paradigm (Menon et al., 2001). Impaired verbal working memory also showed a significant correlation with negative symptoms of schizophrenia in the study by Silver et al. (2003). A significant correlation between the negative symptoms and visual object working memory impairment was found in schizophrenia patients during partial remission (Park et al., 2002).

Increasing evidence also supports a correlation between working memory deficits and positive symptoms of schizophrenia. For example, Nestor et al. (1998) found a relationship between thought disorder and tests of verbal memory and working memory in schizophrenia patients. Findings by Menon et al. (2001) suggested an association between thinking disturbance symptoms, particularly unusual thoughts content, and disrupted working memory processing in schizophrenia. In another study, reduced spatial working memory in clinically stable patients with schizophrenia was correlated with symptoms of disorganization (Takahashi et al., 2005). Finally, semantic memory dysfunction has been theoretically and empirically tied to the symptoms of formal thought disorder (Kerns and Berenbaum, 2002) and hallucinations (DeFreitas et al., 2009; Kerns et al., 1999). In other studies, altered frontal lobe function in executive cognitive tasks has been linked to positive symptoms (Morrison-Stewart et al., 1992; Zakzanis, 1998).

Working memory deficits have also been correlated with other schizophrenia symptoms. For example, spatial working memory in schizophrenia patients correlated significantly with social functioning such as self-care skills, community skills and speech disturbance (Takahashi et al., 2005). Silver et al. (2007) found that a substantial proportion (56.9%) of the variance in performance of schizophrenia patients on an abstraction task was predicted by three measures: task latency, verbal working memory, and spatial working memory. An impact of executive function on emotion recognition in patients with schizophrenia was also reported. For example, emotion recognition performance was correlated with performance on the WCST (Kohler et al., 2000). Similarly, Bryson et al. (1997) found associations in patients with schizophrenia between the emotion recognition task score and WCST variables such as categories completed and perseverative errors. Sachs et al. (2004) also reported happy facial emotion recognition to be correlated with the WCST in schizophrenics. Finally, it was recently shown that variables in the WCST correlated with the total correct score of the Facial Affect Identification Task (FAIT), one of the most frequently used tasks to measure affective domains (Lee et al., 2009). Taken one with another, these studies strongly support the idea that deficits in executive function in schizophrenia can affect performance on facial emotion recognition.

Cognitive deficits contribute to poor functional outcome in patients with schizophrenia. General measures of memory have been associated with a poor global symptomatic outcome at 1 year (Moritz et al., 2000). Poor visual memory has been related to poor outcome in the form of persistent psychotic symptoms and more hospitalizations over 2 years (Verdoux et al., 2002). Perhaps not surprisingly, deficits in visual memory and working memory have been negatively associated with occupational functioning (Hofer et al., 2005). Speed of processing in the Trail Making Test A and poor executive functioning in the Trail Making

Test B have been related to higher negative symptoms over a 3-year period in individuals with first-episode psychosis (Addington et al., 2005) and in non-remitted patients (Helldin et al., 2006). Moreover, specific deficits in verbal memory and working memory in first-episode psychosis have been found to be viable markers of poor outcome after 6 months of treatment (Bodnar et al., 2008).

NEUROBIOLOGICAL CORRELATES OF THE WORKING MEMORY IMPAIRMENTS IN PATIENTS WITH SCHIZOPHRRENIA

As was reviewed above, working memory deficits are a core feature of schizophrenia. The identification of the alterations in brain function underlying these deficits has therefore become a major topic for schizophrenia research. Comprehensively reviewing all the literature relating to the neural correlates of working memory deficits in schizophrenia is beyond the scope of this chapter. In the following sections we will selectively review some important findings relating the contributions of prefrontal dysfunction, disturbed functional connectivity within brain networks and dysregulation of the dopaminergic system to the working memory deficits seen in schizophrenia. Evidence for a role for white matter alterations is also evaluated.

Prefrontal Dysfunction in Schizophrenia

There is strong evidence supporting prefrontal dysfunction as the primary neural substrate for the working deficits in patients with schizophrenia. Early studies repeatedly reported the observation that patients compromised by frontal lobe lesions and schizophrenia patients are similarly impaired on the Continuous Performance Task (Buchsbaum et al., 1990), WCST (Franke et al., 1992; Heaton et al., 1993; Seidman et al., 1991; Weinberger et al., 1986), the Stroop Test (Abramczyk et al., 1983; Everett et al., 1989; Schooler et al., 1997; Stroop, 1935), the TOL task (Andreasen et al., 1992), and on oculomotor delayed-response paradigms (Currie et al., 1993; Fukushima et al., 1988; Hommer et al., 1991; Park and Holzman, 1992). Each of these tasks requires working memory (e.g., keeping a running record of recent events or instructions). Therefore, working memory deficits in humans are believed to be markers of prefrontal dysfunction in patients with schizophrenia (Goldman-Rakic and Selemon, 1997).

Evidence from single unit recordings in nonhuman primates and from neuroimaging studies of humans (Goldman-Rakic, 1999; Petrides et al., 1993) has demonstrated the participation of the DLPFC in working memory. Individuals with schizophrenia show abnormalities in DLPFC activation during working memory performance. The most frequent pattern of abnormal DLPFC activation in schizophrenic brains is the notable task-related "hypofrontality", a reduced activation compared to healthy control participants. For example, Barch et al. (2001) reported that first-episode, medication-naïve patients with schizophrenia showed deficits in DLPFC activation in task conditions requiring context processing. The same group also found that participants with schizophrenia failed to show activation of right DLPFC in response to working memory tasks demands, whereas those with major depression showed clear activation of right and left DLPFC as well as bilateral activation of inferior and superior frontal cortex (Barch et al., 2003). Moreover, individuals with schizophrenia failed to show activation of right DLPFC during performance of the N-back task (Perlstein et al., 2001; Weinberger et al., 1986). These results suggest that the hypofrontality during cognitive task performance is specific to schizophrenia and that the deficit is not simply secondary to the administration of antipsychotic medication.

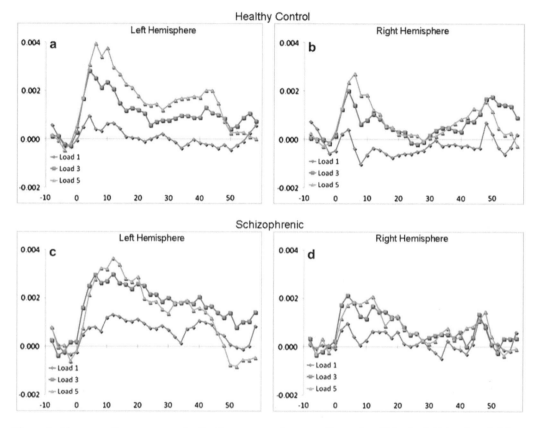

Figure 1. The mean time courses of activation averaged across all voxels within the left (a, c) and right (b, d) hemisphere DLPFC regions of interest for healthy controls (a, b) and schizophrenic (c, d) subjects. The horizontal axis represents time in seconds relative to the onset of thememorandumat time zero (0) formemory loads of 1 (blue line), 3 (red line), and 5 (green line) items. The firstmemory probe was presented at 7 sec and the last memory probe occurred at 38 sec. This figure was reproduced from figure 4 of the article by Potkin et al. (Schizophrenia Bullet. 35: 19-31), permitted by the publisher.

The task-related hypofrontality during working memory paradigms in patients with schizophrenia is, however, not a consistent observation. Several recent fMRI studies reported either equal (Honey et al., 2002; Walter et al., 2003) or increased activation (hyperfrontality) of the DLPFC (Callicott et al., 2000; Manoach et al., 1999, 2000) in schizophrenia during working memory performance. This difference was interpreted to be related to task parameters, including the level of task demand, the requirement that subjects adopt a DLPFC-mediated strategy, the expectation that subjects respond to every item, and the reward for correct responses (Manoach et al., 1999, 2003). In support of this interpretation, DLPFC activation appears to be strongly affected by memory load (Altamura et al., 2007). However, the relationship between DLPFC activation [blood oxygen level-dependent (BOLD) signal change] and memory load changed in patients with schizophrenia relative to controls. In healthy volunteers, BOLD signals in the DLPFC increased with increasing memory load (Altamura et al., 2007) until the highest load level (Callicott et al., 1999), while patients with schizophrenia reached peak activation in DLPFC at a lower processing load than did healthy controls (Callicott et al., 2000, 2003; Jansma et al., 2004). This finding was elegantly reinforced in a more recent fMRI study (Potkin et al., 2009). In this work, which involved a large, multisite sample, the mean BOLD signal in the DLPFC was significantly greater in the schizophrenic group than the healthy group, particularly in the intermediate load condition (Figure 1). However, enhanced activation of DLPFC in schizophrenics was not linked to better performance, suggesting an inefficient DLPFC function. Thus, it appears that there is reduced functional efficiency of prefrontal processing in schizophrenia; the enhanced BOLD signal during less difficult working memory tasks may be an attempt to compensate for this deficit.

Disturbed Functional Connectivity in Schizophrenia

In addition to DLPFC, other brain regions also engage in working memory processes. For example, articulatory rehearsal is particularly dependent on Brodman's areas 44 and 45 (Chein and Fiez, 2001; Fiez et al., 1996), and lesions to these regions impair rehearsal but not the ability to use phonological representation (Vallar et al., 1997). Spatial attention processing is linked to the right posterior parietal cortex (Postle et al., 2004) as this region is activated during spatial working memory processing and lesions to this region lead to selective deficits in spatial working memory. In addition, tasks involving spatial working memory also activate the frontal eye fields and the supplementary eye fields (Curtis et al., 2004). Many processes associated with the central executive function have been assumed to be supported by DLPFC. However, some regions of the parietal cortex are also important for central executive processing (Corbetta et al., 2002; Marshuetz et al., 2000; Peers et al., 2005; Ravizza et al., 2004; Sohn et al., 2000). In addition, a region of left VLPFC is involved in the resolution of proactive interference (Jonides et al., 1998), a process requiring central executive functioning. Therefore, it is not difficult to imagine how working memory deficits in schizophrenia implicate many connected brain regions. In fact, there is increasing evidence suggesting the existence of disturbed functional connectivity within the brain networks subserving domain-specific components of working memory in schizophrenia, as will be reviewed below.

Recent neuroimaging studies show altered patterns of interregional functional connectivity in patients with schizophrenia during working memory task performance. For example, Meyer-Lindenberg et al. (2001) provided evidence for abnormal cortical functional connectivity during working memory in schizophrenia using positron emission tomography (PET) scanning. Using the same method, functional disconnection between the prefrontal and parietal cortices during working memory processing was found in schizophrenia patients (Kim et al., 2003).

To better define the anatomical components of the networks hypothesized to subserve working memory and how they may function differently in schizophrenia, recent studies have employed independent component analysis (ICA). This is a powerful statistical and computational data-driven technique to discover hidden factors underlying sets of random variables, measurements, or signals (Calhoun et al., 2001; McKeown et al., 1998). In a study by Kim et al. (2009), ICA revealed six networks that showed significant differences between patients with schizophrenia and healthy controls. In addition, they found that DLPFC dysfunction in schizophrenia was lateralized to the left hemisphere and intrinsically tied to other regions such as the inferior parietal lobule and cingulate gyrus. In another study (Meda et al., 2009), schizophrenia patients showed decreased functionality and anomalous behavior of the left fronto-cingulate-parietal-basal ganglia neurocognitive network. This network likely plays a crucial role in attention and executive control during working memory (Bunge et al., 2000; Smith and Jonides, 1999). These authors also observed a right fronto-parietal circuit, containing the DLPFC, which engaged abnormally in schizophrenia. The third significant encoding-related network that was abnormal in schizophrenia consists of the anterior/posterior cingulate, medial frontal gyrus and inferior parietal regions. Very recently, Henseler et al. (2010) found that schizophrenia patients showed reduced connectivity of the PFC with the intraparietal cortex and the hippocampus and abnormal negative interactions between the VLPFC and DLPFC during the non-articulatory maintainance of phonological information (Figure 2). During the maintenance of visuospatial information, patients presented reduced connectivity between regions in the superior parietal and occipital cortex, as well as enhanced connectivity of the frontal eye field with visual processing areas (Figure 3). These results indicate complex dysfunction within the networks supporting working memory functions in schizophrenia.

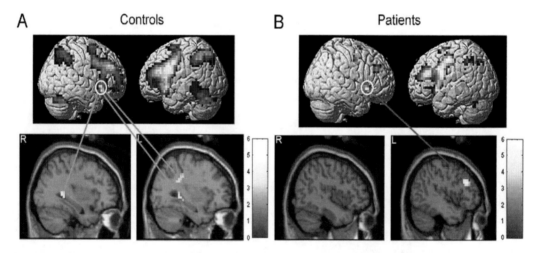

Figure 2. Working memory-related functional connectivity of the right frontal opercular cortex (white circle) during the non-articulatory maintenance task. Healthy subjects showed positive connectivity with the left intraparietal cortex and the bilateral posterior hippocampus (A), whereas patients showed significantly reduced task-related positive connectivity of the frontal operculum with other parts of the brain and presented negative interactions between this region and the left dorsolateral prefrontal cortex (B). Green arrows: positive connectivity. Red arrows: negative connectivity. This figure was reproduced from figure 1 of the article by Henseler et al. (J Neuropsychiatric Res. 44: 364-372), permitted by the publisher.

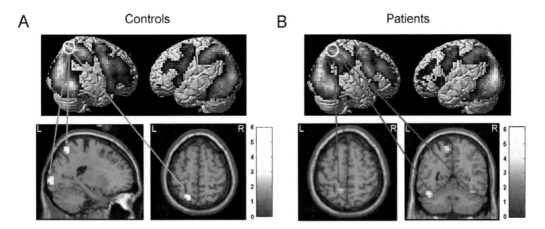

Figure 3. Working memory-related functional connectivity of the right superior parietal cortex (white circle) during the visuospatial maintenance task. Healthy subjects showed positive connectivity with the left superior parietal cortex and the left occipital cortex (A), whereas patients showed significantly reduced task-related positive connectivity of the right superior parietal cortex with the contralateral parietal and occipital cortices and presented negative interactions between the right and left superior parietal cortex, as well as between the right superior parietal cortex and the bilateral fusiform gyrus (B). Green arrows: positive connectivity. Red arrows: negative connectivity. This figure was reproduced from figure 2 of the article by Henseler et al. (J Neuropsychiatric Res. 44: 364-372), permitted by the publisher.

Thus, disrupted functional connectivity is an important neuropathological feature of schizophrenia. It is highly unlikely that this defect can be accounted for by any single factor. At a minimum, dysfunctional neurotransmitter systems as well as white matter abnormalities are likely to be involved, since these two elements are critical for coordination of subcortical to cortical, and of intra-cortical, information processing. Literature relevant to these two issues is reviewed below.

DYSREGULATION OF THE DOPAMINERGIC SYSTEM IN SCHIZOPHRENIA

Dysregulation of dopamine (DA) is centrally implicated in the pathophysiology and treatment of schizophrenia. Animal studies have strongly suggested that schizophrenia symptoms may be modulated by prefrontal D1 and D2, as well as by striatal D2, receptors (Drew et al., 2007; Kellendonk et al., 2006; Seamans and Yang, 2004; Wang et al., 2004). Several lines of evidence have suggested that the PFC of schizophrenia patients may be hypodopaminergic and that this decreased mesocortical dopaminergic activity contributes to poor performance in frontally-mediated cognitive tasks (Weinberger et al., 1988). Some of the evidence for this includes: local depletion of DA in the PFC of monkeys produces an impairment in spatial delayed alternation performance, a deficit that can be reversed by a DA agonist (Brozoski et al., 1979); administration of DA stimulant ameliorates the cognitive performance deficit in frontally-mediated tasks and improves task-dependent activation of regional blood flow in the PFC in patients with schizophrenia (Daniel et al., 1991); and a PET study has revealed that an impaired cognitive-task-induced activation of the anterior cingulated cortex in schizophrenics can be effectively mitigated by dopaminergic manipulation (Dolan et al., 1995).

Dopaminergic D1 receptors play an important role in the cognitive dysfunction present in schizophrenia (Gray and Roth, 2007). A decreased level of D1 receptor-like binding in the PFC of drug-naïve patients with schizophrenia, measured with PET, was found to be correlated with performance on the WCST (Okubo et al., 1997). This is consistent with a previous study showing a reduction in D1 receptors in drug-naïve schizophrenics (Sedvall and Fared, 1996). These results clearly cannot be attributed to the effects of antipsychotic medications. However, antipsychotics do affect the expression of D1-like receptors in the brain. Lidow et al. (1997) reported that chronic treatment with antipsychotic drugs (D2 antagonists) produced a down-regulation of the levels of D1 and D5 receptor mRNAs in the monkey PFC, although no changes were observed in neostriatal samples for any of the drugs examined. This result is consistent with previous studies showing that most D2 antagonists do not regulate subcortical D1 receptors (Fox et al., 1994; Hess et al., 1988; Lappalainen et al., 1990; MacKenzie and Zigmond, 1985).

Interestingly, Abi-Dargham et al. (2002) reported that the binding of the PET ligand $[^{11}C]$ NNC 112, a selective D1 receptor antagonist, was significantly elevated in the DLPFC of patients with schizophrenia compared with control subjects. Further, increased DLPFC $[^{11}C]$ NNC 112 binding was a strong predictor of poor performance at the N-back test of working memory in schizophrenic patients, but not in healthy controls. The authors explained that the increased $[^{11}C]$ NNC 112 binding reflects increased concentration of D1 receptors in DLPFC of patients with schizophrenia. This increased concentration might represent a compensatory (but ineffective) upregulation secondary to chronic deficiency in D1 receptor stimulation by DA. This explanation is consistent with the observation that chronic DA depletion is also associated with increased in vivo binding of $[^{11}C]$ NNC 112 in the PFC (Guo et al., 2001).

Thus, at this point there is not a complete consensus concerning the effect of schizophrenia on cortical D1 receptors. Although the apparent discrepancy in the above-described studies necessitates further investigation, Goldman-Rakic et al. (2000) have proposed a useful hypothesis to explain the relationship between working memory performance and D1 receptor activation. According to their theory, the spatial tuning of prefrontal neurons engaged in spatial working memory is enhanced at moderate levels of D1 occupancy and reduced at both lower and higher levels of occupancy. In support of this view, low doses of D1 agonists, such as dihydrexidine, A77636, and SKF81297, have cognition-enhancing actions in nonhuman primates (Arnsten et al., 1994; Cai et al., 1997; Schneider et al., 1994). Further, low, but not high, doses of typical antipsychotic drugs generate cognitive benefits in patients with schizophrenia (Weickert and Goldberg, 2005), although this effect is perhaps not as great as those produced by atypical antipsychotic drugs (discussed below).

D2 receptors are far less abundant in the cerebral cortex and difficult to measure within the cortical neuropil, but have a prominent presence and influence within the basal ganglia (Lidow et al., 1991). Although some studies found no significant changes in baseline D2 receptor availability in patients with schizophrenia (Abi-Dargham et al., 1998; Breier et al., 1997; Laruelle et al., 1996), a meta-analysis has suggested that schizophrenia is accompanied by a somewhat increased density of D2 receptors (Laruelle, 1998). After the meta-analysis was published, Abi-Dargham et al. (2000) demonstrated that baseline striatal postsynaptic D_2 occupancy was increased in a group of 18 schizophrenic patients that were not taking antipsychotic medication at the time of the study. An increase in striatal postsynaptic D2 receptor availability to the radioligand was also demonstrated in the group of 18 schizophrenic patients (Abi-Dargham et al., 2000). This increase in striatal D2 receptors may contribute to working memory deficits in schizophrenia patients. In support of this notion, developmentally regulated over-expression of striatal D2 receptors has been associated with working memory deficits and with altered activity of the PFC in animals (Kellendonk et al., 2006).

More evidence for the involvement of D2 receptors in working memory performance comes from studies with pharmacological agonists and antagonists. For example, Luciana et al. (1992) investigated the effect of an acute oral dose of 2.5 mg bromocriptine (a D2 receptor agonist) on a sample of 8 young, healthy females, in their performance of a visuospatial delayed response task. The authors observed a 44% improvement in the accuracy of identifying the cue location in the 8-s bromocriptine condition, compared to placebo. In a subsequent study with a larger sample of 66 young adults (Luciana et al., 1997), the performance accuracy of the subjects was improved following administration of a smaller dose of bromocriptine (1.24 mg). This effect was confirmed by the same group, who observed a facilitating effect of 1.35 mg bromocriptine on spatial working memory when behavioral testing occurred between 3.5 and 5.5 h after administration of the drug. In contrast, administration of haloperidol, a D_2 receptor antagonist, decreased performance in a spatial working memory task (Luciana and Collins, 1998). Sulpiride, a more selective D_2 receptor antagonist, has also been shown to cause spatial working memory impairments (Mehta et al., 1999, 2004). Similarly, raclopride (another D_2 antagonist) was shown to reduce spatial working memory accuracy in rhesus monkeys (Von Huben et al., 2006).

White Matter Abnormalities in Schizophrenia

Abnormalities in white matter could play a critical role in disturbed functional connectivity observed in the brains of schizophrenic patients. Indeed, several lines of evidence indicate that the disease is accompanied by profound alterations in white matter morphology and organization as summarized below.

Recent postmortem studies have reported reductions in density and size of oligodendrocytes (OLs) in PFC, striatal regions, superior frontal regions, thalamic nucleus, and the anterior principal thalamic nucleus of patients with schizophrenia as compared with controls (Byne et al., 2006; Hof et al., 2003; Uranova et al., 2004). In addition, ultrastructural alterations, including reduced nuclear euchromatin and mitochondrial number, were found in OLs in frontal cortex of schizophrenics. These alterations were associated with myelin damage (Orlovskaya et al., 1997). Levels of the myelin marker, myelin basic protein (MBP), are decreased in the anterior frontal cortex and hippocampus of patients with schizophrenia (Honer et al., 1999; Chambers et al., 2004). Also, two OL-associated proteins, myelin-associated glycoprotein (MAG) and 2', 3'-cyclonucleo-tide, 3'-phosphodiesterase (CNP), have been reported to be reduced in schizophrenia (Chambers et al., 2004; Flynn et al., 2003).

Conventional MRI studies have shown reductions in total white matter volume in schizophrenia (Antonova et al., 2005; Cannon et al., 1998; Hulshoff Pol et al., 2004). Regional white matter reductions have been seen in the frontal lobe (Paillere-Martinot et al., 2001; Sanfilipo et al., 2000), temporal lobe (Sanfilipo et al., 2000; Mitelman et al., 2003), anterior commissure (Hulshoff Pol et al., 2004), corpus callosum (McDonald et al., 2005), and internal capsule (McIntosh et al., 2005; Zhou et al., 2003). In addition, reductions have also been found in the white matter underlying left frontal and temporal cortex (Spalletta et al., 2003) and in fronto-temporal and fronto-parietal connections such as the arcuate, uncinate, longitudinal and frontooccipital fasciculi (Antonova et al., 2005; McDonald et al., 2005; Spalletta et al., 2003; Sigmundsson et al., 2001).

The application of new MRI techniques such as magnetic transfer imaging (MTI) and diffusion tensor imaging (DTI) in recent research has provided further evidence for white matter abnormalities in schizophrenia. For example, wide-spread MTR (magnetization transfer ratio) reductions were revealed in the cortex, predominantly in the frontal and temporal regions, in schizophrenic brains (Foong et al., 2000, 2001). Reduced MTR reflects reductions in axonal density and/or loss of myelin in the white matter (Barker et al., 1996; Van Waesberghe et al., 1999). MTR reductions in bilateral parieto-occipital cortex and the genu of the corpus callosum have been associated with the severity of negative symptoms in the schizophrenic patients. Subsequent work showed that MTR was also reduced in the medial PFC and the white matter incorporating the fasciculus uncinatus in schizophrenia patients (Bagary et al., 2003).

DTI provides information about the organization of fibers in white matter tracts in vivo. Fractional anisotropy (FA), a quantitative index of white matter coherence and integrity, is a most frequently used measure to evaluate water diffusion in the white matter (Kubicki et al., 2007). Lesions to white matter structures generally produce reductions in FA (Walterfang et al., 2006). Patients with schizophrenia show decreased FA in PFC, temporo-parietal and parieto-occipital regions, splenium, cingulum, posterior capsule, and adjacent occipital white matter of their brains (Agartz et al., 2001; Buchsbaum et al., 1998; Lim et al., 1999).

White Matter Abnormality Related Cognitive Impairments

Based on the above literature review, it is reasonable to infer that the loss of white matter integrity in patients with schizophrenia may be an important factor contributing to the cognitive dysfunction. In support of this speculation, cognitive impairments in attention, recent memory, information processing speed, executive functions, verbal intellectual ability, and visuospatial perception have been correlated with white matter lesion volume in frontal and parietal regions of patients with multiple sclerosis, a white matter disease (Sperling er al., 2001). Patients with the late-onset form (adolescent to young adulthood) of metachromatic leukodystrophy, another white matter disease, often present with symptoms of acute schizophrenia (Alves et al., 1986; Cerizza et al., 1987; Finelli et al., 1985; Hagemen et al., 1995). Another example is provided by individuals with chromosome 22q11-deletion syndrome (22qDS), a disease that was often indistinguishable from schizophrenia until the recent discovery of its genetic basis. 22qDS subjects show reductions in white matter volume twice as large as their gray matter volume reductions (Bearden et al., 2001; Eliez et al., 2000; 2001; Kates, 2001).

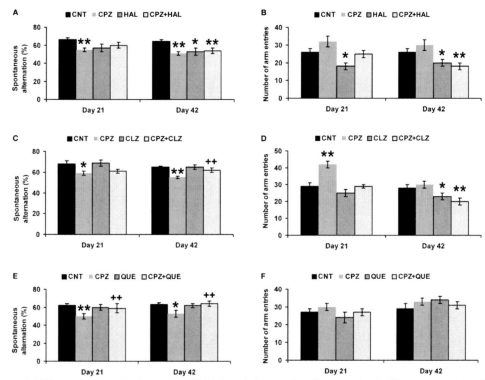

Figure 4. Effects of antipsychotics on the CPZ-induced abnormal performance in the Y-maze test. Control and experimentally treated C57BL/6 mice were subjected to Y-maze test on the same days (21st and 42nd days after CPZ-exposure). (A) The data of the spontaneous alternation in the HAL experiment. (B) The data of the number of arm entries in the HAL experiment. (C) The data of the spontaneous alternation in the CLZ experiment. (D) The data of the number of arm entries in the CLZ experiment. (E) The data of the spontaneous alternation in the QUE experiment. (F) The data of the number of arm entries in the QUE experiment. Data were expressed as M ± SEM ($n = 6$ to 12/group). *p $\leq$ 0.05, **p< 0.01, compared to the CNT group; ++ p <0.01, compared to the CPZ group. This figure was reproduced from figure 2 of the article by Xu et al. (Front Behav Neurosci. 2010 Mar 18; 4:8).

White matter abnormalities have also been associated with cognitive impairments in animal studies. The white matter alterations can be induced by dietary administration of cuprizone to C57BL/6 mice (Yang et al., 2009). Cuprizone is a copper chelator that has been shown to specifically damage the myelin sheath and OLs, but not to cause lesions in other cell types in the central nervous system (Matsushima & Morell, 2001; Remington et al., 2007; Selvaraju et al., 2004). It was demonstrated that cuprizone-exposed mice showed brain demyelination as well as a working memory deficit manifested by lower spontaneous alternation in a Y-maze test (Xu et al., 2009). Similar results have been reported by other investigators using rats. Adolescent rats exposed to cuprizone showed decreased expression of mRNA transcripts encoding oligodendroglial proteins within the medial PFC. These rats also displayed a specific deficit in the ability to shift between perceptual dimensions in the attention set-shifting task (Gregg et al., 2009), a PFC-mediated behavioral paradigm modeled after the WCST (Franke et al., 1992). Interestingly, the working memory deficit in cuprizone-exposed mice was reduced by clozapine and quetiapine (Figure 4), but not haloperidol (Xiao et al., 2008; Xu et al., 2010). These animal models have provided useful platforms for future studies to explore the role of white matter abnormalities in the pathophysiology of schizophrenia.

Treatment of Working Memory Deficits in Patients with Schizophrenia

As was mentioned above, the cognitive deficits that accompany schizophrenia are debilitating, and represent a major hurdle to adequately treating the illness. A number of pharmacological agents have been explored for their potential as tools to relieve cognitive deficits in patients with schizophrenia. Because of the space limitations, we will focus on the effects of atypical antipsychotic medications which have shown some promise for cognitive difficulties in patients with schizophrenia. We will also review studies involving nonpharmacological treatments for cognitive rehabilitation.

Cognitive Benefits of atypical Antipsychotics

Studies comparing atypical antipsychotics to low doses of typical (conventional) antipsychotics usually show greater cognitive benefits for atypical drugs (Weickert and Goldberg, 2005). For example, patients who were treated with atypicals (clozapine, olanzapine, quetiapine, risperidone, or amisulpride) showed better performance in the digit ordering test when compared to a group of patients who received conventional antipsychotics (flupenthixol, haloperidol, pimozide, or levomepromazine). This difference was not due to disease severity, age, or education (Muller et al., 2005). Similarly, impairments in spatial working memory, learning efficiency and error monitoring in schizophrenia patients were improved after one month of treatment with therapeutic doses of atypical antipsychotics (Snyder et al., 2008). Moreover, risperidone improved, while haloperidol worsened, spatial working memory performance in a 4-week, double-blind, randomized trial (McGurk et al., 2005). In an ealier fMRI study, Honey et al. (1999) measured n-back performance of schizophrenia patients after switching from conventional antipsychotics to oral risperidone and found a normalization of the patients, i.e., an increase in the activation in DLPFC and parietal cortex by risperidone. Long-acting injectable risperidone (LAIR) also showed cognitive benefits for patients with schizophrenia, as indicated by significant improvements in cognitive function observed in the backward Digit Span Test, Verbal Learning Test, WCST, correct responses on the Continuous Performance Test, and Trail Making Test part B following a switch to LAIR from oral atypical antipsychotics (Kim et al., 2009). Moreover, LAIR may also contribute to normalization of brain activation in regions involved in working memory function in people with schizophrenia (Surguladze et al., 2007).

Quetiapine also appears to have cognitive benefits. For example, the positive effects of quetiapine on cognitive functions like verbal fluency, memory and executive function were superior to those of haloperidol (Purdon et al., 2001; Velligan et al., 2002). In a task involving emotional stimuli, increased prefrontal activity after antipsychotic treatment with quetiapine was demonstrated in schizophrenic patients (Fahim et al., 2005; Stip et al., 2005). In an fMRI study, both quetiapine-treated patients and healthy control subjects showed a significantly increased activation in the left inferior frontal cortex compared to the drug-naïve group (Jones et al., 2004). In a recent study, after 12 weeks of treatment with quetiapine monotherapy, patients showed significant clinical improvement and increased BOLD activity in the VLPFC during a working memory task (Meisenzahl et al., 2006). Similarly, activation of both bilateral PFC as well as bilateral temporal cortex changed in patients with schizophrenia after 7-8 weeks of treatment with atypical antipsychotics including olanzapine, risperidone, quetiapine and amisulpiride (Wolf et al., 2007). Aripiprazole has also been shown to improve working memory performance in schizophrenia patients (Schlagenhauf et al, 2010). In this study, the beneficial effect was correlated with normalization of BOLD hypoactivity observed in the anterior cingulate cortex.

Initial reports indicated that clozapine, in addition to controlling psychotic symptoms, improved cognition in schizophrenic patients (Hagger et al., 1993). However, many subsequent studies have produced mixed results (Meltzer and McGurk, 1999; Rajji et al., 2010). It has been suggested that these mixed outcomes may be the result of individual differences in drug metabolism. It should be noted that clozapine is a potent antagonist at several types of muscarinic cholinergic receptors (Bolden et al., 1992; Snyder et al., 1974). As such, this drug would be expected to impair cognition. However, clozapine's primary metabolite, N-desmethylclozapine, is a partial agonist at these receptors (Rajji et al., 2010). Further work will be necessary to confirm that N-desmethylclozapine is a cognitive enhancer.

Neurocognitive Rehabilitation for Schizophrenia

Cognitive rehabilitation is an alternative approach to the pharmacological treatment of cognitive deficits in schizophrenia patients. This rehabilitation includes cognitive remediation and cognitive adaptation, each of which comprises different types of cognitive programs. One cognitive rehabilitation approach is the Neuropsychological Education Approach to Remediation (NEAR) program. The NEAR program involves a combination of "drill and practice" exercises and teaching strategies to improve cognitive functioning (Medalia and Choi, 2009). In an early NEAR study (Medalia et al., 2000), inpatients who received 6 hours of problem solving remediation showed significantly greater improvement in verbal problem solving than did the control subjects with psychiatric illness who just received typing instruction. In a subsequent study (Medalia et al., 2002), patients who participated in NEAR showed significant improvements in problem solving relative to a control group of individuals with schizophrenia who received treatment as usual and no remediation. More impressively, a recent randomized controlled multisite study demonstrated that the NEAR program is associated with broad cognitive improvement (including improvements in verbal and visual memory, sustained attention and executive functioning) after 15 weeks of cognitive remediation (Hodge et al., 2010).

Other cognitive rehabilitation programs have also generated encouraging results. For example, Delahunty and Morice (1996) developed a rehabilitation training program to improve deficits in cognitive flexibility, working memory and planning ability that produced significant improvements in neurocognitive performance. In a randomized trial of an intensive cognitive remediation program targeting deficits in cognitive flexibility, working memory and planning, Wykes et al (1999) found a clear benefit versus intensive occupational therapy. In a later study, the same group (Wykes et al., 2002) reported that patient groups who received cognitive remediation therapy showed significantly increased brain activation in regions associated with working memory, particularly the frontocortical areas, while the control group showed decreased activation.

A few studies have focused on effects of cognitive rehabilitation programs on specific types of cognitive deficits in patients with schizophrenia. For example, in a study by Wexler et al. (2000), patients did daily verbal memory exercises that became progressively more difficult over a 10-week training period. The authors found that verbal, but not nonverbal, memory performance was improved in patients after training and that performance gains were correlated with increases in task-related activation of the left inferior frontal cortex. In a more recent case study, a cognitive rehabilitation program designed to improve the updating subcomponent of working memory was administered to a schizophrenia patient. The training protocol, described by Duval and Coyette (2005), significantly improved working memory, and had the additional benefits of decreasing both subjective cognitive complaints and psychiatric symptoms (Levaux et al., 2009).

Computer-assisted cognitive remediation protocols are being increasingly utilized (Bell et al., 2008; Fisher et al., 2009; Grynszpan et al., 2010; Kurtz et al., 2003; McGurk et al., 2007). Computer-based procedures have some advantages, including prolonged multimedia stimulation thought to favour neural plasticity (Hogartly et al., 2004), as well as stimulating and entertaining aspects that may potentially favor the induction of motivation (Medalia et al., 2001). In addition, computer activities are considered helpful for acquiring new compensatory strategies, which is viewed as an important component of cognitive remediation (Kurtz et al., 2007). Several computer-assisted cognitive remediation studies have shown significant cognitive improvements in schizophrenic subjects (Bell et al., 2001; Hogarty et al., 2004; Sartory et al., 2005). A recent example is a study by Fisher et al. (2009). These investigators randomly assigned 55 clinically stable schizophrenia subjects to either 50 hours of computerized auditory training or a control condition using computer games. Those in the auditory training group engaged in daily computerized exercises that placed implicit, increasing demands on auditory perception through progressively more difficult auditory-verbal working memory and verbal learning tasks. The authors found that subjects who received active training showed significant gains in global cognition, verbal working memory, and verbal learning and memory relative to the control group.

Not all studies employing cognitive rehabilitation have produced cognitive improvements (Benedict et al., 1994; Field et al., 1997; Medalia et al., 2000; Dickinson et al., 2010). A number of reasons have been proposed to explain this lack of consistent success (Levaux et al., 2009; McGurk et al., 2007). First, the cognitive programs used in some cognitive rehabilitation studies are not specific to one cognitive function but rather aim to improve several cognitive domains. Second, some of these studies did not take into account the heterogeneity of cognitive deficits characterized in schizophrenia. Third, difficulties in patients' everyday lives have not been given the importance they deserve when designing and proposing cognitive rehabilitation programs. In addition to these, genetic factors should be considered, indicated by the finding that the COMT (catechol-O-methyltransferase) polymorphism influences individual capacity to recover from cognitive deficits through rehabilitation therapy (Bosia et al., 2007). Other genetic differences may also dictate the type of program more likely to be successful with an individual patient.

CONCLUDING REMARKS

There is a great body of literature reporting working memory deficits in patients with schizophrenia. Working memory deficits are a cardinal cognitive impairment which may contribute to the other schizophrenia symptoms. Exploring the relationship between working memory deficits and other symptoms of schizophrenia deserves further study, particularly since working memory impairments may predict increased risk for the disease.

Among the neurobiological correlates of working memory deficits in schizophrenia, prefrontal dysfunction and disturbed functional connectivity have received much attention. The disrupted functional connectivity can not be accounted for by a dysfunctional dopaminergic system alone. White matter abnormalities, which have been shown to be a consistent pathological finding in brains of patients with schizophrenia, may also contribute to working memory deficits.

Working memory deficits in schizophrenia can be somewhat improved by atypical antipsychotic treatment and cognitive rehabilitation approaches. Atypical antipsychotics generally show beneficial effects on the working memory of patients with schizophrenia, although the results with clozapine are mixed. Cognitive rehabilitation shows promise as an alternative, or supplemental, approach to the pharmacological treatment of cognitive deficits in patients with schizophrenia. Developing more effective treatments for the working memory impairments that accompany schizophrenia remains an important therapeutic goal.

REFERENCES

Abi-Dargham A, Gil R, Krystal J, Baldwin RM, Seibyl JP, Bowers M, van Dyck CH, Charney DS, Innis RB, Laruelle M. Increased striatal dopamine transmission in schizophrenia: confirmation in a second cohort. *Am J Psychiatry*. 1998; 155:761-767.

Abi-Dargham A, Mawlawi O, Lombardo I, Gil R, Martinez D, Huang Y, Hwang DR, Keilp J, Kochan L, Van Heertum R, Gorman JM, Laruelle M. Prefrontal dopamine D1 receptors and working memory in schizophrenia. *J Neurosci*. 2002; 22:3708-3719.

Abi-Dargham A, Rodenhiser J, Printz D, Zea-Ponce Y, Gil R, Kegeles LS, Weiss R, Cooper TB, Mann JJ, Van Heertum RL, Gorman JM, Laruelle M. Increased baseline occupancy of D2 receptors by dopamine in schizophrenia. *Proc Natl Acad Sci U S A*. 2000; 97:8104-8109.

Abi-Dargham A. Do we still believe in the dopamine hypothesis? New data bring new evidence. *Int J Neuropsychopharmacol*. 2004; 7 Suppl 1: S1-5.

Abramczyk RR, Jordan DE, Hegel M. Reverse" Stroop effect in the performance of schizophrenics. *Percept Mot Skills* 1983; 56:99-106.

Addington J, Saeedi H, Addington D. The course of cognitive functioning in first episode psychosis: changes over time and impact on outcome. *Schizophr Res*. 2005; 78: 35-43.

Agartz I, Andersson JL, Skare S. Abnormal brain white matter in schizophrenia: a diffusion tensor imaging study. *Neuroreport* 2001; 12:2251-2254.

Albus M, Hubmann W, Ehrenberg C, Forcht U, Mohr F, Sobizack N, Wahlheim C, Hecht S. Neuropsychological impairment in first-episode and chronic schizophrenic patients. *Eur Arch Psychiatry Clin Neurosci*. 1996; 246: 249-255.

Albus M, Hubmann W, Mohr F, Hecht S, Hinterberger-Weber P, Seitz NN, Küchenhoff H. Neurocognitive functioning in patients with first-episode schizophrenia : results of a prospective 5-year follow-up study. *Eur Arch Psychiatry Clin Neurosci.* 2006; 256: 442-451.

Altamura M, Elvevåg B, Blasi G, Bertolino A, Callicott JH, Weinberger DR, Mattay VS, Goldberg TE. Dissociating the effects of Sternberg working memory demands in prefrontal cortex. *Psychiatry Res* 2007; 154:103-114.

Alves D, Pires MM, Guimarães A, Miranda MC. Four cases of late onset metachromatic leucodystrophy in a family: clinical, biochemical and neuropathological studies. *J Neurol Neurosurg Psychiatry* 1986; 49:1417-1422.

Andreasen NC, Rezai K, Alliger R, Swayze VW 2nd, Flaum M, Kirchner P, Cohen G, O'Leary DS. Hypofrontality in neuroleptic-naive patients and in patients with chronic schizophrenia. Assessment with xenon 133 single-photon emission computed tomography and the Tower of London. *Arch Gen Psychiatry* 1992; 49: 943-958.

Andreasen NC. Linking mind and brain in the study of mental illnesses: a project for a scientific psychopathology. *Science* 1997; 275:1586-1593.

Antonova E, Kumari V, Morris R, Halari R, Anilkumar A, Mehrotra R, Sharma T. The relationship of structural alterations to cognitive deficits in schizophrenia: a voxel-based morphometry study. *Biol Psychiatry* 2005; 58:457-467.

Arnsten AF, Cai JX, Murphy BL, Goldman-Rakic PS. Dopamine D1 receptor mechanisms in the cognitive performance of young adult and aged monkeys. *Psychopharmacology (Berl)* 1994; 116:143-151.

Baddeley A. *Working memory*. Clarendon Press: Oxford. 1986.

Bagary MS, Symms MR, Barker GJ, Mutsatsa SH, Joyce EM, Ron MA. Gray and white matter brain abnormalities in first-episode schizophrenia inferred from magnetization transfer imaging. *Arch Gen Psychiatry* 2003; 60:779-788.

Barch DM, Carter CS, Braver TS, Sabb FW, MacDonald A 3rd, Noll DC, Cohen JD. Selective deficits in prefrontal cortex function in medication-naive patients with schizophrenia.*Arch Gen Psychiatry* 2001; 58:280-288.

Barch DM, Csernansky JG. Abnormal parietal cortex activation during working memory in schizophrenia: verbal phonological coding disturbances versus domain-general executive dysfunction. *Am J Psychiatry* 2007; 164:1090-1098.

Barch DM, Sheline YI, Csernansky JG, Snyder AZ. Working memory and prefrontal cortex dysfunction: specificity to schizophrenia compared with major depression. *Biol Psychiatry* 2003; 53:376-384.

Barker GJ, Tofts PS, Gass A. An interleaved sequence for accurate and reproducible clinical measurement of magnetization transfer ratio. *Magn Reson Imaging* 1996; 14:403-411.

Bearden CE,van Erp,Glahn D,Wang PP,Monterosso JR,zackai E,EmanuelB,Cannon TD.Structural and functional neuroanatomy in the 22q deletion syndrome. *Biol Psychiatry* 2001; 49:19s

Bell M, Bryson G, Greig T, Corcoran C, Wexler BE. Neurocognitive enhancement therapy with work therapy: effects on neuropsychological test performance. *Arch Gen Psychiatry* 2001; 58:763-768.

Bell MD, Zito W, Greig T, Wexler BE. Neurocognitive enhancement therapy with vocational services: work outcomes at two-year follow-up. *Schizophr Res.* 2008; 105:18-29.

Benedict RH, Harris AE, Markow T, McCormick JA, Nuechterlein KH, Asarnow RF. Effects of attention training on information processing in schizophrenia. *Schizophr Bull.* 1994; 20:537-546.

Bodnar M, Malla A, Joober R, Lepage M. Cognitive markers of short-term clinical outcome in first-episode psychosis. *Br J Psychiatry* 2008; 193: 297-304.

Bolden C, Cusack B, Richelson E. Antagonism by antimuscarinic and neuroleptic compounds at the five cloned human muscarinic cholinergic receptors expressed in Chinese hamster ovary cells. *J Pharmacol Exp Ther.* 1992; 260:576-580.

Bosia M, Bechi M, Marino E, Anselmetti S, Poletti S, Cocchi F, Smeraldi E, Cavallaro R. Influence of catechol-O-methyltransferase Val158Met polymorphism on neuropsychological and functional outcomes of classical rehabilitation and cognitive remediation in schizophrenia. *Neurosci Lett.* 2007; 417:271-274.

Brahmbhatt SB, Haut K, Csernansky JG, Barch DM. Neural correlates of verbal and nonverbal working memory deficits in individuals with schizophrenia and their high-risk siblings. *Schizophr Res.* 2006; 87:191-204.

Braw Y, Bloch Y, Mendelovich S, Ratzoni G, Gal G, Harari H, Tripto A, Levkovitz Y. Cognition in young schizophrenia outpatients: comparison of first-episode with multiepisode patients. *Schizophr Bull.* 2008; 34: 544-554.

Breier A, Su TP, Saunders R, Carson RE, Kolachana BS, de Bartolomeis A, Weinberger DR, Weisenfeld N, Malhotra AK, Eckelman WC, Pickar D. Schizophrenia is associated with elevated amphetamine-induced synaptic dopamine concentrations: evidence from a novel positron emission tomography method. *Proc Natl Acad Sci U S A.* 1997; 94:2569-2574.

Brozoski TJ, Brown RM, Rosvold HE, Goldman PS. Cognitive deficit caused by regional depletion of dopamine in prefrontal cortex of rhesus monkey. *Science* 1979; 205:929-931.

Bryson G, Bell M, Lysaker P. Affect recognition in schizophrenia: a function of global impairment or a specific cognitive deficit. *Psychiatry Res.* 1997; 71:105-113.

Buchsbaum MS, Nuechterlein KH, Haier RJ, Wu J, Sicotte N, Hazlett E, Asarnow R, Potkin S, Guich S. Glucose metabolic rate in normals and schizophrenics during the Continuous Performance Test assessed by positron emission tomography. *Br J Psychiatry* 1990; 156:216-227.

Buchsbaum MS, Tang CY, Peled S, Gudbjartsson H, Lu D, Hazlett EA, Downhill J, Haznedar M, Fallon JH, Atlas SW. MRI white matter diffusion anisotropy and PET metabolic rate in schizophrenia. *Neuroreport* 1998; 9:425-430.

Bunge SA, Klingberg T, Jacobsen RB, Gabrieli JD. A resource model of the neural basis of executive working memory. *Proc Natl Acad Sci U S A.* 2000; 97:3573-3578.

Byne W, Kidkardnee S, Tatusov A, Yiannoulos G, Buchsbaum MS, Haroutunian V. Schizophrenia-associated reduction of neuronal and oligodendrocyte numbers in the anterior principal thalamic nucleus. *Schizophr Res.* 2006; 85:245-253.

Cai JX, Arnsten AF. Dose-dependent effects of the dopamine D1 receptor agonists A77636 or SKF81297 on spatial working memory in aged monkeys. *J Pharmacol Exp Ther.* 1997; 283:183-189.

Calhoun VD, Adali T, Pearlson GD, Pekar JJ. A method for making group inferences from functional MRI data using independent component analysis. *Hum Brain Mapp.* 2001; 14:140-151.

Callicott JH, Bertolino A, Mattay VS, Langheim FJ, Duyn J, Coppola R, Goldberg TE, Weinberger DR. Physiological dysfunction of the dorsolateral prefrontal cortex in schizophrenia revisited. *Cereb Cortex* 2000; 10:1078-1092.

Callicott JH, Egan MF, Mattay VS, Bertolino A, Bone AD, Verchinksi B, Weinberger DR. Abnormal fMRI response of the dorsolateral prefrontal cortex in cognitively intact siblings of patients with schizophrenia. *Am J Psychiatry* 2003;160:709-719.

Callicott JH, Mattay VS, Bertolino A, Finn K, Coppola R, Frank JA, Goldberg TE, Weinberger DR. Physiological characteristics of capacity constraints in working memory as revealed by functional MRI. *Cereb Cortex* 1999; 9: 20-26.

Cannon TD, Glahn DC, Kim J, Van Erp TG, Karlsgodt K, Cohen MS, Nuechterlein KH, Bava S, Shirinyan D. Dorsolateral prefrontal cortex activity during maintenance and manipulation of information in working memory in patients with schizophrenia. *Arch Gen Psychiatry* 2005; 62: 1071-1080.

Cannon TD, Huttunen MO, Lonnqvist J, Tuulio-Henriksson A, Pirkola T, Glahn D, Finkelstein J, Hietanen M, Kaprio J, Koskenvuo M. The inheritance of neuropsychological dysfunction in twins discordant for schizophrenia. *Am J Hum Genet.* 2000; 67: 369-382.

Cannon TD, van Erp TG, Huttunen M, Lönnqvist J, Salonen O, Valanne L, Poutanen VP, Standertskjöld-Nordenstam CG, Gur RE, Yan M. Regional gray matter, white matter, and cerebrospinal fluid distributions in schizophrenic patients, their siblings, and controls. *Arch Gen Psychiatry* 1998; 55:1084-1091

Carter C, Robertson L, Nordahl T, Chaderjian M, Kraft L, O'Shora-Celaya L. Spatial working memory deficits and their relationship to negative symptoms in unmedicated schizophrenia patients. *Biol Psychiatry* 1996; 40: 930-932.

Cerizza M, Nemni R, Tamma F. Adult metachromatic leucodystrophy: an underdiagnosed disease? *J Neurol Neurosurg Psychiatry* 1987; 50:1710-1712.

Cervellione KL, Burdick KE, Cottone JG, Rhinewine JP, Kumra S. Neurocognitive deficits in adolescents with schizophrenia: longitudinal stability and predictive utility for short-term functional outcome. *J Am Acad Child Adolesc Psychiatry* 2007; 46: 867-878.

Chambers JS, Perrone-Bizzozero NI. Altered myelination of the hippocampal formation in subjects with schizophrenia and bipolar disorder. *Neurochem Res.* 2004; 29:2293-2302.

Chein JM, Fiez JA. Dissociation of verbal working memory system components using a delayed serial recall task. *Cereb Cortex* 2001; 11:1003-1014.

Chey J, Lee J, Kim YS, Kwon SM, Shin YM. Spatial working memory span, delayed response and executive function in schizophrenia. *Psychiatry Res.* 2002; 110: 259-271.

Conklin HM, Curtis CE, Calkins ME, Iacono WG. Working memory functioning in schizophrenia patients and their first-degree relatives: cognitive functioning shedding light on etiology. *Neuropsychologia* 2005; 43: 930-942.

Conklin HM, Curtis CE, Katsanis J, Iacono WG. Verbal working memory impairment in schizophrenia patients and their first-degree relatives: evidence from the digit span task. *Am J Psychiatry* 2000; 157: 275-277.

Corbetta M, Burton H, Sinclair RJ, Conturo TE, Akbudak E, McDonald JW. Functional reorganization and stability of somatosensory-motor cortical topography in a tetraplegic subject with late recovery. *Proc Natl Acad Sci U S A*. 2002; 99:17066-17071.

Currie J, Joyce S, Maruff P, Ramsden B, McArthur-Jackson C, Malone V. Selective impairment of express saccade generation in patients with schizophrenia. *Exp Brain Res.* 1993; 97: 343-348.

Curtis CE, D'Esposito M. The effects of prefrontal lesions on working memory performance and theory. *Cogn Affect Behav Neurosci.* 2004; 4:528-539.

Daniel DG, Weinberger DR, Jones DW, Zigun JR, Coppola R, Handel S, Bigelow LB, Goldberg TE, Berman KF, Kleinman JE. The effect of amphetamine on regional cerebral blood flow during cognitive activation in schizophrenia. *J Neurosci.* 1991; 11:1907-1917.

DeFreitas CM, Dunaway LA, Torres IJ. Preferential semantic fluency impairment is related to hallucinations, but not formal thought disorder. *Schizophr Res.* 2009; 107: 307-312.

Delahunty A, Morice R. Rehabilitation of frontal/executive impairments in schizophrenia. *Aust N Z J Psychiatry* 1996; 30: 760-767.

Dickinson D, Tenhula W, Morris S, Brown C, Peer J, Spencer K, Li L, Gold JM, Bellack AS. A randomized, controlled trial of computer-assisted cognitive remediation for schizophrenia. *Am J Psychiatry* 2010; 167:170-180.

Diforio D, Walker EF, Kestler LP. Executive functions in adolescents with schizotypal personality disorder. *Schizophr Res.* 2000; 42: 125-134.

Dolan RJ, Fletcher P, Frith CD, Friston KJ, Frackowiak RS, Grasby PM. Dopaminergic modulation of impaired cognitive activation in the anterior cingulate cortex in schizophrenia. *Nature* 1995; 378:180-182.

Drew MR, Simpson EH, Kellendonk C, Herzberg WG, Lipatova O, Fairhurst S, Kandel ER, Malapani C, Balsam PD. Transient overexpression of striatal D2 receptors impairs operant motivation and interval timing. *J Neurosci.* 2007; 27:7731-7739.

Duval J, Coyette F, Seron X. Rehabilitation of the central executive component of working memory: a re-organisation approach applied to a single case. *Neuropsychol Rehabil.* 2008; 18:430-460.

Eliez S, Antonarakis SE, Morris MA, Dahoun SP, Reiss AL. Parental origin of the deletion 22q11.2 and brain development in velocardiofacial syndrome: a preliminary study. *Arch Gen Psychiatry* 2001; 58:64-68.

Eliez S, Schmitt JE, White CD, Reiss AL. Children and adolescents with velocardiofacial syndrome: a volumetric MRI study. *Am J Psychiatry* 2000; 157:409-415.

Elliott R. Executive functions and their disorders. *Br Med Bull.* 2003; 65: 49-59.

Everett J, Laplante L, Thomas J. The selective attention deficit in schizophrenia. Limited resources or cognitive fatigue? *J Nerv Ment Dis.* 1989; 177: 735-738.

Fagerlund B, Pagsberg AK, Hemmingsen RP. Cognitive deficits and levels of IQ in adolescent onset schizophrenia and other psychotic disorders. *Schizophr Res.* 2006; 85:30-39.

Fahim C, Stip E, Mancini-Marïe A, Gendron A, Mensour B, Beauregard M. Differential hemodynamic brain activity in schizophrenia patients with blunted affect during quetiapine treatment. *J Clin Psychopharmacol.* 2005; 25:367-371.

Farmer CM, O'Donnell BF, Niznikiewicz MA, Voglmaier MM, McCarley RW, Shenton ME. Visual perception and working memory in schizotypal personality disorder. *Am J Psychiatry* 2000; 157:781-786.

Field CD, Gallety C, Anderson D, Walker P. Computer-aided cognitive rehabilitation: possible application to the attentional deficit of schizophrenia, a report of negative results. *Percept Mot Skills* 1997; 85:995-1002.

Fiez JA, Raife EA, Balota DA, Schwarz JP, Raichle ME, Petersen SE. A positron emission tomography study of the short-term maintenance of verbal information. *J Neurosci.* 1996; 16:808-822.

Finelli PF. Metachromatic leukodystrophy manifesting as a schizophrenic disorder: computed tomographic correlation. *Ann Neurol.* 1985;18:94-95.

Fisher M, Holland C, Merzenich MM, Vinogradov S. Using neuroplasticity-based auditory training to improve verbal memory in schizophrenia. *Am J Psychiatry* 2009; 166:805-811.

Fleming K, Goldberg TE, Binks S, Randolph C, Gold JM, Weinberger DR. Visuospatial working memory in patients with schizophrenia. *Biol Psychiatry* 1997; 41: 43-49.

Flynn SW, Lang DJ, Mackay AL, Goghari V, Vavasour IM, Whittall KP, Smith GN, Arango V, Mann JJ, Dwork AJ, Falkai P, Honer WG. Abnormalities of myelination in schizophrenia detected in vivo with MRI, and post-mortem with analysis of oligodendrocyte proteins. *Mol Psychiatry* 2003; 8:811-820.

Foong J, Maier M, Barker GJ, Brocklehurst S, Miller DH, Ron MA. In vivo investigation of white matter pathology in schizophrenia with magnetisation transfer imaging. *J Neurol Neurosurg Psychiatry* 2000; 68:70-74.

Foong J, Symms MR, Barker GJ, Maier M, Woermann FG, Miller DH, Ron MA. Neuropathological abnormalities in schizophrenia: evidence from magnetization transfer imaging. *Brain* 2001; 124:882-892.

Forbes NF, Carrick LA, McIntosh AM, Lawrie SM. Working memory in schizophrenia: a meta-analysis. *Psychol Med.* 2009; 39: 889-905.

Fox CA, Mansour A, Watson SJ Jr. The effects of haloperidol on dopamine receptor gene expression. *Exp Neurol.* 1994; 130:288-303.

Frangou S, Hadjulis M, Vourdas A. The Maudsley early onset schizophrenia study: cognitive function over a 4-year follow-up period. *Schizophr Bull.* 2008; 34: 52-59.

Franke P, Maier W, Hain C, Klingler T. Wisconsin Card Sorting Test: an indicator of vulnerability to schizophrenia? *Schizophr Res.* 1992; 6:243-249.

Fukushima J, Fukushima K, Chiba T, Tanaka S, Yamashita I, Kato M. Disturbances of voluntary control of saccadic eye movements in schizophrenic patients. *Biol Psychiatry* 1988; 23: 670-677.

Glahn DC, Therman S, Manninen M, Huttunen M, Kaprio J, Lönnqvist J, Cannon TD. Spatial working memory as an endophenotype for schizophrenia. *Biol Psychiatry* 2003; 53: 624-626.

Gold JM, Carpenter C, Randolph C, Goldberg TE, Weinberger DR. Auditory working memory and Wisconsin Card Sorting Test performance in schizophrenia. *Arch Gen Psychiatry* 1997; 54: 159-165.

Goldman-Rakic PS, Muly EC 3rd, Williams GV. D(1) receptors in prefrontal cells and circuits. *Brain Res Brain Res Rev.* 2000; 31:295-301.

Goldman-Rakic PS, Selemon LD. Functional and anatomical aspects of prefrontal pathology in schizophrenia. *Schizophr Bull.* 1997; 23:437-458.

Goldman-Rakic PS. The physiological approach: functional architecture of working memory and disordered cognition in schizophrenia. *Biol Psychiatry* 1999; 46: 650-661.

Goldman-Rakic PS. Working memory dysfunction in schizophrenia. *J Neuropsychiatry Clin Neurosci.* 1994; 6:348-357.

Gray JA, Roth BL. Molecular targets for treating cognitive dysfunction in schizophrenia. *Schizophr Bull.* 2007; 33:1100-1119.

Green MF, Kern RS, Braff DL, Mintz J: Neurocognitive deficits and functional outcome in schizophrenia: are we measuring the "right stuff?" *Schizophr Bull.* 2000; 26:119–136.

Gregg JR, Herring NR, Naydenov AV, Hanlin RP, Konradi C. Downregulation of oligodendrocyte transcripts is associated with impaired prefrontal cortex function in rats. *Schizophr. Res.* 2009; 113: 277–287.

Grynszpan O, Perbal S, Pelissolo A, Fossati P, Jouvent R, Dubal S, Perez-Diaz F. Efficacy and specificity of computer-assisted cognitive remediation in schizophrenia: a meta-analytical study. *Psychol Med.* 2010; 12:1-11.

Guo N, Hwang D, Abdellhadi S, Abi-Dargham A, Zarahn E, Laruelle M. The effect of chronic DA depletion on D1 ligand binding in rodent brain. *Soc Neurosci Abstr.* 2001; 27: 238.10.

Hageman AT, Gabreëls FJ, de Jong JG, Gabreëls-Festen AA, van den Berg CJ, van Oost BA, Wevers RA. Clinical symptoms of adult metachromatic leukodystrophy and arylsulfatase A pseudodeficiency. *Arch Neurol.* 1995;52:408-413.

Hagger C, Buckley P, Kenny JT, Friedman L, Ubogy D, Meltzer HY. Improvement in cognitive functions and psychiatric symptoms in treatment-refractory schizophrenic patients receiving clozapine. *Biol Psychiatry* 1993; 34:702-712.

Heaton R. In: *Wisconsin Card Sorting Test Manual Revised and Expanded*, Psychological Assessment Resources, Inc., Odessa, Fla. 1993.

Heinrichs RW, Zakzanis KK. Neurocognitive deficit in schizophrenia: a quantitative review of the evidence. *Neuropsychology* 1998; 12:426-445.

Helldin L, Kane JM, Karilampi U, Norlander T, Archer T. Remission and cognitive ability in a cohort of patients with schizophrenia. *J Psychiatr Res.* 2006; 40:738-745.

Henseler I, Falkai P, Gruber O. A systematic fMRI investigation of the brain systems subserving different working memory components in schizophrenia. *Eur J Neurosci.* 2009; 30: 693-702.

Henseler I, Falkai P, Gruber O. Disturbed functional connectivity within brain networks subserving domain-specific subcomponents of working memory in schizophrenia: relation to performance and clinical symptoms. *J Psychiatr Res.* 2010; 44:364-372.

Hess EJ, Norman AB, Creese I. Chronic treatment with dopamine receptor antagonists: behavioral and pharmacologic effects on D1 and D2 dopamine receptors. *J Neurosci.* 1988; 8:2361-2370.

Hill SK, Beers SR, Kmiec JA, Keshavan MS, Sweeney JA. Impairment of verbal memory and learning in antipsychotic-naïve patients with first-episode schizophrenia. *Schizophr Res.* 2004; 68:127-136.

Hodge MA, Siciliano D, Withey P, Moss B, Moore G, Judd G, Shores EA, Harris A. A randomized controlled trial of cognitive remediation in schizophrenia. *Schizophr Bull.* 2010; 36:419-427.

Hof PR, Haroutunian V, Friedrich VL Jr, Byne W, Buitron C, Perl DP, Davis KL. Loss and altered spatial distribution of oligodendrocytes in the superior frontal gyrus in schizophrenia. *Biol Psychiatry* 2003; 53:1075-1085.

Hofer A, Baumgartner S, Bodner T, Edlinger M, Hummer M, Kemmler G, Rettenbacher MA, Fleischhacker WW. Patient outcomes in schizophrenia II: the impact of cognition. *Eur Psychiatry* 2005; 20: 395-402.

Hogarty GE, Flesher S, Ulrich R, Carter M, Greenwald D, Pogue-Geile M, Kechavan M, Cooley S, DiBarry AL, Garrett A, Parepally H, Zoretich R. Cognitive enhancement therapy for schizophrenia: effects of a 2-year randomized trial on cognition and behavior. *Arch Gen Psychiatry* 2004; 61:866-876.

Hommer DW, Clem T, Litman R, Pickar D. Maladaptive anticipatory saccades in schizophrenia. *Biol Psychiatry* 1991; 30:779-794.

Honer WG, Falkai P, Chen C, Arango V, Mann JJ, Dwork AJ. Synaptic and plasticity-associated proteins in anterior frontal cortex in severe mental illness. *Neuroscience* 1999; 91:1247-1255.

Honey GD, Bullmore ET, Sharma T. De-coupling of cognitive performance and cerebral functional response during working memory in schizophrenia. *Schizophr Res.* 2002; 53:45-56.

Honey GD, Bullmore ET, Soni W, Varatheesan M, Williams SC, Sharma T. Differences in frontal cortical activation by a working memory task after substitution of risperidone for typical antipsychotic drugs in patients with schizophrenia. *Proc Natl Acad Sci U S A.* 1999; 96:13432-13437.

Hulshoff Pol HE, Brans RG, van Haren NE, Schnack HG, Langen M, Baaré WF, van Oel CJ, Kahn RS. Gray and white matter volume abnormalities in monozygotic and same-gender dizygotic twins discordant for schizophrenia. *Biol Psychiatry* 2004; 55:126-130.

Jansma JM, Ramsey NF, Van Der Wee NJA, Kahn RS. Working memory capacity in schizophrenia: A parametric fMRI study. *Schizophr Res.* 2004; 68: 159-171.

Johnson MR, Morris NA, Astur RS, Calhoun VD, Mathalon DH, Kiehl KA, Pearlson GD. A functional magnetic resonance imaging study of working memory abnormalities in schizophrenia. *Biol Psychiatry* 2006; 60: 11-21.

Jones HM, Brammer MJ, O'Toole M, Taylor T, Ohlsen RI, Brown RG, Purvis R, Williams S, Pilowsky LS. Cortical effects of quetiapine in first-episode schizophrenia: a preliminary functional magnetic resonance imaging study. *Biol Psychiatry* 2004; 56: 938-942.

Jonides J, Schumacher EH, Smith EE, Koeppe RA, Awh E, Reuter-Lorenz PA, Marshuetz C, Willis CR. The role of parietal cortex in verbal working memory. *J Neurosci.* 1998; 18:5026-5034.

Kates WR, Burnette CP, Jabs EW, Rutberg J, Murphy AM, Grados M, Geraghty M, Kaufmann WE, Pearlson GD. Regional cortical white matter reductions in velocardiofacial syndrome: a volumetric MRI analysis. *Biol Psychiatry* 2001; 49:677-684.

Kellendonk C, Simpson EH, Polan HJ, Malleret G, Vronskaya S, Winiger V, Moore H, Kandel ER. Transient and selective overexpression of dopamine D2 receptors in the striatum causes persistent abnormalities in prefrontal cortex functioning. *Neuron* 2006; 49:603-615.

Kerns JG, Berenbaum H, Barch DM, Banich MT, Stolar N. Word production in schizophrenia and its relationship to positive symptoms. *Psychiatry Res.* 1999; 87: 29-37.

Kerns JG, Berenbaum H. Cognitive impairments associated with formal thought disorder in people with schizophrenia. *J Abnorm Psychol.* 2002; 111: 211-224.

Kim DII, Manoach DS, Mathalon DH, Turner JA, Mannell M, Brown GG, Ford JM, Gollub RL, White T, Wible C, Belger A, Bockholt HJ, Clark VP, Lauriello J, O'Leary D, Mueller BA, Lim KO, Andreasen N, Potkin SG, Calhoun VD. Dysregulation of working memory and default-mode networks in schizophrenia using independent component analysis, an fBIRN and MCIC study. *Hum Brain Mapp.* 2009; 30:3795-3811.

Kim JJ, Kwon JS, Park HJ, Youn T, Kang DH, Kim MS, Lee DS, Lee MC. Functional disconnection between the prefrontal and parietal cortices during working memory processing in schizophrenia: a[15(O)]H2O PET study. *Am J Psychiatry* 2003; 160:919-923.

Kindermann SS, Brown GG, Zorrilla LE, Olsen RK, Jeste DV. Spatial working memory among middle-aged and older patients with schizophrenia and volunteers using fMRI. *Schizophr Res.* 2004; 68: 203-216.

Kohler CG, Bilker W, Hagendoorn M, Gur RE, Gur RC. Emotion recognition deficit in schizophrenia: association with symptomatology and cognition. *Biol Psychiatry* 2000; 48: 127-136.

Kubicki M, McCarley R, Westin CF, Park HJ, Maier S, Kikinis R, Jolesz FA, Shenton ME. A review of diffusion tensor imaging studies in schizophrenia. *J Psychiatr Res.* 2007; 41:15-30.

Kumra S, Wiggs E, Bedwell J, Smith AK, Arling E, Albus K, Hamburger SD, McKenna K, Jacobsen LK, Rapoport JL, Asarnow RF. Neuropsychological deficits in pediatric patients with childhood-onset schizophrenia and psychotic disorder not otherwise specified. *Schizophr Res.* 2000; 42: 135-144.

Kurtz MM, Seltzer JC, Shagan DS, Thime WR, Wexler BE. Computer-assisted cognitive remediation in schizophrenia: what is the active ingredient? *Schizophr Res.* 2007; 89:251-260.

Kurtz MM. Neurocognitive rehabilitation for schizophrenia. *Curr Psychiatry Rep.* 2003; 5:303-310.

Lappalainen J, Hietala J, Koulu M, Seppälä T, Sjöholm B, Syvälahti E. Chronic treatment with SCH 23390 and haloperidol: effects on dopaminergic and serotonergic mechanisms in rat brain. *J Pharmacol Exp Ther.* 1990; 252:845-852.

Laruelle M, Innis RB. Images in neuroscience. SPECT imaging of synaptic dopamine. *Am J Psychiatry* 1996; 153:1249.

Laruelle M. Imaging dopamine transmission in schizophrenia. A review and meta-analysis. *Q J Nucl Med.* 1998; 42: 211-221.

Lee SJ, Lee HK, Kweon YS, Lee CT, Lee KU. The impact of executive function on emotion recognition and emotion experience in patients with schizophrenia. *Psychiatry Invest.* 2009; 6:156-162.

Levaux MN, Vezzaro J, Larøi F, Offerlin-Meyer I, Danion JM, Van der Linden M. Cognitive rehabilitation of the updating sub-component of working memory in schizophrenia: a case study. *Neuropsychol Rehabil.* 2009; 19:244-273.

Lidow MS, Elsworth JD, Goldman-Rakic PS. Down-regulation of the D1 and D5 dopamine receptors in the primate prefrontal cortex by chronic treatment with antipsychotic drugs. *J Pharmacol Exp Ther.* 1997; 281:597-603.

Lidow MS, Goldman-Rakic PS, Gallager DW, Rakic P. Distribution of dopaminergic receptors in the primate cerebral cortex: quantitative autoradiographic analysis using [3H]raclopride, [3H]spiperone and [3H]SCH23390. *Neuroscience* 1991; 40:657-671.

Lieberman JA, Perkins D, Belger A, Chakos M, Jarskog F, Boteva K, Gilmore J. The early stages of schizophrenia: speculations on pathogenesis, pathophysiology, and therapeutic approaches. *Biol Psychiatry* 2001; 50: 884-897.

Lim KO, Hedehus M, Moseley M, de Crespigny A, Sullivan EV, Pfefferbaum A. Compromised white matter tract integrity in schizophrenia inferred from diffusion tensor imaging. *Arch Gen Psychiatry* 1999; 56:367-374.

Luciana M, Collins PF, Depue RA. Opposing roles for dopamine and serotonin in the modulation of human spatial working memory functions. *Cereb Cortex* 1998; 8:218-226.

Luciana M, Collins PF. Dopaminergic modulation of working memory for spatial but not object cues in normal humans. *J Cogn Neurosci.* 1997; 9: 330-347.

Luciana M, Depue RA, Arbisi P, Leon A. Facilitation of working memory in humans by a D2 dopamine receptor agonist. 1992; *J Cogn Neurosci.* 4:58-68.

MacKenzie RG, Zigmond MJ. Chronic neuroleptic treatment increases D-2 but not D-1 receptors in rat striatum. *Eur J Pharmacol.* 1985; 113:159-165.

Mahurin RK, Velligan DI, Miller AL. Executive-frontal lobe cognitive dysfunction in schizophrenia: a symptom subtype analysis. *Psychiatry Res* 1998; 79: 139-149.

Manoach DS, Gollub RL, Benson ES, Searl MM, Goff DC, Halpern E, Saper CB, Rauch SL. Schizophrenic subjects show aberrant fMRI activation of dorsolateral prefrontal cortex and basal ganglia during working memory performance. *Biol Psychiatry* 2000; 48:99-109.

Manoach DS, Greve DN, Lindgren KA, Dale AM. Identifying regional activity associated with temporally separated components of working memory using event-related functional MRI. *Neuroimage* 2003; 20:1670-1684.

Manoach DS, Press DZ, Thangaraj V, Searl MM, Goff DC, Halpern E, Saper CB, Warach S. Schizophrenic subjects activate dorsolateral prefrontal cortex during a working memory task, as measured by fMRI. *Biol Psychiatry* 1999; 45:1128-1137.

Marshuetz C, Smith EE, Jonides J, DeGutis J, Chenevert TL. Order information in working memory: fMRI evidence for parietal and prefrontal mechanisms. *J Cogn Neurosci.* 2000; 12 Suppl 2:130-144.

Matsushima GK, Morell P. The neurotoxicant, cuprizone, as a model to study demyelination and remyelination in the central nervous system. *Brain Pathology* 2001; 11: 107–116.

McDonald C, Bullmore E, Sham P, Chitnis X, Suckling J, MacCabe J, Walshe M, Murray RM. Regional volume deviations of brain structure in schizophrenia and psychotic bipolar disorder: computational morphometry study. *Br J Psychiatry* 2005; 186:369-377.

McGurk SR, Carter C, Goldman R, Green MF, Marder SR, Xie H, Schooler NR, Kane JM. The effects of clozapine and risperidone on spatial working memory in schizophrenia. *Am J Psychiatry* 2005; 162:1013-1016.

McGurk SR, Twamley EW, Sitzer DI, McHugo GJ, Mueser KT. A meta-analysis of cognitive remediation in schizophrenia. *Am J Psychiatry* 2007; 164:1791-1802.

McIntosh AM, Job DE, Moorhead TW, Harrison LK, Lawrie SM, Johnstone EC. White matter density in patients with schizophrenia, bipolar disorder and their unaffected relatives. *Biol Psychiatry* 2005; 58:254-257.

McKeown MJ, Sejnowski TJ. Independent component analysis of fMRI data: examining the assumptions. *Hum Brain Mapp.* 1998; 6:368-372.

Meda SA, Bhattarai M, Morris NA, Astur RS, Calhoun VD, Mathalon DH, Kiehl KA, Pearlson GD. An fMRI study of working memory in first-degree unaffected relatives of schizophrenia patients.*Schizophr Res.* 2008; 104:85-95.

Meda SA, Stevens MC, Folley BS, Calhoun VD, Pearlson GD. Evidence for anomalous network connectivity during working memory encoding in schizophrenia: an ICA based analysis. *PLoS One* 2009; 4:e7911.

Medalia A, Choi J. Cognitive remediation in schizophrenia. *Neuropsychol Rev*. 2009; 19: 353-364.

Medalia A, Revheim N, Casey M. Remediation of memory disorders in schizophrenia. *Psychol Med*. 2000; 30:1451-1459.

Medalia A, Revheim N, Casey M. Remediation of problem-solving skills in schizophrenia: evidence of a persistent effect. *Schizophr Res*. 2002; 57:165-171.

Medalia A, Revheim N, Casey M. The remediation of problem-solving skills in schizophrenia. *Schizophr Bull*. 2001; 27:259-267.

Mehta MA, Manes FF, Magnolfi G, Sahakian BJ, Robbins TW. Impaired set-shifting and dissociable effects on tests of spatial working memory following the dopamine D2 receptor antagonist sulpiride in human volunteers. *Psychopharmacology*. 2004; 176: 331-342.

Mehta MA, Sahakian BJ, McKenna PJ, Robbins TW. Systemic sulpiride in young adult volunteers simulates the profile of cognitive deficits in Parkinson's disease. *Psychopharmacology (Berl)*. 1999; 146: 162-174.

Mehta MA, Swainson R, Ogilvie AD, Sahakian J, Robbins TW. Improved short-term spatial memory but impaired reversal learning following the dopamine D(2) agonist bromocriptine in human volunteers. *Psychopharmacology (Berl)* 2001; 159:10-20.

Meisenzahl EM, Scheuerecker J, Zipse M, Ufer S, Wiesmann M, Frodl T, Koutsouleris N, Zetzsche T, Schmitt G, Riedel M, Spellmann I, Dehning S, Linn J, Brückmann H, Möller HJ. Effects of treatment with the atypical neuroleptic quetiapine on working memory function: a functional MRI follow-up investigation. *Eur Arch Psychiatry Clin Neurosci*. 2006; 256: 522-531.

Meltzer HY, McGurk SR. The effects of clozapine, risperidone, and olanzapine on cognitive function in schizophrenia. *Schizophr Bull*. 1999; 25: 233-255.

Menon V., Anagnoson R.T., Mathalon D.H., Glover G.H., Pfefferbaum A. Functional neuroanatomy of auditory working memory in schizophrenia: Relation to positive and negative symptoms. *NeuroImage* 2001; 13 : 433-446.

Meyer-Lindenberg A, Poline JB, Kohn PD, Holt JL, Egan MF, Weinberger DR, Berman KF. Evidence for abnormal cortical functional connectivity during working memory in schizophrenia. *Am J Psychiatry* 2001; 158:1809-1817.

Mitelman SA, Shihabuddin L, Brickman AM, Hazlett EA, Buchsbaum MS. MRI assessment of gray and white matter distribution in Brodmann's areas of the cortex in patients with schizophrenia with good and poor outcomes. *Am J Psychiatry* 2003; 160:2154-2168.

Mitropoulou V, Harvey PD, Maldari LA, Moriarty PJ, New AS, Silverman JM, Siever LJ. Neuropsychological performance in schizotypal personality disorder: evidence regarding diagnostic specificity. *Biol Psychiatry* 2002; 52:1175-1182.

Mitropoulou V, Harvey PD, Zegarelli G, New AS, Silverman JM, Siever LJ. Neuropsychological performance in schizotypal personality disorder: importance of working memory. *Am J Psychiatry* 2005; 162:1896-1903.

Morice R, Delahunty A. Frontal/executive impairments in schizophrenia. *Schizophr Bull*. 1996; 22:125-137.

Morice R. Cognitive inflexibility and pre-frontal dysfunction in schizophrenia and mania. *Br J Psychiatry* 1990; 157: 50-54.

Moritz S, Krausz M, Gottwalz E, Lambert M, Perro C, Ganzer S, Naber D. Cognitive dysfunction at baseline predicts symptomatic 1-year outcome in first-episode schizophrenics. *Psychopathology* 2000; 33:48-51.

Morrison-Stewart SL, Williamson PC, Corning WC, Kutcher SP, Snow WG, Merskey H. Frontal and non-frontal lobe neuropsychological test performance and clinical symptomatology in schizophrenia. *Psychol Med.* 1992; 22:353-359.

Müller U, Werheid K, Hammerstein E, Jungmann S, Becker T. Prefrontal cognitive deficits in patients with schizophrenia treated with atypical or conventional antipsychotics. *Eur Psychiatry* 2005; 20:70-73.

Nestor P.G., Shenton M.E., Wible C., Hokama H., O'Donnell B.F., Law S., McCarley R.W. A neuropsychological analysis of schizophrenic thought disorder. *Schizophr Res.* 1998; 29: 217-225.

Oie M, Rund BR. Neuropsychological deficits in adolescent-onset schizophrenia compared with attention deficit hyperactivity disorder. *Am J Psychiatry* 1999; 156: 1216-1222.

Oie M, Sundet K, Rund BR. Neurocognitive decline in early-onset schizophrenia compared with ADHD and normal controls: evidence from a 13-year follow-up study. *Schizophr Bull.* 2010; 36: 557-565.

Okubo Y, Suhara T, Suzuki K, Kobayashi K, Inoue O, Terasaki O, Someya Y, Sassa T, Sudo Y, Matsushima E, Iyo M, Tateno Y, Toru M. Decreased prefrontal dopamine D1 receptors in schizophrenia revealed by PET. *Nature* 1997; 385:634-636.

Orlovskaya DD, Denisov DV, Uranova NA.The ultrastructural pathology of myelinated fibers and oligodendroglial cells in autopsied caudate nucleus of schizophrenics. *Schizophr Res.*1997; 24:39-40.

Paillère-Martinot M, Caclin A, Artiges E, Poline JB, Joliot M, Mallet L, Recasens C, Attar-Lévy D, Martinot JL. Cerebral gray and white matter reductions and clinical correlates in patients with early onset schizophrenia. *Schizophr Res.* 2001; 50:19-26.

Park S, Holzman PS, Goldman-Rakic PS. Spatial working memory deficits in the relatives of schizophrenic patients. *Arch Gen Psychiatry* 1995; 52: 821-828.

Park S, Holzman PS. Association of working memory deficit and eye tracking dysfunction in schizophrenia. *Schizophr Res.* 1993; 11: 55-61.

Park S, Holzman PS. Schizophrenics show spatial working memory deficits. *Arch Gen Psychiatry* 1992; 49:975-982.

Park S, Püschel J, Sauter BH, Rentsch M, Hell D. Spatial working memory deficits and clinical symptoms in schizophrenia: a 4-months follow-up study. *Biol Psychiatry* 1999; 46: 392-400.

Park S, Püschel J, Sauter BH, Rentsch M, Hell D. Visual object working memory function and clinical symptoms in schizophrenia. *Schizophr Res.* 2002; 59: 261-268.

Peers PV, Ludwig CJ, Rorden C, Cusack R, Bonfiglioli C, Bundesen C, Driver J, Antoun N, Duncan J. Attentional functions of parietal and frontal cortex. *Cereb Cortex* 2005; 15:1469-1484.

Perlstein WM, Carter CS, Noll DC, Cohen JD. Relation of prefrontal cortex dysfunction to working memory and symptoms in schizophrenia. *Am J Psychiatry* 2001; 158:1105-1113.

Perry W, Heaton RK, Potterat E, Roebuck T, Minassian A, Braff DL.Working memory in schizophrenia: transient "online" storage versus executive functioning. *Schizophr Bull.* 2001; 27:157-176.

Petrides M, Alivisatos B, Evans AC, Meyer E. Dissociation of human mid-dorsolateral from posterior dorsolateral frontal cortex in memory processing. *Proc Natl Acad Sci U S A* 1993; 90: 873-877.

Plum F, Mountcastle V(Eds). Handbook of physiology. Betheda, MD: *American Physiological Society*, pp. 373-417, 1987.

Postle BR, Awh E, Jonides J, Smith EE, D'Esposito M. The where and how of attention-based rehearsal in spatial working memory. *Brain Res Cogn Brain Res.* 2004; 20:194-205.

Potkin SG, Turner JA, Brown GG, McCarthy G, Greve DN, Glover GH, Manoach DS, Belger A, Diaz M, Wible CG, Ford JM, Mathalon DH, Gollub R, Lauriello J, O'Leary D, van Erp TG, Toga AW, Preda A, Lim KO; FBIRN. Working memory and DLPFC inefficiency in schizophrenia: the FBIRN study. *Schizophr Bull.* 2009; 35:19-31.

Purdon SE, Malla A, Labelle A, Lit W. Neuropsychological change in patients with schizophrenia after treatment with quetiapine or haloperidol. *J Psychiatry Neurosci.* 2001; 26:137-149.

Rajji TK, Uchida H, Ismail Z, Ng W, Mamo DC, Remington G, Pollock BG, Mulsant BH. Clozapine and global cognition in schizophrenia. *J Clin Psychopharmacol.* 2010; 30:431-436.

Ravizza SM, Delgado MR, Chein JM, Becker JT, Fiez JA. Functional dissociations within the inferior parietal cortex in verbal working memory. *Neuroimage* 2004; 22:562-573.

Remington LT, Babcock AA, Zehntner SP, Owens T. Microglial recruitment, activation, and proliferation in response to primary demyelination. *American Journal of Pathology* 2007; 170: 1713–1724.

Sachs G, Steger-Wuchse D, Kryspin-Exner I, Gur RC, Katschnig H. Facial recognition deficits and cognition in schizophrenia. *Schizophr Res.* 2004; 68:27-35.

Sanfilipo M, Lafargue T, Rusinek H, Arena L, Loneragan C, Lautin A, Feiner D, Rotrosen J, Wolkin A. Volumetric measure of the frontal and temporal lobe regions in schizophrenia: relationship to negative symptoms. *Arch Gen Psychiatry* 2000; 57:471-480.

Sartory G, Zorn C, Groetzinger G, Windgassen K. Computerized cognitive remediation improves verbal learning and processing speed in schizophrenia. *Schizophr Res.* 2005; 75:219-223.

Saykin AJ, Gur RC, Gur RE, Mozley PD, Mozley LH, Resnick SM, Kester DB, Stafiniak P. Neuropsychological function in schizophrenia. Selective impairment in memory and learning. *Arch Gen Psychiatry* 1991; 48: 618-624.

Saykin AJ, Shtasel DL, Gur RE, Kester DB, Mozley LH, Stafiniak P, Gur RC. Neuropsychological deficits in neuroleptic naive patients with first-episode schizophrenia. *Arch Gen Psychiatry* 1994; 51:124-131.

Schlagenhauf F, Dinges M, Beck A, Wüstenberg T, Friedel E, Dembler T, Sarkar R, Wrase J, Gallinat J, Juckel G, Heinz A. Switching schizophrenia patients from typical neuroleptics to aripiprazole: effects on working memory dependent functional activation. *Schizophr Res.* 2010; 118:189-200.

Schlosser R, Gesierich T, Kaufmann B, Vucurevic G, Hunsche S, Gawehn J, Stoeter P. Altered effective connectivity during working memory performance in schizophrenia: A study with fMRI and structural equation modeling. *NeuroImage* 2003; 19: 751-763.

Schneider JS, Sun ZQ, Roeltgen DP. Effects of dihydrexidine, a full dopamine D-1 receptor agonist, on delayed response performance in chronic low dose MPTP-treated monkeys. *Brain Res.* 1994; 663:140-144.

Schooler C, Neumann E, Caplan LJ, Roberts BR. A time course analysis of Stroop interference and facilitation: comparing normal individuals and individuals with schizophrenia. *J Exp Psychol Gen.* 1997; 126:19-36.

Seamans JK, Yang CR. The principal features and mechanisms of dopamine modulation in the prefrontal cortex. *Prog Neurobiol.* 2004; 74:1-58.

Sedvall G, Farde L. Dopamine receptors in schizophrenia. *Lancet* 1996; 347:264.

Seidman LJ, Talbot NL, Kalinowski AG, McCarley RW, Faraone SV, Kremen WS, Pepple JR, Tsuang MT. Neuropsychological probes of fronto-limbic system dysfunction in schizophrenia. Olfactory identification and Wisconsin Card Sorting performance. *Schizophr Res.* 1991; 6:55-65.

Selvaraju R, Bernasconi L, Losberger C, Graber P, Kadi L, Avellana-Adalid V, et al. Osteopontin is upregulated during in vivo demyelination and remyelination and enhances myelin formation in vitro. *Mol Cell Neurosci.* 2004; 25: 707–721.

Siever LJ, Koenigsberg HW, Harvey P, Mitropoulou V, Laruelle M, Abi-Dargham A, Goodman M, Buchsbaum M. Cognitive and brain function in schizotypal personality disorder. *Schizophr Res.* 2002; 54:157-167.

Sigmundsson T, Suckling J, Maier M, Williams S, Bullmore E, Greenwood K, Fukuda R, Ron M, Toone B. Structural abnormalities in frontal, temporal, and limbic regions and interconnecting white matter tracts in schizophrenic patients with prominent negative symptoms. *Am J Psychiatry* 2001; 158:234-243.

Silver H, Goodman C, Bilker WB, Knoll G, Gur R, Povar G. Suboptimal processing strategy and working-memory impairments predict abstraction deficit in schizophrenia. *J Clin Exp Neuropsychol.* 2007; 29:823-830.

Silver H., Feldman P., Bilker W., Gur R. C. Working memory deficit as a core neuropsychological dysfunction in schizophrenia. *Am J Psychiatry* 2003; 160: 1809-1816.

Smith EE, Jonides J. Storage and executive processes in the frontal lobes. *Science* 1999; 283:1657-1661.

Snyder PJ, Jackson CE, Piskulic D, Olver J, Norman T, Maruff P. Spatial working memory and problem solving in schizophrenia: the effect of symptom stabilization with atypical antipsychotic medication. *Psychiatry Res.* 2008; 160: 316-326.

Snyder SH, Greenberg D, Yamumura HI. Antischizophrenic drugs: affinity for muscarinic cholinergic receptor sites in the brain predicts extrapyramidal effects. *J Psychiatr Res.* 1974; 11:91-95.

Sohn MH, Ursu S, Anderson JR, Stenger VA, Carter CS. Inaugural article: the role of prefrontal cortex and posterior parietal cortex in task switching. *Proc Natl Acad Sci U S A.* 2000; 97:13448-13453.

Spalletta G, Tomaiuolo F, Marino V, Bonaviri G, Trequattrini A, Caltagirone C. Chronic schizophrenia as a brain misconnection syndrome: a white matter voxel-based morphometry study. *Schizophr Res.* 2003; 64:15-23.

Sperling RA, Guttmann CR, Hohol MJ, Warfield SK, Jakab M, Parente M, Diamond EL, Daffner KR, Olek MJ, Orav EJ, Kikinis R, Jolesz FA, Weiner HL. Regional magnetic resonance imaging lesion burden and cognitive function in multiple sclerosis: a longitudinal study. *Arch Neurol.* 2001; 58:115-121.

Stip E, Fahim C, Mancini-Marïe A, Bentaleb LA, Mensour B, Mendrek A, Beauregard M. Restoration of frontal activation during a treatment with quetiapine: an fMRI study of blunted affect in schizophrenia. *Prog Neuropsychopharmacol Biol Psychiatry* 2005; 29:21-26.

Stroop J.R.Studies of interference in serial verbal reactions . *J Exp Psychology* 1935; *18*:643-662.

Surguladze SA, Chu EM, Evans A, Anilkumar AP, Patel MX, Timehin C, David AS. The effect of long-acting risperidone on working memory in schizophrenia: a functional magnetic resonance imaging study. *J Clin Psychopharmacol.* 2007; 27: 560-570.

Takahashi H, Iwase M, Nakahachi T, Sekiyama R, Tabushi K, Kajimoto O, Shimizu A, Takeda M. Spatial working memory deficit correlates with disorganization symptoms and social functioning in schizophrenia. *Psychiatry Clin Neurosci.* 2005; 59:453-460.

Tan HY, Choo WC, Fones CS, Chee MW. fMRI study of maintenance and manipulation processes within working memory in first-episode schizophrenia. *Am J Psychiatry* 2005; 162:1849-1858.

Tek C, Gold J, Blaxton T, Wilk C, McMahon RP, Buchanan RW. Visual perceptual and working memory impairments in schizophrenia. *Arch Gen Psychiatry* 2002; 59:146-153.

Thermenos HW, Seidman LJ, Breiter H, Goldstein JM, Goodman JM, Poldrack R, Faraone SV, Tsuang MT. Functional magnetic resonance imaging during auditory verbal working memory in nonpsychotic relatives of persons with schizophrenia: a pilot study. *Biol Psychiatry* 2004; 55:490-500.

Uranova NA, Vostrikov VM, Orlovskaya DD, Rachmanova VI. Oligodendroglial density in the prefrontal cortex in schizophrenia and mood disorders: a study from the Stanley Neuropathology Consortium. *Schizophr Res.* 2004; 67:269-275

Vallar G, Di Betta AM, Silveri MC. The phonological short-term store-rehearsal system: patterns of impairment and neural correlates. *Neuropsychologia* 1997; 35:795-812.

van Waesberghe JH, Kamphorst W, De Groot CJ, van Walderveen MA, Castelijns JA, Ravid R, Lycklama à Nijeholt GJ, van der Valk P, Polman CH, Thompson AJ, Barkhof F. Axonal loss in multiple sclerosis lesions: magnetic resonance imaging insights into substrates of disability. *Ann Neurol.* 1999; 46: 747-754.

Vance A, Hall N, Bellgrove MA, Casey M, Karsz F, Maruff P. Visuospatial working memory deficits in adolescent onset schizophrenia. *Schizophr Res.* 2006; 87: 223-227.

Velligan DI, Newcomer J, Pultz J, Csernansky J, Hoff AL, Mahurin R, Miller AL. Does cognitive function improve with quetiapine in comparison to haloperidol? *Schizophr Res.* 2002; 53:239-248.

Verdoux H, Liraud F, Assens F, Abalan F, van Os J. Social and clinical consequences of cognitive deficits in early psychosis: a two-year follow-up study of first-admitted patients. *Schizophr Res.* 2002; 56:149-159.

Voglmaier MM, Seidman LJ, Salisbury D, McCarley RW. Neuropsychological dysfunction in schizotypal personality disorder: a profile analysis. *Biol Psychiatry* 1997; 41: 530-540.

von Huben SN, Davis SA, Lay CC, Katner SN, Crean RD, Taffe MA. Differential contributions of dopaminergic D1- and D2-like receptors to cognitive function in rhesus monkeys. *Psychopharmacology* 2006; 188: 586-596.

Walter H, Wunderlich AP, Blankenhorn M, Schäfer S, Tomczak R, Spitzer M, Grön G. No hypofrontality, but absence of prefrontal lateralization comparing verbal and spatial working memory in schizophrenia. *Schizophr Res.* 2003; 61:175-184.

Walterfang M, Wood SJ, Velakoulis D, Pantelis C. Neuropathological, neurogenetic and neuroimaging evidence for white matter pathology in schizophrenia. *Neurosci Biobehav Rev.* 2006; 30:918-948.

Wang Y, Goldman-Rakic PS. D2 receptor regulation of synaptic burst firing in prefrontal cortical pyramidal neurons. *Proc Natl Acad Sci U S A.* 2004; 101: 5093-5098.

Weickert TW, Goldberg TE. First- and second-generation antipsychotic medication and cognitive processing in schizophrenia. *Curr Psychiatry Rep.* 2005; 7: 304-310.

Weinberger DR, Berman KF, Chase TN. Mesocortical dopaminergic function and human cognition. *Ann N Y Acad Sci.* 1988; 537:330-338

Weinberger DR, Berman KF, Zec RF. Physiologic dysfunction of dorsolateral prefrontal cortex in schizophrenia. I. Regional cerebral blood flow evidence. *Arch Gen Psychiatry* 1986; 43:114-125.

Wexler BE, Anderson M, Fulbright RK, Gore JC. Preliminary evidence of improved verbal working memory performance and normalization of task-related frontal lobe activation in schizophrenia following cognitive exercises. *Am J Psychiatry* 2000; 157:1694-1697.

Wolf RC, Vasic N, Höse A, Spitzer M, Walter H. Changes over time in frontotemporal activation during a working memory task in patients with schizophrenia. *Schizophr Res.* 2007; 91:141-150.

Wykes T, Brammer M, Mellers J, Bray P, Reeder C, Williams C, Corner J. Effects on the brain of a psychological treatment: cognitive remediation therapy: functional magnetic resonance imaging in schizophrenia. *Br J Psychiatry* 2002; 181:144-152.

Wykes T, Reeder C, Corner J, Williams C, Everitt B. The effects of neurocognitive remediation on executive processing in patients with schizophrenia. *Schizophr Bull.* 1999; 25: 291-307.

Xiao L, Xu H, Zhang Y, Wei Z, He J, Jiang W, Li X, Dyck LE, Devon RM, Deng Y, Li XM. Quetiapine facilitates oligodendrocyte development and prevents mice from myelin breakdown and behavioral changes. *Mol Psychiatry* 2008; 13: 697-708.

Xu H, Yang HJ, McConomy B, Browning R, Li XM. Behavioral and neurobiological changes in C57BL/6 mouse exposed to cuprizone: effects of antipsychotics. *Front Behav Neurosci.* 2010; 4:8.

Xu H, Yang HJ, Zhang Y, Clough R, Browning R, Li XM. Behavioral and neurobiological changes in C57BL/6 mice exposed to cuprizone. *Behav Neurosci.* 2009; 123: 418-429.

Yang HJ, Wang H, Zhang Y, Xiao L, Clough RW, Browning R, Li XM, Xu H. Region-specific susceptibilities to cuprizone-induced lesions in the mouse forebrain: Implications for the pathophysiology of schizophrenia. *Brain Res.* 2009; 1270:121-130.

Zakzanis KK. Neuropsychological correlates of positive vs. negative schizophrenic symptomatology. *Schizophr Res.* 1998; 29: 227-233.

Zhou SY, Suzuki M, Hagino H, Takahashi T, Kawasaki Y, Nohara S, Yamashita I, Seto H, Kurachi M. Decreased volume and increased asymmetry of the anterior limb of the internal capsule in patients with schizophrenia. *Biol Psychiatry* 2003; 54:427-436.

In: Working Memory: Capacity, Developments and…
Editor: Eden S. Levin

ISBN: 978-1-61761-980-9
© 2011 Nova Science Publishers, Inc.

Chapter 14

TOBACCO, NICOTINE AND COTININE: FOR MEMORY, NEUROLOGICAL, AND PSYCHIATRIC DISORDERS

V. Echeverria[1,2], P. Rajeev[3] and R. Zeitlin[1]

[1] Research and Development, Department of Veterans Affairs,
Bay Pines VA Healthcare System, Bay Pines, FL, USA
[2] Department of Molecular Medicine, University of South Florida, Tampa, FL, USA,
[3] Department of Chemistry, University of Miami, FL, USA

ABSTRACT

Epidemiological studies have associated tobacco consumption with a lower incidence of Alzheimer's disease (AD) and Parkinson's disease (PD). The neuroprotective effect of tobacco has been mainly attributed to the stimulation by nicotine of the α7 nicotinic acetylcholine receptors (nAChRs), which are implicated in neuronal survival, attention, and memory. A reduction in cholinergic function including lower levels of the expression of nAChRs in the hippocampus correlates with memory impairment in AD and schizophrenia. Although nicotine improves memory, sensory gating, and attention, its toxicity and undesired effects such as negative cardiovascular effects have terminated its therapeutic applications. Interestingly, its main metabolite cotinine shows similar neuroprotective and mnemonic properties but has a ten-fold longer half-life than nicotine and a good safety profile in humans. In neurodegenerative conditions including AD and PD, the accumulation of aggregated forms of the β-amyloid peptide correlates with cognitive impairment. Cotinine has been shown to reduce Aβ aggregation *in vitro*. Additionally, since cotinine is a weak agonist of the nAChRs, we postulate that cotinine improves neuronal survival and memory at least in part by acting as a positive modulator of the α7 nAChRs. The potentiation of α7 nAChRs by cotinine can be beneficial in a broad range of neurological disorders such as schizophrenia, AD, attention-deficit hyperactivity disorder, and PD in which the modulation of these receptors can ameliorate working memory and attention. Based on actual evidence and these ideas, the relevance and potential therapeutic use of cotinine in several neurological disorders are discussed in this chapter.

"Only do not forget, if I wake up crying it's only because in my dream I'm a lost child hunting through the leaves of the night for your hands...." — *Pablo Neruda* [1]

INTRODUCTION

Smoking prevalence is much higher in individuals suffering from mental health conditions such as schizophrenia, depression, posttraumatic stress disorder (PTSD), attention-deficit hyperactivity disorder (ADHD), and bipolar disorder than in the general population [2-5]. Although smoking has dramatically decreased in the general population as a result of public restrictions to tobacco use and better knowledge of the deleterious consequences of its consumption, there is still a high rate of smoking behavior among persons with psychiatric disorders. As a consequence, research studies aimed at understanding its basis have increased over the past several years [6].

Notably, deficits in attention, concentration, and working memory are common in individuals suffering from mental conditions associated with tobacco dependency such as depression [7-9], schizophrenia [10-12], and PTSD [13-17], and are currently undertreated in most patients [18]. Cognitive impairment in patients with schizophrenia includes deficits in several cognitive abilities including executive function, memory and learning, and social knowledge. These cognitive deficits negatively affect their employability, treatment adherence, and social skills [19]. Unfortunately, current behavioral and pharmacological therapies for schizophrenia, PTSD, and other psychiatric conditions have been mostly ineffective in reducing these deficits and can even potentiate them [20-23].

As a potential therapeutic avenue, the use of tobacco-derived compounds to improve cognitive deficits in psychiatric conditions and neurodegenerative diseases has been investigated for several years. In this respect, the administration by nasal spray of nicotine (3-(1-methyl-2-pyrrolidinyl) pyridine), an agonist of the nicotinic acetylcholine receptors (nAChRs), ameliorated working memory in individuals with schizophrenia [24]. In another study, nicotine has been shown to ameliorate several symptoms present in PTSD patients including sensory deficits, attention, and anxiety [25]. This and other evidence *in vivo* clearly suggest that stimulation of the cholinergic system can be beneficial in these conditions [26, 27]. The importance of stimulating the cholinergic system resides in the fact that the nAChRs are down-regulated in many psychiatric conditions and are majorly involved in the aforementioned processes of attention and memory [28].

Regarding dementia and the stimulation of the cholinergic system, a negative correlation between tobacco use and the incidence of Alzheimer's disease (AD) and Parkinson's disease (PD) has been reported [29]. Most of these studies have been focused on the use of nicotine, which has positive effects on attention and memory in animal models of aging [30, 31] and neurological diseases such as AD [32, 33]. Despite its beneficial effects, the inherent toxicity and short half-life (2-3h) of nicotine have limited its therapeutic value. On the other hand, cotinine ((5S)-1-methyl-5-(3-pyridyl)-pyrrolidin-2-one), the main metabolite of nicotine, is one hundred-fold less toxic than nicotine [34], has a longer half-life (20–24h), has been proven to cross the blood-brain barrier in rodents [35, 36], and has memory-enhancing effects in a transgenic mouse model of AD [37].

The potential use of cotinine, the major metabolite of nicotine, in protecting against working memory loss in individuals with neurological conditions is discussed in this chapter.

Rather than to solely present a review of these topics, this chapter also aims to promote discussion about the use of cotinine in conditions presenting cholinergic deficits.

METABOLISM OF COTININE

More than 80% of nicotine is metabolized to cotinine in mammals. The physiologically active form of cotinine, the (-)-isomer, accumulates in the body as a result of tobacco exposure and its levels depend on the rates of metabolism and clearance. In humans and mice, nicotine is metabolized by cytochrome P450 2A6 (CYP2A6) [38] and cytochrome P450 2A5 (CYP2A5) enzymes [39][40]. The major metabolite of cotinine recovered in urine is the trans-3'-hydroxycotinine that is metabolized by CYP2A5 (90% of cotinine) and its glucuronide [41-43]. Some evidence suggests that the heritable variation in the sequence of the CYP2A6 gene can affect both nicotine metabolism and smoking behaviors [44, 45]. Thus, the degree of the ability to synthesize cotinine from nicotine seems to affect our susceptibility to smoke and become tobacco-dependent. For example, individuals that only express a shorter form of CYP2A6 (*i.e.,* CYP2A6*4) produced low levels of cotinine and smoke fewer cigarettes [46]. This evidence suggests that cotinine may produce distinct pleasing effects in comparison with nicotine, making people more prone toward smoking.

The presence of polymorphic alleles of the CYP2A6 gene may explain the differences in the metabolism of cotinine in people of different ethnic backgrounds [47]. For instance, the alleles that express CYP2A forms with low enzymatic activity are represented differently in different ethnic groups with about 9.1%, 21.9%, 42.9%, and 50.5% in white, black, Korean, and Japanese subjects, respectively [47]. Other studies showed that African Americans have a lower average clearance of cotinine (18% reduction) than Caucasians. Also, the half-life of cotinine and its clearance differs significantly among Caucasians (16.1 ± 5.2), Latinos (14.6 ± 5.2), and Chinese Americans (18.3 ± 5.4) [48]. Therefore, the clearance and half-life of cotinine is determined in part by the individual's ethnicity. In addition to genetic and ethnicity factors, individual variability including food preference can also influence the rate of metabolism of nicotine [47]. It has been demonstrated that several compounds extracted from grapefruit juice can inhibit the activity of the CYP enzymes such as sesquiterpene nootkatone which inhibits CYP2A6 [49, 50].

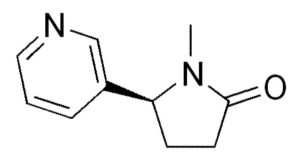

Figure 1. Structural formula of cotinine.

EFFECT OF COTININE AS TESTED IN ANIMAL MODELS

Similar to humans, different strains of mice have a different metabolism of cotinine as a result of the genetic differences in the structure and function of the CYP2A5. For example, the acute administration of cotinine 1 mg/kg induces similar plasma concentrations of cotinine in C57BL/6 (760 ng/ml) and DBA/2 (748 ng/ml) mice; however, after injections DBA/2 mice had a slower clearance of cotinine [51]. Despite these differences, animal models can be very useful in characterizing the potential of cotinine as a new psychiatric drug.

Additionally, it has been discovered using animal models that cotinine has cognitive-enhancing properties in normal and pathological conditions. One study reported that cotinine (0.3, 3, and 10 mg/kg) improved performance of eight adult rhesus monkeys (*Macaca mulatta*) in the delayed matching-to-sample (DMTS) cognitive task that measures working memory [52]. Briefly, this test consists of presenting different color stimuli on a touch-sensitive screen. One color stimulus remains in the view of the monkey until it touches the screen, initiating a delay in its presentation (the retention interval). After this retention interval, two new colors are presented, one of which matches the previous stimulus color. If the individual chooses the matching color, it receives a reward (food pellets). With cotinine treatment, the improvement in DMTS task accuracies was achieved after 10 minutes and 24 hours post-injection, indicating that both short-term and long-term effects were involved. This was one of the first preliminary findings suggesting that cotinine can be useful in improving working memory.

We have recently performed studies using a transgenic (Tg) mouse model of AD, to investigate the effect of cotinine on senile plaque pathology and working and reference memories [37]. The results suggest that cotinine may have potential value as a drug to prevent Aβ-induced memory loss when administered at early or middle stages of the disease. The memory-enhancing properties of cotinine may be the result of the potentiation of the α7 nAChRs, which are primary therapeutic targets for improving memory and attention abilities in individuals with these cognitive impairments due to neurological disorders [53, 54]. We are currently investigating this possibility in our laboratory.

COTININE USE IS SAFE IN HUMANS

Cotinine has been characterized in terms of its safety profile and investigated in previous studies for its potential to reduce tobacco withdrawal symptoms. However, clinical studies assessing cotinine's potential as a drug for neurodegenerative or other psychiatric conditions have not yet been performed. In several seminal studies, the pharmacokinetic profiles and effects of intravenous and orally administered cotinine were investigated in humans [55-61]. These studies revealed that cotinine was almost completely absorbed orally [62]; also, doses up to 1,800 mg of cotinine per day during a 4-day period did not induce detectable negative effects and are well tolerated in humans [55]. In one of these studies, the effect and safety of several doses of oral cotinine fumarate (40, 80, or 160 mg) or placebo were tested in an inpatient, 10-day human study in abstinent cigarette smokers [61]. The data show that short-term treatment with cotinine to reach plasma levels ten-fold higher than the concentrations attained from heavy cigarette smoking had no withdrawal effects or other significant physiologic (*e.g.*, heart rate and blood pressure) or behavioral effects in individuals between 21-42 years of age [61]. In another study, the effect of three doses of cotinine and placebo on cigarette self-administration during 10 days period was investigated. In the conditions and population studied, cotinine did not affect the number of cigarettes smoked at all doses tested, suggesting that cotinine does not help with tobacco cessation [59]

In a third study, the same group found that cotinine at doses 3-4 times higher than during *ad libitum* smoking not only does not reduce craving or withdrawal symptoms but also antagonized the beneficial effects of the nicotine patch in decreasing withdrawal symptoms [60]. Although highly speculative at this point, we hypothesize that by modulating the α7 nAChRs, cotinine may be able to inhibit the desensitization of the receptor induced by nicotine administered through the nicotine patch, thereby affecting its beneficial effects. A different study performed with cotinine alone showed that when administered intravenously to abstinent smokers, this drug reduced self-reported irritability and the desire to smoke [57]. The inhibitory effect of cotinine over the reduction in cigarette cravings induced by nicotine patches suggests that cotinine has behavioral effects and consequently may cross the blood-brain barrier (BBB); however, well-controlled studies need to be performed to determine the extent of cotinine's ability to cross the BBB.

Nevertheless, a reduced ability to cross the BBB may not be an insurmountable problem as a new delivery system to the brain has been proven to be successful for drugs that poorly cross this barrier. Intranasal delivery is a practical non-invasive procedure that bypasses the BBB to deliver drugs to the central nervous system (CNS) and is becoming popular for the treatment of neurological disorders. Developed by Frey in 1989 to deliver nerve growth factor and fibroblast growth factor-2 to the CNS [63], this method is rapid (less than 10 minutes) and reduces systemic exposure to the drugs in comparison with oral or intravenous administration [64]. This method exploits the capacity of trigeminal and olfactory nerves that innervate the nasal cavity to deliver drugs to the brain [64, 65]. Extracellular delivery rather than axonal transport is proposed to occur by diffusion throughout perivascular space as well as the lymphatic and perineuronal channels [66]. We consider that cotinine may ideally be investigated in humans by using both oral and intranasal administration.

TOBACCO CONSUMPTION AND THE POTENTIAL BENEFITS OF COTININE IN MENTAL HEALTH DISORDERS

Posttraumatic Stress Disorder

PTSD is an anxiety disorder induced by exposure to a life-threatening traumatic event [67]. Compared with non-traumatized individuals, PTSD patients have a higher utilization of medical services and are at an increased risk for developing cardiovascular and cancer diseases [68, 69]. Using imaging techniques such as magnet resonance imaging (MRI), functional MRI (fMRI), positron emission tomography (PET), and single-photon emission computed tomography (SPECT), it has been discovered that PTSD is accompanied by morphological and functional changes of the brain, especially in the hippocampus and prefrontal cortex [70-72]. These structural changes in the brain are present concurrently with symptoms such as high levels of anxiety, cognitive decline, hyperarousal, numbing (emotional non-responsiveness), and sleep disorders. These changes have been associated with hormonal changes including the overactivation of the hypothalamus-pituitary-adrenal axis [73] and the dysregulation of several neurotransmitter systems observed in patients with PTSD. Furthermore, the dysregulation of other factors released by the brain such as the opiates (endorphins and enkephalins [74, 75]) and BDNF [76, 77] can also explain some of the aforementioned symptoms (*e.g.*, emotional numbing and amnesia).

Several types of antidepressants are currently used to treat PTSD. These include, but are not limited to, monoamine oxidase inhibitors, selective norepinephrine reuptake inhibitors, tricyclic antidepressants, antiepileptic drugs, and selective serotonin reuptake inhibitors (SSRIs). Depletion of serotonin may be one of the causes of irritability and violent or angry outbursts and the SSRIs are effective in more than 30% of patients with PTSD. SSRIs are the first-line treatments for PTSD [78, 79] and several of these drugs including paroxetine and sertraline have received US Food and Drug Administration (FDA) approval [80-82]. Some of these drugs can ameliorate PTSD symptoms and the cardiovascular disturbances associated with them [83] but are not able to target or can worsen cognitive deficits [14]. Since available therapies including behavioral and pharmacological approaches do not help a large percentage of PTSD patients, it is imperative to find new drugs that can be used alone or in conjunction with current therapies in order to reduce PTSD symptoms and reestablish their cognitive abilities.

It is believed that PTSD patients smoke to alleviate their symptoms, as an association between tobacco dependence and traumatic experiences and PTSD has been reported [84]. In a cross-sectional study of 157 patients with PTSD, severity of nicotine dependence was positively correlated with PTSD symptoms such as hyperarousal and avoidance [3]. The hyperarousal and aggressiveness in PTSD seems at least in part to be related to a decrease in the serotoninergic neurotransmission and an increase in noradrenergic neurotransmission [85].

The effect of cotinine on the turnover, uptake, and release of serotonin in serotoninergic neurons has been determined in the brains of rats [86]. In this study, it has been found that treatment of cotinine 2 mg/kg in rats reduced cerebral serotonin turnover by a mechanism independent of the cholinergic system, as it was not blocked by pretreatment with mecamylamine (general cholinergic system inhibitor) [86]. Extracellular levels of serotonin in the brain are regulated by the modulation of the release and uptake of serotonin [87]. Cotinine inhibited serotonin uptake and retention and increased its spontaneous release. As serotonin promotes acetylcholine release, a decrease in cerebral serotonin may also induce a deficit of the cholinergic system [88]. Since cotinine seems to enhance the cholinergic and serotoninergic systems, it is possible that cotinine is self-administered by traumatized individuals in order to reduce their anxiety and amnesic symptoms by potentiating these neurotransmitter systems. Further investigation is required to confirm this hypothesis.

Schizophrenia

Schizophrenia is a complex neuropsychiatric disorder characterized by cognitive deficits with both positive and negative symptoms. Patients with schizophrenia die approximately 15 years younger than those of the normal population, mainly due to their higher exposure to risk factors contributing to an unhealthy life style including poor diet, modest exercise, obesity, and smoking behavior [89]. Positive symptoms include delusions, difficulty in speaking and organizing thoughts, and hallucinations; the negative symptoms include reduced attention and motivation, social withdrawal, and emotional numbness [90].

All antipsychotics currently used in clinical practice are dopamine D2 receptor antagonists. Chronic treatment with nicotine has been shown to improve cognitive abilities in schizophrenic patients treated with antipsychotics [91, 92]. Based on this evidence, it has been hypothesized that individuals with psychiatric conditions smoke to improve memory and attention and to reduce anxiety levels with tobacco-derived compounds such as nicotine and its long-lasting metabolite cotinine.

The investigation of new compounds to ameliorate cognitive deficits in schizophrenia has been facilitated by the discovery that administration of the N-methyl D-aspartate (NMDA) antagonist dizocilpine to rodents induces psychotic states in the animals closely resembling schizophrenic symptoms [93]. Using this model, it was discovered that the administration of nicotine to rats attenuated the dizocilpine-induced deficit in both working and reference memories [94, 95]. Similarly, chronic treatment with nicotine improved memory in schizophrenic patients treated with antipsychotics such as clozapine, which also stimulates the cholinergic system [91]. It is feasible that the benefits observed with nicotine treatment are due to the potentiation by its metabolite, cotinine, of the activity of the $\alpha7$ nAChRs.

The $\alpha7$ nAChRs are decreased in the hippocampus and neocortex of people with schizophrenia and play a key role supporting sensory gating or filtering of irrelevant stimuli, attention, and memory [96, 97]. For these reasons, these receptors are considered a preferential target to improve cognitive abilities in individuals with this condition [98]. Many compounds that modulate directly (partial or full agonists) or indirectly (allosteric modulators) the nicotinic receptors are under intense scrutiny. Recently, the results of a phase 2 clinical study of the effect of the partial agonist of the $\alpha7$ receptors DMXB-A (GTS-21) on schizophrenia symptoms in several individuals showed that this drug can improve some of the negative symptoms of the disease. However, DMXB-A did not improve cognitive abilities in this population [98]. Other compounds such as TC-5619, EVP-6124, and SS-R180711 are under investigation [53].

Additionally, several psychiatric disorders such as schizophrenia, PTSD, ADHD, borderline personality disorder, and bipolar disorder have a deficit in sensorimotor gating [99, 100]. This deficiency is responsible for the increased startle response (hyperarousal) observed in individuals with these conditions. Since this is a cross-species phenomenon, rodent models of prepulse inhibition (PPI) have been used to investigate at the preclinical level the utility of antipsychotic drugs over sensory-information processing deficits [101]. This test consists of exposing the rodent to a weak acoustic stimulus (the prepulse) and measures the decrease in the reflexive flinching response (startle) as a result of a second stimulus of higher intensity (the pulse). In these animal models, effective antipsychotic agents are able to disrupt the inhibition of PPI induced by dopamine agonists such as apomorphine and glutamate antagonists. Cotinine has been shown to ameliorate apomorphine-induced deficits in PPI of acoustic startle response in rats [52, 102]. It has also been reported that cotinine as well as GTS-21 can completely reverse the cognitive deficit induced by ketamine [103]. These results suggest that cotinine may be useful in decreasing the startle response in conditions leading to hyperarousal.

Since cotinine may modulate the nAChRs and has been shown to improve memory and PPI in animal models, we predict that cotinine can have good therapeutic potential to be able to ameliorate hyperarousal, attention, and working memory deficits in psychiatric disorders including AD.

Alzheimer's Disease

Alzheimer's Disease, the Deterioration of the Cholinergic Neurotransmission, and Memory Loss

AD is a progressive neurodegenerative condition and the main cause of dementia in the elderly [104, 105]. The main neuropathological hallmarks of the disease include the senile plaques mainly composed of aggregated forms of the amyloid-beta peptide (Aβ) and the neurofibrillary tangles consisting of modified forms of the microtubule-associated protein tau [104]. AD is also characterized by synaptic dysfunction, memory loss, neuroinflammation, and neurodegeneration that parallels with a progressive accumulation of Aβ in the brain [106, 107].

According to the amyloid cascade hypothesis, AD pathology is mainly caused by the neurotoxicity of soluble forms of Aβ aggregated into oligomers and protofibrils [108-111]. Therefore, a great effort has been directed at inhibiting the aggregation of the peptide [112-115]. The toxic forms of Aβ preferentially target the more "plastic" regions of the brain such as the cortex and hippocampus, which are associated with higher-order cognitive abilities including working and episodic memories [116]. It has been postulated that the early degeneration of the cholinergic nucleus basalis of Meynert [117] of the cerebral basal forebrain (CBF) results in a deficit of the cortical cholinergic system that greatly contributes to the cognitive deficits in AD [118, 119]. Post-mortem studies have shown that the cholinergic deficit involves a significant reduction in the expression of nAChRs and the choline acetyltransferase (ChAT) activity in the temporal cortex and other regions of the AD brains [120, 121].

It has been found that in AD brains the expression of $\beta 2$, $\alpha 3$, $\alpha 4$, and $\alpha 7$ nAChRs is reduced [121, 122], but the causes of this deficit are not well understood. In this respect, the dysfunction of the nerve growth factor (NGF) signaling has been postulated to be at least in part responsible for the degeneration of the cholinergic neurons [123, 124]. For example, in the brains of normal aged humans, most neurons of the CBF stain for NGF. On the contrary, the CBF displayed markedly less (32%) or undetectable NGF immunoreactivity in AD brains. Based on this evidence, it has been hypothesized that there is a defect in the retrograde transport of NGF which may likely mediate the degeneration of CBF neurons in AD brains [123]. These discoveries have motivated the search for safe strategies of delivering NGF to the brain to reestablish cholinergic function and as a treatment against memory impairment [125-128].

In addition to the use of memantine to decrease glutamate excitotoxicity, current therapies for AD have been mainly directed at reestablishing cholinergic function by inhibiting the clearance of acetylcholine using several acetylcholinesterase inhibitors [129-131]. Unfortunately, these drugs have only marginally ameliorated cognitive and behavioral deficits in AD patients and present only short-term usefulness [132-135].

In the search for drugs able to restore cholinergic function in the brains of AD patients, several tobacco-derived compounds such as nicotine and its derivatives have attracted a great deal of attention. Nicotine is an alkaloid present in tobacco leaves that is the most well-known psychoactive compound derived from this plant. This molecule is neuroprotective against Aβ toxicity and binds to Aβ, blocking its aggregation into fibrils [136].

Nicotine also has attention-enhancing effects [27, 137] and its administration to AD patients attenuates memory decline and attention deficits [138, 139]. Clinical studies have not been very conclusive in showing a beneficial effect of nicotine in improving memory in AD [140, 141]. However, a clear positive effect over attention has been reported in studies using transdermal patches of nicotine in AD [141] and Parkinson's disease patients [33, 142]. It has been hypothesized that nicotine improves attention by targeting the nAChRs, which play a key role in memory and attention abilities [143-145]. Unfortunately, due to its inherent toxicity, its ability to induce tachyphylaxis, and addictive side effects, nicotine is not an optimal therapeutic agent for use against AD [98].

In the search for alternatives to nicotine, several agonists of the nAChRs such as the derivatives from the naturally occurring nicotinic agonist anabaseine [146] and its derivatives such as GTS-21 have been investigated to improve attention and working memory in animal models. These studies showed that activation of the cerebral nAChRs enhances the cognitive abilities in animal models of AD [31, 137, 147] and schizophrenia [98, 103, 148]. Based on these results, several of these compounds are currently being tested in clinical trials as drugs to treat cognitive impairment for schizophrenia [92, 98, 149, 150] and AD [151, 152].

The consistent failure to find effective drugs against AD [153, 154] has encouraged the search for new drugs having multiple therapeutic effects. An ideal drug against AD may inhibit Aβ production and/or its aggregation as well as have a normalizing effect on the cholinergic or glutamatergic system; cotinine seems to fulfill these expectations [55].

Cotinine is an Anti-Aβ$_{1-42}$ Aggregation Compound

When Aβ is dissolved in an aqueous solution, it undergoes a time- and temperature-dependent conformational transition from a more soluble α-helical structure, to an insoluble β-sheet conformation. It has been proposed that the conformational transitions of Aβ are from monomers to oligomeric, protofibrillar, and finally fibrillar insoluble forms of the peptide. However, in some Aβ preparations it has been described that protofibrils can persist for days when incubated in PBS at 37°C, with a slow transition to fibrillar structures that are apparent only after several weeks [155].

It has also been postulated that the oligomerization and fibrillation processes are pathways that can occur independently of each other and can be targeted separately by anti-aggregation compounds [156]. In this regard, anti-aggregation molecules have been divided into three classes [156, 157]. Class I compounds inhibit oligomerization but not fibrillation such as curcumin [158] and *Ginkgo biloba* [159]. Class II compounds inhibit the peptide aggregation into both oligomers and fibrils such as *o*-vanillin [160], and Class III molecules inhibit fibrillation but not oligomerization such as the naphthalene sulfonates AMNS (1-amino-5-naphthalene sulfonate), 1,8-ANS (1-anilinonaphthalene-8-sulfonate), and bis-ANS (4,4'-dianilino-1,1'-binaphthyl-5,5'-disulfonate) [157]. Nonetheless, few compounds that can inhibit both aggregation processes have been tested *in vivo* [161, 162].

It was previously shown that cotinine may reduce the extent of hydrogen-bonding and fiber growth of the fibrillogenic peptide $A\beta_{12-28}$ using x-ray fiber diffraction [163]. Moreover, previous reports showed that both nicotine and cotinine bind to Aβ with high affinity [164] inhibiting its aggregation into fibrils *in vitro* [136]. We are currently expanding these studies by investigating the effect of cotinine *in vivo* on plaque deposition and examining *in vitro* its effects on the formation of Aβ oligomers and fibrils.

Effects of Tobacco-Derived Compounds on the Nicotinic Receptors

The study of the interaction of the nAChRs with their ligands including agonist and allosteric modulators is fundamental for drug design and the modulation of their activities. In addition to their endogenous ligand acetylcholine, nAChRs are reactive toward chemically diverse pharmaceuticals and naturally occurring compounds such as nicotine, alcohol, and different toxins [165-167]. Originally, the refined model of the membrane-associated Torpedo α1β1δγ nAChR was resolved at 4 Å resolution from electron microscopy [168]. This structure provided significant insights into the architecture of the extracellular ligand binding domain (LBD) and the channel pore but the distortion in the binding site made it difficult to obtain information about the binding of ligands. Recently, an high resolution crystal structure of the extracellular domain of the mouse nAChR α1 subunit bound to α-bungarotoxin at 1.94 Å has been determined (PDB ID: 2QC1) [169]. Additionally, in the last few years, numerous x-ray structures of the acetylcholine-binding protein (AChBP) in different agonist/antagonist-bound states have been resolved [165, 170]. Particularly, nicotine agonist-bound structure of AChBP has been determined at 2.2 Å resolution (PDB ID: 1UW6) [165].

In this structure, nicotine is bound in the interface between two subunits (principal and complementary) interacting with Tyr89, Trp143, Cys188, and Tyr192 residues of the principal subunit and Trp53, Leu102, and Met114 of complementary subunit (Figure 2). AChBP shares ~24% sequence homology with LBD of nAChR and has the same pentameric assembly [169]. The x-ray structures of agonist bound AChBP has been broadly used as a model of LBD of nAChR to study the mechanism of receptor-ligand interactions in a number of experimental [165, 170-172] and computational studies [173-175]. However, in contrast to the global conformational change in LBD and quaternary twist induced by the binding of ligand in the nAChR, no such structural changes were observed in various AChBP/ligand complexes. These results suggest that AChBP may represent an "imperturbable homologue" of the nAChR that lacks the necessary structural elements to undergo large-scale conformational changes in response to neurotransmitter binding [176]. Furthermore, a key structural feature of LBD of nAChR observed in the α-bungarotoxin bound structure (2QC1) is the presence of a hydrophilic patch consists of two highly conserved hydrophilic residues and a molecule of water in its hydrophobic interior. This patch has been reported to be important for agonist-induced channel opening [169]. However, this hydrophilic patch is missing in AChBP, which contains hydrophobic residues at the corresponding positions.

We are currently investigating the interactions of cotinine with the Aβ peptide using docking and molecular dynamics approaches and plan to investigate the interaction of cotinine and nicotine with the α7 nAChR subunit by using both nicotine-bound structure of AChBP (1UW6) and α-bungarotoxin-bound structure of the α1 subunit of nAChR (2QC1). These studies will help to elucidate differences in the interactions of these ligands and determine the roles of specific residues of AChBP and nAChR in the binding of nicotine and cotinine.

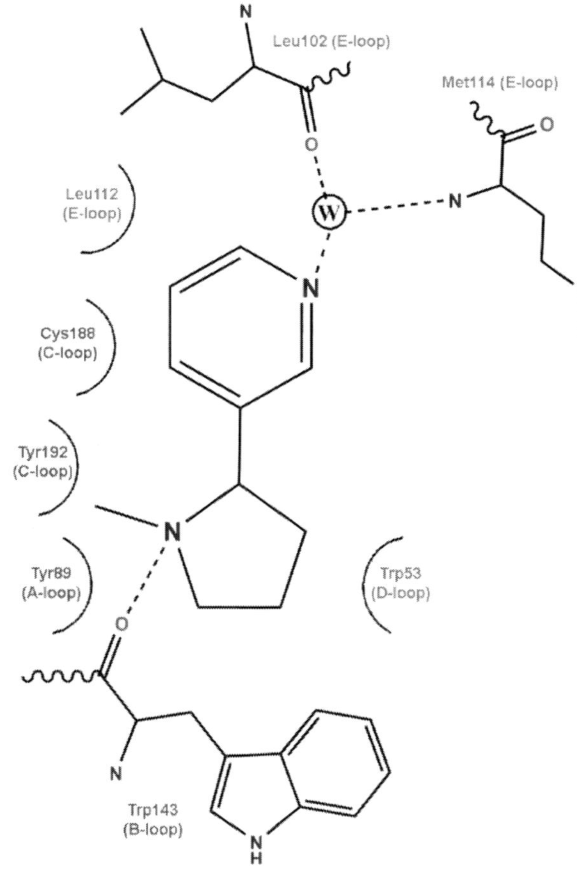

Figure 2. The interactions of nicotine with the principal and complementary subunits of AChBP.

CONCLUSION

Although tobacco consumption is highly deleterious and is responsible for millions of deaths around the world every year, it negatively correlates with the incidence of AD and PD and is higher in people with psychiatric disorders. Nicotine, the more studied psychoactive compound derived from tobacco, attracted considerable attention due to its capacity to stimulate the α7 nAChRs, which when activated, support attention, learning, and memory processes in humans under normal and pathological conditions. Nicotine is toxic and has a short half-life making it unsuitable for pharmacological therapy. However, nicotine metabolizes into cotinine, a compound with approximately a ten-fold longer half-life than nicotine, a good safe profile, and a molecule that we predict may potentiate the α7 nAChRs. Since these receptors are down-regulated in the brains of people with AD, PD, and other psychiatric conditions such as schizophrenia, it is possible that cotinine can ameliorate the cognitive deficits induced by the diseases. As cotinine also stimulates serotonin release in the brain, we hypothesize that cotinine can be an alternative to smoking to alleviate the anxiety, attention, and memory impairments in those with psychiatric conditions. Importantly, cotinine also inhibits the aggregation of the amyloidogenic Aβ_{42} peptide, a process that is considered to induce neurodegeneration leading to dementia. The ongoing investigation by us and other research groups about cotinine's molecular mechanisms of action in the brain gives light to a new understanding of cotinine's potential for the treatment of neurological disorders. The investigation of cotinine derivatives is also a necessary step in the search for new compounds to stop neurodegeneration and memory loss in several neurological conditions.

ACKNOWLEDGMENTS

This material is the result of work supported with resources and the use of facilities at the Bay Pines Veterans Affairs Healthcare System. The authors thank Professor David Sattelle (University of Oxford) and Professor Gary W. Arendash (University of South Florida) for their valuable comments as well as the Bay Pines Foundation, Inc. and our families for their constant support.

REFERENCES

[1] Neruda, P., *100 love sonnets = Cien sonetos de amor* / by Pablo Neruda ; translated by Stephen Tapscott. University of Texas Press: Austin, 1986; p 17.
[2] Buggia-Prevot, V.; Sevalle, J.; Rossner, S.; Checler, F., NFkappaB-dependent control of BACE1 promoter transactivation by Abeta42. *J Biol Chem* 2008, 283, (15), 10037-47.
[3] Thorndike, F. P.; Wernicke, R.; Pearlman, M. Y.; Haaga, D. A., Nicotine dependence, PTSD symptoms, and depression proneness among male and female smokers. *Addict Behav* 2006, 31, (2), 223-31.
[4] Leonard, S.; Adler, L. E.; Benhammou, K.; Berger, R.; Breese, C. R.; Drebing, C.; Gault, J.; Lee, M. J.; Logel, J.; Olincy, A.; Ross, R. G.; Stevens, K.; Sullivan, B.; Vianzon, R.; Virnich, D. E.; Waldo, M.; Walton, K.; Freedman, R., Smoking and mental illness. *Pharmacol Biochem Behav* 2001, 70, (4), 561-70.
[5] Weaver, T. L.; Etzel, J. C., Smoking patterns, symptoms of PTSD and depression: preliminary findings from a sample of severely battered women. *Addict Behav* 2003, 28, (9), 1665-79.
[6] Rasmusson, A. M.; Picciotto, M. R.; Krishnan-Sarin, S., Smoking as a complex but critical covariate in neurobiological studies of posttraumatic stress disorders: a review. *J Psychopharmacol* 2006, 20, (5), 693-707.

[7] Baune, B. T.; Miller, R.; McAfoose, J.; Johnson, M.; Quirk, F.; Mitchell, D., The role of cognitive impairment in general functioning in major depression. *Psychiatry Res.*

[8] Burriss, L.; Ayers, E.; Ginsberg, J.; Powell, D. A., Learning and memory impairment in PTSD: relationship to depression. *Depress Anxiety* 2008, 25, (2), 149-57.

[9] Hinkelmann, K.; Moritz, S.; Botzenhardt, J.; Riedesel, K.; Wiedemann, K.; Kellner, M.; Otte, C., Cognitive impairment in major depression: association with salivary cortisol. *Biol Psychiatry* 2009, 66, (9), 879-85.

[10] Bowie, C. R.; Harvey, P. D., Cognition in schizophrenia: impairments, determinants, and functional importance. *Psychiatr Clin North Am* 2005, 28, (3), 613-33, 626.

[11] Gray, J. A.; Roth, B. L., Molecular targets for treating cognitive dysfunction in schizophrenia. *Schizophr Bull* 2007, 33, (5), 1100-19.

[12] Luck, S. J.; Gold, J. M., The construct of attention in schizophrenia. *Biol Psychiatry* 2008, 64, (1), 34-9.

[13] Tapia, G.; Clarys, D.; El Hage, W.; Belzung, C.; Isingrini, M., PTSD psychiatric patients exhibit a deficit in remembering. *Memory* 2007, 15, (2), 145-53.

[14] Veltmeyer, M. D.; Clark, C. R.; McFarlane, A. C.; Moores, K. A.; Bryant, R. A.; Gordon, E., Working memory function in post-traumatic stress disorder: an event-related potential study. *Clin Neurophysiol* 2009, 120, (6), 1096-106.

[15] Elzinga, B. M.; Bremner, J. D., Are the neural substrates of memory the final common pathway in posttraumatic stress disorder (PTSD)? *J Affect Disord* 2002, 70, (1), 1-17.

[16] Johnsen, G. E.; Asbjornsen, A. E., Verbal learning and memory impairments in posttraumatic stress disorder: the role of encoding strategies. *Psychiatry Res* 2009, 165, (1-2), 68-77.

[17] Horner, M. D.; Hamner, M. B., Neurocognitive functioning in posttraumatic stress disorder. *Neuropsychol Rev* 2002, 12, (1), 15-30.

[18] Terry, A. V., Jr.; Buccafusco, J. J.; Wilson, C., Cognitive dysfunction in neuropsychiatric disorders: Selected serotonin receptor subtypes as therapeutic targets. *Behav Brain Res* 2008.

[19] Matsui, M.; Sumiyoshi, T.; Arai, H.; Higuchi, Y.; Kurachi, M., Cognitive functioning related to quality of life in schizophrenia. *Prog Neuropsychopharmacol Biol Psychiatry* 2008, 32, (1), 280-7.

[20] Levin, E. D.; Rezvani, A. H., Nicotinic-antipsychotic drug interactions and cognitive function. *Exs* 2006, 98, 185-205.

[21] Chung, Y. C.; Lee, C. R.; Park, T. W.; Yang, K. H.; Kim, K. W., Effect of donepezil added to atypical antipsychotics on cognition in patients with schizophrenia: an open-label trial. *World J Biol Psychiatry* 2009, 10, (2), 156-62.

[22] Riedel, M.; Schennach-Wolff, R.; Musil, R.; Dehning, S.; Cerovecki, A.; Opgen-Rhein, M.; Matz, J.; Seemuller, F.; Obermeier, M.; Engel, R. R.; Muller, N.; Moller, H. J.; Spellmann, I., Neurocognition and its influencing factors in the treatment of schizophrenia-effects of aripiprazole, olanzapine, quetiapine and risperidone. *Hum Psychopharmacol* 25, (2), 116-25.

[23] Krakowski, M. I.; Czobor, P.; Nolan, K. A., Atypical antipsychotics, neurocognitive deficits, and aggression in schizophrenic patients. *J Clin Psychopharmacol* 2008, 28, (5), 485-93.

[24] Smith, R. C.; Warner-Cohen, J.; Matute, M.; Butler, E.; Kelly, E.; Vaidhyanathaswamy, S.; Khan, A., Effects of nicotine nasal spray on cognitive function in schizophrenia. *Neuropsychopharmacology* 2006, 31, (3), 637-43.

[25] Buckley, T. C.; Holohan, D. R.; Mozley, S. L.; Walsh, K.; Kassel, J., The effect of nicotine and attention allocation on physiological and self-report measures of induced anxiety in PTSD: a double-blind placebo-controlled trial. *Exp Clin Psychopharmacol* 2007, 15, (2), 154-64.

[26] Cincotta, S. L.; Yorek, M. S.; Moschak, T. M.; Lewis, S. R.; Rodefer, J. S., Selective nicotinic acetylcholine receptor agonists: potential therapies for neuropsychiatric disorders with cognitive dysfunction. *Curr Opin Investig Drugs* 2008, 9, (1), 47-56.

[27] Rezvani, A. H.; Levin, E. D., Cognitive effects of nicotine. *Biol Psychiatry* 2001, 49, (3), 258-67.

[28] Levin, E. D., Nicotinic receptor subtypes and cognitive function. *J Neurobiol* 2002, 53, (4), 633-40.

[29] Graves, A. B.; van Duijn, C. M.; Chandra, V.; Fratiglioni, L.; Heyman, A.; Jorm, A. F.; Kokmen, E.; Kondo, K.; Mortimer, J. A.; Rocca, W. A.; et al., Alcohol and tobacco consumption as risk factors for Alzheimer's disease: a collaborative re-analysis of case-control studies. EURODEM Risk Factors Research Group. *Int J Epidemiol* 1991, 20 Suppl 2, S48-57.

[30] Arendash, G. W.; Sanberg, P. R.; Sengstock, G. J., Nicotine enhances the learning and memory of aged rats. *Pharmacol Biochem Behav* 1995, 52, (3), 517-23.

[31] Arendash, G. W.; Sengstock, G. J.; Sanberg, P. R.; Kem, W. R., Improved learning and memory in aged rats with chronic administration of the nicotinic receptor agonist GTS-21. *Brain Res* 1995, 674, (2), 252-9.

[32] Shim, S. B.; Lee, S. H.; Chae, K. R.; Kim, C. K.; Hwang, D. Y.; Kim, B. G.; Jee, S. W.; Lee, S. H.; Sin, J. S.; Bae, C. J.; Lee, B. C.; Lee, H. H.; Kim, Y. K., Nicotine leads to improvements in behavioral impairment and an increase in the nicotine acetylcholine receptor in transgenic mice. *Neurochem Res* 2008, 33, (9), 1783-8.

[33] Vidal, C., Nicotinic receptors in the brain. Molecular biology, function, and therapeutics. *Mol Chem Neuropathol* 1996, 28, (1-3), 3-11.

[34] Riah, O.; Dousset, J. C.; Courriere, P.; Stigliani, J. L.; Baziard-Mouysset, G.; Belahsen, Y., Evidence that nicotine acetylcholine receptors are not the main targets of cotinine toxicity. *Toxicol Lett* 1999, 109, (1-2), 21-9.

[35] Riah, O.; Courriere, P.; Dousset, J. C.; Todeschi, N.; Labat, C., Nicotine is more efficient than cotinine at passing the blood-brain barrier in rats. *Cell Mol Neurobiol* 1998, 18, (3), 311-8.

[36] Lockman, P. R.; McAfee, G.; Geldenhuys, W. J.; Van der Schyf, C. J.; Abbruscato, T. J.; Allen, D. D., Brain uptake kinetics of nicotine and cotinine after chronic nicotine exposure. *J Pharmacol Exp Ther* 2005, 314, (2), 636-42.

[37] Echeverria, V.; Burgess, S.; Zeitlin, R.; Barman, A.; Thakur, G.; Inouye, H.; Feris, E.; Buckingham, S.; Kirschner, D.; Mori, T.; Leblanc, R.; Prabhakar, R.; Sattelle, D.; Arendash, G., Cotinine: A dual-action drug with multiple benefits against *Alzheimer's disease Alzheimer's & Dementia: The Journal of the Alzheimer's Association* 2010, 6, (4), S536-S537.

[38] Lewis, D. F.; Dickins, M.; Lake, B. G.; Eddershaw, P. J.; Tarbit, M. H.; Goldfarb, P. S., Molecular modelling of the human cytochrome P450 isoform CYP2A6 and investigations of CYP2A substrate selectivity. *Toxicology* 1999, 133, (1), 1-33.

[39] Visoni, S.; Meireles, N.; Monteiro, L.; Rossini, A.; Pinto, L. F., Different modes of inhibition of mouse Cyp2a5 and rat CYP2A3 by the food-derived 8-methoxypsoralen. *Food Chem Toxicol* 2008, 46, (3), 1190-5.

[40] Donato, M. T.; Viitala, P.; Rodriguez-Antona, C.; Lindfors, A.; Castell, J. V.; Raunio, H.; Gomez-Lechon, M. J.; Pelkonen, O., CYP2A5/CYP2A6 expression in mouse and human hepatocytes treated with various in vivo inducers. *Drug Metab Dispos* 2000, 28, (11), 1321-6.

[41] Caldwell, W. S.; Greene, J. M.; Byrd, G. D.; Chang, K. M.; Uhrig, M. S.; deBethizy, J. D.; Crooks, P. A.; Bhatti, B. S.; Riggs, R. M., Characterization of the glucuronide conjugate of cotinine: a previously unidentified major metabolite of nicotine in smokers' urine. *Chem Res Toxicol* 1992, 5, (2), 280-5.

[42] Ghosheh, O.; Hawes, E. M., N-glucuronidation of nicotine and cotinine in human: formation of cotinine glucuronide in liver microsomes and lack of catalysis by 10 examined UDP-glucuronosyltransferases. *Drug Metab Dispos* 2002, 30, (9), 991-6.

[43] Kuehl, G. E.; Murphy, S. E., N-glucuronidation of trans-3'-hydroxycotinine by human liver microsomes. *Chem Res Toxicol* 2003, 16, (12), 1502-6.

[44] Malaiyandi, V.; Goodz, S. D.; Sellers, E. M.; Tyndale, R. F., CYP2A6 genotype, phenotype, and the use of nicotine metabolites as biomarkers during ad libitum smoking. *Cancer Epidemiol Biomarkers Prev* 2006, 15, (10), 1812-9.

[45] Strasser, A. A.; Malaiyandi, V.; Hoffmann, E.; Tyndale, R. F.; Lerman, C., An association of CYP2A6 genotype and smoking topography. *Nicotine Tob Res* 2007, 9, (4), 511-8.

[46] Yamanaka, H.; Nakajima, M.; Nishimura, K.; Yoshida, R.; Fukami, T.; Katoh, M.; Yokoi, T., Metabolic profile of nicotine in subjects whose CYP2A6 gene is deleted. *Eur J Pharm Sci* 2004, 22, (5), 419-25.

[47] Nakajima, M.; Fukami, T.; Yamanaka, H.; Higashi, E.; Sakai, H.; Yoshida, R.; Kwon, J. T.; McLeod, H. L.; Yokoi, T., Comprehensive evaluation of variability in nicotine metabolism and CYP2A6 polymorphic alleles in four ethnic populations. *Clin Pharmacol Ther* 2006, 80, (3), 282-97.

[48] Bramer, S. L.; Kallungal, B. A., Clinical considerations in study designs that use cotinine as a biomarker. *Biomarkers* 2003, 8, (3-4), 187-203.

[49] Hukkanen, J.; Jacob, P., 3rd; Benowitz, N. L., Effect of grapefruit juice on cytochrome P450 2A6 and nicotine renal clearance. *Clin Pharmacol Ther* 2006, 80, (5), 522-30.

[50] Tassaneeyakul, W.; Guo, L. Q.; Fukuda, K.; Ohta, T.; Yamazoe, Y., Inhibition selectivity of grapefruit juice components on human cytochromes P450. *Arch Biochem Biophys* 2000, 378, (2), 356-63.

[51] Siu, E. C.; Tyndale, R. F., Characterization and comparison of nicotine and cotinine metabolism in vitro and in vivo in DBA/2 and C57BL/6 mice. *Mol Pharmacol* 2007, 71, (3), 826-34.

[52] Terry, A. V., Jr.; Hernandez, C. M.; Hohnadel, E. J.; Bouchard, K. P.; Buccafusco, J. J., Cotinine, a neuroactive metabolite of nicotine: potential for treating disorders of impaired cognition. *CNS Drug Rev* 2005, 11, (3), 229-52.

[53] Taly, A.; Corringer, P. J.; Guedin, D.; Lestage, P.; Changeux, J. P., Nicotinic receptors: allosteric transitions and therapeutic targets in the nervous system. *Nat Rev Drug Discov* 2009, 8, (9), 733-50.

[54] Kem, W. R., The brain alpha7 nicotinic receptor may be an important therapeutic target for the treatment of Alzheimer's disease: studies with DMXBA (GTS-21). *Behav Brain Res* 2000, 113, (1-2), 169-81.

[55] Bowman, E. R.; Mc, K. H., Jr., Studies on the metabolism of (-)-cotinine in the human. *J Pharmacol Exp Ther* 1962, 135, 306-11.

[56] Borzelleca, J. F.; Bowman, E. R.; Mc, K. H., Jr., Studies on the respiratory and cardiovascular effects of (-)-cotinine. *J Pharmacol Exp Ther* 1962, 137, 313-8.

[57] Benowitz, N. L.; Kuyt, F.; Jacob, P., 3rd; Jones, R. T.; Osman, A. L., Cotinine disposition and effects. *Clin Pharmacol Ther* 1983, 34, (5), 604-11.

[58] Benowitz, N. L.; Sharp, D. S., Inverse relation between serum cotinine concentration and blood pressure in cigarette smokers. *Circulation* 1989, 80, (5), 1309-12.

[59] Hatsukami, D.; Lexau, B.; Nelson, D.; Pentel, P. R.; Sofuoglu, M.; Goldman, A., Effects of cotinine on cigarette self-administration. *Psychopharmacology* (Berl) 1998, 138, (2), 184-9.

[60] Hatsukami, D.; Pentel, P. R.; Jensen, J.; Nelson, D.; Allen, S. S.; Goldman, A.; Rafael, D., Cotinine: effects with and without nicotine. *Psychopharmacology* (Berl) 1998, 135, (2), 141-50.

[61] Hatsukami, D. K.; Grillo, M.; Pentel, P. R.; Oncken, C.; Bliss, R., Safety of cotinine in humans: physiologic, subjective, and cognitive effects. *Pharmacol Biochem Behav* 1997, 57, (4), 643-50.

[62] De Schepper, P. J.; Van Hecken, A.; Daenens, P.; Van Rossum, J. M., Kinetics of cotinine after oral and intravenous administration to man. *Eur J Clin Pharmacol* 1987, 31, (5), 583-8.

[63] Frey, W., *Neurologic Agents for Nasal Administration to the Brain*. World Intellectual Property Organization: Geneva, 1991.

[64] Hanson, L. R.; Frey, W. H., 2nd, Intranasal delivery bypasses the blood-brain barrier to target therapeutic agents to the central nervous system and treat neurodegenerative disease. *BMC Neurosci* 2008, 9 Suppl 3, S5.

[65] Costantino, H. R.; Leonard, A. K.; Brandt, G.; Johnson, P. H.; Quay, S. C., Intranasal administration of acetylcholinesterase inhibitors. *BMC Neurosci* 2008, 9 Suppl 3, S6.

[66] Dhuria, S. V.; Hanson, L. R.; Frey, W. H., 2nd, Intranasal drug targeting of hypocretin-1 (orexin-A) to the central nervous system. *J Pharm Sci* 2009, 98, (7), 2501-15.

[67] Martenyi, F.; Brown, E. B.; Caldwell, C. D., Failed efficacy of fluoxetine in the treatment of posttraumatic stress disorder: results of a fixed-dose, placebo-controlled study. *J Clin Psychopharmacol* 2007, 27, (2), 166-70.

[68] Boscarino, J. A., Posttraumatic stress disorder and physical illness: results from clinical and epidemiologic studies. *Ann N Y Acad Sci* 2004, 1032, 141-53.

[69] Dobie, D. J.; Maynard, C.; Kivlahan, D. R.; Johnson, K. M.; Simpson, T.; David, A. C.; Bradley, K., Posttraumatic stress disorder screening status is associated with increased VA medical and surgical utilization in women. *J Gen Intern Med* 2006, 21 Suppl 3, S58-64.

[70] Werner, N. S.; Meindl, T.; Engel, R. R.; Rosner, R.; Riedel, M.; Reiser, M.; Fast, K., Hippocampal function during associative learning in patients with posttraumatic stress disorder. *J Psychiatr Res* 2009, 43, (3), 309-18.

[71] Yehuda, R.; Golier, J. A.; Tischler, L.; Harvey, P. D.; Newmark, R.; Yang, R. K.; Buchsbaum, M. S., Hippocampal volume in aging combat veterans with and without post-traumatic stress disorder: relation to risk and resilience factors. *J Psychiatr Res* 2007, 41, (5), 435-45.

[72] Francati, V.; Vermetten, E.; Bremner, J. D., Functional neuroimaging studies in posttraumatic stress disorder: review of current methods and findings. *Depress Anxiety* 2007, 24, (3), 202-18.

[73] Yehuda, R.; Giller, E. L.; Southwick, S. M.; Lowy, M. T.; Mason, J. W., Hypothalamic-pituitary-adrenal dysfunction in posttraumatic stress disorder. *Biol Psychiatry* 1991, 30, (10), 1031-48.

[74] Merenlender-Wagner, A.; Dikshtein, Y.; Yadid, G., The beta-endorphin role in stress-related psychiatric disorders. *Curr Drug Targets* 2009, 10, (11), 1096-108.

[75] Hoffman, L.; Burges Watson, P.; Wilson, G.; Montgomery, J., Low plasma beta-endorphin in post-traumatic stress disorder. *Aust N Z J Psychiatry* 1989, 23, (2), 269-73.

[76] Zhang, H.; Ozbay, F.; Lappalainen, J.; Kranzler, H. R.; van Dyck, C. H.; Charney, D. S.; Price, L. H.; Southwick, S.; Yang, B. Z.; Rasmussen, A.; Gelernter, J., Brain derived neurotrophic factor (BDNF) gene variants and Alzheimer's disease, affective disorders, posttraumatic stress disorder, schizophrenia, and substance dependence. *Am J Med Genet B Neuropsychiatr Genet* 2006, 141B, (4), 387-93.

[77] Dell'osso, L.; Carmassi, C.; Del Debbio, A.; Dell'osso, M. C.; Bianchi, C.; da Pozzo, E.; Origlia, N.; Domenici, L.; Massimetti, G.; Marazziti, D.; Piccinni, A., Brain-derived neurotrophic factor plasma levels in patients suffering from post-traumatic stress disorder. *Prog Neuropsychopharmacol Biol Psychiatry* 2009, 33, (5), 899-902.

[78] Stein, D. J.; Ipser, J.; McAnda, N., Pharmacotherapy of posttraumatic stress disorder: a review of meta-analyses and treatment guidelines. *CNS Spectr* 2009, 14, (1 Suppl 1), 25-31.

[79] Corchs, F.; Nutt, D. J.; Hood, S.; Bernik, M., Serotonin and Sensitivity to Trauma-Related Exposure in Selective Serotonin Reuptake Inhibitors-Recovered Posttraumatic Stress Disorder. *Biol Psychiatry* 2009.

[80] Brady, K.; Pearlstein, T.; Asnis, G. M.; Baker, D.; Rothbaum, B.; Sikes, C. R.; Farfel, G. M., Efficacy and safety of sertraline treatment of posttraumatic stress disorder: a randomized controlled trial. *Jama* 2000, 283, (14), 1837-44.

[81] Davidson, J.; Pearlstein, T.; Londborg, P.; Brady, K. T.; Rothbaum, B.; Bell, J.; Maddock, R.; Hegel, M. T.; Farfel, G., Efficacy of sertraline in preventing relapse of posttraumatic stress disorder: results of a 28-week double-blind, placebo-controlled study. *Am J Psychiatry* 2001, 158, (12), 1974-81.

[82] Brady, K. T.; Clary, C. M., Affective and anxiety comorbidity in post-traumatic stress disorder treatment trials of sertraline. *Compr Psychiatry* 2003, 44, (5), 360-9.

[83] Cohen, H.; Kotler, M.; Matar, M.; Kaplan, Z., Normalization of heart rate variability in post-traumatic stress disorder patients following fluoxetine treatment: preliminary results. *Isr Med Assoc J* 2000, 2, (4), 296-301.

[84] Hapke, U.; Schumann, A.; Rumpf, H. J.; John, U.; Konerding, U.; Meyer, C., Association of smoking and nicotine dependence with trauma and posttraumatic stress disorder in a general population sample. *J Nerv Ment Dis* 2005, 193, (12), 843-6.

[85] Nutt, D. J., The psychobiology of posttraumatic stress disorder. *J Clin Psychiatry* 2000, 61 Suppl 5, 24-9; discussion 30-2.

[86] Fuxe, K.; Everitt, B. J.; Hokfelt, T., On the action of nicotine and cotinine on central 5-hydroxytryptamine neurons. *Pharmacol Biochem Behav* 1979, 10, (5), 671-7.

[87] Chojnacka-Wojcik, E., 5-Hydroxytryptamine in the central nervous system. *Pol J Pharmacol* 1995, 47, (3), 219-35.

[88] Buhot, M. C.; Martin, S.; Segu, L., Role of serotonin in memory impairment. *Ann Med* 2000, 32, (3), 210-21.

[89] van Os, J.; Kapur, S., Schizophrenia. *Lancet* 2009, 374, (9690), 635-45.

[90] Van Snellenberg, J. X., Working memory and long-term memory deficits in schizophrenia: is there a common substrate? *Psychiatry Res* 2009, 174, (2), 89-96.

[91] McEvoy, J. P.; Freudenreich, O.; Wilson, W. H., Smoking and therapeutic response to clozapine in patients with schizophrenia. *Biol Psychiatry* 1999, 46, (1), 125-9.

[92] Freedman, R.; Olincy, A.; Buchanan, R. W.; Harris, J. G.; Gold, J. M.; Johnson, L.; Allensworth, D.; Guzman-Bonilla, A.; Clement, B.; Ball, M. P.; Kutnick, J.; Pender, V.; Martin, L. F.; Stevens, K. E.; Wagner, B. D.; Zerbe, G. O.; Soti, F.; Kem, W. R., Initial phase 2 trial of a nicotinic agonist in schizophrenia. *Am J Psychiatry* 2008, 165, (8), 1040-7.

[93] Seillier, A.; Giuffrida, A., Evaluation of NMDA receptor models of schizophrenia: divergences in the behavioral effects of sub-chronic PCP and MK-801. *Behav Brain Res* 2009, 204, (2), 410-5.

[94] Levin, E. D.; Bettegowda, C.; Weaver, T.; Christopher, N. C., Nicotine-dizocilpine interactions and working and reference memory performance of rats in the radial-arm maze. *Pharmacol Biochem Behav* 1998, 61, (3), 335-40.

[95] Ciamei, A.; Aversano, M.; Cestari, V.; Castellano, C., Effects of MK-801 and nicotine combinations on memory consolidation in CD1 mice. *Psychopharmacology* (Berl) 2001, 154, (2), 126-30.

[96] Woodruff-Pak, D. S.; Gould, T. J., Neuronal nicotinic acetylcholine receptors: involvement in Alzheimer's disease and schizophrenia. *Behav Cogn Neurosci Rev* 2002, 1, (1), 5-20.

[97] Leiser, S. C.; Bowlby, M. R.; Comery, T. A.; Dunlop, J., A cog in cognition: how the alpha7 nicotinic acetylcholine receptor is geared towards improving cognitive deficits. *Pharmacol Ther* 2009, 122, (3), 302-11.

[98] Olincy, A.; Stevens, K. E., Treating schizophrenia symptoms with an alpha7 nicotinic agonist, from mice to men. *Biochem Pharmacol* 2007, 74, (8), 1192-201.

[99] Braff, D. L.; Grillon, C.; Geyer, M. A., Gating and habituation of the startle reflex in schizophrenic patients. *Arch Gen Psychiatry* 1992, 49, (3), 206-15.

[100] Swerdlow, N. R.; Light, G. A.; Cadenhead, K. S.; Sprock, J.; Hsieh, M. H.; Braff, D. L., Startle gating deficits in a large cohort of patients with schizophrenia: relationship to medications, symptoms, neurocognition, and level of function. *Arch Gen Psychiatry* 2006, 63, (12), 1325-35.

[101] Geyer, M. A., Are cross-species measures of sensorimotor gating useful for the discovery of procognitive cotreatments for schizophrenia? *Dialogues Clin Neurosci* 2006, 8, (1), 9-16.

[102] Risner, M. E.; Goldberg, S. R.; Prada, J. A.; Cone, E. J., Effects of nicotine, cocaine and some of their metabolites on schedule-controlled responding by beagle dogs and squirrel monkeys. *J Pharmacol Exp Ther* 1985, 234, (1), 113-9.

[103] Buccafusco, J. J.; Terry, A. V., Jr., A reversible model of the cognitive impairment associated with schizophrenia in monkeys: potential therapeutic effects of two nicotinic acetylcholine receptor agonists. *Biochem Pharmacol* 2009, 78, (7), 852-62.

[104] Braak, H.; de Vos, R. A.; Jansen, E. N.; Bratzke, H.; Braak, E., Neuropathological hallmarks of Alzheimer's and Parkinson's diseases. *Prog Brain Res* 1998, 117, 267-85.

[105] Mott, R. T.; Hulette, C. M., Neuropathology of Alzheimer's disease. *Neuroimaging Clin N Am* 2005, 15, (4), 755-65, ix.

[106] Rowan, M. J.; Klyubin, I.; Wang, Q.; Hu, N. W.; Anwyl, R., Synaptic memory mechanisms: Alzheimer's disease amyloid beta-peptide-induced dysfunction. *Biochem Soc Trans* 2007, 35, (Pt 5), 1219-23.

[107] Weisman, D.; Hakimian, E.; Ho, G. J., Interleukins, inflammation, and mechanisms of Alzheimer's disease. *Vitam Horm* 2006, 74, 505-30.

[108] Hardy, J.; Selkoe, D. J., The amyloid hypothesis of Alzheimer's disease: progress and problems on the road to therapeutics. *Science* 2002, 297, (5580), 353-6.

[109] Ferreira, S. T.; Vieira, M. N.; De Felice, F. G., Soluble protein oligomers as emerging toxins in Alzheimer's and other amyloid diseases. *IUBMB Life* 2007, 59, (4-5), 332-45.

[110] Haass, C.; Selkoe, D. J., Soluble protein oligomers in neurodegeneration: lessons from the Alzheimer's amyloid beta-peptide. *Nat Rev Mol Cell Biol* 2007, 8, (2), 101-12.

[111] Echeverria, V.; Berman, D. E.; Arancio, O., Oligomers of beta-amyloid peptide inhibit BDNF-induced arc expression in cultured cortical Neurons. *Curr Alzheimer Res* 2007, 4, (5), 518-21.

[112] Nakagami, Y.; Nishimura, S.; Murasugi, T.; Kaneko, I.; Meguro, M.; Marumoto, S.; Kogen, H.; Koyama, K.; Oda, T., A novel beta-sheet breaker, RS-0406, reverses amyloid beta-induced cytotoxicity and impairment of long-term potentiation in vitro. *Br J Pharmacol* 2002, 137, (5), 676-82.

[113] Walsh, D. M.; Townsend, M.; Podlisny, M. B.; Shankar, G. M.; Fadeeva, J. V.; Agnaf, O. E.; Hartley, D. M.; Selkoe, D. J., Certain inhibitors of synthetic amyloid beta-peptide (Abeta) fibrillogenesis block oligomerization of natural Abeta and thereby rescue long-term potentiation. *J Neurosci* 2005, 25, (10), 2455-62.

[114] Sapra, M.; Kim, K. Y., Anti-amyloid treatments in Alzheimer's disease. *Recent Pat CNS Drug Discov* 2009, 4, (2), 143-8.

[115] Doig, A. J., Peptide inhibitors of beta-amyloid aggregation. *Curr Opin Drug Discov Devel* 2007, 10, (5), 533-9.

[116] Savioz, A.; Leuba, G.; Vallet, P. G.; Walzer, C., Contribution of neural networks to Alzheimer disease's progression. *Brain Res Bull* 2009, 80, (4-5), 309-14.

[117] Engelborghs, S.; De Deyn, P. P., The neurochemistry of Alzheimer's disease. *Acta Neurol Belg* 1997, 97, (2), 67-84.

[118] Mufson, E. J.; Counts, S. E.; Perez, S. E.; Ginsberg, S. D., Cholinergic system during the progression of Alzheimer's disease: therapeutic implications. *Expert Rev Neurother* 2008, 8, (11), 1703-18.

[119] Jacobs, R. W.; Duong, T.; Scheibel, A. B., Immunohistochemical analysis of the basal forebrain in Alzheimer's disease. *Mol Chem Neuropathol* 1992, 17, (1), 1-20.
[120] Svensson, A. L.; Warpman, U.; Hellstrom-Lindahl, E.; Bogdanovic, N.; Lannfelt, L.; Nordberg, A., Nicotinic receptors, muscarinic receptors and choline acetyltransferase activity in the temporal cortex of Alzheimer patients with differing apolipoprotein E genotypes. *Neurosci Lett* 1997, 232, (1), 37-40.
[121] Nordberg, A., Nicotinic receptor abnormalities of Alzheimer's disease: therapeutic implications. *Biol Psychiatry* 2001, 49, (3), 200-10.
[122] Burghaus, L.; Schutz, U.; Krempel, U.; de Vos, R. A.; Jansen Steur, E. N.; Wevers, A.; Lindstrom, J.; Schroder, H., Quantitative assessment of nicotinic acetylcholine receptor proteins in the cerebral cortex of Alzheimer patients. *Brain Res Mol Brain Res* 2000, 76, (2), 385-8.
[123] Mufson, E. J.; Conner, J. M.; Kordower, J. H., Nerve growth factor in Alzheimer's disease: defective retrograde transport to nucleus basalis. *Neuroreport* 1995, 6, (7), 1063-6.
[124] Coulson, E. J.; May, L. M.; Sykes, A. M.; Hamlin, A. S., The role of the p75 neurotrophin receptor in cholinergic dysfunction in Alzheimer's disease. *Neuroscientist* 2009, 15, (4), 317-23.
[125] Covaceuszach, S.; Capsoni, S.; Ugolini, G.; Spirito, F.; Vignone, D.; Cattaneo, A., Development of a non invasive NGF-based therapy for Alzheimer's disease. *Curr Alzheimer Res* 2009, 6, (2), 158-70.
[126] Tuszynski, M. H.; Sang, H.; Yoshida, K.; Gage, F. H., Recombinant human nerve growth factor infusions prevent cholinergic neuronal degeneration in the adult primate brain. *Ann Neurol* 1991, 30, (5), 625-36.
[127] Koliatsos, V. E.; Price, D. L.; Clatterbuck, R. E.; Markowska, A. L.; Olton, D. S.; Wilcox, B. J., *Neurotrophic strategies for treating Alzheimer's disease: lessons from basic neurobiology and animal models.* Ann N Y Acad Sci 1993, 695, 292-9.
[128] Ebendal, T.; Lonnerberg, P.; Pei, G.; Kylberg, A.; Kullander, K.; Persson, H.; Olson, L., Engineering cells to secrete growth factors. *J Neurol* 1994, 242, (1 Suppl 1), S5-7.
[129] Nordberg, A., Mechanisms behind the neuroprotective actions of cholinesterase inhibitors in Alzheimer disease. *Alzheimer Dis Assoc Disord* 2006, 20, (2 Suppl 1), S12-8.
[130] Munoz-Torrero, D., Acetylcholinesterase inhibitors as disease-modifying therapies for Alzheimer's disease. *Curr Med Chem* 2008, 15, (24), 2433-55.
[131] Nikolov, R., Alzheimer's disease therapy - an update. *Drug News Perspect* 1998, 11, (4), 248-55.
[132] Tsuno, N., Donepezil in the treatment of patients with Alzheimer's disease. *Expert Rev Neurother* 2009, 9, (5), 591-8.
[133] Umegaki, H.; Itoh, A.; Suzuki, Y.; Nabeshima, T., Discontinuation of donepezil for the treatment of Alzheimer's disease in geriatric practice. *Int Psychogeriatr* 2008, 20, (4), 800-6.
[134] Raina, P.; Santaguida, P.; Ismaila, A.; Patterson, C.; Cowan, D.; Levine, M.; Booker, L.; Oremus, M., Effectiveness of cholinesterase inhibitors and memantine for treating dementia: evidence review for a clinical practice guideline. *Ann Intern Med* 2008, 148, (5), 379-97.

[135] Gongadze, N.; Antelava, N.; Kezeli, T.; Okudjava, M.; Pachkoria, K., The mechanisms of neurodegenerative processes and current pharmacotherapy of Alzheimer's disease. *Georgian Med News* 2008, (155), 44-8.

[136] Salomon, A. R.; Marcinowski, K. J.; Friedland, R. P.; Zagorski, M. G., Nicotine inhibits amyloid formation by the beta-peptide. *Biochemistry* 1996, 35, (42), 13568-78.

[137] Nordberg, A.; Hellstrom-Lindahl, E.; Lee, M.; Johnson, M.; Mousavi, M.; Hall, R.; Perry, E.; Bednar, I.; Court, J., Chronic nicotine treatment reduces beta-amyloidosis in the brain of a mouse model of Alzheimer's disease (APPsw). *J Neurochem* 2002, 81, (3), 655-8.

[138] Lawrence, A. D.; Sahakian, B. J., Alzheimer disease, attention, and the cholinergic system. *Alzheimer Dis Assoc Disord* 1995, 9 Suppl 2, 43-9.

[139] Lawrence, A. D.; Sahakian, B. J., The cognitive psychopharmacology of Alzheimer's disease: focus on cholinergic systems. *Neurochem Res* 1998, 23, (5), 787-94.

[140] Howe, M. N.; Price, I. R., Effects of transdermal nicotine on learning, memory, verbal fluency, concentration, and general health in a healthy sample at risk for dementia. *Int Psychogeriatr* 2001, 13, (4), 465-75.

[141] White, H. K.; Levin, E. D., Four-week nicotine skin patch treatment effects on cognitive performance in Alzheimer's disease. *Psychopharmacology* (Berl) 1999, 143, (2), 158-65.

[142] Kelton, M. C.; Kahn, H. J.; Conrath, C. L.; Newhouse, P. A., The effects of nicotine on Parkinson's disease. *Brain Cogn* 2000, 43, (1-3), 274-82.

[143] Lukas, R. J.; Changeux, J. P.; Le Novere, N.; Albuquerque, E. X.; Balfour, D. J.; Berg, D. K.; Bertrand, D.; Chiappinelli, V. A.; Clarke, P. B.; Collins, A. C.; Dani, J. A.; Grady, S. R.; Kellar, K. J.; Lindstrom, J. M.; Marks, M. J.; Quik, M.; Taylor, P. W.; Wonnacott, S., International Union of Pharmacology. XX. Current status of the nomenclature for nicotinic acetylcholine receptors and their subunits. *Pharmacol Rev* 1999, 51, (2), 397-401.

[144] Jensen, A. A.; Frolund, B.; Liljefors, T.; Krogsgaard-Larsen, P., Neuronal nicotinic acetylcholine receptors: structural revelations, target identifications, and therapeutic inspirations. *J Med Chem* 2005, 48, (15), 4705-45.

[145] Linert, W.; Bridge, M. H.; Huber, M.; Bjugstad, K. B.; Grossman, S.; Arendash, G. W., In vitro and in vivo studies investigating possible antioxidant actions of nicotine: relevance to Parkinson's and Alzheimer's diseases. *Biochim Biophys Acta* 1999, 1454, (2), 143-52.

[146] Kem, W. R., A study of the occurrence of anabaseine in Paranemertes and other nemertines. *Toxicon* 1971, 9, (1), 23-32.

[147] Wang, D.; Noda, Y.; Zhou, Y.; Mouri, A.; Mizoguchi, H.; Nitta, A.; Chen, W.; Nabeshima, T., The allosteric potentiation of nicotinic acetylcholine receptors by galantamine ameliorates the cognitive dysfunction in beta amyloid25-35 i.c.v.-injected mice: involvement of dopaminergic systems. *Neuropsychopharmacology* 2007, 32, (6), 1261-71.

[148] Araki, H.; Suemaru, K.; Gomita, Y., Neuronal nicotinic receptor and psychiatric disorders: functional and behavioral effects of nicotine. *Jpn J Pharmacol* 2002, 88, (2), 133-8.

[149] Olincy, A.; Harris, J. G.; Johnson, L. L.; Pender, V.; Kongs, S.; Allensworth, D.; Ellis, J.; Zerbe, G. O.; Leonard, S.; Stevens, K. E.; Stevens, J. O.; Martin, L.; Adler, L. E.;

Soti, F.; Kem, W. R.; Freedman, R., Proof-of-concept trial of an alpha7 nicotinic agonist in schizophrenia. *Arch Gen Psychiatry* 2006, 63, (6), 630-8.

[150] Tregellas, J. R.; Olincy, A.; Johnson, L.; Tanabe, J.; Shatti, S.; Martin, L. F.; Singel, D.; Du, Y. P.; Soti, F.; Kem, W. R.; Freedman, R., Functional magnetic resonance imaging of effects of a nicotinic agonist in schizophrenia. *Neuropsychopharmacology* 35, (4), 938-42.

[151] Kadir, A.; Almkvist, O.; Wall, A.; Langstrom, B.; Nordberg, A., PET imaging of cortical 11C-nicotine binding correlates with the cognitive function of attention in Alzheimer's disease. *Psychopharmacology* (Berl) 2006, 188, (4), 509-20.

[152] Galvin, J. E.; Cornblatt, B.; Newhouse, P.; Ancoli-Israel, S.; Wesnes, K.; Williamson, D.; Zhu, Y.; Sorra, K.; Amatniek, J., Effects of galantamine on measures of attention: results from 2 clinical trials in Alzheimer disease patients with comparisons to donepezil. *Alzheimer Dis Assoc Disord* 2008, 22, (1), 30-8.

[153] Thomsen, M. S.; Hansen, H. H.; Timmerman, D. B.; Mikkelsen, J. D., Cognitive improvement by activation of alpha7 nicotinic acetylcholine receptors: from animal models to human pathophysiology. *Curr Pharm Des* 16, (3), 323-43.

[154] Gauthier, S.; Scheltens, P., Can we do better in developing new drugs for Alzheimer's disease? *Alzheimers Dement* 2009, 5, (6), 489-91.

[155] Williams, A. D.; Sega, M.; Chen, M.; Kheterpal, I.; Geva, M.; Berthelier, V.; Kaleta, D. T.; Cook, K. D.; Wetzel, R., Structural properties of Abeta protofibrils stabilized by a small molecule. *Proc Natl Acad Sci U S A* 2005, 102, (20), 7115-20.

[156] Necula, M.; Kayed, R.; Milton, S.; Glabe, C. G., Small molecule inhibitors of aggregation indicate that amyloid beta oligomerization and fibrillization pathways are independent and distinct. *J Biol Chem* 2007, 282, (14), 10311-24.

[157] Ferrao-Gonzales, A. D.; Robbs, B. K.; Moreau, V. H.; Ferreira, A.; Juliano, L.; Valente, A. P.; Almeida, F. C.; Silva, J. L.; Foguel, D., Controlling {beta}-amyloid oligomerization by the use of naphthalene sulfonates: trapping low molecular weight oligomeric species. *J Biol Chem* 2005, 280, (41), 34747-54.

[158] Yang, F.; Lim, G. P.; Begum, A. N.; Ubeda, O. J.; Simmons, M. R.; Ambegaokar, S. S.; Chen, P. P.; Kayed, R.; Glabe, C. G.; Frautschy, S. A.; Cole, G. M., Curcumin inhibits formation of amyloid beta oligomers and fibrils, binds plaques, and reduces amyloid in vivo. *J Biol Chem* 2005, 280, (7), 5892-901.

[159] Yao, Z.; Drieu, K.; Papadopoulos, V., The Ginkgo biloba extract EGb 761 rescues the PC12 neuronal cells from beta-amyloid-induced cell death by inhibiting the formation of beta-amyloid-derived diffusible neurotoxic ligands. *Brain Res* 2001, 889, (1-2), 181-90.

[160] De Felice, F. G.; Vieira, M. N.; Saraiva, L. M.; Figueroa-Villar, J. D.; Garcia-Abreu, J.; Liu, R.; Chang, L.; Klein, W. L.; Ferreira, S. T., Targeting the neurotoxic species in Alzheimer's disease: inhibitors of Abeta oligomerization. *Faseb J* 2004, 18, (12), 1366-72.

[161] Zhao, W.; Wang, J.; Ho, L.; Ono, K.; Teplow, D. B.; Pasinetti, G. M., Identification of antihypertensive drugs which inhibit amyloid-beta protein oligomerization. *J Alzheimers Dis* 2009, 16, (1), 49-57.

[162] Hou, Y.; Aboukhatwa, M. A.; Lei, D. L.; Manaye, K.; Khan, I.; Luo, Y., Antidepressant natural flavonols modulate BDNF and beta amyloid in neurons and hippocampus of double TgAD mice. *Neuropharmacology* 58, (6), 911-20.

[163] Kirschner, D. A.; Gross, A. A.; Hidalgo, M. M.; Inouye, H.; Gleason, K. A.; Abdelsayed, G. A.; Castillo, G. M.; Snow, A. D.; Pozo-Ramajo, A.; Petty, S. A.; Decatur, S. M., Fiber diffraction as a screen for amyloid inhibitors. *Curr Alzheimer Res* 2008, 5, (3), 288-307.

[164] Szymanska, I.; Radecka, H.; Radecki, J.; Kaliszan, R., Electrochemical impedance spectroscopy for study of amyloid beta-peptide interactions with (-) nicotine ditartrate and (-) cotinine. *Biosens Bioelectron* 2007, 22, (9-10), 1955-60.

[165] Celie, P. H. N. v. R.-F., S.E; van Dijk, W.J; Brejc, K; Smit ,A.B and Sixma, T. K, Nicotine and Carbamylcholine Binding to Nicotinic Acetylcholine Receptors as Studied in AChBP Crystal Structures. *Neuron* 2004, 41, (6), 907-914.

[166] Karlin, A., Emerging structure of the nicotinic acetylcholine receptors. *Nat Rev Neurosci* 2002, 3, (2), 102-14.

[167] Le Novere, N.; Grutter, T.; Changeux, J. P., *Models of the extracellular domain of the nicotinic receptors and of agonist- and Ca2+-binding sites.* Proc Natl Acad Sci U S A 2002, 99, (5), 3210-5.

[168] Unwin, N., Refined structure of the nicotinic acetylcholine receptor at 4A resolution. *J Mol Biol* 2005, 346, (4), 967-89.

[169] Dellisanti, C. D.; Yao, Y.; Stroud, J. C.; Wang, Z. Z.; Chen, L., Crystal structure of the extracellular domain of nAChR alpha1 bound to alpha-bungarotoxin at 1.94 A resolution. *Nat Neurosci* 2007, 10, (8), 953-62.

[170] Hansen, S. B.; Sulzenbacher, G.; Huxford, T.; Marchot, P.; Taylor, P.; Bourne, Y., Structures of Aplysia AChBP complexes with nicotinic agonists and antagonists reveal distinctive binding interfaces and conformations. *Embo J* 2005, 24, (20), 3635-46.

[171] Talley, T. T.; Yalda, S.; Ho, K. Y.; Tor, Y.; Soti, F. S.; Kem, W. R.; Taylor, P., Spectroscopic analysis of benzylidene anabaseine complexes with acetylcholine binding proteins as models for ligand-nicotinic receptor interactions. *Biochemistry* 2006, 45, (29), 8894-902.

[172] Hibbs, R. E.; Radic, Z.; Taylor, P.; Johnson, D. A., Influence of agonists and antagonists on the segmental motion of residues near the agonist binding pocket of the acetylcholine-binding protein. *J Biol Chem* 2006, 281, (51), 39708-18.

[173] Huang, X.; Zheng, F.; Stokes, C.; Papke, R. L.; Zhan, C. G., Modeling binding modes of alpha7 nicotinic acetylcholine receptor with ligands: the roles of Gln117 and other residues of the receptor in agonist binding. *J Med Chem* 2008, 51, (20), 6293-302.

[174] Taly, A.; Corringer, P. J.; Grutter, T.; Prado de Carvalho, L.; Karplus, M.; Changeux, J. P., *Implications of the quaternary twist allosteric model for the physiology and pathology of nicotinic acetylcholine receptors.* Proc Natl Acad Sci U S A 2006, 103, (45), 16965-70.

[175] Taly, A.; Delarue, M.; Grutter, T.; Nilges, M.; Le Novere, N.; Corringer, P. J.; Changeux, J. P., Normal mode analysis suggests a quaternary twist model for the nicotinic receptor gating mechanism. *Biophys J* 2005, 88, (6), 3954-65.

[176] Cheng, X.; Lu, B.; Grant, B.; Law, R. J.; McCammon, J. A., Channel opening motion of alpha7 nicotinic acetylcholine receptor as suggested by normal mode analysis. *J Mol Biol* 2006, 355, (2), 310-24.

In: Working Memory: Capacity, Developments and... ISBN: 978-1-61761-980-9
Editor: Eden S. Levin © 2011 Nova Science Publishers, Inc.

Chapter 15

WORKING MEMORY AND FUNCTIONAL OUTCOME IN PATIENTS WITH MAJOR DEPRESSIVE DISORDER

Yasuhiro Kaneda[*]
Department of Psychiatry, Iwaki Clinic, Tokushima, Japan

ABSTRACT

Objective

Patients with major depressive disorder (MDD) have been reported to perform less well in neurocognitive tests than normal control subjects. The author tested the hypotheses that a specific type of cognitive function, namely verbal working memory (WM), in patients with MDD is predictive of the functional outcome.

Study 1

In this naturalistic cross-sectional study, the subjects consisted of 54 clinic adult out-patients. The assessments were performed using the 7-item Hamilton Rating Scale for Depression (HAM-D7) for the severity of depression, and the Digit Sequencing Task (DST) for evaluation of verbal WM. Functional outcome was rated on a scale of 0 (non-impaired) to 3 (severely impaired). The author found that, in the patients with current episode of MDD, functional outcome was significantly correlated with HAM-D7 scores, but not with DST scores. Meanwhile, in a sample of full remitted or partial remitted (mildly depressed) patients, functional outcome was significantly correlated with both DST and HAM-D7 scores. Moreover, in a sample of full remitted or partial remitted (mildly depressed) patients, the DST scores significantly contributed to the prediction of the functional outcome, but the HAM-D7scores did not.

---

[*] Corresponding author: Yasuhiro Kaneda, M.D., Ph.D., Dept. of Psychiatry, Iwaki Clinic, 11-1 Kamimizuta, Gakubara, Anan, Tokushima 774-0014, Japan, Tel: +81-884-23-5600, Fax: +81-884-22-1780, E-mail: kaneday-tsh@umin.ac.jp

Study 2

In this naturalistic longitudinal study, the subjects consisted of 24 adult outpatients. Significant decrease of the HAM-D7 scores was observed during the 12-week study period, whereas the DST scores showed no significant increase. At baseline, the functional outcome was significantly correlated with the scores on HAM-D7, but, at 12 weeks, it was significantly correlated with both HAM-D7 and DST scores. According to a multiple regression analysis, the DST scores at baseline significantly contributed to prediction of the functional outcome at 12 weeks.

Conclusion

These studies suggest the existence of a correlation between a deficit of verbal WM and the functional outcome after treatment in patients with MDD. Enhancement of verbal WM function may be useful to achieve normalization of functioning as an important component of remission in addition to symptomatic remission.

Keywords: depression, functional outcome, symptomatlogy, working memory

INTRODUCTION

Major depressive disorder (MDD) is a significant health problem, with major economic implications, and estimates of the economic burden of depression range from $52 billion in 1990 to $83 billion in 2000 [12]. Among others, the effect on employment is considered to have a great impact on the societal costs of depression, due to lost income, lost productivity, and disability income payments.

In previous studies [8, 9], the author demonstrated that neurocognitive performance was more important than the clinical symptoms in predicting the future employment status in patients with schizophrenia, and among the neurocognitive functions, verbal working memory (WM) was found to be the most important for determining the employment outcome. Patients with MDD also have been reported to perform less well in neurocognitive tests than normal control subjects, even after their depression is successfully treated with newer-generation antidepressants [4, 18]. In a recent report, Gualtieri and Morgan [5] reported that substantial numbers of patients with depression exhibit cognitive impairment.

The author also demonstrated that the deficit of verbal WM existed even after remission [7]. In this naturalistic cross-sectional study, the subjects consisted of 54 clinic adult outpatients and 54 age- and sex-equated healthy comparison subjects. The Digit Sequencing Task (DST; methodological details are described below) scores as verbal WM were significantly less in both patients with current episode of MDD and in full remitted or partial remitted (mildly depressed) patients than in controls. Also there were no significant correlations between DST scores and the dose of antidepressants or benzodiazepines in full remitted or partial remitted (mildly depressed) patients.

However, until date, little attention has been paid to the relation between neurocognitive performance and the psychosocial or functional outcomes in studies of depression.

Thus, the author tested the hypothesis that verbal WM in MDD would predict functional outcome [6]. In this naturalistic cross-sectional study, the subjects consisted of 54 clinic adult outpatients. The assessments were performed using the 7-item Hamilton Rating Scale for Depression (HAM-D7) [14] for the severity of depression, and the DST for evaluation of verbal WM. Functional outcome was rated on a scale of 0 (non-impaired) to 3 (severely impaired). The author found that, in the patients with current episode of MDD, functional outcome was significantly correlated with HAM-D7 scores, but not with DST scores. Meanwhile, in a sample of full remitted or partial remitted (mildly depressed) patients, functional outcome was significantly correlated with both DST and HAM-D7 scores. Moreover, in a sample of full remitted or partial remitted (mildly depressed) patients, the DST scores significantly contributed to the prediction of the functional outcome, but the HAM-D7 scores did not.

Since verbal WM was suggested to be more important than depressive symptoms in determining the functional outcome in full remitted or partial remitted (mildly depressed) patients, a further longitudinal study was conducted to verify the suggestion that verbal WM is predictive of the functional outcome in patients with MDD after remission.

SUBJECTS AND METHODS

In this prospective, open-label study, consecutive 31 adult outpatients (aged 21-59 years) who satisfied the DSM-IV [1] criteria for a current episode of unipolar MDD (non-psychotic) were recruited. Patients had no comorbid psychiatric disorders, or any medical, neurological, or developmental conditions that could affect cognition (e.g., ADHD, brain injury, MCI, chronic pain). The investigation was carried out in accordance with the Declaration of Helsinki and informed consent was obtained from all subjects.

The assessments were performed using the following instruments: 1) the HAM-D7 to determine the severity of depression and status of remission; full remission was defined as a score of 3 or less, and partial remission (mild depression) as a score of 10 or less on the HAM-D7, and 2) the Brief Assessment of Cognition in Schizophrenia (BACS) [10] DST to assess verbal WM (the patients were presented with clusters of numbers in random order of increasing length, and asked to recount the numbers in the right order, from lowest to highest, to the experimenter). The BACS DST has been validated in normal control subjects [10]. The scores on the DST in each depression group were normalized for the respective age- and sex-matched control groups (data available on request). The functional outcome (productivity), including the ability to go to work, doing household chores, or going to school was assessed by the author based on the interviews with the patients and their family, and was graded on a scale of 0-3, as follws: 0=non-impaired, 1=mildly impaired, 2=moderately impaired, 3=severely impaired.

The clinical assessments were performed on two occasions (1) on the day of entry and (2) after approximately 12 weeks (a mean period of 88.0 days, SD=10.5). Seven out of the 31 (23%) patients with a current episode of MDD did not report for the second assessment, i.e., they dropped out of the study.

The JMI software (Version 8.0.1) for Macintosh was used to perform the analyses. For numerical variables, the *t*-test procedures for independent group comparisons were used to compare the differences in the variables between two groups. The clinical assessment scores were compared between the two assessments by repeated-measures analysis of variance (ANOVA). Pearson's correlation was used to examine the relationships between two numerical variables. A logistic regression model with forward selection criteria was used to predict the functional outcome using the demographic variables, and the HAM-D7 and verbal WM scores. The level of significance was set at $p<0.05$.

RESULTS

The demographic characteristics at baseline are presented in Table 1. At baseline, four out of the 24 patients (17%) were on paroxetine (mean dose, 22.5mg) and one (4%) was on sulpiride (100mg). No of the patients was receiving more than one antidepressant drug. And eight of the 24 patients (33%) were on benzodiazepines. At the time of the second assessment, 22 out of the 24 patients were under treatment with the following antidepressant drugs: paroxetine (n=14; mean dose, 28.6mg), fluvoxamine (n=2; 37.5mg), sertraline (n=3; 75.0mg), and milnaciprane (n=3; 86.7mg); one patient was receiving two antidepressant drugs, while the remaining two patients were receiving no antidepressant drugs. Seventeen of the 24 patients (71%) were on benzodiazepines.

At the second assessment conducted after 12 weeks, according to the symptom severity scores, nine out of 24 patients (38%) with a current episode of MDD were in full remission. In addition, among these nine full remitted patients, normalization of the work function was seen in six patients (67%).

Significant decrease of the HAM-D7 scores from 13.2±3.3 to 6.3±4.3 ($p<0.0001$) was observed during the 12-week study period; on the other hand, the DST score (z-score) increased numerically during the same period (from -0.9±1.3 to -0.6±1.2), although the difference did not reach statistical significance.

At baseline, the functional outcome was significantly correlated with the HAM-D7 scores (r=0.43, $p<0.05$), but not with the DST scores, whereas at 12 weeks, the functional outcome was significantly correlated with both DST (r=-0.55, $p<0.01$) and the HAM-D7 scores (r=0.49, $p<0.05$). When we looked at only patients with full remission or partial remission (mild depression), the functional outcome was significantly correlated with the DST scores (r=-0.50, $p<0.05$), but not with the HAM-D7 scores.

Table 1. Demographic Data

N (F/M)	Age (yr.)	Education (yr.)	Age at onset (yr.)	Dose of antidepressants (mg/d)[a]	Dose of benzodiazepines (mg/d)[b]
24 (9/15)	35.5 (12.1)	12.6 (3.1)	34.0 (12.0)	4.3 (8.9)	2.3 (3.8)

Data are expressed as mean (SD).
[a]Paroxetine equivalent
[b]Diazepam equivalent

In regard to the relationship between the DST scores and the HAM-D7 scores, there was no significant relation between the two either at the baseline or at 12 weeks.

According to a multiple regression analysis with a forward stepwise procedure, the DST scores, but not the HAM-D7 scores, at baseline, significantly contributed to prediction of the functional outcome at 12 weeks (F=6.0, df=1, $p<0.05$). On the other hand, the HAM-D7 scores, but not the DST scores, at baseline, significantly contributed to prediction of the HAM-D7 scores at 12 weeks (F=9.8, df=1, $p<0.01$).

CONCLUSION

The findings of this study suggest the existence of a correlation between a deficit of verbal WM associated with MDD, and the functional outcome after treatment. The findings are consistent with those of a previous study carried out by the author [6], but not with those of the study reported by Kennedy et al. [11], who reported in their review that residual symptomatology after remission from depression may lead to enduring psychosocial impairment, as may subtle neurocognitive deficits. While the findings in this study do not underscore the importance of clinical remission from depression, a defined objective outcome indicated by a quantifiable score with a depressive symptom measurement tool, symptomatic full remission should always be the primary goal of treatment, since it is the optimal outcome in patients with depression [15]. However, the findings of this sturdy do suggest that enhancement of the verbal WM function, e.g., by cognitive rehabilitation, may be useful to achieve normalization of functioning of the important component of remission [21].

In terms of predictive factors, some previous studies have reported the predictive value of neurocognitive functions for symptomatic improvement, mainly in geriatric patients with depression [13]. However, in this study, the HAM-D7 scores were more important to predict symptomatic improvement than the scores on the DST used to assess verbal VM, a finding well in line with that reported by Biringer et al. [2], who showed that neurocognitive function at the baseline was not predictive of improvement in depressive symptoms over time in younger adult patients. Meanwhile, this study suggested that verbal VM was more important to predict the functional outcome than depressive symptoms. Therefore, in order to obtain a better functional outcome, it may be important to place more emphasis on the pretreatment verbal VM than depressive symptoms.

The findings of this study also suggest again that MDD-associated deficit in verbal WM exists both in acute depression and after treatment of depression. These findings are consistent with those of a previous study conducted by the author [7] and by Nebes et al. [16], who found that verbal VM dysfunction persisted in older depressed patients even after their mood disorder had responded to antidepressant medications. The observations in this study may be explained by an impairment of WM/central executive functions in MDD, as suggested by Rose and Ebmeier [19], since executive function impairment is considered to be, at least to a degree, trait-related [17].

However, the possibility of the influence of antidepressants [3] / benzodiazepines [20] on the verbal WM function cannot completely be ruled out. Another limitation of this study was that patients with full and partial remission were included together for the statistical analyses, mainly because there were few patients with full remission. Also, we may need a longer observation period to allow sufficient recovery of the verbal WM function. Therefore, a further long-term study on remitted patients of depression who are no longer on medication might be necessary to confirm the results of the present study.

ACKNOWLEDGMENTS

This work was supported in part by grants from Daido Life Welfare Foundation (2009), the Japanese Association of Neuro-Psychiatric Clinics (Ken TANAKA Memorial Grant, 2008), and the Charitable Trust Kimi IMAI Memorial Stress Associated Diseases Research Aid Fund (2009). This study was presented in part at the 15th Annual Meeting of the Japanese Association of Neuro-Psychiatric Clinics, Chiba, Japan, and the 1st Meeting of the Asian College of Neuropsychopharmacology (AsCNP), Kyoto, Japan.

REFERENCES

[1] *American Psychiatric Association Diagnostic and Statistical Manual of Mental Disorders,* Fourth Edition (DSM-IV). Washington, D.C., American Psychiatric Association, 1994.

[2] Biringer, E; Mykletun, A; Sundet, K; et al. A longitudinal analysis of neurocognitive function in unipolar depression. *J Clin Exp Neuropsychol*, 2007, 29, 879-91.

[3] Gorenstein, C; de Carvalho, SC; Artes, R; et al. Cognitive performance in depressed patients after chronic use of antidepressants. *Psychopharmacol*, (Berl), 2006, 185, 84-92.

[4] Gualtieri, CT; Johnson, LG; Benedict, KB. Neurocognition in depression: patients on and off medication versus healthy comparison subjects. *J Neuropsychiatry Clin Neurosci*, 2006, 18, 217-25.

[5] Gualtieri, CT; Morgan, DW. The frequency of cognitive impairment in patients with anxiety, depression, and bipolar disorder: an unaccounted source of variance in clinical trials. *J Clin Psychiatry*, 2008, 69, 1122-30.

[6] Kaneda, Y. Verbal working memory and functional outcome in patients with unipolar major depressive disorder. *World J Biol Psychiatry*, 2009, 10, 591-4.

[7] Kaneda, Y. Verbal working memory impairment in patients with current episode of unipolar major depressive disorder and in remission. *Clin Neuropharmacol*, 2009, 32, 346-7.

[8] Kaneda, Y; Jayathilak, K; Meltzer, H. Determinants of work outcome in neuroleptic-resistant schizophrenia and schizoaffective disorder: Cognitive impairment and clozapine treatment. *Psychiatry Res*, 2010, 178, 57-62.

[9] Kaneda, Y; Jayathilak, K; Meltzer, HY. Determinants of work outcome in schizophrenia and schizoaffective disorder: role of cognitive function. *Psychiatry Res*, 2009, 169, 178-9.

[10] Keefe, RS; Goldberg, TE; Harvey, PD; et al. The Brief Assessment of Cognition in Schizophrenia: reliability, sensitivity, and comparison with a standard neurocognitive battery. *Schizophr Res*, 2004, 68, 283-97.

[11] Kennedy, N; Foy, K; Sherazi, R; et al. Long-term social functioning after depression treated by psychiatrists: a review. *Bipolar Disord*, 2007, 9, 25-37.

[12] Malone, DC. A budget-impact and cost-effectiveness model for second-line treatment of major depression. *J Manag Care Pharm*, 2007, 13, S8-18.

[13] Marcos, T; Portella, MJ; Navarro, V; et al. Neuropsychological prediction of recovery in late-onset major depression. *Int J Geriatr Psychiatry*, 2005, 20, 790-5.

[14] McIntyre, R; Kennedy, S; Bagby, RM; et al. Assessing full remission. *J Psychiatry Neurosci*, 2002, 27, 235-9.

[15] McIntyre, RS; Konarski, JZ; Mancini, DA; et al. Measuring the severity of depression and remission in primary care: validation of the HAMD-7 scale. *CMAJ*, 2005, 173, 1327-34.

[16] Nebes, RD; Pollock, BG; Houck, PR; et al. Persistence of cognitive impairment in geriatric patients following antidepressant treatment: a randomized, double-blind clinical trial with nortriptyline and paroxetine. *J Psychiatr Res*, 2003, 37, 99-108.

[17] Porter, RJ; Gallagher, P; Thompson, JM; et al. Neurocognitive impairment in drug-free patients with major depressive disorder. *Br J Psychiatry*, 2003, 182, 214-20.

[18] Reppermund, S; Ising, M; Lucae, S; et al. Cognitive impairment in unipolar depression is persistent and non-specific: further evidence for the final common pathway disorder hypothesis. *Psychol Med*, 2009, 39, 603-14.

[19] Rose, EJ; Ebmeier, KP. Pattern of impaired working memory during major depression. *J Affect Disord*, 2006, 90, 149-61.

[20] Stewart, SA. The effects of benzodiazepines on cognition. *J Clin Psychiatry*, 2005, 66 Suppl 2, 9-13.

[21] Zimmerman, M; McGlinchey, JB; Posternak, MA; et al. How should remission from depression be defined? The depressed patient's perspective. *Am J Psychiatry*, 2006, 163, 148-50.

In: Working Memory: Capacity, Developments and ...
Editor: Eden S. Levin

ISBN: 978-1-61761-980-9
© 2011 Nova Science Publishers, Inc.

Chapter 16

CONTROL OF WORKING MEMORY CONTENTS DURING TASK-SWITCHING

James A. Grange[*]
Centre for Cognitive Neuroscience, Bangor University, UK

Abstract

Every day life requires frequent switches between tasks in order to achieve goal-directed behaviour. For example, driving presents us with a complicated environment wherein many sub-tasks—speed monitoring, steering, recollection of directions from memory etc.—must be switched between in order to arrive safely at our destination. However, as working memory is limited in capacity, the question arises as to how a new task is implemented in working memory in the face of conflicting activation from the now-irrelevant task.

The mechanisms that allow such fluid switching are measured by utilising the so-called task-switching paradigm. Within this paradigm, participants switch between two or three simple cognitive tasks (e.g. odd/even; higher/lower than 5 judgements on number stimuli). Recent research from the task-switching paradigm has suggested that task performance is afforded by activation of task-relevant representations in working memory. Such an established representation guides behaviour by directing attention to task-relevant stimuli and actions whilst filtering out task-irrelevant information.

The present chapter provides a critical review of behavioural results in the task-switching paradigm, outlining the controversies that have surrounded this popular paradigm in recent years. This chapter also reviews the concept of inhibitory mechanisms in task-switching, serving to suppress the activation levels of the previously relevant task. Inhibition is inferred by slower reaction times returning to a recently executed task after one intervening trial (an AB*A* sequence) compared to returning to a task not recently executed (a CB*A* sequence, where A, B, & C are arbitrary labels for tasks). This reaction time cost is thus an important phenomenon for exploring the dynamics of inhibitory processes of working memory contents during task-switching.

---

[*] Please address all correspondence to James A. Grange, who is now at Keele University, School of Psychology, Dorothy Hodgkin Building, Keele University, Keele, Staffordshire, UK (email: j.a.grange@psy.keele.ac.uk).

Introduction

It is a well-established finding that working memory is limited in capacity. Due to this limitation, it is imperative that the contents of working memory at any one time are relevant to the current goals of an individual. Control of working memory contents can become problematic, as at any time there are many cognitive processes that an individual can engage in, most of which are irrelevant for current goals. Some control mechanism is therefore required; but how is this control implemented?

The question as to how humans organise and control their ongoing cognitive processes is fundamental in cognitive psychology. The question is fundamental as humans live in an extremely rich, multi-task environment, which often requires selecting and switching between relevant operations in order to achieve goal-directed behaviour. For example, the simple act of making a cup of coffee requires many cognitive processes that need to be implemented: walking to the kitchen (which requires attentional resources), retrieval from memory where the coffee is stored, mental rotation to read the coffee label to assure you don't select the de-caf, coordination of both hands to open the coffee jar, and so on. Despite our impressive knowledge of how individual processes such as these are implemented [1, 2, 3, 4], much less is known about how they are controlled and selected appropriately [5].

The problem of how humans select appropriate cognitive processes is compounded when stimuli afford several actions, many of which are irrelevant to the current task. For example, there are many operations that can be performed on a printed word: it can be read aloud, read silently, translated into another language, categorised semantically etc. [6]. However, all of these operations would be totally inappropriate if the task were to name the colour the word was printed in [7, 8]. In order not to allow behaviour to be stimulus-driven in this manner, top-down control mechanisms are required to select the goal-relevant action [9]. Selection failure is often seen in every day action slips (such as putting a tea bag in your mug instead of coffee; Reason, 1984[10]). Pathologically, damage to the prefrontal cortex is sometimes associated with "utilisation behaviour" [11], where patients are unable to inhibit goal-irrelevant actions afforded by stimuli presented to them.

Selection is not the only problem the cognitive system has to overcome. Once selection has occurred, the system needs to ensure that the selected task dominates behaviour, preventing intrusion from competing tasks. Thus, the system needs to ensure *stability* of tasks once selection has occurred. Somewhat paradoxically, this stability needs to be *flexible*, in that tasks must be removed and replaced when goals change. The tension between these competing demands has been called the *stability-flexibility dilemma* [12], and understanding the mechanisms that allow this balance to occur is a major challenge to researchers of cognitive control.

1. The Task-switching Paradigm

One tool to investigate the control of cognitive processes that has garnered much attention in the literature over the past decade is the task-switching paradigm (see, for reviews; c.f. [13, 14, 15]). The first empirical study of task-switching was introduced by [16]. Jersild presented participants with two lists of stimuli (e.g. numbers), and compared the time it required for participants to work through each list. One list required participants to perform the same task on each stimulus (e.g. addition), and the second list required participants to switch between two tasks (addition on first stimulus, subtraction on second stimulus etc.). Jersild found that list completion times were longer for lists requiring task-switching compared to repetitions (an effect the reader can replicate in figure 1; see also[17].

$$\boxed{19, 33, 26, 58, 11, 73, 78}$$

Figure 1. Example of list-based task switching paradigm, a variant of which was used by Jersild (1927). Initially, work through the list by adding 3 to each number (example of task repetition). After this, work through the list again, adding 3 to the first number, subtracting 3 from the next, and repeating this pattern until the list is complete (example of task-switching). List completion should take longer when task-switching compared to repeating the same task throughout.

Based on this finding, [16] suggested that in order to perform the correct task, participants must collate in working memory a set of task-relevant rules that allow correct performance of the task, which takes time to implement. This "mental-set" guides behaviour in situations where stimuli afford more than one task (i.e. when stimuli are *bivalent*). During the alternating list, participants must update their mental-set at every stimulus, unlike in the repetition list where only one mental-set is relevant throughout. The concept of mental set has been somewhat updated (now called a *task-set*), and is typically now defined as *"the configuration of perceptual, attentional, mnemonic, and motor processes critical for a particular task goal"* [18, p.5.]. Establishment of a relevant task-set has been suggested as being one key way that the cognitive system shields itself from interference in multi-task situations [19, 20], ensuring stability during task performance.

1.1. Alternating-runs Procedure

Although the list paradigm is sometimes used today [21, 22, 23], there are certain flaws within its design that suggest it is not a clean measure of cognitive control. The main concern with the list paradigm is that in the alternating condition, two task-sets must be held accessible in memory, whereas only one is required for the repetition list (see, for a related finding [24, 25, 26, 27]). Related to this, the alternating lists require memory for where in the sequence one is, a problem not relevant in the repetition lists. Thus the difference in list completion times are likely due to memory-load differences rather than task-switching operations.

Rogers & Monsell [28] addressed this problem by introducing the alternating runs procedure. In this paradigm, participants switch between two tasks every second trial in a predictable manner (e.g. AABBAABB...). This paradigm allows a measure of the time taken for task-repetitions and task-switches within the same block (e.g. A*A* and A*B* respectively), thus overcoming the memory-load problems inherent in the design of [16]. To reduce the impact of memory-load for where participants were in the sequence of tasks, stimuli were presented within a 2 x 2 grid, with the stimulus location rotating between each quadrant clockwise after every trial. Stimuli were mostly bivalent, consisting of a number and a letter. The two relevant tasks were a parity judgement on the number stimulus (odd/even) or a consonant/vowel judgement on the letters. The relevant task was signalled by the location of the stimulus within the 2 x 2 grid: one task was relevant when the stimuli were in the upper-two quadrants, and the task switched to the alternative task when the stimuli location rotated into the lower two quadrants (thus producing the AABBAA... structure).

Rogers & Monsell [28] replicated and extended the findings of [16] by finding that RTs to a task-switch were slower and more error-prone than task-repetitions, an effect they called the "switch cost". Rogers & Monsell suggested that this switch cost was the behavioural manifestation of a time-consuming reconfiguration process that enabled a switch from one task-set to another. This endogenous reconfiguration occurs on task-switch trials as the previously relevant task-set is no longer relevant, and needs to be altered; task-repetitions do not require reconfiguration as the system is supposedly configured to the correct task already. Thus, by this logic[1], the switch cost provides a useful window into the temporal dynamics of cognitive control processes in operation.

Besides the advantage of reducing memory load for which task is relevant, the alternating runs paradigm allows some degree of control over how much time a participant has to engage in readying themselves for the switch in task-set. Rogers & Monsell [28] argued that if reconfiguration processes are the source of the switch cost, and if reconfiguration is an endogenous control mechanism, then some degree of reconfiguration might be able to occur in advance of the task stimulus. By manipulating the time between a response on the previous trial (n-1) and the onset of the stimuli for the current trial (n), Rogers & Monsell [28] were able to manipulate preparation time (this interval is called the response-stimulus interval, or RSI). Rogers & Monsell proposed that extended preparation intervals, especially intervals longer than an assumed reconfiguration process might take, should reduce the switch cost, as much of the reconfiguration can occur in advance. They tested this hypothesis in their Experiments 2-5 by manipulating the RSI between 150 milliseconds (ms) and 1,200ms. Despite a significant reduction of the switch cost at RSI , of up to half a second, no further improvement was observed, and a significant cost still remained at the longest RSI. Rogers & Monsell suggested this "residual switch cost" may reflect an exogenous influence of stimuli, impervious to endogenous control.

The suggestion of an exogenous influence of stimuli was sensible given Roger's & Monsell's [28] design, as stimulus display consisted of stimuli from both possible tasks. Therefore on any given trial, the stimulus from the irrelevant task might activate the irrelevant task-set [32, 33, 34, 35, 36, 37, 9] much like interference from Stroop stimuli [7, 8] activates the task-set of word reading despite its inappropriateness. Stimulus-induced interference between task-sets may be increased as the tasks in Rogers & Monsell [28] share response-keys, and thus a decision on the correct stimulus-response (SR) mapping might be part of any putative reconfiguration process (e.g. if number is odd, press left key). If stimuli activate their relevant SR mapping, then irrelevant stimuli in the bivalent display will increase interference during selection of the appropriate SR mapping. Indeed, Rogers & Monsell [28] suggested that only part of reconfiguration can occur in advance; the remainder is only completed upon presentation of the stimuli. Although this hypothesis serves to

---

[1] A logic, we will come to discover, that has not met universal acceptance in the literature [15, 29, 30, 31]

explain the experimental findings, one might ask what functionality this delayed process might provide the cognitive system [38].

1.2. Task-set Inertia

A similar account of the residual switch cost was provided by Allport, Styles & Hisieh [32]. Rather than appealing to a homunculun reconfiguration metaphor, Allport and colleagues (see also [33]) explained switch costs as arising from familiar memory based processes such as priming and interference (a path continued by [39, 40, 15, 41, 42, 29]). Specifically, Allport and colleagues suggest that when a task switches, the activation of the now-irrelevant task persists and hinders activation of the relevant task. Implementation of the relevant task thus involves its activation, and the suppression of the activation levels of the irrelevant task [43, 18]. Thus, the switch cost arises as a by-product of positive priming of the irrelevant task, and negative priming (or inhibition) of the relevant task, rather than a specific switching mechanism.

To examine this proposal, [32] presented participants with incongruent Stroop stimuli (e.g. the word "Yellow" written in blue ink), and participants had to name either the word or the colour of the ink. In terms of switching between these tasks, the reconfiguration hypothesis suggests that switching to word reading (e.g. Colour—*Word*) should be fast, likely as word reading is a well practiced task and configuration of this task-set should be straightforward. Conversely, switching to colour naming should be slower, as it is a less-well practiced task. Despite overall RTs being slower for colour naming (the typical Stroop effect), switch costs were much larger for word naming than for colour naming, a "reverse-stroop effect" [32, 33]. Allport and colleagues explained this effect by suggesting that in order to perform the more difficult colour naming task, the easier task of word naming would interfere, and thus must be negatively primed (inhibited). At the same time, the more difficult task of colour naming must be activated. When a switch occurs from colour naming to word naming, the positive priming (activation) of the colour task persists, as does the negative priming (inhibition) of the word task. These combined conditions of greater activation of the irrelevant task and inhibition of the relevant task make switching to the easier task more difficult. Conversely, switching from word naming to colour naming (an easy task switching to a more difficult task) would produce less interference, as there would be less negative priming of the difficult task and less positive priming of the easy task. This effect has been replicated in a number of studies [44, 45, 46, 47, but see Schneider & Anderson, in press, for an alternative explanation], and is a challenge to the reconfiguration metaphor [28], as this theory posits no carry-over of previous task-activation once a switching operation has been triggered.

Allport, Styles & Hisieh [32] called this persistence of task activation "task-set inertia" (TSI). To explain reduction of switch costs at longer RSI intervals, TSI posits that at extended intervals, the irrelevant (to-be switched away from) tasks activation levels have time to dissipate somewhat. At shorter intervals, the previous task is still highly active, and the relevant task is still negatively primed, thus making switching more difficult. TSI explains residual switch costs as the positive priming of the irrelevant task and the negative priming of the relevant task persisting over a long period [33, 48].

The TSI hypotheses does not automatically assume that cognitive control is not required in the task-switching procedure [30], as it is likely that proactive interference from irrelevant tasks is reduced by inhibitory control [18, 49]. It does however argue that the switch cost is not a valid measure of cognitive control operations being executed [50, 28]. The cognitive system faces the same problem on switch trials *and* repetition trials of ensuring that the relevant task is the most active among competing representations [29].

1.3. Explicit-cuing Paradigm

There exists a certain degree of conflict between the two theories in deciding whether the switch cost reflects control processes. The best evidence for cognitive control during task switching is the reduction of switch cost when there exists an opportunity for advanced preparation. However, the TSI explains the reduction of switch cost at prolonged preparation intervals in a more elementary fashion. The alternating runs procedure is unable to distinguish between these two hypotheses. A solution to this impasse was provided by Meiran [50], who introduced the explicitly-cued task switching paradigm (see also [51]). Within this paradigm trials are presented randomly; participants know which task to perform on a given trial as a valid pre-cue is provided. For example, Meiran [50] presented participants with a 2 x 2 grid in which a smiley face symbol would appear within one of the four quadrants. Participants had to decide whether the symbol was in the upper- or lower-half of the grid, or whether it was on the left or the right side. Cues used were a pair of arrows, either pointing up and down (cuing the upper/lower judgement) or left and right.

Trials were orgaised post-hoc into repetition and switch trials by comparing the cue used on trial n-1 to that on n. The elegance of this paradigm lies in its ability to separate preparation and proactive interference interpretations of the switch cost. Specifically, preparation time can now be manipulated independently of the effects of proactive interference by varying the temporal distance between the onset of the cue and the onset of the stimulus (the cue-stimulus interval, or CSI), whilst keeping the RSI constant (which is still defined in the same manner as in the alternating runs procedure, i.e. the time between the response on one trial and the stimulus for the next trial). The constant RSI ensured that any modulation of switch cost due to CSI was due to preparation processes only, as any proactive interference from trial n-1 to n would be equivalent in all cases. The CSI was manipulated independently of the RSI in [50, ; Experiments 2-3] by placing the cue for the current trial close to the response on trial n-1 (and hence further away from the stimulus on the current trial, allowing for greater preparation) or further from the response on n-1 (closer to the stimulus on current trial, not allowing much preparation time). Meiran predicted that if the reduction of switch cost found by Rogers & Monsell (1995) was due to active preparation processes, switch costs should be reduced at prolonged CSIs. However, if TSI was the primary explanation of switch costs [32], switch costs should be equivalent between CSI conditions (as the remoteness of n from n-1 is equivalent in all conditions).

Meiran [50] found switch costs in this paradigm, demonstrating such costs were not unique to the alternating runs procedure. Additionally, Meiran reported that the switch costs were significantly reduced at extended CSIs, consistent with Rogers & Monsell's (1995) account. However, despite very long CSIs (up to 1,908ms in Experiment 5), a significant residual switch cost remained. This suggests that some part of the switch cost may be due to proactive interference from the preceding trial [32]. This possibility was investigated by Meiran[52], who controlled for preparation intervals whilst varying the degree of interference from trial n-1 (Experiments 1 & 2). This was achieved by varying the temporal distance between the response on trial n-1, and the cue for trial n. This response-cue interval (RCI) allows passive decay of the previously executed task, as no specific preparation can be performed during this interval due to the randomness of task presentation. [52] manipulated the RCI between 132-3,032ms with a constant CSI of 117ms, and found that switch cost reduced at longer RCIs, consistent with the idea that some proportion of the switch cost is caused by non-preparation processes such as TSI. With this empirical separation of CSI and RCI, we can see that in the alternating runs procedure, the RSI is an inseparable mixture of both CSI and RCI [52].

To unequivocally examine the role of preparation processes in reducing the switch cost, [52, Experiment 3] varied the CSI whilst using a constant, but long, RCI. As the switch cost was drastically reduced when RCI was extended up to 500ms, and only a smaller drop in cost was found for RCIs from 500ms up to 3,000ms, [52] suggested that proactive interference from the preceding trial has dissipated to an acceptable level with an RCI of 1,000ms. Therefore, to investigate preparatory processes independent of proactive interference, Meiran et al. used an RCI of 1,017ms. Results showed the predicted reduction of switch cost at longer CSIs. Despite this, a residual cost of 40ms was still evident with a CSI of 3,000ms.

Based on these findings Meiran [52] suggested that the switch cost consisted of three independent components: the passive dissipation of previously executed tasks (and possibly the dissipation of suppression of the relevant task), a preparatory component that readies the system for changing task demands, and a residual component.

For the remainder of the introduction, and this thesis, we will focus on the preparatory component of task performance, as this element seems the most related to the study of cognitive control. In the explicitly cued task switching paradigm, preparation is initiated by the cue, and so relevant theories of cue encoding will be discussed. Preparatory processes are also closely related to the other two components. Specifically, proactive interference from the preceding task may be overcome by the preparation of the current task, possibly by employing inhibitory mechanisms to irrelevant (but active) representations [53, 54, 55, 18, 56, 49]. Additionally, the residual component has been explained in terms of failure to employ preparatory processes [57, 58, 59].

2. Cue-based Preparation

Cues that guide behaviour are not unique to the task switching paradigm; indeed, we encounter cues frequently in our daily lives, which must be successfully translated into relevant actions. For example, when driving, we are presented with many cues in the guise of road signs. Sometimes these cues are explicit (such as a number, which represents the maximum speed limit), and sometimes the cues are more abstract, and rely on a pre-learned association with an action (e.g. a red circle with a horizontal white rectangle placed within it means "No-Entry"). Cues are incredibly important when there are multiple actions available. For example, when approaching a traffic light, you can decide to carry on driving or stop. However, the most appropriate action is cued by the colour of the light. Likewise, in the task switching paradigm with random task sequences, it is impossible to decipher the relevant task with bivalent stimuli unless provided with a cue. This is the critical distinction between cues and primes, which are often used in attentional research (see for example inhibition of return,[60]). Primes are useful for performance, but not necessary, whereas cues are necessary for performance [61, 51]. How one translates cues into relevant actions, especially if the cue triggers a change of what you are currently engaged in (e.g. a phone ringing whilst you are writing your PhD), is paramount to our understanding of cognitive control.

That task cues aid performance even when they are not necessary for performance was demonstrated by Koch [62]. Koch combined the alternating runs procedure with the explicit cuing paradigm by having participants alternate between two tasks in a predictable sequence (e.g., AABBAA...). However, unlike Roger's & Monsell's [28] paradigm where position of stimuli served as a cue for which task to perform, stimuli in Koch's study were presented centrally. One group had to recall the sequence from memory, whereas another group received a task cue in addition to the predictable sequence. This allowed investigation of the difference between cue-based performance and performance from memory recall alone. Results showed that at extended preparation intervals (here manipulated by RSI), the switch cost was reduced to a greater extent in the group with the task cue compared to the no-cue group. These results show that purely memory based reconfiguration is much weaker than cue-based preparation (see also [63]).

However there still remained a residual switch cost. Indeed, the presence of such costs in the explicitly-cued task switching paradigm suggest that the reduction of switch cost given extended preparation intervals is not due to cognitive control processes [32], or at least that advanced reconfiguration is in some way limited [28, 50]. DeJong [57] proposed that perhaps advanced reconfiguration was not limited (see also[64]), but rather participants did not fully prepare themselves on all trials. This *Failure to Engage* (FTE) theory posits that task preparation is an all-or-none process, and that participants have the capacity to be fully prepared for a task switch. By this notion, participants should perform equivalently on task-switch trials and task-repetition trials, especially given sufficient preparation time.

The transient failure to fully prepare (a situation DeJong and colleagues also call *Goal Neglect*)[64] is suggested to be driven by one (or a combination of) three factors: i) a lack of goal-driven intention (i.e. lack of motivation), ii)reduced environmental support (i.e. no task cue or insufficient feedback on task performance), and iii) fatigue. In the cued task-switching paradigm, environmental support is relatively strong, so [57] suggested that in this scenario, FTE emerged from a combination of a lack of motivation and fatigue.

To demonstrate his hypothesis, DeJong [57] suggested that analysing the whole RT distribution would highlight the dynamics of prepared and unprepared trials. Specifically, at long preparation intervals, DeJong suggested that RTs consisted of a mixture of fully prepared trials and fully un-prepared trials. By this logic, fully prepared task-switch RTs at long preparation intervals should be as fast as task-repetition trials (in which full preparation is assumed to be present), and that fully un-prepared task-switch RTs at long intervals should be just as slow as task-switch RTs from very short preparation intervals (where preparation is assumed to be zero). To analyse this mixture model, DeJong constructed cumulative distribution functions (CDFs) for task-switch and task-repetition trials at long and short preparation intervals. CDFs are constructed by rank ordering individual participants raw RTs for all conditions. Then for each condition and each participant separately, quantile cut-off points are calculated at various degrees of separation (e.g. 10th percentile, 20th percentile, 30th...etc.). Once these are calculated, quantiles for each condition are averaged across participants [65]. This procedure provides a clear picture of the dynamics of all RTs across the whole distribution (i.e. from fastest RTs to slowest), and comparisons between conditions across these distributions can be made.

The hypothesis of DeJong [57] was confirmed with the CDFs. RTs for task-repetition trials were faster than task-switch trials at short preparation intervals across the entire RT distribution. However, RTs for switch-trials given longer preparation time were closer to repetition RTs at the faster end of the RT distribution, and closer to switch-trials given no preparation time at the slower end of the RTs. This suggests that when participants were fully prepared, performance was as good as task-repetition trials (where full preparation is likely), and that residual switch costs likely are a product of the tail-end of the RT distribution, which reflects a proportion of trials where participants are fully un-prepared.

However, Nieuwenhuis & Monsell [58] directly attempted to reduce the proportion of FTE trials by adding motivational incentives to participants. Nieuwenhuis and Monsell provided financial incentives for improvement of RTs and error rates throughout the experiment. Additionally, block length was kept very short in order to avoid fatigue. Despite this additional incentive to engage in preparation (and despite improved RTs), residual switch costs were still evident (although statistically smaller than in conditions with no incentive). Based on these findings, Nieuwenhuis and Monsell concluded that although FTE may explain some portion of the residual switch cost, the residual does reflect a limitation of advanced reconfiguration. In a similar vein, Lien et al. [66] proposed that residual costs, instead of reflecting full preparation some of the time (FTE), they reflect the preparation of some of the task all of the time. By this explanation, residual costs emerge as a steady-state (but partial) preparation process.

Verbruggen et al. [59] however provided an answer to the impasse. They noted that in the cuing paradigm, the cue is often retained on the screen, co-present with the imperative stimulus. In this instance, participants need not engage in advanced preparation as it is not essential to perform the task; indeed they can just wait for stimulus onset to engage in any putative preparatory process. To investigate this issue, Verbruggen and colleagues compared conditions in which the cue at longer preparation intervals either remained on the screen or disappeared after a very short presentation. The results of this manipulation were clear: when the cue was presented for a short period during long preparation intervals, the residual switch cost disappeared. This finding is consistent with the FTE theory [57], and inconsistent with the idea that task preparation is limited [58], and that participants prepare some of the task all of the time [66]. However, these latter cases may still be viable when the cue remains on the screen as it is likely that the strategy participants adopt between experiments differs.

It remains an open question what work the cognitive system is doing when presented with a task cue [41]. One natural assumption, given the above reviewed literature, is that task cues allow implementation of a relevant task-set. Logan & Gordon [67] described, in their theory of ECTVA[2], a task-set as a collection of parameters required to perform one task over all possibilities; such parameters include attention-setting and attentional bias to

---

[2]Executive Control of the Theory of Visual Attention

relevant aspects of stimulus display. These parameters are explained to be part of the cognitive control system, and that these parameters feed-forward and set lower-level parameters that allow execution of subordinate (i.e. single) tasks. When a task set changes, new parameters are fed into the system which allows selection of a new task. Switch costs from this perspective arise as more task-set parameters change on switch trials than on repetition trials. Advanced preparation aids performance as many of these parameters can change ahead of stimulus presentation.

The idea that switch costs reflect to a certain degree the time required to update task-set parameters was supported by Arrington, Altmann & Carr [68], who suggested that switching between similar tasks would require less parameter alterations than switching between tasks that are very different from one another. According to Logan & Gordon [67], the fewer parameters that require updating, the less time required for the system to switch tasks. To test this, Arrington and colleagues had participants switch between four tasks, each one being a judgement on a presented rectangle: height, width, hue, and brightness. Arrington and colleagues argued that height and width tasks are very similar, as they both require a spatial judgement attentional setting [67]; similarly, hue and brightness may be considered to share the attentional setting of "colour". By this logic, Arrington and colleagues found greater switch costs for switching between tasks of limited similarity (e.g. Width - Brightness) than for switching between tasks that share task-set components (e.g. Hue - Brightness).

Mayr & Kliegl [56] suggested that task preparation processes involve retrieval of relevant task rules from long-term memory (LTM), and their installation into working memory (WM). They suggested that it was un-parsimonious to assume that switching between two tasks requires holding both tasks ready for selection in WM. This would require the selected task to be activated, and at the same time be co-present with an activated competitor task in WM (albeit at an activation level below selection threshold). Such a scenario could leave the system prone to selection errors, requiring an extra mechanism to overcome the interference between tasks. Mayr & Kliegl [56] proposed that selection of a task and its activation in WM are concurrent processes, and that a non-selected task is not in WM. Evidence for this suggestion is also provided by the backward inhibition paradigm [18], which shows that selection of a task requires the inhibition of WM contents. By holding only one task active in WM would also resolve any potential interference that the system may experience due to multiple tasks in WM activated below selection threshold.

Based on this proposal, to select a task requires its retrieval from LTM. To test this hypothesis, Mayr & Kliegl [56] manipulated the difficulty of a tasks retrieval from LTM and seeing whether it interacted with switch costs. They proposed that if some (or all) of the switch cost reflected a time consuming process of LTM retrieval of task rules, switch costs should be greater for tasks with more involved LTM processing. Difficulty of LTM retrieval was manipulated by comparing two conditions: the semantic condition required judging a presented word on its size (i.e. bigger or smaller than a football) or whether it was living or non-living; the episodic condition required recalling a recently learned association during a learning phase between the word and a)its position on the computer screen, and b)the colour of the font. During the experimental phase all words were presented centrally and in white font. It was proposed that episodic retrieval from LTM should be harder than semantic retrieval, as the former is recently learned.

Mayr & Kliegl [56] found the predicted pattern of larger switch costs when switching to an episodic task (e.g. size-*position*) than switching to a semantic task. This pattern was true even when *n*-1 was also an episodic task (e.g. colour-*position* compared to size-*living*). This effect was determined to be due to LTM retrieval difficulty rather than overall task difficulty (Experiment 2), and that this retrieval could be accomplished with extended preparation intervals (i.e. the CSI reduced the switch cost for episodic retrieval; Experiment 3). The precise nature of the task representation that is retrieved via the cue is unclear, but must clearly involve some specification of the desired stimulus-response mapping (or "rule"). For instance, [69] simply state that "task rules" are retrieved. [70] state that "retrieval results in a relatively abstract description of what has to be done with the next stimulus" (p.75). Mayr & Kliegl (2000, Experiment 3) suggested that the rules are specific stimulus-response mappings (e.g., if stimulus is small animal then press left, if large animal then press right) rather than more abstract task specifications (e.g., respond according to stimulus size).

This model of task-rule retrieval for performance in the explicitly-cued paradigm is similar to that offered by [71]. However, Rubinstein and colleagues suggested that rule activation occurs after stimulus identification c.f.[56], and that cue-based preparation involves goal-setting (or goal-switching if the cue indicates a switch). [56, see also Mayr & Kliegl, 2003] alternatively suggest that stimulus onset triggers the application of the retrieved rules to the stimulus. This second stage of the model offers an alternative explanation for why residual switch costs are still evident at prolonged preparation intervals in the explicit cuing paradigm, as complete reconfiguration must await stimulus onset however, there is some evidence that this process can begin earlier [70, 72]. No clear explanation has been provided for why the cognitive system benefits from awaiting stimulus onset to complete reconfiguration. One suggestion provided by [38] is that waiting for stimulus onset may allow the system to "hedge its bets" (p.603) and await evidence from the stimulus that a new task is required. However, this seems rather uneconomic in task-switching situations where the cue is 100% valid, and therefore no uncertainty should be present. More likely, residual switch costs within Mayr & Kliegl's model might reflect sporadic retrieval failures from LTM due to insufficient preparation [57]. As this is a more parsimonious assumption, the second stage of Mayr & Kliegl's model might be called into question.

2.1. Altmann & Gray's Model

Altmann's approach to explaining task-switching effects is rooted in well defined and established memory processes that are integral to performance in other situations outside of task-switching, (e.g. activation & interference;)[39, 15, 41, 42, 40, 29]), without the need for reconfiguration mechanisms during switch trials. For example, [41] suggested that the same processes run on repetition as on switch trials, processes that ensure the desired task is the most active. The switch cost from this perspective is seen as repetition priming, rather than a cost emerging from a dedicated switching mechanism (c.f. Rogers & Monsell, 1995). There are several pieces of evidence that support this view, the two most prominent being that firstly CSI affects repetition trials as well as switch trials [41, 42, 63] and secondly when a cue is followed by a run of a number of stimuli upon which the cued task is to be performed, there is a reaction time cost on the cued trial (trial 1) compared to other cue-less trials in the run (e.g. trials 2-6) even if the cue indicated a repeat of task (Allport & Wylie, 2000; Altmann, 2002; 2006; 2007; Altmann & Gray, 2002; Gopher, Armony, & Greenshpan, 2000; Poljac, Koch, & Bekkering, 2008). This "restart cost" has been attributed by Altmann to the time taken to re-activate task representations, which will have decayed since the last cue exposure. The restart cost is important theoretically, as it suggests that encoding and activation processes run on repetition trials as well as switch trials, a view not compatible with the reconfiguration view of a dedicated set of processes that run on switch trials only.

Altmann & Gray (2008) utilised the cognitive architecture of ACT-R [74, 75] to model task-switching performance utilising these activation-based memory processes. Altmann & Gray suggest that cue encoding results in a retrieval of a task code from episodic memory, from which the meaning of the cue is retrieved. After this, the stimulus is encoded, and its meaning is retrieved. Once this encoding is complete, the meaning of the cue and the meaning of the stimulus are used to retrieve the correct response. Thus, cue encoding is the first stage of a general encoding episode, and if the meaning of the cue is different from that most recently attended to (i.e. if it is a switch trial), the now relevant task cue meaning must be activated over and above the old cue meaning to achieve selection. The extra time taken to achieve this required activation is reflected in the task-switch cost. From the examples given by Altmann & Gray, it appears that the cue meaning retrieved during encoding is used to probe semantic memory to retrieve specific S-R mappings (i.e. if Even then left, if Odd then right, Altmann & Gray, p.608).

3. Problems with the Cuing Paradigm

A critical problem with the explicitly cued task-switching paradigm was identified by two labs concurrently. Both Logen & Bundesen [76] and Mayr & Kliegl [69] reported that using one cue per task confounds cue-switching with task-switching. Specifically, they noted that every time a task repeats, so too does the cue; conversely, a task-switch always requires a switch of cue. Therefore the possibility exists that switch costs within this paradigm reflect cue-related processing rather than cognitive control processes. To overcome this problem, both labs introduced the two-cue per task paradigm (hereafter a 2:1 mapping), where each task is cued by one of two cues. This new manipulation allows three types of sequence, two of which are familiar: *Cue-Repetition* (both cue and task repeat; e.g. Magnitude - Magnitude), *Task-Switch* (both cue and task switches; e.g. (Parity - Magnitude), and the new sequence possibility of *Cue-Switch* (task repeats but cue switches; e.g. High/Low - Magnitude). This paradigm allows separation of cue-related processes to the switch cost. Specifically, task-switch costs are measured within this paradigm by subtracting cue-switch RT from task-switch RT, as in both cases the cue has switched from n-1 to n, and therefore the effects of cue-switching are controlled. Additionally, the time taken to encode a new cue without the additional burden of switching tasks can be measured by subtracting cue-repetition RT from cue-switch RT.

Both Logen & Bundesen [76] and Mayr & Kliegl [69] found substantial costs of switching cues in the absence of a task switch. These *cue-switch costs* suggest that a significant component of the switch cost with one cue per task is due to the extra processes required to encode a new cue. Mayr & Kliegl [69] additionally found a task-switch cost over and above that explained by cue-switching. They took this as evidence for supporting their two stage model of task-switching [56]. Specifically, they suggested that the cue-switch cost reflected utilisation of a new retrieval route to obtain task rules from LTM. When the cue repeats, the retrieval path is primed and thus speeds responses. Mayr & Kliegl (2003) found that the cue-switch cost was reduced given extended preparation intervals, consistent with their earlier work [56] suggesting that cue-based preparation involves retrieval of task rules from LTM. The task-switch cost in their paradigm was insensitive to preparation, consistent with the second stage of their model (application of retrieved rules to the stimulus display) which must await stimulus onset, but see [59].

However, Both Logen & Bundesen [76] found no difference between cue-switching and task-switching. By this formulation, they questioned the presence of cognitive control processes in the explicitly-cued task-switching paradigm, and suggested that the switch cost with one cue per task reflected priming of cue-encoding processes on task repetition trials. They developed their theory (and competing "reconfiguration" theories) into explicit mathematical models, which I detail below. To anticipate their findings, they found that the model with no cognitive control built into its assumptions fit the data better than reconfiguration models.

3.1. Logan and colleagues' Models

The models initially presented in [76] have been a serious challenge to the notion that cognitive control processes can be measured by the cued task-switching paradigm. Instead, they suggested that participants adopt a "compound cue" strategy whereby the cue and the stimulus are combined to retrieve the correct response from LTM. For example, the cue "Odd/Even" and the stimulus "7" uniquely retrieve the response "Odd" from LTM. By this notion, no switch of task is required, as on every trial participants encode the cue, encode the stimulus, and use them together to retrieve the response. Switch costs from this perspective are seen as repeated cue-encoding benefits when the cue switches (regardless of "task"). To explain the preparation effects found in the literature, which had been taken to reflect cognitive control operations, Logan and Bundesen suggested that longer cuing intervals mean cue encoding on cue-switch trials can be completed before stimulus onset.

Model 1 [76] initially modeled the reconfiguration metaphor of [28] and [50], which assumes an endogenous act of control. In this model, the cue is encoded, which takes $\mu_c$ms to complete. If the cue that is encoded is identical to the cue on the previous trial, no further executive control is required, as the correct task-set is assumed to be already implemented. If however the cue differs, as in a task-switch scenario, the cognitive system must retrieve the correct task-set and install it, which Logan and Bundesen state takes $\mu_s$ms to complete. Based on these assumptions, and given no preparation time (i.e. CSI = 0ms), reaction time for a repetition trial is formalised as:

$$RT = RT_{Base} + \mu_c \quad (1)$$

and reaction time for a task-switch is:

$$RT = RT_{Base} + \mu_c + \mu_s \quad (2)$$

In both cases, RT_{Base} is the estimated time to encode the stimulus and respond. The authors assume, in this model and the following, that cue encoding time is exponentially distributed, so the probability that cue encoding is complete before stimulus onset increases as a function of the CSI. To model the effects of extended preparation intervals on performance, model 1 now estimates RT for task repetition trials as:

$$RT = RT_{Base} + \mu_c \cdot exp\left(\frac{-CSI}{\mu_c}\right) \quad (3)$$

and RTs for task-switches as:

$$RT = RT_{Base} + exp\left(\frac{-CSI}{\mu_c}\right) \cdot (\mu_c + \mu_s) + \frac{\frac{1}{\mu_c}}{\frac{1}{\mu_c} - \frac{1}{\mu_s}}$$
$$\cdot \left[exp\left(\frac{-CSI}{\mu_s}\right) - exp\left(\frac{-CSI}{\mu_c}\right)\right] \cdot \mu_s \quad (4)$$

Note that model 1, and indeed the reconfiguration metaphor as it originally stood [28, 50, 77, 52], makes no allowance for cue-switch RT to be any different from task-repetition RT, as in both cases no reconfiguration (μ_s) is required. Qualitatively, we can already see that model 1 will provide a poor fit to new data from the 2:1 mapping paradigm due to this.

Model 2 Model 2 is the "compound-cue model", and it assumes no cognitive control process (μ_s). Rather it suggests that task-switching performance can be explained by differential cue-encoding times. The authors explain this approach in terms of short-term- (STM) and long-term-memory comparisons between the presented cue and the desired compound stimulus (a stored amalgamation of cue-stimulus-response compounds). They describe this comparison as a race, and whichever process finishes first determines performance. In the case of a cue-repetition, the comparison between the presented cue and STM traces finishes before the comparison between the presented cue and LTM (as the cue from the previous trial is still active in STM), thus producing faster encoding time (see [31, 61]for a more detailed overview of this process). In the case of a task (cue) switch, the current cue does not match representations in STM, and so has to rely on retrieving from LTM, a longer process. Cue-encoding time for cue-repetitions (μ_r) can be expressed as:

$$\mu_r = \frac{1}{V_{STM} + V_{LTM}} \quad (5)$$

and cue-encoding time for cue-switches (μ_a) as:

$$\mu_a = \frac{1}{V_{LTM}} \quad (6)$$

where V_{STM} and V_{LTM} are parameters estimating comparison rates to short-term and long-term memory respectively. As a result of these expressions, μ_r ¡ μ_a, formalising the unique prediction that task repetitions are faster due to a *benefit* from cue encoding and comparisons to STM traces rather than a *cost* of switching tasks. This benefit should appear at smaller CSI's, as cue encoding will not have had time to complete before the stimulus is presented.

Based on these assumptions, model 2 makes no distinction between cue-switch trials and task-switch trials, as in both cases the cue on trial n has switched from n-1. Therefore, estimated RT for cue-repetitions are formalised as:

$$RT = RT_{Base} + \mu_r \cdot exp\left(\frac{-CSI}{\mu_r}\right) \tag{7}$$

and RT for cue-switch and task-switch trials as:

$$RT = RT_{Base} + \mu_a \cdot exp\left(\frac{-CSI}{\mu_a}\right) \tag{8}$$

Model 2+1 The final model expressed by Logan and Bundesen attempts to integrate the above two models. It assumes repeated cue-encoding benefits and an act of reconfiguration. RT for cue-repetitions is the same as before:

$$RT = RT_{Base} + \mu_r \cdot exp\left(\frac{-CSI}{\mu_r}\right) \tag{9}$$

For cue-switches, cue-encoding does not benefit from repetition priming, and thus must be encoded anew (as per model 2):

$$RT = RT_{Base} + \mu_a \cdot exp\left(\frac{-CSI}{\mu_a}\right) \tag{10}$$

For task-switches, again cue-encoding does not benefit from repetition priming, but additionally it requires reconfiguration processes. This is expressed formally:

$$RT = RT_{Base} + exp\left(\frac{-CSI}{\mu_a}\right) \cdot (\mu_a + \mu_c) + \frac{\frac{1}{\mu_a}}{\frac{1}{\mu_a} - \frac{1}{\mu_s}}$$
$$\cdot \left[exp\left(\frac{-CSI}{\mu_s}\right) - exp\left(\frac{-CSI}{\mu_a}\right)\right] \cdot \mu_s \tag{11}$$

Across their experiments, [76] consistently found that model 2 fit their 2:1 mapping data better than either of the competing models. This is hardly surprising, as they found no difference between cue-switching and task-switching. This pattern of results (and thus the model fits) was inconsistent with the data of [69]. To address these differences, [78] investigated procedural differences between the two labs. Logan and Bundesen (2004) suggested that the difference in cue-types used between the two sets of reports could explain the differences found. For instance, whilst Logan and Bundesen (2003) used cues that have a pre-experimental association with the tasks they were associated with (e.g. Odd/Even), [69] used abstract cues with no pre-experimental association with the tasks (e.g. the letter "G" signalled a colour discrimination).

Pre-experimental associations between cues and their respective tasks has been called *cue-transparency* in the literature [79], and has been found to affect switch costs. For example, [80] found that non-transparent cues (cues that have little pre-experimental association with the task) produce greater switch costs than transparent cues (which have strong pre-experimental association with the task). [79] suggested that when a cue is relatively non-transparent, a verbal mediator is retrieved which aids performance. For example, when presented with the cue "G", the participant will retrieve the mediator "Colour", which can then be used like a transparent cue to perform the task. To explain the results of [69], [81] suggested that participants retrieve such a mediator. Once retrieved, this mediator is then employed much like a transparent cue, i.e. it is used jointly with the stimulus to act as a compound retrieval cue to select the correct response from LTM.

The notion of mediator retrieval can explain why [69] found significant task-switch costs without appealing to cognitive control (or application of stimulus-response rule). On cue-repetition trials, the non-transparent cue requires retrieval of a mediator, which is used with the stimulus to select a unique response. On cue-switch trials, the cue is different, so has to be encoded anew, but the mediator it retrieves is primed from the previous trial, as participants are assumed to use the same mediator for both cues. On a task-switch trial, neither the cue nor the mediator is primed from recency, and both must be encoded anew. Therefore, the priming of mediator retrieval explains why RTs are faster to cue-switch trials than task-switch trials for [69]. Conversely, [76] found no difference between cue-switch and task-switch RT as they used transparent cues; therefore, no mediator is retrieved, leading to no benefits of priming for cue-switch trials compared to task-switch trials.

Model 3 [81] formalised their thesis by comparing performance of their model (model 2) with that of a new model based on the two-stage process of [69]. This model assumes a benefit of repeated cue-encoding (explaining the cue-switch cost), but unlike model 2, assumes an extra set of processes that run when the stimulus is presented (their rule-application stage). In the models of [76], stimulus-based processes are estimated using the parameter RT_{Base}. Thus, a shift in this parameter was used to conceptualise the second stage of Mayr & Kliegl's model. RT for cue-repetitions is expressed formally as:

$$RT = RT_{BaseRep} + \mu_r \cdot exp\left(\frac{-CSI}{\mu_r}\right) \quad (12)$$

and for cue-switches as:

$$RT = RT_{BaseRep} + \mu_a \cdot exp\left(\frac{-CSI}{\mu_a}\right) \quad (13)$$

both identical to model 2. However, for task-switches, as a new rule is being applied to the target display, a shift occurs for estimation of RT_{Base}. RT for task-switches is expressed as:

$$RT = RT_{BaseAlt} + \mu_a \cdot exp\left(\frac{-CSI}{\mu_a}\right) \quad (14)$$

All models were fit to a conceptual replication of [69], and results showed that model 2 again was the better fit to the data. Based on these results, [81] concluded that no cognitive control processes were captured in the task-switch cost (see also [82, 83, 84, 31, 85, 61] for further vindications of this model). Despite the bleak outlook for the task-switching paradigm in measuring cognitive control processes, there is evidence that suggests not all data can be explained by Logan and colleagues' models.

3.2. Challenges to Logan's Models

A series of direct challenges to Logan's modeling was presented by [72]. By manipulating the probability of a task switch, Monsell & Mizon found under certain circumstances a significant task-switch cost was present, which reduced with increased preparation. The other critical difference between the studies of [76] and [69] was the probabilities of a task-switch. Given no constraints, selection between two tasks produces a p(task-switch)=.5, which is what Logan and Bundesen used; however, Mayr & Kliegl used a p(task-switch)=.3, so that cue-repetitions, cue-switches, and task-switches were equally likely on each trial. Monsell

& Mizon argued that with a high probability of a task-switch, participants may engage in some form of switching reconfiguration before cue-onset (even if they have no foreknowledge of the upcoming trial). By preparing for a switch before cue-onset, participants may be fully ready for the switch task before the cue signals such a switch, and thus no switch cost in RT will be evident. Keeping the p(task-switch) low discourages this reconfiguration until the cue actually signals a switch is required, ensuring switch related processes are captured within the RT.

However, Logan et al. [84] countered this proposal theoretically and empirically. They highlighted that manipulating the probability of a task-switch also manipulates the probability of one cue following another. Specifically, if p(task-switch) is low, then the probability of a cue for task B will follow a cue for task A is also lower. Logan and colleagues thus suggested that the "true" task-switch cost found by [72] might actually reflect infrequency effects, whereby participants respond slower to infrequent stimuli. Logan and colleagues also found that a slightly modified version of their model fit Monsell & Mizon's data without the assumption of cognitive control processes. Thus, based on this evidence, Logan's models still hold quite strong explanatory power.

However, empirical evidence has been forthcoming that suggests limitations in Logan's models. Altmann [86] presented an experiment to examine whether the task-switching procedure produces behavioural effects not explained by Logan's models. We have already reviewed several effects found in the task-switching literature that can not be explained sufficiently by the model (e.g. residual switch costs, within-run slowing, full-run error switch cost), but Altmann was particularly interested in two main questions. Firstly, if cue encoding explains switch cost then no switch cost should be evident on cue-less trials within extended runs designs, e.g. [39]. Altmann [86] tested this by adding an extra trial following an instructive cue, within a 2:1 mapping paradigm. Results showed that task-switch costs were evident on trial 2 of the run, but cue-switch costs were zero. If task-switching was merely the cost of switching cues, then no task-switch cost should be evident on trial 2, as cue-encoding must have been completed on trial 1. Thus, this data suggests the switch cost is not entirely due to the effects of switching cues. Although the model of Altmann and Gray (2008) does not explicitly address paradigms with two cues per task, the cue-switch cost can be explained by the ACT-R architecture by repetition priming of perceptual identification of the task cue on cue-repetition trials [74, 75].

Additionally, Altmann [86] noted that reduction of switch cost at extended preparation intervals is not as pervasive as the literature might suggest, see e.g. [14, 30]. In earlier work, Altmann had shown that reduction in switch cost at extended preparation intervals was particular to a within-subjects manipulation of CSI, (see also [63, 41, 42]). When CSI is manipulated between-subjects, the CSI by Switch cost interaction was null. Altmann [41, 42] has suggested that the system needs to be exposed to varying preparation intervals to appreciate the benefits of advanced preparation. The modeling of Logan and colleagues says that the reduction of switch cost given preparation is due to a pervasive cue-encoding process. However, this stance cannot explain the null interaction given a between-subjects design.

Arrington, Logan & Schneider [87] sought to separate cue-encoding processes from task-switching empirically in order to investigate whether task-switching in isolation produces switch costs. To achieve this, Arrington and colleagues had participants make separate responses to the cue and the stimulus. The logic of the design assumes that cue and stimulus processing are serial. If the type of response made to the cue is completed after successful cue-encoding, then all cue-switch costs should only appear in cue-RT, with no cue-switch costs in stimulus RT. If however the type of response to the cue is not a result of complete cue encoding, then cue processing will spill over into RT to targets, resulting in cue-switch costs to both cues and targets. The additional appeal of this design is that one can assess the final representation gained from cue encoding by comparing cue responses that resulted in successful separation to cue responses that were not successful.

Across experiments, two cues were used for each task, and the type of response required for the cue varied between experiments, either indicating which cue was presented (i.e. a separate response for each cue, resulting in a 1:1 mapping of cues to responses) or which task was presented (one response for each task, resulting in a 2:1 cue-response mapping). The results showed that with a 1:1 cue-response mapping, cue switch effects were still apparent in stimulus RT, suggesting cue encoding had not been separated from target processing. However, a successful separation did occur when a 2:1 response-cue mapping was utilised, with all cue-switch costs observable in cue RT only; stimulus RT only showed task-switch costs. The presence of these task-switch costs after cue encoding is complete suggests that task-switch costs cannot be explained in their entirety by cue-switching c.f.[30, 31]. Additionally, these results suggest that cue encoding results in a semantic representation of the task to be performed, and not a representation of the cue itself.

Additional evidence for the dissociation of cue-switching from task-switching came from Jost et al. [70]. These authors investigate event-related potentials (ERPs) of cue-switching and task-switching performance, and found distinct neural responses to cue-switching and task-switching. Cue-switching affected negative ERP components about 300ms after cue-onset, with task-switching affecting negativity potentials around 400ms. Both of these responses had distinct topography, suggesting that they were emerging from distinct underlying neural responses.

4. Inhibitory Mechanisms in Task Switching

One established task-switching phenomenon that cannot be adequately explained by Logan's models (nor by Altmann & Gray's, 2008, model) is the evidence for inhibitory mechanisms being employed during switching. Inhibition in task-switching implies that some task-specific component is being altered, and this cannot be explained by a model that assumes no cognitive control is in operation. Thus, inhibition might be the best evidence yet for supporting the notion task-switching requires cognitive control processes.

4.1. Backward Inhibition

The concept of behavioural inhibition in cognitive psychology has been a controversial topic for many years (see [88, 89, 90, 91] for recent discussions on the arguments for and against inhibition). The concept that task-switching requires inhibition has been popular since the studies of Allport and colleagues [32, 33, 48], who argued that switch costs to some degree reflect persisting inhibition of the switched-to task. But definitive evidence for inhibition was absent until the study of [18]. In this study, Mayr & Keele highlighted that it is impossible to investigate inhibition in task-switching using only two tasks. By introducing a third task, Mayr & Keele contrasted two switching sequences. In one sequence, participants performed three different tasks in succession (e.g. a CBA sequence, where A, B, & C are arbitrary labels for tasks); in the other sequence, participants were required to return to a recently performed task after one intermediate trial (e.g. ABA sequence). The tasks were simple perceptual discrimination tasks, where participants were presented with a screen with one rectangle in each quadrant of the screen. The participants task was to respond to the location of a odd-item out rectangle whose perceptual properties differed from the other rectangles based on a cued dimension. For example, the cue "Colour" required participants to respond to the rectangle whose colour was different to the others (e.g. a purple rectangle among blue rectangles). The other two relevant dimensions were orientation (one rectangle was tilted to the left or to the right) and movement (one rectangle was moving from left-to-right or up and down). Responses were to be made to which quadrant the odd rectangle occupied by making a spatially compatible key press.

They suggested that if inhibition is applied during task-switching, then inhibition of a recently performed task should persist and hinder its reactivation if the task is to be performed relatively soon again (for example task A in an ABA sequence). During a CBA sequence, task A was inhibited longer ago, and thus has more time to overcome the inhibition applied to it. By this logic, Mayr & Keele (2000) predicted slower RTs to ABA sequences than to CBA sequences. Note that if task-switching merely requires activation of the relevant task (e.g. Altmann & Gray, 2008), ABA sequences should be faster than CBA sequences due to positive priming of task A. Indeed repetition priming is a fundamental psychological construct, and is observed in many different fields of research. Despite this, Mayr & Keele did find slower RTs to ABA than CBA sequences, thus supporting their notion of inhibition. They called this inhibitory mechanism "Backward Inhibition" (BI). For the remainder of this thesis, I shall use the more theoretically neutral term "n-2 repetition cost" to refer to the reaction time deficit in ABA sequences, retaining the term BI to refer to the mechanism postulated to be behind the cost [92, 89].

Mayr & Keele [18] proposed that BI is an inhibitory mechanism that is deployed proactively to remove the no-longer relevant task-set. In support of this, in their Experiment 3 they contrasted two situations: a "bottom-up" condition versus a "top-down" condition. In both, the stimulus display consisted of one deviant object among three identical distractors (plain rectangles), so that the relevant target could be gleaned from stimulus display alone. However, in the top-down condition, participants were presented with a valid cue that signalled the relevant dimension, whereas in the bottom-up condition, a line of asterisk (******) were used instead of a cue. Mayr & Keele posited that if BI is a top-down mechanism, then n-2 repetition costs should only be observed in the top-down condition, as this is the only condition that allows for advanced task preparation. However, if n-2 repetition costs reflect a more reactive form of inhibition that is triggered during stimulus onset, costs should be equivalent between the two conditions. Despite this, Mayr & Keele only found n-2 repetition costs in the top-down condition, and suggested that preparation for a specific task triggers backward inhibition of the previously executed task.

N-2 repetition costs have been replicated in a number of studies using various different task demands [93, 94, 95, 96, 43, 80, 97, 98, 99, 100, 101, 54, 53, 55, 102, 103, 104, 105,

106, 107, 108, 109, 110, 111, 112, 113, 114, 115, 116, 117, 118], and are a promising empirical marker for inhibitory mechanisms as they are (to-date) immune from non-inhibitory accounts [92, 107, 49]. Additionally, n-2 repetition costs increase when inter-trial conflict is increased by reducing the interval between successive trials, as measured by the RCI [99, 54]. Reduction of the RCI means that when a new task is switched-to, the previous task is still very active and therefore requires greater inhibitory control to reduce its activation allowing selection of the relevant task; a greater RCI allows passive decay of the previous tasks activation levels [32], reducing conflict when the new task is selected.

4.2. Response-related Inhibition

However, it remains unclear what is exactly inhibited during task-switching. [18] suggested that it is the task-set as a whole that is inhibited. As task-sets comprise of many components [119], a more fine-grained approach might suggest that inhibition targets those aspects of the task-set that generates the greatest inter-trial conflict, as this is where conflict resolution mechanisms are most needed [120, 53, 54, 55, 121]. Evidence for such a view comes from the work of Koch and colleagues, who have provided much evidence that inhibition might target response processes of the task-set [100, 92, 110, 111, 116].

Philipp & Koch [110] demonstrated that n-2 repetition costs are to some degree generated by response processes. They had participants perform a magnitude judgement on number stimuli, but were cued to use one of three response modalities: their hands (i.e. typical finger key press), their feet (using left/right foot pedals), or a vocal response. In this instance, ABA and CBA sequences were constructed not based on task sequencing, but response modality sequences (e.g. foot-vocal-foot is an ABA sequence). Philipp & Koch found n-2 modality-repetition costs, suggesting that when response modalities switch, the previously irrelevant modality is inhibited.

Schuch & Koch [116] demonstrated the importance of response processes in generating n-2 repetition costs by combining the backward inhibition paradigm with a go/no-go manipulation. In an otherwise normal cued task-switching experiment, a go or a no-go signal was presented shortly after the presentation of the task cue. If presented with a go signal, participants had to respond to the stimulus in a regular fashion. However, on the small proportion of trials in which a no-go signal was presented, participants had to withhold their response to the stimulus (see [122, 123]for a related design). In all cases, participants could prepare for the relevant task, but the relevant stimulus-response (SR) rule was only selected and executed on go trials. Therefore, if n-2 repetition costs reflect an inhibitory mechanism targeting response selection/execution aspects of a trial structure, then n-2 repetition costs should be absent from an ABA sequence where the task for n-1 was a no-go trial. In this instance, the SR rule for task A should not be inhibited as no SR selection occurred for the intermediate trial. [116] found significant n-2 repetition costs, but only when trial n-1 was a go trial (i.e. response selection & execution occurred). When a no-go trial was present on n-1, n-2 repetition costs were absent. These results (see also[122, 123]) strongly support the hypothesis that BI targets response related processes in task-switching[3].

---

[3]However, on a more theoretical note, one might ask that if no inhibition of task A occurred in an ABA sequence when n-1 was a no-go trial, why is there not a significant n-2 repetition *prime*, as presumably task A retains its activation levels somewhat and should prime performance when task A is required again. Thus, in

However, the study of Schuch & Koch [116] left open the question whether it was the absence of response selection or response execution that led to the reduction of n-2 repetition costs. To disentangle these processes, [113] used a "go-signal" paradigm in conjunction with a typical BI design. In this paradigm, participants are presented with a cue, followed by the stimulus, but uniquely, participants must not respond to the stimulus until a go signal is presented (a high tone). Similar to [116], a small proportion of trials presented a no-go signal (a low tone). The critical difference between this manipulation and that of [116] is that on some trials the go/no-go signal is presented up to a 1,500ms after stimulus onset (unlike Schuch & Koch, where the signal was presented simultaneously with stimulus onset). In cases where the go/no-go signal delay (GSD) is long, participants are able to select a response because the stimulus is presented long before execution is required. However, when the GSD signals a no-go response, no response execution occurs (c.f. Schuch & Koch).

Using these manipulations, Philipp et al. [113] predicted to replicate the findings of Schuch & Koch [116], with no n-2 repetition costs when there was a no-go signal on n-1 in an ABA sequence. The unique prediction was that if inhibition affects response selection processes, then in an ABA sequence, if trial n involves a long go-signal delay, then no n-2 repetition costs should be present as the inhibition can be overcome in during the GSD when response selection can occur. However, if inhibition affects response execution processes, then a long GSD should not allow overcoming residual inhibition of task A, and n-2 repetition costs should remain. The results clearly showed however that with a long GSD indicating a go response on trial n, no n-2 repetition costs were evident (indeed a significant n-2 repetition prime was evident). The results therefore support the suggestion that n-2 repetition costs reflect persisting inhibition of response selection processes, which can be overcome given enough time to select an appropriate response.

Response selection is likely to induce conflict (and hence, inhibition), as typically multiple tasks are mapped onto the same response sets. For example, a left key press in an experiment can be associated with an "Odd" or "Lower than 5" judgement, depending on the currently relevant task. Indeed, such overlapping response sets have been shown to contribute to n-2 repetition costs. For example, [100] had participants switch between four tasks, three of which had overlapping response sets (vocal responses "left" or "right"). The fourth task however did not overlap with the response set for the other three tasks, and required a vocal response of "up" or "down". The overlapping response-set tasks were referred to as "trivalent" (T) tasks, and the single non-overlapping response-set task as a "univalent" (U) task. ABA sequences were constructed to contrast TTT transitions with TUT transitions. During TTT transitions, response-set conflict should occur at n-1, triggering inhibition of task A, generating n-2 repetition costs. Conversely, a TUT sequence should generate no conflict at n-1 as the U task does not conflict with the response set for T tasks, thus no n-2 repetition costs should be present. The predicted pattern of results was confirmed, suggesting overlapping response sets contribute to BI (see also[115]for a related finding). However, it should be noted that this finding stands in contradiction to the observation of significant n-2 repetition costs in many of Abrbuthnott's studies [94, 95, 96, 43, 80] despite the fact her tasks all use univalent response-sets.

---

the absence of a cost, it remains an open question why there is not a benefit (see e.g. [124].

4.3. Inhibition at Earlier Stages of Trial Processing

Despite the considerable evidence that inhibition is triggered by response-related processes of the trial structure, there is some evidence that it is not exclusively tied to these processes. Indeed, response competition should not have played a significant role in generating n-2 repetition costs in the original BI study of Mayr & Keele [18], as response sets were not unique to each task. Participants merely had to respond to the location of the deviant rectangle on each trial, and thus the response-set is constant throughout the whole experiment. Therefore earlier components of the trial structure could be a source of inhibition.

For example, Sdoia & Ferlazzo [117] have provided some evidence that inhibition can be triggered during stimulus presentation, and critically at a distinct time before response selection [112]. They found n-2 repetition costs even when the task for n-1 required stimulus encoding for later comparison, but critically no response selection was required.

Stimulus encoding [117] and response selection Philipp et al. [112] occurs quite late in the typical trial structure, and it is somewhat surprising that conflict during earlier, preparatory processes stages of task performance does not trigger inhibition. This is especially surprising, as some models of task-switching performance suggest that task cues initiate retrieval of task rules from LTM and installation into WM [69], a process that might benefit from inhibition of the previous contents of WM [18, 56]. Despite the dominance of a response-locus of BI, there is some evidence that it can be triggered earlier.

Huebner et al. [125] developed a variant of the BI paradigm with the goal of investigating positive effects of backward inhibition (i.e. reduced interference from the previous task during current task performance) rather than on negative side-effects of inhibition (i.e. n-2 repetition costs). They used a version of the Eriksen flanker paradigm [126], where the unique stimulus sets were used for each task, and the stimulus for the current task was flanked by either stimuli from the previous task or stimuli from a task not recently completed. The flanker effect refers to slowed RTs when the flanking stimuli are from a different task to the central, relevant stimulus. However, if the flanking stimuli on trial n are from the task performed on n-1, then they should induce less interference because of backward inhibition. Flanking stimuli from a task performed less recently should interfere more as they are less inhibited. As such a finding would suggest stimulus-based inhibition [117], [125] presented participants with pre-cues. In their Experiment 2, the task cue either informed participants of which task was going to be relevant on the next trial (i.e. a task-specific cue), of the cue merely signalled a switch would occur, with no specific information as to which task would be relevant. In the latter case, participants can not prepare for an upcoming task, unlike with task-spcific cues.

Huebner et al. [125] found less interference from flanking stimuli, demonstrating for the first time some of the positive effects of BI. Importantly, they only found reduced flanker interference when participants were presented with a task-specific cue. This suggests that when preparing for a specific task, inhibition of the previous task can occur, unlike when a mere "Switch" cue appears. So although the reduced interference occurred at the stimulus level, this could only be achieved with task-specific preparation. This finding is in agreement with the top-down/bottom-up distinction of [18, Experiment 3], finding n-2 repetition costs only when a task was prepared endogenously.

4.4. Cue-target Translation & Inhibition

Recent work in our laboratory has been concerned with the role of inhibition at earlier stages of the trial structure. We have suggested that inhibition should be employed where there is the greatest need to reduce inter-trial conflict [120], and it is possible that other parts of the trial-structure may also be found to play a role, if the locus of conflict is shifted onto them [55]. As the cue signals a change of task-set, we have suggested that there must be some degree of conflict present during cue encoding. Additionally, [55] suggested that the manner in which a task is cued should modulate n-2 repetition costs, if the nature of the cue affects the degree of conflict with recent task performance. Thus, if a task-set is installed into WM after cue presentation [56, 69], and the mechanism underlying n-2 repetition costs serves to clear WM of components from recently performed tasks (Bao et al., 2007; Mayr & Keele, 2000), then the previous task must undergo some form of inhibition during preparatory stages.

The way in which a task is cued has been shown to influence n-2 repetition costs [94, 80]. The authors contrasted spatial with verbal cues when performing judgment tasks on number stimuli. The spatial cues consisted of a row of asterisks presented at any one of the vertices of a triangle, with each of the three positions cuing a different task. The verbal cues described the task to be performed (e.g. "Odd/Even"), and were presented centrally. While the verbal cues produced robust n-2 repetition costs, the spatial cues did not. Arbuthnott attributed lack of BI with the spatial cues to increased discrimination between the three tasks category-response rules, and also proposed that in the spatial cueing condition, competing task-sets remain active to some degree during task performance (Arbuthnott, 2005, Experiment 2). However, in the spatially cued condition, the stimuli appeared at the cued location and hence changed position from trial to trial (unlike in the verbally cued condition). Thus one must be wary of attributing the attenuation of BI to differences in the cues alone, but see [95, 96].

However, Arbuthnotts (2005) study does present a challenge to the suggestion that BI is exclusively generated by the use of overlapping response sets (Gade & Koch, 2007). In particular, Experiment 1 of Arbuthnott (2005) utilized univalent response sets and trivalent stimuli (i.e. a single digit that affords all three possible tasks), a condition which should not generate n-2 repetition costs according to Gade & Koch [100]. This may be construed as evidence that components of the task-set other than response processes are targeted by inhibitory mechanisms when the locus of conflict is placed upon them.

To further investigate the role of task cues in generating n-2 repetition costs, Houghton et al. [55] used a paradigm very similar to that of Mayr & Keele (2000). Participants were required to respond to the location of a relevant target. Targets were four ovals presented with one centralised to each quadrant of the screen. Ovals differed on visual properties: one was angled, one had a thick border, one was shaded in, and one was neutral. Responses were spatially compatible to the location of the correct oval on the screen (four keys, top-left [D], top-right [J], bottom-left [C], & bottom-right [N]). Participants knew which oval was relevant on a given trial due to a valid pre-cue. In one condition, the cues were verbal, describing which oval to search for (e.g. "Border", "Angled", and "Shaded"). In this instance, [55] suggested that participants needed to translate the cue into an active WM representation of the target to search for (a process they called "cue-target translation").

When a cue signals a switch (e.g. "Border"-"*Shaded*"), participants must engage in a new episode of cue-target translation. Instantiation of the new target representation in WM should generate conflict due to the still-active representation from the previous trial. Thus, inhibition is required to overcome this conflict, leading to *n*-2 repetition costs in an AB*A* sequence (see figure 2 for an example trial sequence).

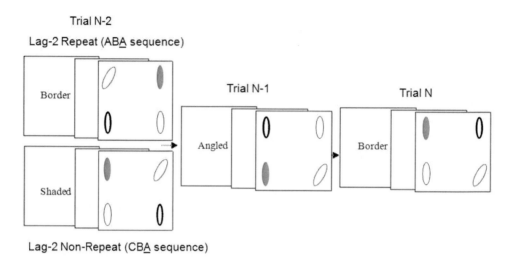

Figure 2. Example of AB*A* and CB*A* sequences with word cues from Houghton et al., (2009; Experiment 1).

However, Houghton and colleagues [55] suggested that if the cue eased the burden on WM during cue-target translation, then less conflict should be present during switching as less work is being done by WM. Easing cue-target translation was accomplished by using so-called iconic cues, which were rectangles that provided a relevant sample of the to-be-attended oval. For example, to cue the target with a thick border, the cue was a rectangle with a thick borer (see figure 3. In this instance, cue-target translation is less involved than the word cues (which provided no sample of the relevant target). Houghton and colleagues predicted that this scenario would produce no *n*-2 repetition costs, as less conflict is present in WM during cue-target translation when the relevant target switches.

Houghton and colleagues [55] found the predicted pattern, with significant *n*-2 repetition costs for word cues, but none for iconic cues. Importantly, this effect cannot be explained due to primary task–difficulty (see their Experiment 2). In their Experiment 3, Houghton and colleagues used arbitrary iconic cue-target relationships (for example a triangle cue indicated to search for the angled oval). In this instance, cue-target translation is even more difficult than for the word cues, and thus should induce greater inter-trial conflict when a new cue-target translation process is required. Indeed, the experiment showed greater *n*-2 repetition costs for arbitrary cue-target relationships than for word cues, further supporting the cue-target translation hypothesis of BI.

This difference in inhibition due to cue-transparency [80, 127, 79] is important theoretically, as for all cue-types, stimulus display and response-processes are identical. Additionally, responses were required on every trial, which requires response selection and

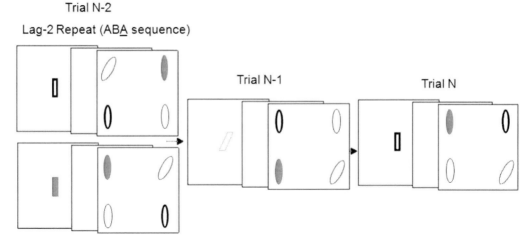

Figure 3. Example of AB*A* and CB*A* sequences with iconic cues from Houghton et al., (2009; Experiment 1).

execution c.f.[116]. Thus the difference in *n*-2 repetition costs between cue-types can only be explained by cue-based preparatory processes c.f. [100, 92, 110, 111, 116, 117]. Indeed, from trial to trial, all that changes is the relevant cue-target relationship. By holding all aspects of the trial structure constant in this manner, apart from the component of interest (cue-processing), is a powerful tool in determining the role of that component in switching performance (see also [128, 119]).

It must be noted that the finding of Houghton and colleagues [55] does not automatically assume that cue-trasnlation processes are subject to inhibition in other BI paradigms. This is especially true for paradigms where the greatest source of inter-trial conflict is response selection,i.e. when tasks share response-sets [100, 112, 116]. In this instance, cue-transparency might have little effect on n-2 repetition costs, as reducing interference during cue-processing may have little effect on the interference still inherent during response selection (although this needs to be empirically demonstrated). As response processes are the major source of inter-trial conflict in these studies, it is unsurprising that manipulation of response difficulty effects BI in these studies (see e.g. Koch et al., 2004; Philipp et al., 2007; Schuch & Koch, 2003 [102, 112, 116]).

Based on these findings, we suggest that backward inhibition is an active cognitive control mechanism that serves to suppress those aspects of the trial structure that generates the greatest inter-trial conflict [54, 53, 55].

5. Conclusion

The present chapter has reviewed behavioural findings from the task-switching literature. Despite the controversies reviewed, the task-switching paradigm remains an effective way to measure the mechanisms that allow flexible control of working memory contents.

References

[1] J. Diedrichsen, R. Shadmehr, and R. B. Ivry, "The coordination of movement. optimal feedback control and beyond," *Trends in Cognitive Science*, vol. 14, pp. 31–39, 2010.

[2] K.-C. Siu, L. S. Chou, U. Mayr, P. vanDonkelaar, and M. H. Woollacott, "Attentional mechanisms contributing to balance constraints during gait: The effects of balance impairments," *Brain Research*, vol. 1248, pp. 59–67, 2009.

[3] K. L. Vilberg and M. D. Rugg, "Memory retrieval and the parietal cortex: A review of evidence from a dual-process perspective." *Neuropsychologia*, vol. 46, pp. 1787–1799, 2008.

[4] J. M. Zacks, "Neuroimaging studies of mental rotation: A meta-analysis and review," *Journal of Cognitive Neuroscience*, vol. 20, pp. 1–19, 2008.

[5] S. Monsell and J. Driver, Eds., *Control of Cognitive Processes: Attention and Performance XVIII*. Cambridge, MA: MIT Press, 2000.

[6] S. Monsell and J. Driver, "Banishing the control homunculus," in *Control of Cognitive Processes: Attention and Performance XVIII*, S. Monsell and J. Driver, Eds. Cambridge, MA: MIT Press, 2000, pp. 3–32.

[7] C. M. MacLeod, "Half a century of research on the stroop effect: an integrative review." *Psychological Bulletin*, vol. 109, pp. 163–203, 1991.

[8] J. R. Stroop, "Studies of interference in serial verbal reactions," *Journal of Experimental Psychology*, vol. 18, pp. 643–662, 1935.

[9] F. Waszak, "Across-task long-term priming: Interaction of task readiness and automatic retrieval," *Quarterly Journal of Experimental Psychology*, in press.

[10] J. T. Reason, "Lapses of attention," in *Varieties of attention*, R. Parasuraman, R. Davies, and J. Beatty, Eds. Orlando, FL: Academic Press, 1984, pp. 515–549.

[11] F. Lhermitte, "Utlization behaviour and its relation to the frontal lobes," *Brain*, vol. 106, pp. 237–255, 1983.

[12] T. Goschke, "Intentional reconfiguration and involuntary persistence in task set switching," in *Control of Cognitive Processes: Attention and Performance XVIII*, S. Monsell and J. Driver, Eds. Cambridge, MA: MIT Press, 2000, pp. 331–356.

[13] N. Meiran, "Task switching: Mechanisms underlying rigid vs. flexible self control," in *Social Cognition and Social Neuroscience*, R. Hassin, K. Ochsner, and Y. Trope, Eds. NY: Oxford University Press, in press.

[14] S. Monsell, "Task switching." *Trends in Cognitive Sciences*, vol. 7, pp. 134–140, 2003.

[15] E. M. Altmann, "Task switching and the pied homunculus: where are we being led?" *Trends in Cognitive Science*, vol. 7, pp. 340–341, 2003.

[16] A. T. Jersild, *Mental set and shift.*   Archives of Psychology, whole No. 89, 1927.

[17] A. Spector and I. Biederman, "Mental set and mental shift revisited," *American Journal of Psychology*, vol. 89, pp. 669–679, 1976.

[18] U. Mayr and S. W. Keele, "Changing internal constraints on action: the role of backward inhibition." *Journal of Experimental Psychology: General*, vol. 129, pp. 4–26, 2000.

[19] G. Dreisbach and H. Haider, "That's what task sets are for: shielding against irrelevant information." *Psychological Research*, vol. 72, pp. 355–361, 2008.

[20] ——, "How task representations guide attention: further evidence for the shielding function of task sets." *Journal of Experimental Psychology: Learning, Memory, and Cognition*, vol. 35, pp. 477–486, 2009.

[21] A. Baddeley, D. Chincotta, and A. Adlam, "Working memory and the control of action: Evidence from task switching," *Journal of Experimental Psychology: General*, vol. 130, pp. 641–657, 2001.

[22] R. L. Bryck and U. Mayr, "On the role of verbalization during task set selection: switching or serial order control?" *Memory & Cognition*, vol. 33, pp. 611–623, 2005.

[23] M. J. Emerson and A. Miyake, "The role of inner speech in task switching: A dual-task investigation," *Journal of Memory and Language*, vol. 148-168, 2003.

[24] S. A. Los, "On the origin of mixing costs: Exploring information processing in pure and mixed blocks of trials," *Acta Psychologica*, vol. 94, pp. 145–188, 1996.

[25] A. M. Philipp, C. Kalinich, I. Koch, and R. I. Schubotz, "Mixing costs and switch costs when switching stimulus dimensions in serial predictions." *Psychological Research*, vol. 72, pp. 405–414, 2008.

[26] E. Poljac, I. Koch, and H. Bekkering, "Dissociating restart cost and mixing cost in task switching." *Psychological Research*, vol. 73, no. 3, pp. 407–416, 2009.

[27] O. Rubin and N. Meiran, "On the origins of the task mixing cost in the cuing task-switching paradigm." *Journal of Experimental Psychology: Learning, Memory, and Cognition*, vol. 31, pp. 1477–1491, 2005.

[28] R. D. Rogers and S. Monsell, "The cost of a predictable switch between simple cognitive tasks," *Journal of Experimental Psychology: General*, vol. 124, pp. 207–231, 1995.

[29] E. M. Altmann and W. D. Gray, "An integrated model of cognitive control in task switching." *Psychological Review*, vol. 115, pp. 602–639, 2008.

[30] G. D. Logan, "Executive control of thought and action: In search of the wild homunculus," *Current Directions in Psychological Science*, vol. 12, pp. 45–48, 2003.

[31] D. W. Schneider and G. D. Logan, "Modeling task switching without switching tasks: a short-term priming account of explicitly cued performance." *Journal of Experimental Psychology: General*, vol. 134, pp. 343–367, 2005.

[32] A. Allport, E. Styles, and S. Hisieh, "Shifting intentional set: Exploring the dynamic control of tasks," in *Consciousness and nonconscious information processing: Attention and Performance XV*, C. Ulmita and M. Moscovitch, Eds. Cambridge, MA: MIT Press, 1994, pp. 421–452.

[33] A. Allport and G. R. Wylie, "Task switching, stimulus-response bindings, and negative priming," in *Control of Cognitive Processes: Attention and Performance XVIII*, S. Monsell and J. Driver, Eds. Cambridge, MA: MIT Press, 2000, pp. 35–70.

[34] I. Koch and A. Allport, "Cue-based preparation and stimulus-based priming of tasks in task switching." *Memory & Cognition*, vol. 34, pp. 433–444, 2006.

[35] F. Waszak, B. Hommel, and A. Allport, "Task-switching and long-term priming: Role of episodic stimulus-task bindings in task-shift costs," *Cognitive Psychology*, vol. 46, pp. 361–413, 2003.

[36] ——, "Semantic generalization of stimulus-task bindings." *Psychonomic Bulletin & Review*, vol. 11, pp. 1027–1033, 2004.

[37] ——, "Interaction of task readiness and automatic retrieval in task switching: negative priming and competitor priming." *Memory & Cognition*, vol. 33, pp. 595–610, 2005.

[38] E. M. Altmann, "Think globally, ask functionally," *Behavioral & Brain Sciences*, vol. 26, pp. 602–603, 2003.

[39] ——, "Functional decay of memory for tasks." *Psychological Research*, vol. 66, pp. 287–297, 2002.

[40] E. M. Altmann and W. D. Gray, "Forgetting to remember: the functional relationship of decay and interference." *Psychological Science*, vol. 13, pp. 27–33, 2002.

[41] E. M. Altmann, "Advance preparation in task switching: what work is being done?" *Psychological Science*, vol. 15, pp. 616–622, 2004.

[42] ——, "The preparation effect in task switching: carryover of soa." *Memory & Cognition*, vol. 32, pp. 153–163, 2004.

[43] K. D. Arbuthnott and J. Frank, "Executive control in set switching: Residual switch cost and task-set inhibition," *Canadian Journal of Experimental Psychology*, vol. 54, pp. 33–41, 2000.

[44] K. D. Arbuthnott, "Asymmetric switch cost and backward inhibition: Carryover activation and inhibition in switching between tasks of unequal difficulty." *Canadian Journal of Experimental Psychology*, vol. 62, pp. 91–100, 2008.

[45] R. F. I. Meuter and A. Allport, "Bilingual language switching in naming: Asymmetrical costs of language selection," *Journal of Memory and Language*, vol. 40, pp. 25–40, 1999.

[46] S. Monsell, N. Yeung, and R. Azuma, "Reconfiguration of task-set: Is it easier to switch to the weaker task?" *Psychological Research*, vol. 63, pp. 250–264, 2000.

[47] N. Yeung and S. Monsell, "The effects of recent practice on task switching." *Journal of Experimental Psychology: Human Perception and Performance*, vol. 29, pp. 919–936, 2003.

[48] G. R. Wylie and A. Allport, "Task switching and measurement of "switch costs"," *Psychological Research*, vol. 63, pp. 212–233, 2000.

[49] U. Mayr, "Inhibition of task sets," in *Inhibition in Cognition*, D. S. Gorfein and C. M. MacLeod, Eds. Washington D.C.: American Psychological Association, 2007, pp. 27–44.

[50] N. Meiran, "Reconfiguration of processing mode prior to task performance," *Journal of Experimental Psychology: Learning, Memory, and Cognition*, vol. 22, pp. 1423–1442, 1996.

[51] P. Sudevan and D. A. Taylor, "The cuing and priming of cognitive operations," *Journal of Experimental Psychology: Human Perception and Performance*, vol. 13, pp. 89–103, 1987.

[52] N. Meiran, Z. Chorev, and A. Sapir, "Component processes in task switching." *Cognitive Psychology*, vol. 41, pp. 211–253, 2000.

[53] J. A. Grange and G. Houghton, "Heightened conflict in cue-target translation increases backward inhibition in set switching," *Journal of Experimental Psychology: Learning, Memory, and Cognition*, in press.

[54] ——, "Temporal cue-target overlap is not essential for backward inhibition in task switching." *Quarterly Journal of Experimental Psychology*, vol. 62, pp. 2069–2080, 2009.

[55] G. Houghton, R. Pritchard, and J. A. Grange, "The role of cue-target translation in backward inhibition of attentional set." *Journal of Experimental Psychology: Learning, Memory, and Cognition*, vol. 35, pp. 466–476, 2009.

[56] U. Mayr and R. Kliegl, "Task-set switching and long-term memory retrieval." *Journal of Experimental Psychology: Learning, Memory, and Cognition*, vol. 26, pp. 1124–1140, 2000.

[57] R. DeJong, "An intention-activation account of residual switch costs," in *Attention & Performance XVIII: Control of Cognitive Processes*, S. Monsell and J. Driver, Eds. Cambridge, MA: MIT Press, 2000.

[58] S. Nieuwenhuis and S. Monsell, "Residual costs in task switching: testing the failure-to-engage hypothesis." *Psychonomic Bulletin & Review*, vol. 9, pp. 86–92, 2002.

[59] F. Verbruggen, B. Liefooghe, A. Vandierendonck, and J. Demanet, "Short cue presentations encourage advance task preparation: a recipe to diminish the residual switch cost." *Journal of Experimental Psychology: Learning, Memory, and Cognition*, vol. 33, pp. 342–356, 2007.

[60] R. M. Klein, "Inhibition of return," *Trends in Cognitive Sciences*, vol. 4, pp. 138–147, 2000.

[61] D. W. Schneider and G. D. Logan, "Selecting a response in task switching: Testing a model of compound cue retrieval." *Journal of Experimental Psychology: Learning, Memory, and Cognition*, vol. 35, pp. 122–136, 2009.

[62] I. Koch, "The role of external cues for endogenous advance reconfiguration in task switching." *Psychonomic Bulletin & Review*, vol. 10, pp. 488–492, 2003.

[63] ——, "Automatic and intentional activation of task-sets," *Journal of Experimental Psychology: Learning, Memory, and Cognition*, vol. 27, pp. 1474–1486, 2001.

[64] R. DeJong, E. Berendsen, and R. Cools, "Goal neglect and inhibitory limitations: dissociable causes of interference effects in conflict situations," *Acta Psychologica*, vol. 101, pp. 379–394, 1999.

[65] R. Ratcliff, "Group reaction time distributions and an analysis of distribution statistics," *Psychological Bulletin*, vol. 86, pp. 446–461, 1979.

[66] M.-C. Lien, E. Ruthruff, R. W. Remington, and J. C. Johnston, "On the limits of advance preparation for a task switch: Do people prepare all the task some of the time or some of the task all the time?" *Journal of Experimental Psychology: Human Perception and Performance*, vol. 31, pp. 299–315, 2005.

[67] G. D. Logan and R. D. Gordon, "Executive control of visual attention in dual-task situations," *Psychological Review*, vol. 108, pp. 393–434, 2001.

[68] C. M. Arrington, E. M. Altmann, and T. H. Carr, "Tasks of a feather flock together: similarity effects in task switching." *Memory & Cognition*, vol. 31, pp. 781–789, 2003.

[69] U. Mayr and R. Kliegl, "Differential effects of cue changes and task changes on task-set selection costs." *Journal of Experimental Psychology: Learning, Memory, and Cognition*, vol. 29, pp. 362–372, 2003.

[70] K. Jost, U. Mayr, and F. Rsler, "Is task switching nothing but cue priming? evidence from erps." *Cognitive, Affective, and Behavioral Neuroscience*, vol. 8, pp. 74–84, 2008.

[71] J. S. Rubinstein, D. E. Meyer, and J. E. Evans, "Executive control of cognitive processes in task switching," *Journal of Experimental Psychology: Human Perception and Performance*, vol. 27, pp. 763–797, 2001.

[72] S. Monsell and G. A. Mizon, "Can the task-cuing paradigm measure an endogenous task-set reconfiguration process?" *Journal of Experimental Psychology: Human Perception and Performance*, vol. 32, pp. 493–516, 2006.

[73] D. Gopher, L. Armony, and Y. Greenshpan, "Switching tasks and attention policies," *Journal of Experimental Psychology: Oeneral*, vol. 129, pp. 308–339, 2000.

[74] J. R. Anderson, *How can the human mind occur in the physical universe?* Oxford: University Press, 2007.

[75] J. R. Anderson, D. Bothell, M. D. Byrne, S. Douglass, C. Lebiere, and Y. Qin, "An integrated theory of mind," *Psychological Review*, vol. 111, pp. 1036–1060, 2004.

[76] G. D. Logan and C. Bundesen, "Clever homunculus: is there an endogenous act of control in the explicit task-cuing procedure?" *Journal of Experimental Psychology: Human Perception and Performance*, vol. 29, pp. 575–599, 2003.

[77] N. Meiran, "Modeling cognitive control in task-switching." *Psychological Research*, vol. 63, pp. 234–249, 2000.

[78] G. D. Logan, "Working memory, task switching, and executive control in the task span procedure." *Journal of Experimental Psychology: General*, vol. 133, pp. 218–236, 2004.

[79] G. D. Logan and D. W. Schneider, "Interpreting instructional cues in task switching procedures: the role of mediator retrieval." *Journal of Experimental Psychology: Learning, Memory, and Cognition*, vol. 32, pp. 347–363, 2006.

[80] K. D. Arbuthnott and T. S. Woodward, "The influence of cue-task association and location on switch cost and alternating-switch cost," *Canadian Journal of Experimental Psychology*, vol. 56, pp. 18–29, 2002.

[81] G. D. Logan and C. Bundesen, "Very clever homunculus: compound stimulus strategies for the explicit task-cuing procedure." *Psychonomic Bulletin & Review*, vol. 11, pp. 832–840, 2004.

[82] C. M. Arrington and G. D. Logan, "Episodic and semantic components of the compound-stimulus strategy in the explicit task-cuing procedure." *Memory & Cognition*, vol. 32, pp. 965–978, 2004.

[83] G. D. Logan and D. W. Schneider, "Priming or executive control? associative priming of cue encoding increases "switch costs" in the explicit task-cuing procedure." *Memory & Cognition*, vol. 34, pp. 1250–1259, 2006.

[84] G. D. Logan, D. W. Schneider, and C. Bundesen, "Still clever after all these years: searching for the homunculus in explicitly cued task switching." *Journal of Experimental Psychology: Human Perception and Performance*, vol. 33, pp. 978–994, 2007.

[85] D. W. Schneider and G. D. Logan, "Priming cue encoding by manipulating transition frequency in explicitly cued task switching." *Psychonomic Bulletin & Review*, vol. 13, pp. 145–151, 2006.

[86] E. M. Altmann, "Task switching is not cue switching." *Psychonomic Bulletin & Review*, vol. 13, pp. 1016–1022, 2006.

[87] C. M. Arrington, G. D. Logan, and D. W. Schneider, "Separating cue encoding from target processing in the explicit task-cuing procedure: are there "true" task switch effects?" *Journal of Experimental Psychology: Learning, Memory, and Cognition*, vol. 33, pp. 484–502, 2007.

[88] D. S. Gorfein and C. M. MacLeod, Eds., *Inhibition in cognition*. Washington D.C.: American Psychological Association, 2007.

[89] C. M. MacLeod, M. D. Dodd, E. D. Sheard, D. E. Wilson, and U. Bibi, "In opposition to inhbition," *Psychology of Learning & Motivation*, vol. 43, pp. 163–214, 2003.

[90] J. T. Nigg, "On inhibition/disinhibition in developmental psychopathology: Views from cognitive and personality psychology and a working inhibition taxonomy," *Psychological Bulletin*, vol. 126, pp. 220–246, 2000.

[91] S. P. Tipper, "Does negative priming reflect inhibitory mechanisms: A review and integration of conflicting views," *Quarterly Journal of Experimental Psychology*, vol. 54A, pp. 321–343, 2001.

[92] I. Koch, M. Gade, S. Schuch, and A. M. Philipp, "The role of inhibition in task switching - a review," *Psychonomic Bulletin & Review*, in press.

[93] E. M. Altmann, "Cue-independent task-specific representations in task switching: evidence from backward inhibition." *Journal of Experimental Psychology: Learning, Memory, and Cognition*, vol. 33, pp. 892–899, 2007.

[94] K. D. Arbuthnott, "The influence of cue type on backward inhibition." *Journal of Experimental Psychology: Learning, Memory, and Cognition*, vol. 31, pp. 1030–1042, 2005.

[95] ——, "The effect of task location and task type on backward inhibition." *Memory & Cognition*, vol. 36, pp. 534–543, 2008.

[96] ——, "The representational locus of spatial influence on backward inhibition," *Memory & Cognition*, vol. 37, pp. 522–528, 2009.

[97] M. Bao, Z.-H. Li, X.-C. Chen, and D.-R. Zhang, "Backward inhibition in a task of switching attention within verbal working memory." *Brain Research Bulletin*, vol. 69, pp. 214–221, 2006.

[98] J.-C. Dreher and K. F. Berman, "Fractioning the neural substrate of cognitive control processes," *Proceedings of the National Academy of Sciences of the United States of America*, pp. 14 595–14 600, 2002.

[99] M. Gade and I. Koch, "Linking inhibition to activation in the control of task sequences." *Psychonomic Bulletin & Review*, vol. 12, pp. 530–534, 2005.

[100] ——, "The influence of overlapping response sets on task inhibition." *Memory & Cognition*, vol. 35, pp. 603–609, 2007.

[101] ——, "Dissociating cue-related and task-related processes in task inhibition: evidence from using a 2:1 cue-to-task mapping." *Canadian Journal of Experimental Psychology*, vol. 62, pp. 51–55, 2008.

[102] I. Koch, M. Gade, and A. M. Philipp, "Inhibition of response mode in task switching." *Experimental Psychology*, vol. 51, pp. 52–58, 2004.

[103] I. Koch, A. M. Philipp, and M. Gade, "Chunking in task sequences modulates task inhibition." *Psychological Science*, vol. 17, pp. 346–350, 2006.

[104] D. Kuhns, M.-C. Lien, and E. Ruthruff, "Proactive versus reactive task-set inhibition: evidence from flanker compatibility effects." *Psychonomic Bulletin & Review*, vol. 14, pp. 977–983, 2007.

[105] M.-C. Lien and E. Ruthruff, "Inhibition of task set: converging evidence from task choice in the voluntary task-switching paradigm." *Psychonomic Bulletin & Review*, vol. 15, pp. 1111–1116, 2008.

[106] M. E. J. Masson, D. N. Bubb, T. S. Woodward, and J. C. K. Chan, "Modulation of word-reading procesees in task switching," *Journal of Experimental Psychology: General*, vol. 132, pp. 400–418, 2003.

[107] U. Mayr, "Inhibition of action rules." *Psychonomic Bulletin & Review*, vol. 9, pp. 93–99, 2002.

[108] ——, "Sticky plans: Inhibition and binding during serial task control," *Cognitive Psychology*, vol. 59, pp. 123–153, 2009.

[109] ——, "What matters in the cued task-switching paradigm: tasks or cues?" *Psychonomic Bulletin & Review*, vol. 13, pp. 794–799, 2006.

[110] A. M. Philipp and I. Koch, "Switching of response modalities." *Quarterly Journal of Experimental Psychology: A*, vol. 58, no. 7, pp. 1325–1338, 2005.

[111] ——, "Task inhibition and task repetition in task switching," *European Journal of Cognitive Psychology*, vol. 18, pp. 624–639, 2006.

[112] A. M. Philipp, M. Gade, and I. Koch, "Inhibitory processes in language switching: Evidence from switching language-defined response sets," *European Journal of Cognitive Psychology*, vol. 19, pp. 395–416, 2007.

[113] A. M. Philipp, P. Jolicoeur, M. Falkenstein, and I. Koch, "Response selection and response execution in task switching: evidence from a go-signal paradigm." *Journal of Expimental Psychology: Learning, Memory, and Cognition*, vol. 33, pp. 1062–1075, 2007.

[114] D. W. Schneider, "Task-set inhibition in chunked task sequences," *Psychonomic Bulletin & Review*, vol. 14, pp. 970–976, 2007.

[115] D. W. Schneider and F. Verbruggen, "Inhibition of irrelevant category-response mappings," *Quarterly Journal of Experimental Psychology*, vol. 61, pp. 1629–1640, 2008.

[116] S. Schuch and I. Koch, "The role of response selection for inhibition of task sets in task shifting." *Journal of Experimental Psychology: Human Perception and Performance*, vol. 29, pp. 92–105, 2003.

[117] S. Sdoia and F. Ferlazzo, "Stimulus-related inhibition of task set during task switching," *Experimental Psychology*, vol. 55, pp. 322–327, 2008.

[118] M. Sinai, P. Goffaux, and N. A. Phillips, "Cue- versus response-locked processes in backward inhibition: evidence from erps." *Psychophysiology*, vol. 44, pp. 596–609, 2007.

[119] D. W. Schneider and G. D. Logan, "Defining task-set reconfiguration: the case of reference point switching." *Psychonomic Bulletin & Review*, vol. 14, pp. 118–125, 2007.

[120] M. M. Botvinick, T. S. Braver, D. M. Barch, C. S. Carter, and J. D. Cohen, "Conflict monitoring and cognitive control," *Psychological Review*, vol. 108, pp. 624–652, 2001.

[121] G. Houghton and S. P. Tipper, "Inhibitory mechanisms of neural and cognitive control: applications to selective attention and sequential action." *Brain & Cognition*, vol. 30, no. 1, pp. 20–43, 1996.

[122] F. Verbruggen, B. Liefooghe, A. Szmalec, and A. Vandierendonck, "Inhibiting responses when switching: Does it matter?" *Experimental Psychology*, vol. 52, pp. 125–130, 2005.

[123] F. Verbruggen, B. Liefooghe, and A. Vandierendonck, "Selective stopping in task switching: The role of response selection and response execution." *Experimental Psychology*, vol. 53, pp. 48–57, 2006.

[124] J. Jonides and R. Mack, "On the cost and benefit of cost and benefit," *Psychological Bulletin*, vol. 96, pp. 29–44, 1983.

[125] M. Huebner, G. Dreisbach, H. Haider, and R. H. Kluwe, "Backward inhibition as a means of sequential task-set control: evidence for reduction of task competition." *Journal of Experimental Psychology: Learning, Memory, and Cognition*, vol. 29, pp. 289–297, 2003.

[126] B. A. Eriksen and C. W. Eriksen, "Effects of noise letters upon the identification of a target letter in a nonsearch task," *Perception & Psychophysics*, vol. 16, pp. 143–149, 1974.

[127] J. A. Grange and G. Houghton, "Cue-switch costs in task-switching: Cue-priming or control processes?" *Psychological Research*, in press.

[128] S. Cooper and P. Mari-Beffa, "The role of response repetition in task switching." *Journal of Experimental Psychology: Human Perception and Performance*, vol. 34, pp. 1198–1211, 2008.

In: Working Memory: Capacity, Developments and… ISBN: 978-1-61761-980-9
Editor: Eden S. Levin © 2011 Nova Science Publishers, Inc.

Chapter 17

DEVELOPMENT OF NEURAL MECHANISMS OF WORKING MEMORY

V. Vuontela[1] and S. Carlson[1,2,3]

[1]Neuroscience Unit, Institute of Biomedicine/Physiology,
University of Helsinki, Helsinki, Finland
[2]Brain Research Unit, Low Temperature Laboratory,
Aalto University School of Science and Technology, Espoo, Finland
[3]Medical School, University of Tampere, Tampere, Finland

ABSTRACT

Working memory (WM), the ability to hold and manipulate information online, improves during childhood as shown by an increase in WM capacity and a positive correlation between age and measures of WM performance. Intact function of WM is essential in many forms of complex cognition such as learning, reasoning, problem solving and language comprehension. WM function has a strong impact on academic achievement and is related to adaptive functioning at school. Children with deficits in WM have learning difficulties that are often accompanied by behavioural problems.

The neural processes subserving WM performance and brain structures supporting this system continue to develop throughout childhood till adolescence and early adulthood. The prefrontal cortex (PFC), that is one of the last brain regions to mature, has a central role in the function of WM. WM network involves also distributed areas in parietal, temporal and striatal regions. It has been suggested that neuroanatomical brain development occurs in parallel with behavioural and cognitive maturation during childhood and adolescence. In this chapter, we focus on the neural mechanisms that support the function of WM, their developmental trajectories and relation of their development to the maturation of cognitive abilities. We will also discuss the development of the brain's "default-mode" network that is active in the absence of cognitive task performance, i.e. during a resting state and shows attenuation of activation (deactivation) when the brain becomes engaged in attention requiring cognitive task performance. Deactivation mechanisms are important in the performance of WM tasks: inability to deactivate is associated with impaired task performance and is evident in patients with certain neuropsychological disorders.

INTRODUCTION

WM refers to a cognitive system that allows us to temporarily maintain and manipulate just experienced information or information just retrieved from the long-term memory and to use this information for goal-directed behaviour [Baddeley, 1992, 1996]. This system has a protracted developmental trajectory and it plays a critical role in many forms of complex cognition such as learning, reasoning, problem solving, and language comprehension. In several models attempting to explain the function of WM, this system is proposed to be composed of both storage and executive control functions. It has been shown that although WM with simple response demands develops early, the development of the ability to implement WM is protracted compared to other forms of memory [Nelson 1995]. Simple encoding, maintenance and retrieval of information are established already in early childhood and even in infancy, but coordination and integration of functions, so called executive WM continues to develop until young adulthood [Diamond 1990; Luna et al., 2004; Nelson 1995].

In addition to division to storage and executive functions, WM has further been fractionated into subcomponents e.g. according to cognitive processes needed in the task performance (maintenance vs. manipulation) or according to the type of information being processed (spatial vs. nonspatial) [Curtis and D'Esposito, 2006]. Currently there is very little information available of the development of the fractionation of WM into subcomponents. The ability to maintain information in WM has been shown to reach functional maturity considerably earlier than the ability to manipulate information in WM [Crone et al., 2006]. Functional fractionation of WM into spatial and nonspatial processing domains has been shown in adults [Belger et al., 1998; Courtney et al., 1996; Mottaghy et al., 2002; Sala et al., 2003; Ventre-Dominey et al., 2005], but is not evident in children [Vuontela et al., 2009].

The use of advanced neuroimaging techniques has led to the identification of distinct cortical brain structures underpinning the proposed principal components of WM [Gathercole, 1999]. Functional magnetic resonance imaging (fMRI) has provided a specifically useful non-invasive method for developmental studies allowing assessment of brain function relevant for specific behaviour also in non-clinical pediatric populations.

MATURE NEURAL NETWORKS OF WM

Neuroimaging studies have shown that mature WM involves a widely distributed network of brain areas including ventrolateral PFC (vlPFC), dorsolateral PFC (dlPFC), medial PFC, posterior parietal, temporal, striatal and cerebellar regions [Carlson et al., 1998; Courtney et al., 1998; D'Esposito et al., 1998; Martinkauppi et al., 2000; Rämä et al., 2001]. However, several lines of evidence from different experimental disciplines suggest that the PFC is the most important brain region supporting WM. Based on observations on patients with PFC lesions [Milner, 1982; Fuster, 1989; Vilkki and Holst, 1989; Miotto et al., 1996], the functioning of WM via the executive control system is strongly dependent on the frontal lobes; this notion is also supported by selective lesion studies and electrophysiological recordings in nonhuman primates [Goldman and Rosvold, 1970; Goldman-Rakic 1987; Fuster 1989; Funahashi and Kubota 1994]. Many studies indicate that also posterior parietal cortex plays an important role in the function of WM; these areas have been associated with both mnemonic and executive control processes [Collette et al., 2006; D'Esposito et al., 1999; Wager and Smith, 2003]. Results from several studies show that a frontoparietal network involving several areas in the PFC and posterior parietal cortex (Fig. 2) is especially important to WM function [Owen et al., 2005; Klingberg, 2006].

The indisputable importance of the PFC in WM has produced several models in attempts to explain the functional organization of this cortical area [reviewed e.g. by Curtis and D'Esposito, 2006 and Fletcher and Henson, 2001]. One model suggests that the organization is based on the type of cognitive operation performed. In this model the dlPFC is responsible for monitoring and manipulating and the vlPFC for maintaining (including transferring, rehearsal and matching) information. Neuroimaging studies in adults provide evidence to substantiate this model [Owen et al., 1998; D'Esposito et al., 1999, 2000; Owen, 2000] which has evolved to produce variants that nevertheless support the idea of organization-by-process [Petrides et al., 2002; Petrides, 2005; Rypma, 2006]. Another model emphasizes domain specificity, proposing that the functional organization of the PFC is based on the type of information processed in WM [Wilson et al., 1993; Goldman-Rakic, 1995]. According to this model, WM processing of spatial information is handled in the dlPFC and nonspatial information in the vlPFC, a division also supported by brain imaging studies in adult human subjects [Courtney et al., 1996; Belger et al., 1998; Mottaghy et al., 2002; Sala et al., 2003; Ventre-Dominey et al., 2005]. These two models of WM may not be mutually exclusive as there is evidence that the organization of the PFC is based both on the type of information being processed and the cognitive operation [Johnson et al., 2003; Mohr et al., 2006].

WM and attention, which have been defined as core processes of executive functions, are closely intertwined. Both processes promote goal-directed behavior and show a considerable overlap of the underlying neural circuitry [LaBar et al., 1999; Wager et al., 2004; Awh et al., 2006]. The neural networks subserving WM and spatial attention have been found to intersect at several frontoparietal brain areas [LaBar et al., 1999]. On the other hand, it has been shown that verbal WM and visual attention recruit a common network in the posterior cortical and subcortical areas related to higher level attentional processing, whereas the frontoparietal network is mainly associated with memory processes [Tomasi et al., 2007]. Memory, attention, and inhibitory mechanisms are key components of cognitive control or executive processes that have been suggested to share some mechanisms but to have also separable functions [Miyake et al., 2000; Davidson et al., 2006; Huizinga et al., 2006]. Alternatively, these processes have been suggested to be parts of a single construct of a common underlying neural circuitry [Smith and Jonides, 1999; Casey et al. 2000; Miller and Cohen, 2001].

DEVELOPMENT OF NEURAL NETWORKS OF WM

The developing brain undergoes massive structural and functional changes that reflect a dynamic interplay of simultaneously occurring progressive and regressive events [reviewed in Tau and Peterson, 2010]. The brain regions underlying basic motor and sensory functions are the first ones to mature, whereas neuroanatomical and neurophysiological changes take place in higher-order association cortices well into adolescence and beyond it [Gogtay et al., 2004; Casey et al., 2005a,b]. Neuroanatomical brain development occurs in parallel with behavioral and cognitive maturation during childhood and adolescence [Casey et al., 2005a,b]. Measures of increased brain connectivity have also been linked to improved cognitive abilities [Klingberg, 2006].

Most of the dynamic changes of the cortex and subcortical grey matter nuclei occur during fetal life in a strictly organized sequence of cell proliferation, migration and maturation, but changes in these structures continue also during the postnatal life including regional changes in synaptic density and myelination [Casey et al., 2000, 2005a,b; Toga et al., 2006]. After birth there is a great increase in the dendritic branching and synaptic connections between neurons. This development reaches a plateau phase which is followed by a process of dendritic pruning and synapse elimination leading to more fine-tuned and efficient connections. In the human brain, the time-course of these changes varies enormously by brain region. In the auditory cortex, synaptic overproduction reaches its maximum at about the third postnatal month and, in the visual cortex, it peaks at about the age of four months [Huttenlocher, 1979, 1990, 1997]. The process of synapse elimination begins after this age period and continues until the adult level of synaptic density is reached at about preschool age for primary auditory and visual cortices. In the PFC, the synaptic density peaks at 8-15 months but the plateau and elimination phases are protracted and continue till young adulthood [Huttenlocher, 1979, 1990, 1997; Bourgeois et al., 1994]. The process of myelination that increases neural conduction velocity progresses most rapidly until the age of 1.5 years [Kinney et al., 1988; Ballesteros et al., 1993] but continues well into adulthood. The spatial and temporal pattern of changes related to myelination seem to parallel the developmental changes in synaptic density. Primary sensory and motor cortices myelinate before the temporal and parietal association cortices, and higher-order association areas in the prefrontal and lateral temporal cortices that seem to mature last [Yakovlev and Lecours, 1967; Gogtay et al., 2004; Sowell et al., 2004].

Although the total brain size of a child has reached about 90% of its adult size by the age of 6, the gray and white matter subcomponents of the brain continue to undergo dynamic changes throughout adolescence [Casey et al., 2000, 2005a,b]. Measures of gray matter volume follow an inverted U-shaped pattern with variation in regional changes [Jernigan et al., 1991; Giedd et al., 1999; Gogtay et al., 2004]. Increase in the gray matter volume is followed by gray matter loss which occurs first in the primary sensorimotor regions at about the age of 4-8 years, then in the frontal and parietal cortices at 11-13 years, and last in the PFC and temporal association areas at about the age of 16 continuing till late adolescence [Giedd et al. 1999; Gogtay et al., 2004]. In the PFC, gray matter loss is completed first in the frontal pole followed by the vlPFC while the dlPFC matures last [Gogtay et al., 2004]. Grey matter changes occur also in subcortical regions. For example, grey matter loss has been reported in those portions of the basal ganglia to which the PFC projects [Thompson et al., 2000].

Concurrently with ongoing changes in gray matter, the white matter volume increases in a roughly linear manner until approximately young adulthood with a pattern that seems to proceed from caudal to more rostral areas [Jernigan et al., 1991; Giedd et al., 1999; Paus et al., 1999]. Studies on connectivity between brain structures utilizing diffusion tensor imaging (DTI) technique, which is sensitive to myelination and neuroanatomical changes in the white matter microstructure, have shown progressive maturation of white matter during childhood and adolescence [Klingberg et al., 1999; Mukherjee et al., 2001; Snook et al., 2005]. As measured by an index of fractional anisotropy, there is greater coherence of white matter tracts in adults than in children [Barnea-Goraly et al., 2005]. Maturation of neural networks has also been related to improved connectivity within brain areas in the network [Olesen et al., 2003]. To conclude, dynamic interplay of regressive grey matter and progressive white matter processes underlie neuroanatomical brain development. The brain regions to mature first are the ones related to most basic functions, such as motor and sensory systems, followed by parietal and temporal association areas involved in spatial attention and basic language skills [Gogtay et al., 2004; Sowell et al., 2004]. Higher-order association areas such as the prefrontal and lateral temporal cortices that are involved in more advanced functions, e.g. in integration of primary sensorimotor processes, attentional modulation and language processes, mature last. The sequence of the maturation of brain areas seems to follow the order in which these areas were created so that phylogenetically older areas mature earlier than the more recently evolved higher-order areas [Gogtay et al., 2004].

Cortical development has been found to correlate with measures of behavioral performance. Moreover, gray matter increases and decreases, especially in the PFC, have been associated with differences in intellectual abilities [Shaw et al., 2006]. One study found an association between structural maturation of the PFC and improved memory function using neuropsychological measures [Sowell et al., 2001]. Similarly, white matter maturation in the PFC and in an area between the PFC and posterior parietal cortex has been related to the development of visuospatial WM [Nagy et al., 2004]. In another study, increase in WM capacity with age was associated with increased activity in the frontoparietal network [Klingberg et al., 2002]. Furthermore, age-related joint maturation of white and grey matter has been found in the PFC and posterior parietal cortex [Olesen et al., 2003]. Together these studies [Klingberg et al., 2002; Olesen et al., 2003; Nagy et al., 2004] provide evidence for a frontoparietal network subserving visuospatial WM in which brain activity, myelination and the development of cognitive capacity are tightly coupled. However, age-related functional specialization of specific brain areas in the PFC and PPC has also been found independent of performance changes providing evidence for joint maturation of two neural systems involved in visuospatial WM: a right hemisphere visuospatial attention system and a left hemisphere phonological store and rehearsal system [Kwon et al., 2002].

BEHAVIORAL CORRELATES OF WM IN CHILDHOOD AND ADOLESCENCE

Behavioral and cognitive maturation parallels neuroanatomical brain development during childhood and adolescence [Casey et al., 2005a,b]. WM that depends on the PFC circuitry emerges relatively early in life considering that the PFC is among the last to reach neuroanatomical maturity. Behavioral studies in very young children have shown that 8 to 12-month-old infants are able to correctly retain objects in delayed response (DR) tasks with short delays but lack accurate reaching behavior [Diamond 1990]. From this age onwards, their capacity to retain simple information in WM improves gradually. This result suggests that in very young children, the WM circuits supporting simple encoding, maintenance and retrieval are sufficiently developed by this age, but the neural circuits subserving coordination and integration of functions lack functional maturity [Nelson 1995].

We [Vuontela et al., 2003; Aronen et al., 2005] and others [Hale et al., 1997; Swanson 1999; Brocki and Bohlin, 2004; Gathercole et al., 2004; Luna et al., 2004; Huizinga et al.,

2006] have shown that developmental maturation of WM is characterized by gradual improvement in the performance of WM tasks. During this time executive control over information that is held in WM gains increasing precision. We used audiospatial and visuospatial n-back WM tasks to investigate the development of WM performance in 6-13-year-old school children. In this task, the child is presented with a visual stimulus on a computer display (visuospatial task) or a sound from the headphones (audiospatial task) presented in one of several possible locations. After the presentation of each stimulus, the child has to respond by pressing either the left or right button of the mouse. The difficulty level is lowest in the 0-back task in which the child presses the left button of the mouse whenever the stimulus is presented in a predetermined location and the right button if in any other location. In the 1-back task the child presses the left button of the mouse if the stimulus is presented in the same location as the previous one (two trials back in the 2-back task, etc.) and the right button if in different location (Fig. 1). Thus with this task paradigm it is possible to increase the difficulty level of the task by increasing the memory load just by changing the instructions while maintaining all other features of the task (number of stimuli, number and type of response) constant [Braver et al., 1997; Carlson et al., 1998]. While 2-back and 1-back tasks require on-line monitoring, updating and manipulation of retained information placing great demands on the key processes within WM, the 0-back is an attentional task that requires detection of a predetermined stimulus but does not demand manipulation or memorizing of the stimuli presented earlier [Owen et al., 2005]. Having these properties the n-back tasks are especially well suited for studying children both behaviourally and with neuroimaging methods.

In our studies, auditory and visual WM performance correlated positively with age, however, even the oldest of the 6- to 13-year-old children did not quite reach the level of accuracy and speed reported for adults in audiospatial and visuospatial n-back tasks [Anourova et al., 1999; Vuontela et al., 1999]. This result is consistent with studies showing that WM continues to develop into young adulthood, and a mature level of performance begins only after approximately 15-19 years of age [Luna et al., 2004; Luciana et al., 2005; Huizinga et al., 2006]. As in another experiment [Luciana and Nelson, 1998], the youngest children (aged 6-8 years) of our study expressed both mnemonic and executive failures in the performance of the WM tasks. Children aged 9-10 were better able to manage tasks placing high demands on executive functions and memory capacity than younger children whereas children aged 11-13 performed superior to the other age groups. Several studies have shown that children are more susceptible to interference and less able to withhold inappropriate responses than adults [Casey et al. 1997; Hale et al. 1997; Luna et al. 2001; Bunge et al. 2002]. Younger children are also suggested to be behaviorally more impulsive than older children [Davidson et al., 2006]. In line with these notions, all children in the youngest age group of our study expressed immature cognitive control in their performance of the WM tasks, and interestingly, boys in this age group manifested significantly more impulsive behavior than girls suggesting that the maturation of executive systems including cognitive control takes longer in boys than girls. Memory, attention and inhibition are suggested to be parts of a single construct of a common underlying neural circuitry [Casey et al. 2000]. In WM performance, these processes are not easily separable from each other, as both memory and attention are intertwined and involve also inhibitory processes [Smith and Jonides 1999; Casey et al. 2000; Davidson et al., 2006]. Accordingly, the performance of the n-back tasks of our study required not only memory processes but also attention and the ability to inhibit inappropriate responses and interference of non-target stimuli in the 2-back task. Our results thus give support to the suggestion that the development of WM occurs in parallel with the physiological and developmental changes in the brain networks subserving this cognitive ability [Casey et al. 2000; Luna et al. 2001; Kwon et al., 2002; Klingberg, 2006].

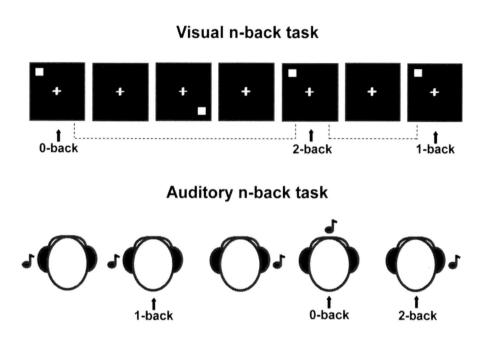

Figure 1. Illustration of four trials of visual and five trials of auditory 0-back, 1-back and 2-back tasks. The left button of the mouse is pressed whenever the stimulus is in the predetermined location (0-back) or when the stimulus is presented in the same location as the previous one (1-back) or in the location two trials back (2-back). In all other cases, the right button of the mouse is pressed.

NEURAL CORRELATES OF WM IN CHILDHOOD AND ADOLESCENCE

Neuroimaging methods including functional magnetic resonance (fMRI) and diffusion tensor (DTI) imaging have provided means to image brain activity and connectivity in children and adolescents and to study brain changes related to the development of WM. Functional MRI studies indicate that brain networks supporting WM in adults are also recruited in children during the performance of WM tasks, although the degree of engagement of different regions may change according to maturational state [Berl et al., 2006].

Using fMRI and n-back WM tasks, we studied brain networks involved in visual spatial and nonspatial WM processing in 11-13-year-old school children [Vuontela et al., 2009]. In the performance of these tasks, the children recruited several areas of the frontoparietal network including regions in the superior frontal cortex, dlPFC, and superior and inferior parietal cortices in similar regions as have been implicated in adults (Fig. 2). This is in line with fMRI studies that have shown frontoparietal activation in children during the WM processing of diverse classes of information [Casey et al., 1995; Thomas et al., 1999; Nelson et al., 2000; Klingberg et al., 2002; Kwon et al., 2002; Ciesielski et al., 2006; Crone et al.,

2006; Scherf et al., 2006; Geier et al., 2009]. In several visuospatial and verbal WM studies children activate similar PFC and parietal regions as adults [Casey et al., 1995; Thomas et al., 1999; Nelson et al., 2000; Klingberg et al., 2002; Kwon et al., 2002] but mnemonic processing of nonspatial information seems to engage at least partly different brain networks in these age groups [Ciesielski et al., 2006; Crone et al., 2006]. Similar activation of the WM network in children and adults may reflect the recruitment of comparable cognitive processes such as executive processes subserving WM and selective attention [Owen, 2000; Collette et al., 2006] or similar cognitive strategies [Casey et al., 2000, 2005b; Berl et al., 2006; Kirchhoff and Buckner, 2006; Rypma, 2006] in the performance of WM tasks.

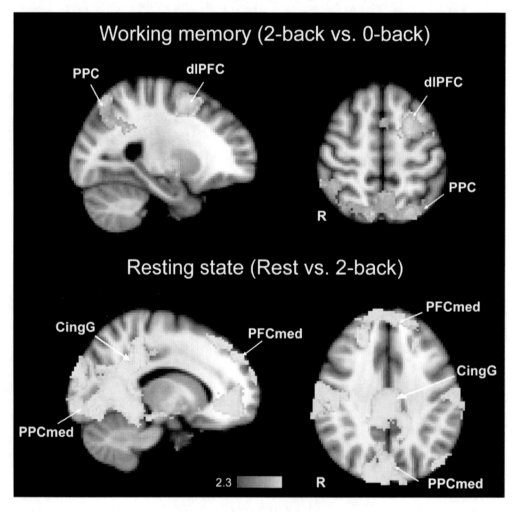

Figure 2. Demonstration of the distribution of memory load (upper row) and resting state (lower row) related activation in 11-13-year-old children. WM task performance recruits brain areas of the frontoparietal network while during resting, areas of the DMN are engaged. dlPFC dorsolateral prefrontal cortex, PFCmed medial parts of the prefrontal cortex, PPC posterior parietal cortex, PPCmed medial parts of the posterior parietal cortex, CingG cingulate gyrus, R right hemisphere.

It has been shown with imaging methods that the basic WM circuitry is in place already in 5- to 6-year-old children [Tsujimoto et al., 2004; Ciesielski et al., 2006] and that this circuitry undergoes qualitative and quantitative changes during maturation from childhood through adolescence till adulthood [Scherf et al., 2006]. During the performance of complex WM tasks, children engage only limited areas of the core WM network involving dlPFC and parietal regions compared to adolescents and adults [Crone et al., 2006; Scherf et al., 2006]. While adolescents recruit spatially more diffuse portions of the prefrontal and parietal cortices with stronger magnitude of right dlPFC participation than adults who engage the most specialized WM network, children rely primarily on ventromedial brain areas in the performance of these tasks. This indicates that from childhood through adolescence till adulthood there are considerable refinements in the WM circuitry including both changes in the recruitment of brain areas and their integration with other areas which reflects neural maturation from early recruitment of childhood compensatory networks to later refinement of functional connectivity among necessary performance enhancing regions [Luna et al., 2010; Scherf et al., 2006].

Some studies on the development of WM have shown a more diffuse, widespread, and greater magnitude of activation in children compared to adults [Casey et al., 1995; Thomas et al., 1999; Nelson et al., 2000] while others have observed increased extent and magnitude of activation with increasing age [Thomas et al., 1999; Klingberg et al., 2002; Kwon et al., 2002]. Some of these differences between the findings concerning the development of visuospatial WM may be related to methodological differences among studies in terms of a wide age range of the children participating the studies, varying maturational status of the tested children, task difficulty differences between children and adults, or differences in problem solving strategies [Berl et al., 2006]. The focal network model of maturation states that during development there is a shift from low power diffuse patterns of brain activation to more focal and greater magnitude of activation [Berl et al., 2006] probably reflecting fine-tuning of relevant neural systems [Johnson et al., 2002]. Studies that show that similar brain regions are activated in adults and children, but the extent of activation is greater in children [Casey et al., 1995; Thomas et al., 1999; Nelson et al., 2000], give some support to this model. Another model of development proposes that the same areas of the distributed network are involved in children and adults, but the degree of engagement of each region systematically changes with maturation [Berl et al., 2006].

When considering the function of the PFC, most often WM processing in adults is suggested to be fractionated into subcomponents according to cognitive operation needed in the task performance (maintenance vs. manipulation) or the type of information being processed (spatial vs. nonspatial). Currently there is very little information available of the fractionation of WM into subcomponents in children. In our fMRI study using n-back WM tasks (0-back and 2-back), we studied brain networks involved in visual spatial and nonspatial WM processing in 11-13-year-old school children [Vuontela et al., 2009]. We found memory load-related activation in areas of the frontoparietal network and occipital cortex during the performance of both spatial and nonspatial WM tasks suggesting that mnemonic visual information processing in 11-13-year-old children is organized by cognitive processes relevant to task performance and not by the type of information being processed. Some neuroimaging studies in adults have suggested process specific organization of WM for the PFC and organization by the type of information for posterior cortical areas [Postle and D'Esposito, 1999; Postle et al., 2000; Hautzel et al., 2002]. The children in our study, however, recruited both the PFC and posterior cortical areas in a similar manner in the performance of the 2-back WM tasks. As areas in the PFC and posterior parietal cortex have been associated with executive processes including manipulation of retained information [Owen, 2000; Wager and Smith, 2003; Collette et al., 2006; Mottaghy, 2006], our result suggests that children employ comparable executive processes in the performance of spatial and nonspatial WM tasks. Similar activation of the dlPFC which has been related to strategic control of WM processing [Owen et al., 2005; Rypma, 2006] suggests comparable use of cognitive strategies in the performance of both tasks. The PFC and posterior parietal areas indicated in executive function were not recruited in 8-12-year-old children performing a task requiring manipulation of mnemonic information [Crone et al., 2006] but the 11-13-year-old children of our study employed these cortical areas in the performance of 2-back tasks that involve both maintenance and manipulation of information in WM. There may be several reasons why we could not observe memory load-dependent segregation of information processing into spatial and nonspatial domains in our study. The n-back task involves multiple processing which may hamper the detection of subtle differences between spatial and nonspatial tasks. In the study of Sala et al. [2003] on adults, the stimuli that contained both spatial and nonspatial features activated areas indicated in the maintenance of object information but the activation overlapped with the brain areas indicated in the maintenance of spatial information. The children of our study may have retained both spatial and nonspatial information while performing either of the tasks because the stimuli were the same in both types of tasks. However, we found indication of partial dissociation of spatial and nonspatial information processing in WM when we compared the activation during the lower memory loads (0-back, attentional task) between spatial and nonspatial tasks. Attention directed to spatial information generated a greater activation in several PFC, parietal and occipital cortical areas, many of which are part of the dorsal visual pathway indicated in the processing of spatial visual information [Mishkin et al., 1983; Van Essen and Maunsell, 1983; Goodale and Milner, 1992]. Although several studies in adults have proposed that attention to spatial or nonspatial stimulus features activates largely overlapping cortical areas [Coull and Frith, 1998; Vanderberghe et al., 2001], it has been shown that selective attention to spatial but not to nonspatial features of the stimulus recruits regions of the frontoparietal attentional network [Giesbrecht et al., 2003] expressing a similar distribution of activation as in the children of our study.

An investigation of developmental changes related to maintenance of information in WM indicate that the core WM processes are established in childhood enabling goal-directed responses based on information stored in WM, but the fidelity of the WM representation and response precision continue to mature through adolescence [Geier et al., 2009]. The developmental trajectory of process specific model of WM function has been investigated in one study [Crone et al., 2006] that showed that the ability to manipulate items in WM develops more slowly than the ability to simply maintain items in WM. During maintenance of items, the PFC and parietal areas were recruited in a similar manner in 8-12-year-old children, 13-17-year-old adolescents and adults. When manipulation of information was required, the children failed to recruit the regions that the adolescents and adults relied on when manipulating the items.

THE DEFAULT MODE NETWORK (DMN) OF THE MATURE BRAIN

The human brain is suggested to be intrinsically organized into distinct functional networks of brain areas [Greicius et al., 2003; Fox et al., 2006; Seeley et al., 2007] that exhibit temporally correlated fluctuation of activity that can be measured during resting state or task-free paradigms using fMRI [for a review see Fox and Raichle, 2007]. It is thought that spontaneous activity of neurons in these networks may be involved in maintaining network integrity by strengthening the synaptic connections that subserve the network's normal functioning during awake states [Fox and Raichle, 2007]. Studies of resting-state functional connectivity that typically measure correlations between signal time courses have detected several distinct intrinsic activity networks, one of which is the default mode network (DMN) [Greicius et al., 2003; Beckmann et al., 2005; Fox et al., 2006; Seeley et al., 2007]. The DMN refers to areas in the medial prefrontal and parietal cortices, cingulate cortex and inferior parietal lobule that are active during the resting state and attenuated (deactivated) during attention demanding cognitive task performance (Fig. 2) [Raichle et al., 2001]. The specific functions of the DMN are currently unclear [Raichle, 2010]. Activity observed in the DMN has been suggested to be related to internally directed processes such as episodic memory [Mazoyer et al., 2001], self-referential processing [Kelley et al., 2002], self-projection [Buckner and Carroll, 2007] and mind wandering [Mason et al., 2007]. The DMN activity is most frequently related to internally directed mental activity but an alternative view relates the function of the DMN to ongoing and recent experiences [Esposito et al., 2006; Fransson, 2006; Garrity et al., 2007; Harrison et al., 2008] and suggests that the DMN plays an important role in higher-level cognitive functions [Hasson et al., 2009]. Resting state activity has not only been reported in awake human participants but also during light sleep in humans [Larson-Prior et al., 2009] and under anesthesia both in infants [Kiviniemi et al., 2000] and macaque monkeys [Vincent et al., 2007], and the signal is reported to be similar across scanners and subjects [Biswal et al., 2010]. Temporally correlated resting state activity does not require direct anatomical connections between the areas in the network [Vincent et al., 2007], but is nevertheless restricted by the physical structure of the network [Johnston et al., 2008].

The physiological mechanisms underlying attenuation of activation i.e. deactivation of the DMN during cognitive task performance are incompletely understood at present. It has been suggested that deactivation seen by fMRI results from a disproportionate decrease in blood flow and glucose utilization in the DMN areas [Raichle and Mintun, 2006] and may reflect a decrease in the activity of the cells that project to the deactivated area rather than increased activity of local inhibitory interneurons in that area [Gusnard and Raichle, 2001]. The deactivation of the DMN increases with task difficulty as shown by larger deactivation with increasing memory load during WM task performance which is suggested to reflect efficient reallocation of processing resources from the DMN to brain areas involved in successful task performance [McKiernan et al., 2003]. A critical role in switching between central executive network needed in the task performance and the DMN activated during rest has been suggested for the right fronto-insular cortex [Sridharan et al., 2008]. Deactivation mechanisms have been shown to be important in the performance of WM and other tasks that require concentrated attention. Failure to deactivate the DMN has been related to impaired task performance so that the extent to which the DMN is attenuated during task engagement is related to successful performance [Otten and Rugg, 2001; Daselaar et al., 2004; Polli et al., 2005; Weissman et al., 2006]. Inability to deactivate is also evident in patients with certain neuropsychological disorders [Kennedy et al., 2006; Fassbender et al., 2009].

THE DMN IN CHILDREN AND ADOLESCENTS

The DMN is fairly well documented in adults, but much less is known about the properties and function of this network in children. In very young children, resting state activity has been reported in primary sensory areas [Kiviniemi et al., 2000]. Resting state activity in young children has also been reported in other cortical areas in networks that resembled but were not equivalent of the DMN observed in adults [Fransson et al., 2007; Gao et al., 2009]. After infancy, the DMN structure still deviates significantly from the adult architecture and the functional connectivity between areas changes over childhood and adolescence. In early school aged children, the DMN areas are shown to be only sparsely functionally connected but during development these areas integrate into a cohesive, interconnected adult-like network [Fair et al., 2008]. In resting state networks, the overall trend for development is that brain regions in children communicate with other regions more locally, i.e. the functional connections between short-range regions are stronger and over age this communication becomes more distributed i.e. the functional connections between long-range regions become stronger [Fair et al., 2007; 2009]. However, in the DMN in children, very few functional short-range connections were found and some of them even showed an increase in correlation strength over development. Although there seems to be a trend towards increased functional connectivity within the DMN over development in some studies [Fair et al., 2007; 2009; Kelly et al., 2009; Supekar et al.,2009, 2010], more comprehensive studies of functional networks are needed to elucidate the course of development of these networks [Power et al., 2010].

There is very little information available of deactivation of the DMN in children and adolescents. Deactivation of the DMN can be studied within the settings of a cognitive task paradigm by using fMRI during cognitive task performance in which the cognitive load is parametrically modulated and activity related to cognitive load contrasted with activity measured during the rest periods (without task performance) within the same fMRI session. In our fMRI study, we used visual spatial and nonspatial n-back WM tasks interleaved with rest-periods to test whether deactivation mechanisms found in adults induced by cognitive task performance are functional in 11-13-year-old children [Vuontela et al., 2009]. As noted before, due to the properties of the n-back task, it is well suited also for studying deactivation in pediatric populations.

The results of our study showed that brain areas of the DMN in the medial PFC and the lateral and medial posterior cortices in children were less active during n-back task performance than rest condition (Fig. 2). Deactivation of the DMN during WM task performance has been shown to increase with task difficulty in adults and has been related to reallocation of processing resources to areas involved in task performance [McKiernan et al., 2003]. The deactivation observed in our study was also memory load dependent: it was larger during 2-back than 0-back tasks. In the same way, deactivation related to increased cognitive load during the performance of spatial and verbal WM tasks has been shown for 7-12-year-old children [Thomason et al., 2008]. Deactivation in children has earlier been reported in a study conducted in infants listening to spoken words but the distribution of the deactivation was not topographically similar to the adult DMN [Dehaene-Lambertz et al., 2006]. In another study, spatial WM task induced deactivation was observed in 12-17-year-olds in DMN areas (medial PFC) and in areas that are not usually reported as part of the DMN (occipital cortex) [Schweinsburg et al., 2005]. Our results indicate that, in 11-13-year-old children, cognitive task performance induces deactivation in cortical areas that have a similar cortical distribution as the DMN in adults. Partly in concordance with our study, both similarities and differences between the DMN in adults and 7-12-year-old children have been observed [Thomason et al., 2008]. Most of the differences in the DMN between adults and children in the study of Thomason et al. [2008] occurred in regions of the PFC so that several regions of the DMN usually reliably associated with task induced decreases in adults were not found in children suggesting immaturities in the functionality of the PFC in children.

The demonstration of deactivation of the DMN during cognitive performance in children may have important clinical implications when assessing abnormal brain functions in children. A study in adults demonstrated that subjects with autism did not show deactivation of the medial cortical network during a counting task contrasted with the rest condition, which was suggested to reflect abnormal internally directed mental processes at rest [Kennedy et al., 2006]. The results of an investigation of the ability of 8-14-year-old children with Attention Deficit Hyperactivity Disorder (ADHD) to deactivate the DMN during cognitive task performance showed deficient deactivation of this network in these children which was suggested to be linked to increased distractibility in ADHD [Fassbender et al., 2009]. We detected attenuation of activation also in primary cortical areas involved in somatosensory and auditory processing i.e. in the postcentral gyrus and Heschl's gyrus during the performance of visual WM tasks compared to rest. This result reflects findings of earlier studies showing that selective attention to one sensory modality reduces activity in cortical areas processing information from other sensory modalities [Haxby et al., 1994; Laurienti et al., 2002]. Significant task-related deactivation of the postcentral gyrus has also been observed in 7-12-year-old children performing spatial and verbal WM tasks [Thomason et al., 2008].

CONCLUSION

Elucidation of the development of neural networks underlying WM with neuroimaging methods has provided accumulating evidence that behavioral and cognitive maturation parallels neuroanatomical and functional brain development during childhood and adolescence. The frontoparietal network of brain areas, especially the areas within the PFC have a central role in the function of WM. The brain networks supporting WM in adults are also recruited in children during the performance of WM tasks, although the degree of engagement of different regions seems to change according to maturational state. The core WM circuitry is in place already at early age but the WM circuitry undergoes qualitative and quantitative changes during maturation from childhood through adolescence till adulthood.

The properties and function of the DMN that expresses activity during the resting state and is attenuated (deactivated) during attention demanding cognitive task performance are not well documented in children. The composition of brain areas in the DMN in early childhood seem to differ from those observed in adulthood. After infancy, the DMN structure still deviates from the adult architecture and the functional connectivity between areas changes over childhood and adolescence. Deactivation mechanisms are important in the performance of WM and other tasks that require concentrated attention and a failure to deactivate the DMN is related to impaired task performance. The demonstration of deactivation of the DMN during cognitive performance in children may have important clinical implications when assessing abnormal brain functions as inability to deactivate has been detected in patients with certain neuropsychological disorders.

REFERENCES

Anourova, I., Rämä, P., Alho, K., Koivusalo, S., Kahnari, J., Carlson, S. (1999). Selective interference reveals dissociation between auditory memory for location and pitch. *NeuroReport* 10, 3543-3547.

Aronen, E.T., Vuontela, V., Steenari, M.-R., Salmi, J., Carlson, S. (2005). Working memory, psychiatric symptoms, and academic performance at school. *Neurobiology of Learning and Memory* 83, 33-42.

Awh, E., Vogel, E.K., Oh, S-H. (2006). Interactions between attention and working memory. *Neuroscience* 139, 201-208.

Baddeley, A.D. (1992). Working memory. *Science*, 255, 556-559.

Baddeley, A.D. (1996). The fractionation of working memory. *Proceedings of the National Academy of Sciences* 93, 13468-13472.

Ballesteros, M.C., Hansen, P.E., Soila, K. (1993). MR imaging of the developing human brain. *Radiographics* 13, 611-622.

Barnea-Goraly, N., Menon, V., Eckert, M., Tamm, L., Bammer, R., Karchemskiy, A., Dant, C.C., Reiss, A.L. (2005). White matter development during childhood and adolescence: a cross-sectional diffusion tensor imaging study. *Cerebral Cortex* 15, 1848-1854.

Beckmann, C.F., DeLuca, M., Devlin, J.T., Smith, S.M. (2005). Investigations into resting-state connectivity using independent component analysis. *Philosophical Transactions of the Royal Society* B: Biological Sciences 360, 1001-1013.

Belger, A., Puce, A., Krystal, H.J., Gore, J.C., Goldman-Rakic, P., McCarthy, G. (1998). Dissociation of mnemonic and perceptual processes during spatial and nonspatial working memory using fMRI. *Human Brain Mapping* 6, 14-32.

Berl, M.M., Vaidya, C.J., Gaillard, W.D. (2006). Functional imaging of developmental and adaptive changes in neurocognition. *NeuroImage* 30, 679-691.

Biswal, B.B., Mennes, M., Zuo, X.N., Gohel, S., Kelly, C., Smith, S.M., Beckmann, C.F., Adelstein, J.S., Buckner, R.L., Colcombe, S. et al. (2010). Toward discovery science of human brain function. *Proceedings of the National Academy of Sciences U.S.A.* 107, 4734-4739.

Bourgeois, J.P., Goldman-Rakic, P.S., Rakic, P. (1994). Synaptogenesis in the prefrontal cortex of rhesus monkeys. *Cerebral Cortex* 4, 78-96.

Braver, T.S., Cohen, J.D., Nystrom, L.E., Jonides, J., Smith, E.E., Noll, D.C. (1997). A parametric study of prefrontal cortex involvement in human working memory. *NeuroImage* 5, 49-62.

Brocki, K.C., Bohlin, G. (2004). Executive functions in children aged 6 to 13: A dimensional study. *Developmental Neuropsychology* 26(2), 571-593.

Buckner, R.L., Carroll, D.C. (2007). Self-projection and the brain. Trends in Cognitive *Sciences* 11, 49-57.

Bunge, S.A., Dudukovic, N.M., Thomason, M.E., Vaidya, C.J., Gabrieli, J.D. (2002). Immature frontal lobe contributions to cognitive control in children: evidence from fMRI. *Neuron* 33, 301-311.

Carlson, S., Martinkauppi, S., Rämä, P., Salli, E., Korvenoja, A., Aronen, H.J. (1998). Distribution of cortical activation during visuospatial n-back tasks as revealed by functional magnetic resonance imaging. *Cerebral Cortex* 8, 743-752.

Casey, B.J., Cohen, J.D., Jezzard, P., Turner, R., Noll, D.C., Trainor, R.J., Giedd, J., Kaysen, D., Hertz-Pannier, L., Rapoport, J.L. (1995). Activation of prefrontal cortex in children during a nonspatial working memory task with functional MRI. *NeuroImage* 2, 221-229.

Casey, B.J., Galvan, A., Hare, T.A. (2005a). Changes in cerebral functional organization during cognitive development. *Current Opinion in Neurobiology* 15, 239-244.

Casey, B.J., Giedd, J.N., Thomas, K.M. (2000). Structural and functional brain development and its relation to cognitive development. *Biological Psychology* 54, 241-257.

Casey, B.J., Tottenham, N., Liston, C., Durston, S. (2005b). Imaging the developing brain: what have we learned about cognitive development? *Trends in Cognitive Science* 9, 104-110.

Casey, B.J., Trainor, R.J., Orendi, J.L., Schubert, A.B., Nystrom, L.E., Giedd, J.N., Castellanos, F.X., Haxby, J.V., Noll, D.C., Cohen, J.D., Forman, S.D., Dahl, R.E., Rapoport, J.L. (1997). A developmental functional MRI study of prefrontal activation during performance of a go-no-go task. *Journal of Cognitive Neuroscience* 9, 835-847.

Ciesielski, K.T., Lesnik, P.G., Savoy, R.L., Grant, E.P., Ahlfors, S.P. (2006). Developmental neural networks in children performing a categorical n-back task. *NeuroImage* 33, 980-990.

Collette, F., Hogge, M., Salmon, E., Van der Linden, M. (2006). Exploration of the neural substrates of executive functioning by functional neuroimaging. *Neuroscience* 139, 209-221.

Coull, J.T., Frith, C.D. (1998). Differential activation of right superior parietal cortex and intraparietal sulcus by spatial and nonspatial attention. *NeuroImage* 8, 176-187.

Courtney, S.M., Petit, L., Maisog, J.M., Ungerleider, L.G., Haxby, J.V. (1998). An area specialized for spatial working memory in human frontal cortex. Science 279, 1347-1351.

Courtney, S.M., Ungerleider, L.G., Keil, K., Haxby, J.V. (1996). Object and spatial visual working memory activate separate neural systems in human cortex. *Cerebral Cortex* 6, 39-49.

Crone, E.A., Wendelken, C., Donohue, S., van Leijenhorst, L., Bunge, S.A. (2006). Neurocognitive development of the ability to manipulate information in working memory. *Proceedings of the National Academy of Sciences U.S.A.* 103, 9315-9320.

Curtis, C.E., D'Esposito, M. (2005). Functional neuroimaging of working memory. In: Cabeza, R. & Kingstone, A. (Eds.), *Handbook of functional neuroimaging of cognition* (2nd edition, pp. 269-306). Cambridge, The MIT Press.

Daselaar, S.M., Prince, S.E., Cabeza, R. (2004). When less means more: deactivations during encoding that predict subsequent memory. *NeuroImage* 23, 921-927.

Davidson, M.C., Amso, D., Anderson, L.C., Diamond, A. (2006). Development of cognitive control and executive functions from 4 to 13 years: Evidence from manipulations of memory, inhibition and task switching. *Neuropsychologia* 44, 2037-2078.

Dehaene-Lambertz, G., Hertz-Pannier, L., Dubois, J., Mériaux, S., Roche, A., Sigman, M., Dehaene, S. (2006). Functional organization of perisylvian activation during presentation of sentences in preverbal infants. *Proceedings of National Academy of Science, U.S.A.* 103, 14240-14245.

D'Esposito, M., Aguirre, G.K., Zarahn, E., Ballard, D., Shin, R.K., Lease, J. (1998). Functional MRI studies of spatial and nonspatial working memory. *Cognitive Brain Research* 7, 1-13.

D'Esposito, M., Postle, B.R., Ballard, D., Lease, J. (1999). Maintenance versus manipulation of information held in working memory: an event-related fMRI study. *Brain and Cognition* 41, 66-86.

D'Esposito, M., Postle, B.R., Rypma, B. (2000). Prefrontal cortical contributions to working memory: evidence from event-related fMRI studies. *Experimental Brain Research* 133, 3-11.

Diamond, A. (1990). The development and neural bases of memory formation as indexed by the AB and delayed response tasks in human infants and infant monkeys. *Annals of the New York Academy of Sciences* 608, 267-317.

Esposito, F., Bertolino, A., Scarabino, T., Latorre, V., Blasi, G., Popolizio, T., Tedeschi, G., Cirillo, S., Goebel, R., Di Salle, F. (2006). Independent component model of the default-mode brain function: Assessing the impact of active thinking. *Brain Research Bulletin* 70, 263-269.

Fair, D.A., Cohen, A.L., Dosenbach, N.U., Church, J.A., Miezin, F.M., Barch, D.M., Raichle, M.E., Petersen, S.E., Schlaggar, B.L. (2008). The maturing architecture of the brain's default network. *Proceedings of National Academy of Science, U.S.A.* 105, 4028-4032.

Fair, D.A., Cohen, A.L., Power, J.D., Dosenbach, N.U., Church, J.A., Miezin, F.M., Schlaggar, B.L., Petersen, S.E. (2009). Functional brain networks develop from a "local to distributed" organization. *PLoS Computational Biology* 5(5), e1000381.

Fair, D.A., Dosenbach, N.U., Church, J.A., Cohen, A.L., Brahmbhatt, S., Miezin, F.M., Barch, D.M., Raichle, M.E., Petersen, S.E., Schlaggar, B.L. (2007). Development of distinct control networks through segregation and integration. *Proceedings of National Academy of Science, U.S.A.* 104, 13507-13512.

Fassbender, C., Zhang, H., Buzy, W.M., Cortes, C.R., Mizuiri, D., Beckett, L., Schweitzer, J.B. (2009). A lack of default network suppression is linked to increased distractibility in ADHD. *Brain Research* 1273, 114-128.

Fletcher, P.C., Henson, R.N. (2001). Frontal lobes and human memory: insights from functional neuroimaging. *Brain* 124, 849-881.

Fox, M.D., Corbetta, M., Snyder, A.Z., Vincent, J.L., Raichle, M.E. (2006). Spontaneous neuronal activity distinguishes human dorsal and ventral attention systems. *Proceedings of the National Academy of Sciences U.S.A.* 103, 10046-10051.

Fox, M.D., Raichle, M.E. (2007). Spontaneous fluctuations in brain activity observed with functional magnetic resonance imaging. *Nature Reviews Neuroscience* 8, 700-711.

Fransson, P. (2006). How default is the default mode of brain function? Further evidence from intrinsic BOLD signal fluctuations. *Neuropsychologia* 44, 2836-2845.

Fransson, P., Skiöld, B., Horsch, S., Nordell, A., Blennow, M., Lagercrantz, H., Åden, U. (2007). Resting-state networks in the infant brain. *Proceedings of National Academy of Science, U.S.A.* 104, 15531-15536.

Funahashi, S., Kubota, K. (1994). Working memory and prefrontal cortex. *Neuroscience Research* 21, 1-11.

Fuster, J.M. (1989). *The Prefrontal Cortex.* Press R ed., New York.

Gao, W., Zhu, H., Giovanello, K.S., Smith, J.K., Shen, D., Gilmore, J.H., Lin, W. (2009). Evidence on the emergence of the brain's default network from 2-week-old to 2-year-old healthy pediatric subjects. *Proceedings of National Academy of Science, U.S.A.* 106, 6790-6795.

Garrity, A.G., Pearlson, G.D., McKiernan, K., Lloyd, D., Kiehl, K.A., Calhoun, V.D. (2007). Aberrant "default mode" functional connectivity in schizophrenia. *American Journal of Psychiatry* 164(3), 450-457.

Gathercole, S.E. (1999). Cognitive approaches to the development of short-term memory. *Trends in Cognitive Sciences* 3(11), 410-419.

Gathercole, S.E., Pickering, S.J., Ambridge, B., Wearing, H. (2004). The structure of working memory from 4 to 15 years of age. *Developmental Psychology* 40(2), 177-190.

Geier, C.F., Garver, K., Terwillinger, R., Luna, B. (2009). Development of working memory maintenance. *Journal of Neurophysiology* 101, 84-99.

Giedd, J.N., Blumenthal, J., Jeffries, N.O., Castellanos, F.X., Liu, H., Zijdenbos, A., Paus, T., Evans, A.C., Rapoport, J.L. (1999). Brain development during childhood and adolescence: a longitudinal MRI study. *Nature Neuroscience* 2(10), 861-863.

Giesbrecht, B., Woldorff, M.G., Song, A.W., Mangun, G.R. (2003). Neural mechanisms of top-down control during spatial and feature attention. *NeuroImage* 19, 496-512.

Gogtay, N., Giedd, J.N., Lusk, L., Hayashi, K.M., Greenstein, D., Vaituzis, A.C., Nugent, III T.F., Herman, D.H., Clasen, L.S., Toga, A.W., Rapoport, J.L., Thompson, P.M. (2004). Dynamic mapping of human cortical development during childhood through early adulthood. *Proceedings of National Academy of Science U.S.A.* 101, 8174-8179.

Goldman, P.S., Rosvold, H.E. (1970). Localization of function within the dorsolateral prefrontal cortex of the rhesus monkey. *Experimental neurology* 27, 291-304.

Goldman-Rakic, P.S. (1987). Circuitry of primate prefrontal cortex and regulation of behavior by representational memory. In: *Handbook of Physiology*, Vol 5, (ed. Bethesda Blum F), Mountcastle VB, MD, American Physiological Society, pp. 373-417.

Goldman-Rakic, P.S. (1995). Cellular basis of working memory. *Neuron* 14, 477-485.

Goodale, M.A., Milner, A.D. (1992). Separate visual pathways for perception and action. *Trends in Neuroscience* 15, 20-25.

Greicius, M.D., Krasnow, B., Reiss, A.L., Menon, V. (2003). Functional connectivity in the resting brain: A network analysis of the default mode hypothesis. *Proceedings of the National Academy of Sciences U.S.A.* 100, 253-258.

Gusnard, D.A., Raichle, M.E. (2001). Searching for a baseline: Functional imaging and the resting human brain. *Nature Reviews Neuroscience* 2, 685-694.

Hale, S., Bronik, M.D., Fry, A.F. (1997). Verbal and spatial working memory in school-age children: Developmental differences in susceptibility to interference. *Developmental Psychology* 33, 364-371.

Harrison, B.J., Pujol, J., López-Solà, M., Hernández-Ribas, R., Deus, J., Ortiz, H., Soriano-Mas, C., Yücel, M., Pantelis, C., Cardoner, N. (2008). Consistency and functional specialization in the default mode brain network. *Proceedings of the National Academy of Sciences U.S.A.* 105, 9781-9786.

Hasson, U., Nusbaum, H.C., Small, S.L. (2009). Task-dependent organization of brain regions active during rest. *Proceedings of the National Academy of Sciences U.S.A.* 106, 10841-10846.

Hautzel, H., Mottaghy, F.M., Schmidt, D., Zemb, M., Shah, N.J., Muller-Gartner, H.W. (2002). Topographic segregation and convergence of verbal, object, shape and spatial working memory in humans. *Neuroscience Letters* 323(2), 156-160.

Haxby, J.V., Horwitz, B., Ungerleider, L.G., Maisog, J.M., Pietrini, P., Grady, C.L. (1994). The functional organization of human extrastriate cortex: a PET-rCBF study of selective attention to faces and locations. *Journal of Neuroscience* 14, 6336-6353.

Huizinga, M., Dolan, C.V., van der Molen, M.W. (2006). Age-related change in executive function: Developmental trends and a latent variable analysis. *Neuropsychologia* 44, 2017-2036.

Huttenlocher, P.R. (1979). Synaptic density in human frontal cortex - developmental changes and effects of aging. *Brain Research* 16, 195-205.

Huttenlocher, P.R. (1990). Morphometric study of human cerebral cortex development. *Neuropsychologia* 28, 517-527.

Huttenlocher, P.R. (1997). Regional differences in in synaptogenesis in human cerebral cortex. *Journal of Comparative Neurology* 387, 167-178.

Jernigan, T.L., Trauner, D.A., Hesselink, J.R., Tallal, P.A. (1991). Maturation of human cerebrum observed in vivo during adolescence. *Brain* 114, 2037-2049.

Johnson, M.H., Halit, H., Grice, S.J., Karmiloff-Smith, A. (2002). Neuroimaging of typical and atypical development: A perspective from multiple levels of analysis. *Development & Psychopathology* 14(3), 521-536.

Johnson, M.K., Raye, K.J., Greene, M.E., Anderson, A.W. (2003). fMRI evidence for an organization of prefrontal cortex by both type of process and type of information. *Cerebral Cortex* 13, 265-273.

Johnston, J.M., Vaishnavi,S.N., Smyth, M.D., Zhang, D., He, B.J., Zempel, J.M., Shimony, J.S., Snyder, A.Z., Raichle, M.E. (2008). Loss of resting interhemispheric functional connectivity after complete section of the corpus callosum. *Journal of Neuroscience* 28, 6453-6458.

Kelley, W.M., Macrae, C.N., Wyland, C.L., Caglar, S., Inati, S., Heatherton, T.F. (2002). Finding the self? An event-related fMRI study. *Journal of Cognitive Neuroscience* 14, 785-794.

Kelly, A.M., Di Martino, A., Uddin, L.Q., Shehzad, Z., Gee, D.G., Reiss, P.T., Margulies, D.S., Castellanos, F.X., Milham, M.P. (2009). Development of anterior cingulate functional connectivity from late childhood to early adulthood. *Cerebral Cortex* 19, 640-657.

Kennedy, D.P., Redcay, E., Courchesne, E. (2006). Failing to deactivate: resting functional abnormalities in autism. *Proceedings of National Academy of Science, U.S.A.* 103, 8275-8280.

Kinney, H., Brody, B., Kloman, A., Gilles, F. (1988). Sequence of central nervous system myelination in human infancy. II. Patterns of myelination in autopsied infants. *Journal of Neuropathology and Experimental Neurology* 47, 217-234.

Kirchhoff, B.A., Buckner, R.L. (2006). Functional-anatomic correlates of individual differences in memory. *Neuron* 51, 263-274.

Kiviniemi, V., Jauhiainen, J., Tervonen, O., Pääkkö, E., Oikarinen, J., Vainionpää, V., Rantala, H., Biswal, B.B. (2000). Slow vasomotor fluctuation in fMRI of anesthetized child brain. *Magnetic Resonance in Medicine* 44, 373-378.

Klingberg, T. (2006). Development of a superior frontal-intraparietal network for visuospatial working memory. *Neuropsychologia* 44, 2171-2177.

Klingberg, T., Forssberg, H., Westerberg, H. (2002). Increased brain activity in frontal and parietal cortex underlies the development of visuospatial working memory capacity during childhood. *Journal of Cognitive Neuroscience* 14, 1-10, 2002.

Klingberg, T., Vaidya, C.J., Gabrieli, J.D., Moseley, M.E., Hedehus, M. (1999). Myelination and organization of the frontal white matter in children: a diffusion tensor MRI study. *NeuroReport* 10, 2817-2821.

Kwon, H., Reiss, A.L., Menon, V. (2002). Neural basis of protracted developmental changes in visuo-spatial working memory. *Proceedings of National Academy of Science, U.S.A.* 99, 13336-13341.

LaBar, K.S., Gitelman, D.R., Parrish, T.B., Mesulam, M.M. (1999). Neuroanatomic overlap of working memory and spatial attention networks: a functional MRI comparison within subjects. *NeuroImage* 10, 695-704.

Larson-Prior, L.J., Zempel, J.M., Nolan, T.S., Prior, F.W., Snyder, A.Z., Raichle, M.E. (2009). Cortical network functional connectivity in the descent to sleep. *Proceedings of the National Academy of Sciences U.S.A.* 106, 4489-4494.

Laurienti, P.J., Burdette, J.H., Wallace, M.T., Yen, Y-F., Field, A.S., Stein, B.E. (2002). Deactivation of sensory-specific cortex by cross-modal stimuli. *Journal of Cognitive Neuroscience* 14, 420-429.

Luciana, M., Conklin, H.M., Hooper, C.J., Yarger, R.S. (2005). The development of nonverbal working memory and executive control processes in adolescents. *Child Development* 76(3), 697-712.

Luciana, M., Nelson, C.A. (1998). The functional emergence of prefrontally-guided working memory systems in four- to eight-year old children. *Neuropsychologia* 36, 273-293.

Luna, B., Garver, K.E., Urban, T.A., Lazar, N.A., Sweeney JA. (2004). Maturation of cognitive processes from late childhood to adulthood. *Child Development* 75(5), 1357-1372.

Luna, B., Padmanabhan, A., O'Hearn, K. (2010). What has fMRI told us about the development of cognitive control through adolescence? *Brain and Cognition* 72, 101-113.

Luna, B., Thulborn, K.R., Munoz, D.P., Merriam, E.P., Garver, K.E., Minshew, N.J., Keshavan. M.S., Genovese, C.R., Eddy, W.F., Sweeney, J.A. (2001). Maturation of widely distributed brain function subserves cognitive development. *NeuroImage* 13, 786-793.

Martinkauppi, S., Rämä, P., Aronen, H.J., Korvenoja, A., Carlson, S. (2000). Working memory of auditory localization. *Cerebral Cortex* 10, 889-898.

Mason, M.F., Norton, M.I., Van Horn, J.D., Wegner, D.M., Grafton, S.T., Macrae, N. (2007). Wandering minds: the default network and stimulus-independent thought. *Science* 315, 393-395.

Mazoyer, B., Zago, L., Mellet, A., Bricogne, S., Etard, H., Houdé, O., Crivello, F., Joliot, M., Petit, L., Tzourio-Mazoyer, N. (2001). Cortical networks for working memory and executive functions sustain the conscious resting state in man. *Brain Research Bulletin* 54, 287-298.

McKiernan, K.A., Kaufman, J.N., Kucera-Thompson, J., Binder, J.R. (2003). A parametric manipulation of factors affecting task-induced deactivation in functional neuroimaging. *Journal of Cognitive Neuroscience* 15, 394-408.

Miller, E.K., Cohen, J.D. (2001). An integrative theory of prefrontal cortex function. *Annual Review in Neuroscience* 24, 167-202.

Milner, B. (1982). Some cognitive effects of frontal lesions in man. *Philosophical Transactions of the Royal Society of London* 298, 211-226.

Miotto, E.C., Bullock, P., Polkey, C.E., Morris, R.G. (1996). Spatial working memory and strategy formation in patients with frontal lobe excisions. *Cortex* 32, 613-630.

Mishkin, M., Ungerleider, L., Macko, K. (1983). Object vision and spatial vision: two cortical pathways. *Trends in Neuroscience* 6, 414-417.

Miyake, A., Friedman, N.P., Emerson, M.J., Witzki, A., Howerter, A. (2000). The unity and diversity of executive functions and their contributions to complex "frontal lobe" tasks: A latent variable analysis. *Cognitive Psychology* 41, 49-100.

Mohr, H.M., Goebel, R., Linden, D.E. (2006). Content- and task-specific dissociations of frontal activity during maintenance and manipulation in visual working memory. *Journal of Neuroscience* 26, 4465-4471.

Mottaghy, F.M. (2006). Interfering with working memory in humans. *Neuroscience* 139, 85-90.

Mottaghy, F.M., Gangitano, M., Sparing, R., Krause, B.J., Pascual-Leone, A. (2002). Segregation of areas related to visual working memory in the prefrontal cortex revealed by rTMS. *Cerebral Cortex* 12, 369-375.

Mukherjee, P., Miller, J.H., Shimony, J.S., Conturo, T.E., Lee, B.C., Almli, C.R., McKinstry, R.C. (2001). Normal brain maturation during childhood: Developmental trends characterized with diffusion-tensor MR imaging. *Radiology* 221, 349-358.

Nagy, Z., Westerberg, H., Klingberg, T. (2004). Maturation of white matter is associated with the development of cognitive functions during childhood. *Journal of Cognitive Neuroscience* 16(7), 1227-1233.

Nelson, C.A. (1995). The ontogeny of human memory: a cognitive neuroscience perspective. *Developmental Psychology* 31(5), 723-738.

Nelson, C.A., Monk, C.S., Lin, J., Carver, L.J., Thomas, K.M., Truwit, C.L. (2000). Functional neuroanatomy of spatial working memory in children. *Developmental Psychology* 36, 109-116.

Olesen, P.J., Nagy, Z., Westerberg, H., Klingberg, T. (2003). Combined analysis of DTI and fMRI data reveals a joint maturation of white and grey matter in a fronto-parietal network. *Cognitive Brain Research* 18, 48-57.

Otten, L.J., Rugg, M.D. (2001). When more means less: neural activity related to unsuccessful memory encoding. *Current Biology* 11, 1528-1530.

Owen, A.M. (2000). The role of the lateral frontal cortex in mnemonic processing: the contribution of functional neuroimaging. *Experimental Brain Research* 133, 33-43.

Owen, A.M., McMillan, K.M., Laird, A.R., Bullmore, E. (2005). N-back working memory paradigm: A meta-analysis of normative functional neuroimaging studies. *Human Brain Mapping* 25, 46-59.

Owen, A.M., Stern, C.E., Look, R.B., Tracey, I., Rosen, B.R., Petrides, M. (1998). Functional organization of spatial and nonspatial working memory processing within the human lateral frontal cortex. *Proceedings of National Academy of Science U.S.A.* 95, 7721-7726.

Paus, T., Zijdenbos, A., Worsley, K., Collins, D.L., Blumenthal, J., Giedd, J.N. (1999). Structural maturation of neural pathways in children and adolescents: in vivo study. *Science* 283, 1908-1911.

Petrides, M. (2005). Lateral prefrontal cortex: architectonic and functional organization. *Philosophical Transactions of the Royal Society of London. Series B* 360, 781-795.

Petrides, M., Alivisatos, B., Frey, S. (2002). Differential activation of the human orbital, mid-ventrolateral, and mid-dorsolateral prefrontal cortex during the processing of visual stimuli. *Proceedings of National Academy of Science, U.S.A.* 99, 5649-5654.

Polli, F.E., Barton, J.J., Cain, M.S., Thakkar, K.N., Rauch, S.L., Manoach, D.S. (2005). Rostral and dorsal anterior cingulate cortex make dissociable contributions during antisaccade error commission. *Proceedings of National Academy of Science, U.S.A.* 102, 15700-15705.

Postle, B.R., D'Esposito, M. (1999). "What" – then "where" in visual working memory: an event-related fMRI study. *Journal of Cognitive Neuroscience* 11(6), 585-597.

Postle, B.R., Stern, C.E., Rosen, B.R., Corkin, S. (2000). An fMRI investigation of cortical contributions to spatial and nonspatial visual working memory. NeuroImage 11, 409-423.

Power, J.D., Fair, D.A., Schlaggar, B.L., Petersen, S.E. (2010). The development of human functional brain networks. *Neuron* 67, 735-748.

Raichle, M.E. (2010). Two views of brain function. *Trends in Cognitive Sciences* 14, 180-190.

Raichle, M.E., MacLeod, A.M., Snyder, A.Z., Powers, W.J., Gusnard, D.A., Shulman, G.L. (2001). A default mode of brain function. *Proceedings of National Academy of Science, U.S.A.* 98, 676-682.

Raichle, M.E., Mintun, M.A. (2006). Brain work and brain imaging. *Annual Review of Neuroscience* 29, 449-476.

Rypma, B. (2006). Factors controlling neural activity during delayed-response task performance: testing a memory organization hypothesis of prefrontal function. *Neuroscience* 139, 223-235.

Rämä, P., Martinkauppi, S., Linnankoski, I., Koivisto, J., Aronen, H.J., Carlson, S. (2001). Working memory of identification of emotional vocal expressions: an fMRI study. *NeuroImage* 13, 1090-1101.

Sala, J.B., Rämä, P., Courtney, S.M. (2003). Functional topography of a distributed neural system for spatial and nonspatial information maintenance in working memory. *Neuropsychologia* 41, 341-356.

Scherf, K.S., Sweeney, J.A., Luna, B. (2006). Brain basis of developmental change in visuospatial working memory. *Journal of Cognitive Neuroscience* 18(7), 1045-1058.

Schweinsburg, A.D., Nagel, B.J., Tapert, S.F. (2005). fMRI reveals alteration of spatial working memory networks across adolescence. *Journal of International Neuropsychological Society* 11, 631-644.

Seeley, W.W., Menon, V., Schatzberg, A.F., Keller, J., Glover, G.H., Kenna, H., Reiss, A.L., Greicius, M.D. (2007). Dissociable intrinsic connectivity networks for salience processing and executive control. *Journal of Neuroscience* 27(9), 2349-2356.

Shaw, P., Greenstein, D., Lerch, J., Clasen, L., Lenroot, R., Gogtay, N., Evans, A., Rapoport, J., Giedd, J. (2006). Intellectual ability and cortical development in children and adolescents. *Nature* 440, 676-679.

Smith, E.E., Jonides, J. (1999). Storage and executive processes in the frontal lobes. *Science* 283, 1657-1661.

Snook, L., Paulson, L.A., Roy, D., Phillips, L., Beaulieu, C. (2005). Diffusion tensor imaging of neurodevelopment in children and young adults. *NeuroImage* 26, 1164-1173.

Sowell, E.R., Delis, D., Stiles, J., Jernigan, T.L. (2001). Improved memory functioning and frontal lobe maturation between childhood and adolescence: a structural MRI study. *Journal of International Neuropsychological Society* 7, 312-322.

Sowell, E.R., Thompson, P.M., Leonard, C.M., Welcome, S.E., Kan, E., Toga, A.W. (2004). Longitudinal mapping of cortical thickness and brain growth in normal children. *Journal of Neuroscience* 24(38), 8223-8231.

Sridharan, D., Levitin, D.J., Menon, V.(2008). A critical role for the right fronto-insular cortex in switching between central-executive and default-mode networks. *Proceedings of National Academy of Science, U.S.A*. 105, 12569-12574.

Supekar, K., Musen, M., Menon, V. (2009). Development of large-scale functional brain networks in children. *PLoS Biology* 7, e1000157.

Supekar, K., Uddin, L.Q., Prater, K., Amin, H., Greicius, M.D., Menon, V. (2010). Development of functional and structural connectivity within the default mode network in young children. *NeuroImage* 52, 290-301.

Swanson, H.L. (1999). What develops in working memory? *A life span perspective. Developmental Psychology* 35(4), 986-1000.

Tau, G.Z., Peterson, B.S. (2010). Normal development of brain circuits. *Neuropsychopharmacology Reviews* 35, 147-168.

Thomas, K.M., King, S.W., Franzen, P.L., Welsh, T.F., Berkowitz, A.L., Noll, D.C., Birmaher, V., Casey, B.J. (1999). A developmental functional MRI study of spatial working memory. *NeuroImage* 10, 327-338.

Thomason, M.E., Chang, C.E., Glover, G.H., Gabrieli, J.D., Greicius, M.D., Gotlib, I.H. (2008). Default-mode function and task-induced deactivation have overlapping brain substrates in children. *NeuroImage* 41, 1493-1503.

Thompson, P.M., Giedd, J.N., Woods, R.P., MacDonald, D., Evans, A.C., Toga, A.W. (2000). Growth patterns in the developing brain detected by using continuum-mechanical tensor maps. *Nature* 404, 190-193.

Toga, A.W., Thompson, P.M., Sowell, E.R. (2006). Mapping brain maturation. *Trends in Neurosciences* 29, 148-159.

Tomasi, D., Chang, L., Caparelli, E.C., Ernst, T. (2007). Different activation patterns for working memory load and visual attention load. *Brain Research* 1132, 158-165.

Tsujimoto, S., Yamamoto, T., Kawaguchi, H., Koizumi, H., Sawaguchi, T. (2004). Prefrontal cortical activation associated with working memory in adults and preschool children: an event-related optical topography study. *Cerebral Cortex* 14, 703-712.

Vandenberghe, R., Gitelman, D.R., Parrish, T.B., Mesulam, M.M. (2001). Location- or feature-based targeting of peripheral attention. *NeuroImage* 14, 37-47.

Van Essen, D.C., Maunsell, J.H.R. (1983). Hierarchial organization and functional streams in the visual cortex. *Trends in Neuroscience* 6, 370-375.

Ventre-Dominey, J., Bailly, A., Lavenne, F., Lebars, D., Mollion, H., Costes, N., Dominey, P.F. (2005). Double dissociation in neural correlates of visual working memory: A PET study. *Cognitive Brain Research* 25, 747-759.

Vilkki, J., Holst, P. (1989). Deficient programming in spatial learning after frontal lobe damage. *Neuropsychologia* 27, 971-976.

Vincent, J.L., Patel, G.H., Fox, M.D., Snyder, A.Z., Baker, J.T., Van Essen, D.C., Zempel, J.M., Snyder, L.H., Corbetta, M., Raichle, M.E. (2007). Intrinsic functional architecture in the anesthetized monkey brain. *Nature* 447, 83-86.

Vuontela, V., Rämä, P., Raninen, A., Aronen, H.J., Carlson, S. (1999). Selective interference reveals dissociation between memory for location and colour. *NeuroReport 10*, 2235-2240.

Vuontela, V., Steenari, M.R., Aronen, E.T., Korvenoja, A., Aronen, H.J., Carlson, S. (2009). Brain activation and deactivation during location and color working memory tasks in 11-13-year-old children. *Brain and Cognition* 69(1), 56-64.

Vuontela, V., Steenari, M.R., Carlson, S., Koivisto, J., Fjällberg, M., Aronen, E.T. (2003). Audiospatial and visuospatial working memory in 6-13 year old school children. *Learning and Memory* 10, 74-81.

Wager, T.D., Jonides, J., Reading, S. (2004). Neuroimaging studies of shifting attention: a meta-analysis. *NeuroImage* 22, 1679-1693.

Wager, T.D., Smith, E.E. (2003). Neuroimaging studies of working memory: a meta-analysis. *Cognitive, Affective and Behavioral Neuroscience* 3, 255-274.

Weissman, D.H., Roberts, K.C., Visscher, K.M., Woldorff, M.G. (2006). The neural bases of momentary lapses in attention. *Nature Neuroscience* 9, 971-978.

Wilson, F.A., Scalaidhe, S.P., Goldman-Rakic, P.S. (1993). Dissociation of object and spatial processing domains in primate prefrontal cortex. *Science* 260, 1955-1958.

Yakovlev, P., Lecours, A. (1967). The myelogenetic cycles of regional maturation of the brain. *In Regional development of the brain in early life*. Minkowski A (ed.), Oxford, Blackwell, pp. 3-70.

INDEX

#

20th century, 44

A

abuse, ix, 109, 111, 113, 119, 121, 125, 126, 127, 134, 137, 138
academic learning, 65
academic performance, 38, 54, 428
academic progress, 17, 192
academic success, 17
access, 15, 57, 74, 153, 173, 207, 217, 226, 231, 251
accessibility, 79, 242
accounting, 148, 228
acetylcholine, xiii, 14, 349, 350, 354, 357, 358, 362, 366, 367, 368, 369, 370, 371
acetylcholinesterase, 357, 364
acetylcholinesterase inhibitor, 357, 364
acid, 112, 139
acquired immunodeficiency syndrome, x, 141, 146
acquisition phase, 119
active thinking, 430
adaptation, 128
adaptations, 111
adaptive functioning, xv, 415
adolescents, vii, 1, 5, 8, 9, 12, 14, 24, 48, 73, 166, 208, 218, 421, 423, 424, 426, 433, 435, 436
adulthood, xv, 4, 5, 7, 13, 23, 92, 155, 167, 180, 288, 415, 416, 418, 420, 423, 427, 428, 431, 432, 433
adults, ix, xii, 18, 19, 20, 24, 25, 50, 53, 54, 62, 64, 71, 73, 75, 78, 81, 92, 97, 99, 101, 105, 106, 145, 152, 153, 154, 155, 161, 167, 170, 180, 195, 202, 204, 205, 218, 222, 240, 245, 252, 253, 255, 282, 287, 288, 289, 292, 293, 294, 295, 297, 416, 417, 418, 420, 421, 423, 424, 426, 427, 437
adverse effects, 191
advertisements, 129

affective disorder, 128, 365
African Americans, 351
aggregation, xiii, 349, 356, 357, 358, 360, 367, 370
aggregation process, 358
aggression, 361
aggressiveness, 354
agnosia, 105
agonist, xiii, 123, 125, 135, 349, 350, 355, 357, 358, 362, 366, 370, 371
AIDS, 147, 150, 159, 161, 169, 171
alcohol consumption, ix, 109, 127
alcohol dependence, 128, 129, 138
alcohol use, 127, 128, 131
alcoholics, ix, 109, 127, 128, 129, 130, 132, 138
alcoholism, 77, 128, 135, 137, 138, 139, 170
allergy, 128
alters, 125
American Psychiatric Association, 378
American Psychological Association, 24, 106, 168, 174
amino, 358
amnesia, 138, 144, 147, 172, 263, 299, 311, 354
amplitude, 130, 131, 132, 274
amygdala, 14, 116, 117, 134, 310
amyloid beta, 367, 370, 371
amyloidosis, 369
analgesic, 127
analgesic agent, 127
anatomy, 24, 95, 134, 179, 194
animal learning, ix, 82, 109
anisotropy, 418
ANOVA, 186, 213, 230, 234, 235, 261, 274, 275, 279, 376
anterior cingulate cortex, 114, 435
anticonvulsant, ix, 109, 127
antidepressant, 128, 376, 377, 379
antidepressant medication, 377
antidepressants, 354, 374, 376, 377, 378
antiepileptic drugs, 354

antihypertensive drugs, 370
antioxidant, 369
antipsychotic, 76, 355, 361
antipsychotic drugs, 355
anxiety, 128, 350, 353, 354, 355, 360, 362, 365, 378
anxiety disorder, 353
apathy, 114
aphasia, 146, 246
aripiprazole, 361
arithmetic, 7, 41, 44, 45, 52, 68, 72, 73, 79, 203, 207, 209, 213, 215, 216, 220, 221, 222, 226, 233, 244
arithmetical learning, 68
arousal, xii, 115, 291, 292, 293, 294, 295, 296, 298, 301, 302, 303, 305, 306, 308, 309, 310, 311
arousal ratings, 292, 293, 294, 295, 296, 303, 306
articulation, xi, 6, 218, 225
aspartate, 137, 355
asphyxia, 193
assessment, viii, xi, 33, 34, 36, 37, 41, 42, 43, 44, 45, 47, 48, 52, 58, 60, 68, 69, 70, 71, 72, 76, 77, 103, 106, 128, 134, 139, 151, 162, 165, 168, 173, 174, 176, 177, 178, 181, 182, 190, 193, 201, 203, 213, 216, 231, 237, 261, 269, 368, 375, 376, 416
assessment tools, 34, 177, 178
asymmetry, 106
asymptomatic, 174
atrophy, 101, 151, 161
attachment, 236, 237, 244, 247
Attention Deficit Hyperactivity Disorder (ADHD), 12, 13, 21, 26, 30, 55, 60, 63, 65, 68, 69, 70, 71, 73, 74, 75, 76, 79, 194, 208, 216, 221, 350, 355, 375, 427, 430
attention to task, xiv
attentional bias, 290, 298
auditory cortex, 418
auditory evoked potentials, 139
autism, vii, 1, 2, 4, 7, 8, 9, 10, 11, 12, 13, 14, 15, 16, 20, 22, 23, 24, 25, 26, 27, 28, 29, 30, 31, 32, 55, 75, 177, 427, 432
autobiographical memory, 51, 74, 75
automatic processes, 231
automaticity, 232
autonomic nervous system (ANS), 115, 358
autonomy, 128, 243, 262
autopsy, 151
avoidance, 354
awareness, 44, 62, 70, 73, 93, 142, 221
axon terminals, 123

B

basal forebrain, 356, 368
basal ganglia, 14, 16, 116, 277, 418

base, 73, 233, 309
battered women, 360
batteries, 36, 37, 41, 43, 44, 46, 48, 60, 203, 205
Beck Depression Inventory, 289
beer, 131
behavioral assessment, 61, 311
behavioral disorders, 128
behaviors, vii, 51, 111, 115, 126, 351
beneficial effect, 350, 353, 357
benefits, 43, 154, 160, 355, 362
beverages, 128, 129, 131
bias, xii, xiii, 13, 22, 260, 287, 288, 289, 291, 292, 294, 296, 297, 298, 299, 301, 303, 306, 307, 308, 309, 310, 311
biomarkers, 162, 363
biopsy, 151
bipolar disorder, 58, 60, 62, 70, 350, 355, 378
birthweight, x, 53, 79, 176, 177, 181, 182, 186, 187, 188, 189, 190, 192, 193, 195, 197, 198
blindness, 98
blood, xii, 229, 267, 270, 303, 350, 353, 362, 364, 425
blood flow, 425
blood pressure, 303, 353, 364
blood-brain barrier (BBB), 350, 353, 362, 364
bonding, 358
borderline personality disorder, 58, 355
brain abnormalities, 15, 24
brain activity, ix, 105, 110, 129, 132, 133, 197, 276, 279, 419, 421, 430, 433
brain damage, 174, 196, 227
brain functions, 111, 280, 427, 428
brain growth, 190, 436
brain size, 418
brain stem, 14
brain structure, xv, 14, 16, 23, 112, 118, 126, 415, 416, 418
branching, 240, 418
breakdown, 153
bronchopulmonary dysplasia, 197
buttons, 304

C

calcium, 126
cancer, 353
career development, 180
case study, 99, 138, 144, 180
catalysis, 363
categorization, 212, 262
category a, 147, 232
category b, 154, 155, 158, 159, 160
caucasians, 351

causality, 281, 282
cell death, 370
central executive, vii, xi, 2, 3, 4, 7, 11, 12, 14, 15, 20, 22, 24, 25, 34, 35, 39, 40, 43, 50, 51, 52, 53, 54, 56, 57, 58, 59, 66, 67, 70, 74, 82, 93, 102, 142, 148, 152, 153, 164, 168, 201, 202, 205, 206, 207, 210, 217, 218, 226, 250, 251, 264, 282, 377, 425
central nervous system (CNS), 111, 149, 169, 179, 181, 190, 191, 353, 363, 364, 365, 366, 367, 433
cerebellum, 14, 16, 94, 277
cerebral blood flow, 194
cerebral cortex, 14, 368
cerebral function, 429
cerebral palsy, 52, 68, 74
cerebrum, 432
challenges, xii, 60, 267, 268
childhood, x, xv, 7, 11, 26, 53, 69, 73, 175, 180, 193, 194, 195, 196, 415, 416, 417, 418, 419, 423, 424, 426, 427, 428, 431, 432, 433, 434, 436
choline, 356, 368
cholinesterase, 368
cholinesterase inhibitors, 368
chronic fatigue syndrome, 58, 66
chunking, 4, 5, 7, 13, 37, 226
cigarette smoke, 352, 364
cigarette smokers, 352, 364
cigarette smoking, 353
civilization, 113
classes, xi, 209, 210, 249, 269, 357, 421
classical conditioning, 266
classification, 138, 272
classroom, 16, 17, 19, 20, 21, 22, 26, 31, 61
classroom environment, 22
clinical assessment, 164, 375, 376
clinical examination, 151
clinical symptoms, 94, 374
clinical syndrome, 157
clinical trials, 357, 370, 378
clozapine, ix, 109, 355, 366, 378
clustering, 147, 148, 150, 154, 155, 157, 158, 159, 160, 163, 165, 166, 169, 172
clusters, 46, 63, 274, 275, 375
cocaine, 53, 71, 125, 126, 138, 367
coding, 18, 25, 51, 99, 136, 149, 192, 208, 241, 251, 261, 262
cognition, vii, xv, 24, 34, 38, 61, 68, 73, 75, 95, 96, 97, 98, 99, 101, 104, 117, 151, 163, 165, 170, 171, 177, 196, 197, 218, 220, 264, 298, 361, 363, 366, 375, 379, 415, 416, 429
cognitive abilities, x, xv, 44, 46, 47, 59, 64, 68, 71, 82, 151, 156, 175, 176, 189, 193, 350, 354, 355, 356, 357, 415, 418
cognitive ability, viii, 33, 35, 46, 151, 421

cognitive capacity, 419
cognitive deficit, xiii, 58, 76, 79, 127, 149, 150, 151, 169, 194, 196, 220, 350, 354, 355, 356, 360, 366
cognitive development, viii, 4, 24, 25, 31, 33, 180, 190, 193, 196, 429, 433
cognitive domains, 94, 95, 239
cognitive dysfunction, 106, 119, 149, 361, 362, 369
cognitive flexibility, 13, 264
cognitive function, viii, ix, xiv, 4, 7, 33, 34, 35, 44, 97, 100, 107, 109, 118, 119, 121, 123, 125, 126, 127, 128, 135, 137, 169, 170, 178, 196, 208, 276, 295, 361, 362, 370, 373, 378, 425, 434
cognitive impairment, xiii, 51, 62, 72, 74, 92, 96, 106, 155, 166, 167, 168, 170, 171, 173, 190, 349, 352, 357, 361, 367, 374, 378, 379
cognitive load, 16, 22, 262, 302, 426
cognitive map, 89, 96, 100, 102, 103, 265
cognitive performance, ix, 109, 157, 369, 427, 428
cognitive process, xiii, 14, 15, 36, 45, 48, 59, 88, 91, 95, 116, 126, 149, 156, 198, 216, 217, 230, 231, 250, 268, 269, 281, 309, 416, 422, 423, 433
cognitive profile, 29, 173
cognitive psychology, xi, 30, 75, 82, 135, 242, 249, 250, 265, 284
cognitive research, 26, 39, 60, 88
cognitive science, 142
cognitive skills, 7, 30, 70, 76, 177
cognitive style, 10
cognitive system, 83, 88, 262, 268, 416
cognitive tasks, xiv, 3, 4, 9, 15, 82, 101, 115, 116, 226, 228, 231, 252, 310
coherence, 280, 418
college students, 129
color, 3, 40, 47, 250, 257, 275, 279, 311, 352, 437
coma, 172
communication, 9, 24, 426
community, viii, 33, 101, 105
comorbidity, 12, 26, 170, 365
compensation, 100, 151
competition, 100, 157
competitors, 218
complement, 236, 238, 240
complexity, vii, 1, 8, 9, 10, 11, 28, 87, 106, 227, 230, 233, 235, 236, 237, 239, 240, 244, 245
complications, x, 175, 176, 180, 181, 182, 186, 187, 189, 190, 198, 230, 235
composites, 43, 44, 46, 47
composition, 205, 428
compounds, 350, 351, 355, 357, 358, 360
comprehension, xi, xv, 39, 57, 65, 71, 77, 97, 118, 204, 205, 207, 213, 215, 223, 225, 226, 227, 228, 234, 235, 239, 241, 242, 243, 245, 247, 251, 253, 268, 283, 415, 416

compulsion, 111, 134
computation, 152, 153
computed tomography, 178, 353
computer, 20, 21, 40, 93, 131, 256, 257, 259, 260, 304, 420
conception, 181
conceptualization, 86, 128, 236, 253
concordance, 427
concussion, 101
conduction, 418
conflict, 115, 128, 227
confounding variables, 186
confrontation, 153
connectivity, xiii, 16, 28, 29, 126, 145, 146, 150, 159, 160, 194, 232, 280, 281, 285, 418, 421, 423, 425, 426, 428, 431, 432, 433, 436
connectivity patterns, 281
conscious awareness, 3, 143, 231
consciousness, 151, 172
consensus, 7, 22, 116, 169, 226
consent, 255, 259
consolidation, 58, 66, 143, 144, 145, 146, 147, 148, 150, 156, 157, 165, 174, 366
constituents, 231, 236
construct validity, 69
construction, 97, 196, 240, 245
consumption, xiii, 131, 349, 350, 359, 362
contour, 236
control condition, 209, 302, 303, 304, 309
control group, 8, 11, 12, 19, 22, 206, 214, 215, 375
controlled studies, 353
controversial, 93, 123, 206
controversies, xii, xiv, 267
convention, 151
convergence, 432
cooling, 178
cooperation, 100
coordination, 55, 60, 61, 150, 160, 416, 419
corpus callosum, 14, 23, 432
correlation, xiv, 39, 41, 48, 60, 74, 78, 98, 171, 215, 234, 235, 239, 240, 350, 374, 376, 377, 426
correlations, 38, 44, 48, 49, 55, 59, 227, 234, 276, 374, 425
cortex, viii, ix, x, 2, 15, 94, 95, 97, 98, 110, 112, 113, 114, 115, 116, 119, 129, 135, 139, 141, 144, 156, 163, 164, 169, 177, 178, 179, 180, 191, 194, 196, 270, 279, 356, 368, 417, 418, 419, 422, 425, 429, 432, 433, 436, 437
cortical pathway, 434
cortisol, 361
cost, xv, 229, 230, 236, 379
cotinine, xiii, 349, 350, 351, 352, 353, 354, 355, 356, 357, 358, 360, 362, 363, 364, 366, 371

CPT, 42, 43, 77
craving, ix, 109, 112, 113, 127, 129, 139, 353
criticism, 227
cross-sectional study, xiv, 138, 354, 373, 374, 375
crystal structure, 358
crystallized intelligence, 49, 67
cues, 3, 45, 89, 94, 95, 98, 103, 105, 115, 129, 149, 165, 173, 237, 253, 255, 260, 262
curcumin, 357
curricula, 27
curriculum, 21, 194, 219
cycles, 437
cytochrome, 351, 363
cytotoxicity, 367

D

daily living, 17, 151, 197
data analysis, 182, 279
data set, 234
database, 63, 68, 72, 76
deaths, 359
decay, 2, 6, 10, 83, 91, 202, 228, 250
decision task, 269
decision-making process, 272
declarative knowledge, 173
declarative memory, 143, 164, 173, 174
deconvolution, 274
deficiencies, 50, 52, 58, 115, 117
deficiency, 56, 78, 122, 125, 135, 138, 295, 355
deficit, vii, xiii, xiv, 1, 7, 13, 17, 19, 24, 26, 52, 53, 54, 55, 56, 58, 59, 61, 62, 65, 66, 69, 70, 71, 74, 76, 79, 92, 93, 95, 99, 102, 103, 106, 125, 147, 149, 150, 152, 156, 157, 162, 163, 164, 167, 169, 177, 219, 349, 350, 354, 355, 356, 361, 374, 377
deflation, 234
delirium, 128
delirium tremens, 128
delusions, 355
dementia, viii, 33, 51, 62, 90, 92, 96, 99, 100, 101, 104, 105, 106, 146, 151, 155, 161, 162, 165, 166, 167, 168, 171, 245, 299, 311, 350, 356, 360, 368, 369
demographic characteristics, 376
demographic factors, 176
demonstrations, 204
dendrites, 123, 126
dendritic spines, 126
Department of Health and Human Services, 169
dependent variable, 181, 214, 261
deposition, 358
depression, xiv, 57, 69, 72, 173, 178, 297, 298, 299, 350, 360, 361, 373, 374, 375, 376, 377, 378, 379

depressive symptoms, 375, 377
depth, 14, 42, 45, 47, 158, 203, 216, 256
derivatives, 357, 360
desensitization, 58, 353
detectable, 352
detection, 31, 115, 193, 272, 420, 424
developing brain, 196, 417, 429, 436
developmental change, 25, 85, 179, 418, 421, 424, 432, 433, 435
developmental disorder, 4, 7, 23, 26, 32, 61, 78, 194
developmental dyslexia, 62, 76, 223
developmental factors, 176
Diagnostic and Statistical Manual of Mental Disorders, 378
diagnostic criteria, 8, 151
diamonds, 271, 276, 277
diet, 355
diffraction, 358, 371
diffusion, 353, 418, 421, 428, 433, 434
directionality, 281
disability, 54, 55, 64, 67, 73, 74, 76, 77, 160, 192, 216, 220, 374
discomfort, 111
discontinuity, 163
discrimination, xiii, 51, 72, 95, 104, 223, 288, 289, 291, 292, 293, 294, 295, 296, 301, 303, 306, 307, 308, 309, 310
discrimination learning, 51, 72
diseases, 169, 195, 353, 360, 367, 369
disgust, 296
disorder, xiii, 2, 24, 25, 26, 28, 29, 30, 31, 32, 55, 58, 60, 61, 62, 65, 66, 69, 71, 72, 74, 76, 125, 164, 169, 177, 196, 207, 349, 350, 355, 361, 364, 365, 366, 374, 378, 379
displacement, 93
disposition, 247, 296, 364
dissociation, xiii, 5, 83, 85, 98, 102, 106, 144, 167, 170, 283, 301, 424, 428, 437
distortions, 86, 260
distracters, 63, 211
distribution, 143, 194, 422, 424, 427
diversity, 189, 221, 434
DNA, 190
dogs, 153, 367
dominance, 253
dopamine, 14, 110, 112, 113, 117, 118, 119, 121, 122, 123, 125, 135, 136, 137, 138, 179, 195, 355
dopamine agonist, 355
dopamine antagonists, 136, 195
dopaminergic, ix, xiii, 109, 119, 123, 127, 133, 135, 136, 137, 369

dorsolateral prefrontal cortex, viii, ix, 2, 15, 109, 114, 130, 131, 132, 133, 136, 179, 180, 191, 283, 422, 431, 435
Down syndrome, 54, 61, 70
drawing, 37, 44, 86, 93, 206, 263
dream, 350
drug abuse, 133, 134
drug action, 111, 113
drug addict, ix, 109, 110, 111, 112, 113, 118, 121, 126, 127, 129, 132, 133, 134, 137
drug addiction, ix, 109, 110, 111, 112, 113, 118, 121, 126, 127, 129, 132, 133, 134, 137
drug consumption, 110, 111
drug dependence, 110, 111
drug design, 358
drug interaction, 361
drugs, ix, 109, 111, 112, 113, 119, 121, 125, 126, 127, 129, 134, 138, 178, 289, 353, 354, 357, 370, 376
dual task, xi, xii, 17, 221, 229, 240, 244, 249, 250, 255, 258, 265
dyslexia, 57, 68, 75, 203, 217, 222
dysthymic disorder, 66

E

editors, 136, 217
education, 37, 104, 105, 147, 177, 193, 289
educational attainment, 219
educational experience, 176
educators, 216
effortful processing, 102
elaboration, viii, 2, 19, 36, 157, 158, 211
electroencephalogram, 151, 156
electron, 358
electron microscopy, 358
elementary school, 193
emission, 178, 353
emotion, 115, 116, 288, 290, 294, 298, 299, 302, 305, 310, 311
emotional experience, 298, 311
emotional information, 288, 299, 302
emotional responses, 311
emotional stimuli, 288, 289, 297, 298, 302, 303, 310
emotionality, xii, 287, 296, 301, 302, 303, 309
empathy, 115
employability, 350
employment, 253, 260, 374
employment status, 374
encapsulation, 253
encephalitis, 161, 166
encoding, x, xi, xii, 2, 3, 4, 11, 18, 25, 34, 39, 49, 53, 92, 95, 103, 141, 143, 144, 145, 146, 147, 148,

149, 150, 152, 153, 154, 155, 156, 157, 158, 159, 160, 161, 163, 165, 166, 167, 168, 170, 171, 172, 174, 227, 238, 242, 249, 254, 255, 263, 264, 267, 268, 269, 270, 272, 275, 276, 279, 280, 281, 282, 285, 290, 295, 299, 304, 361, 416, 419, 430, 434
encouragement, 20, 133
endorphins, 354
enkephalins, 354
enslavement, 115
entorhinal cortex, 119
environment, vii, viii, xi, xiv, 36, 81, 88, 89, 90, 91, 92, 93, 94, 96, 103, 105, 114, 115, 117, 189, 191, 249, 252, 253, 255, 256, 257, 258, 259, 260, 261, 262, 264, 265
environmental factors, 176
environmental influences, 189
environmental stimuli, x, 113, 116, 175, 176, 181, 186, 189
enzymatic activity, 351
enzymes, 351
epidemiologic studies, 364
epilepsy, 144
episodic memory, x, 51, 68, 91, 95, 141, 143, 156, 162, 163, 164, 165, 170, 171, 173, 250, 425
error detection, 115
ethanol, ix, 109, 119, 121, 122, 123, 124, 137
ethical standards, 129
ethics, 290, 304
ethnic background, 351
ethnic groups, 351
ethnicity, 351
etiology, 147, 155, 177
euphoria, 115
event-related potential (ERPs), 131, 139, 156, 166, 361
evidence, vii, ix, xi, xiii, xiv, 1, 3, 4, 5, 6, 9, 10, 11, 13, 15, 16, 17, 18, 20, 21, 26, 27, 29, 32, 56, 57, 61, 71, 81, 86, 92, 97, 102, 104, 105, 106, 110, 111, 123, 125, 126, 134, 143, 144, 145, 147, 153, 156, 157, 158, 166, 167, 168, 178, 179, 182, 191, 194, 196, 198, 203, 205, 206, 215, 218, 219, 220, 221, 223, 228, 230, 235, 238, 240, 241, 245, 249, 253, 263, 265, 268, 269, 282, 285, 311, 349, 350, 351, 355, 356, 368, 379, 416, 417, 419, 427, 429, 430, 431, 432
excitability, 129
excitatory postsynaptic potentials, 123
excitatory synapses, 113
excitotoxicity, 357
execution, 51, 128, 206
executive function, viii, xiii, 3, 7, 11, 14, 26, 28, 29, 31, 33, 48, 52, 54, 62, 64, 65, 68, 94, 100, 114, 115, 117, 126, 127, 129, 132, 135, 136, 146, 155, 156, 157, 194, 199, 217, 221, 223, 246, 350, 377, 416, 417, 420, 424, 429, 430, 432, 434
executive processes, 11, 36, 56, 116, 117, 118, 135, 213, 268, 275, 417, 422, 424, 436
exercise, 355
experimental condition, xi, 85, 204, 209, 210, 213, 249, 257, 260
experimental design, vii, xii, 1, 8, 209, 267
experimental space, 265
explicit memory, 269
exposure, x, 53, 102, 126, 138, 175, 176, 181, 186, 189, 351, 353, 355, 362
external environment, 89, 115
external validation, 169
extraction, 143, 231
eye movement, 6, 10, 58, 67, 247
eye-tracking, 233, 242, 298

F

facial expression, xiii, 288, 290, 291, 294, 295, 296, 301, 302, 303, 304, 305, 308, 309, 310
factor analysis, 69
false alarms, 291, 305
false positive, 216
families, 360
FDA, 354
fear, 296
feelings, 288, 299, 311
fiber, 358
fibers, 119
fibrillation, 357
fibroblast growth factor, 353
fidelity, 424
financial, 51, 66
first degree relative, 58
fish, 252, 265
fixation, 273, 290, 291, 298, 304
flaws, 231, 234
flexibility, 13, 30, 128, 233, 264
flight, 238
fluctuations, 430, 431
fluid, xiv, 4, 49, 54, 60, 64, 66, 71, 75, 76, 78, 135, 218, 282
fluid intelligence, 49, 54, 60, 64, 66, 75, 76, 78, 135, 282
fluoxetine, 364, 365
fluvoxamine, 376
foils, 47, 154
food, 119, 252, 351, 352, 363
force, 79, 158
Ford, 5, 25, 160
forebrain, 136

formal education, 289, 295
formation, 19, 99, 100, 143, 162, 191, 226, 227, 358, 363, 369, 370, 434
formula, 351
foundations, 98
fragment completion, 238
free recall, 31, 149, 150, 164, 165, 166, 168, 169, 174, 211, 212, 246, 251, 283, 295
freedom, 292, 306
frontal cortex, 95, 104, 113, 119, 134, 136, 179, 195, 279, 421, 429, 432, 435
frontal lobe, 6, 114, 127, 128, 135, 144, 150, 165, 177, 178, 179, 180, 192, 194, 195, 196, 222, 282, 284, 416, 429, 434, 436, 437
functional architecture, 437
functional changes, 353, 417
functional imaging, 23, 113
functional MRI, 30, 283, 284, 353, 429, 433, 436

G

GABA, 112
gender differences, 84, 85
gene expression, 111, 126
general intelligence, 16, 46, 48, 49, 60, 63, 64, 65, 268
general knowledge, 90
genes, 126
genetic components, 220
genetic disorders, viii, 33, 35, 52, 54
genetic endowment, 176
genetics, 164, 296
genome, 126
genotype, 299, 363
genre, 245
geometry, 253, 263, 264, 265
Gestalt, 24
gestation, x, 176, 180, 181, 182, 186, 188, 189, 190, 191, 192, 198
gestational age, 198, 199
gestures, 115
gifted, 218
glasses, 289
globus, 112
glucose, 164, 167, 179, 425
glutamate, 112, 113, 117, 123, 355, 357
goal-directed behavior, ix, 109, 117, 127, 129, 156, 417
grading, 160, 165, 297
grants, 378
gray matter, 149, 168, 418, 419
group membership, 11
grouping, 148
growth, 26, 29, 64, 78, 189, 191, 358, 368
growth factor, 368
guidance, 22, 105
guidelines, 365

H

HAART, 149, 150, 169, 171, 174
habituation, 193, 366
half-life, xiii, 349, 350, 351, 359
hallucinations, 355
head injuries, 147, 162
head injury, x, 101, 141, 146, 160, 168, 171, 173, 174, 196
health, 177, 289, 369, 374
heart rate, 303, 353, 365
height, 256, 257
hemisphere, 159
hemorrhage, 193
hepatocytes, 363
heterogeneity, 31, 147, 152, 163
hippocampus, xiii, 14, 16, 23, 91, 94, 95, 97, 99, 101, 107, 116, 117, 144, 153, 157, 165, 173, 277, 349, 353, 355, 356, 370
history, xi, 142, 143, 151, 166, 197, 249
HIV/AIDS, 146, 149, 150, 159, 160, 171
HIV-1, 161, 162, 165, 169, 174
homes, 92
homophones, 228, 248
hormones, 99
host, 142, 151
house, 87
housing, 257, 260
human, ix, x, 17, 18, 67, 75, 81, 82, 94, 95, 97, 99, 100, 101, 102, 103, 104, 106, 107, 109, 111, 125, 129, 135, 141, 146, 161, 163, 164, 165, 166, 169, 170, 172, 177, 179, 180, 194, 195, 196, 199, 226, 250, 253, 257, 262, 263, 264, 265, 281, 283, 284, 285, 311, 352, 363, 364, 368, 370, 417, 418, 425, 428, 429, 430, 431, 432, 433, 434, 435
human behavior, 135
human brain, 129, 179, 196, 199, 284, 311, 418, 425, 428, 431
human cerebral cortex, 196, 432
human cognition, 75, 164, 226, 264
human development, 17, 18
human immunodeficiency virus (HIV), x, 53, 62, 141, 146, 149, 150, 159, 160, 161, 162, 163, 164, 165, 166, 167, 168, 169, 170, 171, 173, 174
human information processing, 226, 250
human subjects, 106, 417
Hunter, 53, 71, 285
hunting, 350

hydrocephalus, 52, 63, 199
hydrogen, 358
hyperactivity, xiii, 12, 24, 26, 55, 62, 65, 66, 69, 71, 74, 76, 125, 156, 349, 350
hyperarousal, 354, 355, 356
hypersensitivity, 156
hypothalamus, 354
hypothesis, xi, 41, 71, 89, 95, 111, 127, 135, 149, 207, 228, 230, 231, 237, 239, 240, 249, 251, 255, 284, 289, 296, 354, 356, 367, 375, 379, 431, 435

I

ideal, xii, 159, 267, 270, 272, 357
identification, 44, 52, 92, 93, 106, 125, 152, 177, 218, 277, 416, 435
identity, xii, 67, 287, 288, 289, 290, 291, 294, 296, 305, 309
illusions, 24
image, 19, 24, 106, 256, 421
imagery, 19, 20, 34, 84, 98, 101, 103, 254, 262
images, 12, 19, 129, 257, 264, 297, 298, 305
imitation, 42, 107, 115
immunoreactivity, 356
impairments, vii, xiii, 1, 4, 6, 7, 8, 9, 10, 13, 22, 24, 27, 50, 51, 52, 53, 54, 55, 56, 57, 58, 64, 65, 67, 70, 71, 72, 77, 79, 80, 98, 100, 128, 151, 152, 153, 155, 156, 158, 161, 168, 170, 172, 180, 195, 197, 221, 360, 361
implicit memory, 167
improvements, 5, 11, 17, 18, 19, 20, 148, 155, 160, 208, 216, 232, 362
impulsive, 125, 128, 420
impulsivity, 12
in utero, 71
in vitro, xiii, 349, 358, 363, 367
in vivo, 137, 161, 350, 358, 363, 369, 370, 432, 435
inattention, 12
incidence, xiii, 171, 177, 190, 349, 350, 359
income, 374
independence, 21
independent variable, 261
indirect measure, 44
individual character, 232, 235, 241
individual differences, viii, 3, 29, 33, 36, 62, 76, 81, 84, 96, 97, 98, 179, 203, 227, 229, 230, 235, 236, 239, 241, 242, 247, 263, 269, 270, 281, 284, 296, 433
individuality, 168
individuals, vii, x, xi, 1, 7, 8, 9, 10, 11, 12, 13, 14, 15, 16, 18, 19, 20, 21, 29, 41, 42, 43, 44, 49, 51, 52, 53, 54, 55, 56, 57, 58, 59, 62, 64, 70, 78, 83, 85, 86, 89, 90, 91, 93, 95, 141, 142, 144, 146, 149, 150, 163, 166, 167, 171, 174, 178, 202, 207, 225, 226, 227, 229, 230, 234, 235, 240, 288, 290, 304, 350, 351, 352, 353, 354, 355
individuation, 203
induction, 305
ineffectiveness, 261
inefficiency, 125, 156, 166
infants, x, xi, 175, 176, 177, 179, 180, 181, 182, 183, 185, 186, 187, 188, 189, 190, 191, 192, 193, 195, 196, 197, 198, 416, 419, 425, 426, 427, 428, 430, 433
infection, 53, 62, 149, 161, 164, 165, 169, 170
inferences, 42
inferior parietal region, 270
inflammation, 367
information processing, 15, 28, 36, 51, 63, 66, 78, 84, 92, 97, 99, 156, 173, 193, 355, 423
information processing speed, 63
informed consent, 182, 290, 304, 375
inhibition, vii, 2, 11, 12, 13, 14, 15, 22, 24, 30, 40, 50, 51, 55, 56, 62, 66, 69, 75, 76, 79, 117, 137, 156, 171, 185, 193, 194, 202, 212, 217, 218, 355, 363, 420, 430
inhibitor, 354
initiation, 113, 115, 125, 126
injections, 125, 136, 138, 195, 352
injuries, 20, 105, 113, 144, 160, 178
injury, 30, 53, 97, 114, 145, 147, 149, 150, 159, 160, 166, 168, 170, 173, 174, 195, 375
inner ear, 217
institutionalized individuals, 35
instruction time, 68
integration, vii, ix, x, xi, 3, 15, 16, 32, 36, 49, 81, 84, 92, 96, 102, 114, 115, 116, 141, 178, 233, 244, 249, 250, 254, 255, 262, 416, 419, 423, 430
integrity, ix, x, 69, 81, 109, 119, 121, 127, 141, 157, 172, 425
intellectual disabilities, 54, 68, 79
intelligence, viii, 16, 17, 33, 35, 37, 45, 47, 48, 49, 51, 53, 60, 64, 65, 66, 68, 69, 71, 73, 78, 147, 180, 193, 253
intelligence tests, 35, 180
interaction effect, 275, 277, 279, 307, 309
interface, 35, 61, 82, 358
interference, xii, 3, 13, 26, 28, 46, 47, 50, 51, 65, 68, 70, 73, 75, 86, 106, 128, 202, 227, 228, 239, 240, 244, 247, 250, 251, 254, 260, 262, 420, 428, 431, 437
interneurons, 425
intervention, vii, 1, 18, 19, 20, 21, 22, 30, 65, 208, 216
intervention strategies, vii, 1
intoxication, 111

intrauterine growth retardation, 190
intravenously, 353
intrusions, 219
invertebrates, 111
invitation to participate, 182
irritability, 115, 353, 354
isolation, 270, 273, 280
issues, xi, 34, 44, 48, 49, 57, 68, 69, 71, 72, 76, 137, 172, 225, 268, 280, 281, 303

J

joints, 93

K

kindergarten, 199, 220
kinetics, 362

L

laboratory tests, 60
laminar, 136
language acquisition, 34
language development, 72
language impairment, 55, 60, 68, 72, 73, 75, 222
language lateralization, 102
language processing, 227, 228, 232, 244
language skills, 419
latency, 132, 239, 272
later life, 50
latinos, 351
lead, xi, xii, 9, 17, 19, 82, 90, 92, 177, 180, 202, 216, 229, 231, 249, 250, 255, 262, 276, 377
learners, 17
learning behavior, 95
learning difficulties, x, xi, xv, 30, 61, 62, 72, 75, 175, 176, 177, 180, 181, 191, 192, 201, 204, 216, 221, 415
learning disabilities, viii, 33, 35, 52, 56, 68, 71, 76, 77, 78, 84, 98, 193, 203, 207, 216, 217, 218, 221, 223
learning environment, 257, 259, 260
learning process, 88
learning skills, 17, 21
learning task, 89, 92, 115, 157, 196
left hemisphere, 115, 144, 145, 151, 153, 159, 196, 419
lesions, 95, 96, 97, 101, 102, 114, 115, 119, 147, 177, 178, 179, 180, 194, 195, 196, 198, 229, 416, 434

leukemia, 53
level of education, 239
lexical processing, 228, 246
life changes, 126
life experiences, 134
lifetime, 53, 126
ligand, 358, 371
light, viii, xi, xii, xiii, 81, 85, 157, 249, 250, 257, 262, 301, 303, 304, 305, 306, 309, 310, 360, 425
limbic system, 110, 115
linear model, 247
linguistic processing, 233, 253
linguistics, 226
lipids, 190
literacy, 62
liver, 363
localization, 72, 93, 103, 136, 433
location information, 26
locomotor, 125
locus, 98, 156, 157
logical reasoning, 226
longitudinal study, xiv, 220, 374, 375
long-term memory, viii, xii, 2, 3, 27, 28, 33, 34, 35, 36, 37, 40, 54, 62, 69, 82, 142, 161, 162, 166, 171, 172, 173, 201, 202, 203, 220, 226, 262, 287, 302, 366, 416
love, 360
low birthweight, 180, 187, 189, 190, 191, 192, 197, 198
low risk, 189
lumbar puncture, 151
Luo, 36, 70, 370

M

machinery, 117
Mackintosh, 48, 69, 71
macrophages, 173
magnet, 353
magnetic resonance, xii, 83, 95, 99, 144, 165, 166, 167, 171, 172, 178, 198, 246, 267, 281, 282, 370, 416, 421, 429, 430
magnetic resonance imaging, (MRI), xii, 24, 27, 31, 83, 101, 135, 144, 165, 166, 171, 172, 174, 178, 198, 246, 267, 281, 353, 370, 416, 421, 429, 430, 431, 433, 436
magnitude, 112, 207, 213, 229, 233, 234, 236, 272, 273, 277, 423
major depression, 361, 379
major depressive disorder, xiv, 373, 378, 379
majority, 18, 148, 150, 277
mammals, 351
man, 70, 72, 96, 103, 194, 195, 196, 238, 364, 434

manic, 70
manipulation, vii, viii, xi, xiii, 3, 24, 33, 34, 36, 45, 52, 62, 63, 83, 84, 116, 144, 154, 156, 157, 159, 168, 202, 205, 207, 212, 225, 268, 269, 272, 280, 282, 284, 309, 416, 420, 423, 424, 430, 434
MAPK/ERK, 126
mapping, 40, 42, 96, 99, 100, 282, 431, 436
Marx, 138
matching-to-sample, 67, 352
materials, 183, 262
mathematical achievement, 205, 209
mathematical disabilities, 69
mathematics, 27, 71, 74, 79, 191, 207, 218, 220
matrix, 38, 42, 44, 51, 75, 85, 87, 199, 211, 212, 236, 258, 272
matter, 146, 149, 150, 151, 153, 166, 171, 233, 418, 419, 428, 434
maturation process, 180
measurement, viii, 33, 35, 36, 40, 41, 44, 45, 47, 48, 49, 55, 59, 60, 156, 168, 202, 222, 234, 377
measurements, 63, 64, 68, 72, 76
median, 234, 235
mediation, ix, 27, 109, 121, 247, 280
medical, viii, x, 33, 35, 52, 53, 132, 175, 176, 180, 181, 182, 186, 187, 189, 190, 191, 192, 193, 197, 353, 364, 375
medication, 62, 76, 128, 150, 378
memorizing, 420
memory capacity, vii, 3, 4, 5, 10, 11, 17, 18, 19, 20, 22, 23, 25, 28, 38, 48, 49, 51, 52, 63, 65, 71, 75, 77, 78, 90, 205, 218, 219, 227, 228, 229, 231, 232, 233, 234, 235, 236, 237, 241, 251, 272, 282, 420
memory formation, 163, 430
memory function, viii, 2, 4, 16, 23, 24, 29, 32, 34, 43, 44, 50, 51, 52, 53, 55, 56, 59, 71, 76, 117, 171, 196, 216, 268, 361, 419, 436
memory loss, 152, 352, 356, 360
memory performance, vii, 1, 3, 4, 13, 16, 20, 22, 31, 48, 51, 57, 62, 70, 90, 91, 98, 117, 146, 160, 161, 170, 196, 208, 295, 366
memory processes, vii, ix, 1, 6, 7, 12, 13, 14, 15, 25, 42, 43, 49, 109, 117, 159, 216, 232, 359, 417, 420
memory retrieval, 35, 135, 149
mental activity, 135, 425
mental age, 9, 10, 54
mental arithmetic, 219, 220, 221, 233
mental disorder, 297
mental energy, 242
mental health, 311, 350
mental illness, 360
mental image, 63, 99, 101, 222
mental processes, 116, 427

mental representation, 207, 260, 269
mental state, 165, 166, 167, 297
meta-analysis, 52, 53, 57, 64, 65, 66, 70, 71, 73, 76, 145, 157, 161, 166, 168, 171, 173, 193, 243, 283, 435, 437
metabolism, 179, 351, 352, 363, 364
metabolites, 363, 367
metacognition, 25
methodology, xi, 235, 249
mice, 125, 351, 352, 362, 363, 366, 369, 370
microsomes, 363
microstructure, 418
midbrain, 136
migration, 418
mildly depressed, xiv, 373, 374, 375
minorities, 47
models, xii, 24, 34, 56, 59, 67, 68, 83, 84, 101, 116, 142, 150, 180, 201, 228, 235, 236, 239, 242, 250, 267, 271, 272, 275, 299, 350, 352, 355, 356, 357, 363, 366, 368, 370, 371, 416, 417
modifications, 2, 39, 280
modules, 266
molecular dynamics, 358
molecular weight, 370
molecules, 357
monoamine oxidase inhibitors, 354
monomers, 357
mood disorder, 65, 377
morality, 115
morbidity, 128
morphine, 126
morphological abnormalities, 127
motivation, 23, 61, 76, 96, 102, 113, 115, 126, 134, 161, 263, 355
motor control, 116
motor skills, 69
motor system, 117
motor task, 115
multidimensional, 14, 23, 71, 138, 251
multi-infarct dementia, 97
multiple regression, xiv, 374, 377
multiple regression analysis, xiv, 374, 377
multiple sclerosis, 52, 57, 61, 70, 146, 161, 162, 163, 168, 170, 171, 172
multiplication, 218, 222
multivariate analysis, 186
multivariate statistics, 299
murder, 303
muscarinic receptor, 368
muscles, 93
music, xii, 301, 302, 309
myelin, 190
myelomeningocele, 63

N

naming, 47, 153, 207, 217
naphthalene, 358, 370
National Institutes of Health, 147, 169, 241
negative consequences, 111
negative effects, 352
negative valence, 302, 310
neocortex, 138, 144, 355
nerve, 353, 356, 368
nerve growth factor, 353, 356, 368
nervous system, 136, 364
neural network, 100, 148, 282, 367, 417, 418, 427, 429
neural physiology, 179
neural systems, 16, 103, 285, 419, 423, 429
neurobiology, 29, 196, 368
neurodegeneration, 155, 169, 356, 360, 367
neurodegenerative diseases, 194, 350
neurodegenerative disorders, 170
neurofibrillary tangles, 151, 356
neuroimaging, 4, 112, 117, 118, 134, 145, 148, 151, 153, 156, 161, 166, 170, 177, 178, 194, 283, 311, 365, 416, 420, 423, 427, 429, 430, 434, 435
neuroinflammation, 356
neurological disease, 350
neuronal cells, 370
neurons, 118, 119, 123, 125, 137, 354, 356, 366, 370, 418, 425
neuropsychological tests, 153
neuropsychology, x, 24, 141, 162, 168, 193, 194, 195, 196, 218, 222
neuroscience, 30, 134, 157, 162, 171, 196, 434
neurosurgery, 144
neurotoxicity, 356
neurotransmission, 135, 354
neurotransmitter, xiii, 119, 121, 179, 354, 358
neurotransmitters, 14, 112
neutral, xii, 287, 288, 289, 290, 292, 293, 294, 295, 296, 297, 301, 302, 303, 304, 306, 307, 308, 309, 311
nicotine, ix, xiii, 109, 119, 121, 126, 349, 350, 351, 353, 354, 355, 357, 358, 359, 362, 363, 364, 366, 367, 369, 370, 371
NMDA receptors, 123, 126, 137
nodes, 156, 238, 280
norepinephrine, 354
normal aging, 24, 61, 68, 79, 91, 101, 167
normal children, 221, 436
normal development, 23, 203
nuclei, 418
nucleus, 95, 101, 107, 111, 112, 137, 138, 157, 356, 368

O

obesity, 125, 355
object permanence, 179
occipital cortex, 423, 427
occipital regions, 14, 15, 23
oculomotor, vii, 1, 6, 10, 11, 14, 15, 22, 123, 125, 136, 195, 280, 281
olanzapine, 361
old age, 25, 67, 70, 73, 239, 298
olfactory nerve, 353
oligomerization, 357, 367, 370
oligomers, 356, 357, 358, 367, 370
omission, 86
one dimension, 264
operations, 8, 39, 40, 116, 207, 226, 230, 232, 239, 268
opiates, 354
opportunities, 37, 158, 231
organ, 113
organism, 111, 113
organize, ix, 109, 114, 158, 275
orthography, 205
outpatients, xiv, 374, 375
overlap, x, 13, 41, 83, 141, 143, 145, 157, 159, 160, 417, 433
overproduction, 418
oxygen, xii, 267, 270

P

pain, 115, 375
parallel, xv, 31, 86, 114, 415, 417, 418, 421
parameter estimates, 272, 274
parenthood, 177
parents, 17, 55, 67, 177
parietal cortex, 94, 116, 178, 279, 416, 419, 422, 424, 433
parietal lobe, 95, 145, 151, 156
parole, 218, 219
paroxetine, 354, 376, 379
participants, xi, xiv, 5, 8, 9, 11, 12, 13, 15, 19, 22, 38, 39, 85, 86, 87, 88, 90, 91, 92, 93, 95, 104, 115, 147, 148, 149, 150, 151, 152, 153, 154, 155, 156, 157, 158, 159, 160, 202, 213, 229, 230, 231, 232, 233, 234, 236, 239, 249, 253, 254, 256, 257, 259, 260, 261, 262, 269, 270, 272, 273, 289, 290, 291, 293, 294, 295, 296, 304, 305, 306, 307, 309, 425
pathological aging, 163
pathology, 134, 146, 149, 150, 151, 152, 155, 157, 158, 159, 160, 168, 352, 356, 371

pathophysiology, 370
pathways, 3, 27, 116, 127, 133, 134, 171, 179, 357, 370, 431, 435
peptide, xiii, 349, 356, 357, 358, 360, 367, 369, 371
perinatal, 176, 180, 181, 182, 186, 187, 189, 190, 191, 198
permit, xi, 88, 133, 249
personal computers, 260
personality, 76, 115, 296
personality disorder, 76
pharmaceuticals, 358
pharmacology, 134
pharmacotherapy, 369
phenotype, 363
phenotypes, 138
phenylketonuria, 54, 79, 179
phonemes, 210
phonological codes, 5, 18, 204
phonological deficit, 203
phonological form, 7, 208
phonology, 248
physical environment, 99
physical structure, 425
physiological, 109, 196, 282, 311, 431
physiological mechanisms, 425
physiology, 156, 194, 371
pigs, 190
pilot study, 74
pitch, 428
placebo, ix, 109, 127, 352, 362, 364, 365
plaque, 352, 358
plasma levels, 352, 365
plasticity, 31, 70, 111, 118, 125, 126, 127, 134, 138, 180
platform, 91
plausibility, 159, 229, 246
playing, 215, 302
polar, 157
polarity, 129
poor performance, 7, 8, 11, 96, 189
poor readers, 220
population, vii, 1, 4, 7, 10, 11, 12, 14, 22, 23, 52, 55, 56, 139, 153, 155, 158, 177, 189, 192, 227, 234, 297, 298, 350, 353, 355, 366
position effect, 174, 283
positive correlation, xv, 415
positive relationship, 5
positron, 83, 104, 115, 144, 167, 178, 179, 196, 353
positron emission tomography (PET), 83, 104, 115, 144, 162, 163, 164, 167, 170, 178, 179, 196, 353, 370, 432, 437
posttraumatic stress, 350, 360, 361, 364, 365, 366

post-traumatic stress disorder (PTSD), 196, 350, 353, 354, 355, 360, 361, 362, 365
poverty, 177
prefrontal cortex, vii, ix, x, xv, 15, 23, 81, 94, 95, 98, 109, 111, 112, 114, 116, 117, 120, 121, 122, 124, 133, 134, 135, 136, 137, 138, 139, 141, 144, 162, 164, 177, 178, 179, 180, 191, 194, 195, 196, 268, 281, 282, 283, 284, 285, 289, 310, 311, 354, 415, 422, 428, 429, □ 431, 432, 434, 435, 437
premature infant, 197, 198
prematurity, x, 175, 186, 189, 190, 192, 194, 198
preparation, 184
preschool, 31, 76, 204, 208, 223, 418, 437
preschool children, 204, 208, 223, 437
preschoolers, 10, 85
preservation, 95, 243
preterm infants, x, 53, 79, 175, 176, 177, 181, 182, 186, 187, 188, 189, 190, 191, 192, 197, 198, 199
prevention, xi, 30, 111, 201
primacy, 150, 262
primacy effect, 150
primary school, 204, 208, 209, 216
primate, 99, 119, 195, 282, 368, 431, 437
priming, 228, 246, 247
priming paradigm, 246
principles, 31
prior knowledge, 59, 60
proactive interference, 28
probability, 292, 306
probe, xii, 269, 270, 271, 272, 273, 274, 275, 276, 277, 279, 280, 287, 290, 292, 295, 296, 304, 306, 307, 309
problem solving, x, xv, 8, 31, 35, 73, 76, 78, 98, 118, 175, 177, 220, 221, 222, 223, 268, 415, 416, 423
procedural knowledge, 173
procedural memory, 146, 168
processing deficits, 174
prognosis, 138, 216
programming, 115, 128, 139, 194, 437
project, 182, 241, 425
proliferation, 418
promoter, 360
pronunciation, 220
protease inhibitors, 150
protective factors, 195
proteins, 368, 371
prototype, 38
pruning, 15, 418
psychiatric diagnosis, 58
psychiatric disorders, 35, 350, 355, 356, 359, 365, 369, 375
psychiatric patients, 361
psychobiology, 366

psychological development, 193
psychological processes, 72, 103, 245
psychology, 23, 35, 37, 60, 66, 82, 96, 102, 161, 226, 250, 263, 265
psychometric approach, 247
psychopharmacology, 369
psychosis, 60, 80, 128, 168
psychosocial factors, 176
psychostimulants, 134

Q

quality of life, 361
questionnaire, 260, 311
quetiapine, 361

R

race, 262
radiation, 53, 76
radiation therapy, 53, 76
radius, 182, 256, 257
rape, 303
rating scale, 44, 61, 193
reaction time, xiv, 72, 233, 234, 236
reactions, 303
reading, xi, 7, 35, 36, 38, 39, 40, 51, 55, 56, 57, 60, 62, 63, 64, 65, 67, 69, 70, 74, 75, 76, 77, 78, 79, 152, 201, 203, 204, 205, 206, 207, 208, 209, 213, 215, 216, 217, 218, 219, 220, 221, 222, 223, 230, 231, 232, 233, 235, 236, 243, 245, 247, 248, 259, 282
reading comprehension, 7, 35, 39, 51, 57, 64, 77, 204, 205, 209, 213, 218, 222, 248, 282
reading difficulties, 57, 75, 204
reading disorder, 203, 220
reading skills, 206
real time, 2
reality, 96, 98, 155, 196, 260, 263
reasoning, ix, xv, 3, 7, 17, 21, 27, 30, 35, 40, 47, 51, 67, 69, 73, 75, 77, 109, 115, 117, 118, 127, 222, 251, 252, 268, 415, 416
recall, 5, 6, 7, 9, 13, 18, 20, 24, 25, 27, 35, 37, 38, 39, 41, 42, 43, 44, 46, 47, 51, 68, 71, 83, 84, 86, 88, 89, 91, 92, 106, 119, 127, 143, 145, 146, 147, 148, 149, 150, 152, 153, 154, 155, 158, 159, 160, 161, 166, 195, 202, 203, 206, 207, 208, 210, 211, 212, 218, 232, 233, 238, 242, 251, 263, 264, 295
recency effect, 150
receptors, xiii, 112, 121, 122, 123, 125, 136, 137, 349, 350, 355, 360, 362, 364, 366, 368, 369, 370, 371

recognition, 24, 46, 86, 88, 89, 90, 92, 93, 95, 97, 103, 107, 147, 149, 154, 161, 170, 174, 193, 203, 269, 288, 295, 297, 299, 303, 307, 310, 311
recognition phase, 86
recognition test, 149, 295
recommendations, 59, 246
reconstruction, 88
recovery, 53, 168, 377, 379
reference frame, 89
regression, xii, 148, 150, 267, 271, 273, 274, 275, 376
regression analysis, 273, 274, 275
regression model, xii, 150, 267, 271, 376
rehabilitation, xiii, 25, 98, 160, 164, 169, 216, 377
rehearsing, 83, 142
reinforcement, 134
relapses, 111
relatives, 62, 232, 233
relevance, xiv, 122, 349, 369
reliability, 234, 248, 378
remediation, viii, 34, 52
remission, xiv, 374, 375, 376, 377, 378, 379
repetition priming, 63
repetitions, 35, 40
replication, 78, 233, 254
reprocessing, 58
reproduction, 69, 111, 203, 250, 289, 303
requirements, xi, 22, 145, 148, 159, 237, 249, 255, 269
researchers, 7, 34, 48, 50, 51, 53, 55, 57, 83, 177, 190, 216, 228, 229, 234, 236, 239, 262
resection, 144, 145
residues, 358, 359, 371
resilience, 365
resolution, 73, 78, 223, 242, 246, 247, 304, 358, 371
resource availability, 295
resources, xi, 3, 6, 7, 9, 12, 16, 19, 49, 67, 84, 89, 90, 92, 142, 196, 197, 201, 221, 222, 226, 228, 230, 231, 232, 233, 237, 244, 249, 255, 269, 303, 360, 425, 426
response, xii, xiii, 12, 13, 15, 25, 30, 47, 64, 70, 85, 86, 87, 115, 116, 118, 119, 122, 123, 125, 135, 136, 137, 156, 172, 185, 195, 197, 198, 231, 256, 257, 259, 260, 261, 267, 270, 271, 272, 273, 274, 276, 280, 281, 282, 283, 284, 287, 288, 289, 290, 291, 292, 294, 296, 301, 303, 304, 306, 307, 308, 309, 310, 311, 355, 358, 366, 416, 419, 420, 424, 430, 435
response time, 12, 231
responsiveness, 354
restrictions, 281, 350
retention interval, xii, 64, 105, 160, 287, 302, 309, 352

retina, 93
rewards, 20
rhythm, 254, 255, 262
right hemisphere, viii, 2, 15, 151, 159, 419, 422
risk, x, 31, 58, 73, 80, 92, 111, 176, 177, 180, 187, 189, 190, 191, 192, 193, 197, 216, 220, 353, 355, 362, 365, 369
risk factors, x, 176, 180, 187, 189, 190, 191, 192, 355, 362
risks, 186, 191, 193, 195, 235
risperidone, 361
rodents, ix, 109, 134, 135, 350, 355
rotations, 86
Rouleau, 8, 24, 51, 62
routes, 88, 89, 94, 102, 212
routines, 178
Royal Society, 61, 220, 428, 434, 435
rules, 12, 43, 198

S

saccades, 11, 195
sadness, 296
safety, xiii, 349, 352, 365
saturation, 272, 303
scaling, 274
schizophrenia, xiii, 58, 62, 63, 64, 66, 67, 69, 70, 71, 73, 74, 75, 76, 77, 80, 137, 155, 161, 162, 163, 164, 165, 166, 167, 168, 169, 170, 171, 172, 173, 174, 349, 350, 355, 357, 360, 361, 362, 365, 366, 367, 370, 374, 378, 431
schizophrenic patients, 77, 163, 355, 361, 366
schizotypal personality disorder, 58, 71
schizotypy, 58, 73
scholastic achievement, 209, 213, 214
school, x, xv, 8, 17, 21, 25, 27, 31, 71, 132, 175, 176, 180, 190, 191, 192, 194, 198, 204, 209, 211, 213, 214, 215, 216, 375, 415, 420, 421, 423, 426, 428, 431, 437
school learning, 17
science, 135, 168, 428
secrete, 368
segregation, 424, 430, 432
selective attention, 157, 422, 424, 427, 432
selective serotonin reuptake inhibitor, 354
selectivity, 152, 294, 297, 363
self-assessment, 310
self-concept, 192
self-monitoring, 115
self-regulation, 76
semantic association, 43, 145, 153, 159
semantic categorization, 43
semantic information, 54, 230, 235, 250
semantic memory, x, 39, 46, 100, 104, 141, 143, 145, 168, 170, 172, 173, 229, 266
semantic networks, 146, 159
semantic processing, 51, 142, 154, 158
semantics, 68, 172, 230
senile dementia, 165
sensitivity, 86, 92, 111, 128, 204, 229, 282, 378
sensitization, 125, 134, 137, 138
sensorimotor gating, 355, 367
sensory memory, 143
sensory modalities, 115, 427
sensory systems, 419
sentence comprehension, xi, 16, 27, 68, 75, 225, 227, 228, 229, 232, 240, 241, 243, 244, 246, 247, 248
sentence processing, xi, 72, 142, 225, 227, 228, 229, 230, 231, 232, 233, 235, 236, 241, 242, 247, 248
sequencing, 43, 44, 45, 68
serotonin, 14, 354, 360, 361, 366
sertraline, 354, 365, 376
serum, 364
services, 353
severity levels, 151
sex, 99, 104, 105, 147, 182, 265, 294, 296, 374, 375
sex differences, 105, 265, 294, 296
shape, 3, 9, 46, 83, 87, 233, 250, 252, 257, 261, 262, 272, 273, 432
short-term memory (STM), vii, viii, ix, xii, 1, 2, 3, 4, 6, 7, 8, 9, 13, 18, 23, 24, 25, 26, 27, 32, 33, 35, 36, 37, 38, 39, 42, 43, 44, 45, 46, 47, 48, 53, 55, 62, 64, 66, 77, 78, 82, 98, 100, 101, 102, 105, 107, 109, 114, 116, 117, 119, 127, 136, 142, 150, 172, 202, 203, 204, 207, 210, 211, 213, 214, 218, 220, 221, 223, 228, 229, 245, 246, 251, 281, 282, 287, 288, 289, 290, 294, 295, 296, 298, 301, 302, 303, 304, 305, 307, 309, 310, 311, 431
showing, ix, 3, 8, 44, 58, 110, 115, 150, 156, 204, 232, 251, 256, 261, 275, 281, 293, 357, 420, 427
sibling, 12
side effects, 178, 357
significance level, 292, 295, 306
signs, 22, 40, 87, 197
simulations, 274
skin, 369
smoking, 125, 350, 351, 353, 355, 360, 363, 366
social behavior, 115
social development, 193
social interactions, 288
social problems, 128
social psychology, 162
social sciences, 299
social skills, 350
social withdrawal, 355
societal cost, 374

socioeconomic status, 177, 193
software, 256, 260, 274, 285, 375
solution, 357
spatial ability, 89, 105
spatial information, 18, 38, 83, 84, 89, 91, 95, 101, 105, 115, 202, 211, 250, 251, 253, 254, 417, 424
spatial learning, 19, 71, 91, 265, 437
spatial location, 3, 11, 15, 38, 40, 41, 67
spatial memory, xi, 5, 6, 10, 16, 47, 69, 85, 91, 93, 94, 95, 96, 97, 98, 99, 100, 101, 103, 104, 105, 136, 208, 213, 215, 219, 249, 264
spatial processing, 64, 102, 106, 233, 264, 437
special education, 23, 191, 197
specialization, 241, 419, 432
species, 111, 255, 264, 355, 367, 370
spectroscopy, 371
speech, 6, 12, 27, 32, 34, 52, 57, 76, 77, 115, 202, 204, 222, 239, 240, 242, 244, 245, 248, 253
spelling, 76, 205, 213, 221
split-half reliability, 234
stability, 76, 111, 167, 218, 248
standard deviation, 306
standard error, 120, 276
standardization, 43, 52, 60
stars, 40
state, xi, xv, 30, 116, 165, 225, 226, 268, 277, 297, 305, 415, 421, 422, 425, 426, 427, 428, 431, 434
states, 40, 294, 355, 358, 423, 425
statistics, 213, 214, 275, 279
stimulant, 62, 136
stimulus, xii, 47, 111, 113, 118, 119, 131, 156, 157, 251, 264, 273, 281, 287, 288, 289, 290, 292, 296, 301, 302, 303, 306, 309, 352, 355, 420, 421, 424, 434
storage, viii, xi, 3, 17, 25, 33, 34, 35, 36, 37, 38, 42, 43, 44, 48, 49, 52, 56, 57, 59, 64, 70, 78, 82, 84, 115, 116, 117, 118, 136, 144, 149, 150, 152, 157, 166, 167, 172, 174, 202, 205, 220, 225, 236, 251, 281, 282, 283, 290, 296, 416
strategy use, 18, 24, 39, 43, 62, 147, 164, 218
stress, 113, 216, 364, 365
structural changes, 354, 358
structure, 22, 23, 26, 59, 72, 73, 82, 84, 95, 103, 106, 112, 117, 126, 136, 142, 155, 205, 208, 216, 218, 222, 231, 233, 238, 239, 240, 242, 244, 245, 256, 263, 352, 357, 358, 359, 371, 426, 428, 431
structuring, 227, 237
style, 355
subgroups, x, 77, 78, 176, 207, 223
substance abuse, 111, 121
substitution, 44
substrate, x, 95, 100, 116, 121, 141, 173, 363, 366
substrates, 135, 136, 159, 160, 164, 361, 429, 436

subtraction, 40, 153, 284
succession, 97
Sun, 281
superior parietal cortex, 277, 429
supervision, 250
suppression, xi, 63, 75, 89, 111, 169, 202, 204, 221, 249, 251, 255, 258, 259, 261, 262, 430
surface area, 164
surgical intervention, 178
surveillance, 112
survival, xiii, 111, 176, 198, 289, 303, 349
survival rate, 176
survivors, 147, 148, 174
susceptibility, 351, 431
symptoms, xiii, 10, 12, 13, 14, 15, 30, 32, 55, 58, 63, 65, 76, 91, 111, 126, 128, 194, 216, 350, 352, 353, 354, 355, 360, 366, 377, 428
synapse, 151, 191, 418
synaptic plasticity, 126
synchronization, 11, 16, 27
syndrome, 24, 31, 54, 55, 68, 70, 73, 105, 111, 114, 115, 125, 135, 138, 155, 168
synergistic effect, 7
synthesis, 29, 96

T

talent, 30
target, xi, 23, 38, 39, 88, 90, 94, 125, 157, 158, 212, 217, 238, 249, 255, 257, 258, 259, 260, 261, 270, 354, 355, 356, 364, 369, 421
target identification, 369
target stimuli, 421
task conditions, 50, 79, 92
task demands, 9, 90
task difficulty, 423, 425, 426
task load, 156
task performance, xiv, xv, 20, 51, 118, 119, 129, 135, 152, 156, 178, 229, 234, 284, 295, 311, 415, 416, 422, 423, 425, 426, 427, 435
tau, 356
taxonomy, 96
TEA-Ch, 12
teachers, 17, 21, 22, 65, 209, 210, 213, 214, 215, 216
techniques, vii, xii, 11, 14, 129, 133, 178, 217, 234, 267, 268, 281, 353, 416
technologies, 262
technology, 176, 180
telephone, 182, 250
television commercial, 129
temperature, 357
temporal lobe, 95, 99, 101, 102, 104, 144, 153, 161, 164, 165, 173

temporal lobe epilepsy, 104, 161, 173
temporal window, 130, 131
terminals, 123
test items, 182
test procedure, 375
test scores, 215
testing, 77, 91, 102, 106, 135, 155, 184, 185, 213, 231, 256, 257, 258, 259, 260, 261, 290, 292, 295, 435
texture, 84, 250
thalamus, 16, 277
therapeutic agents, 364
therapeutic approaches, 133
therapeutic effects, 357, 367
therapeutic interventions, 23
therapeutic targets, 352, 361, 364
therapeutic use, xiv, 349
therapeutics, 362, 367
therapy, 58, 149, 164, 165, 171, 359, 368
thoughts, ix, 109, 114, 355
time constraints, 192
time frame, 2
time series, 285
tissue, 144, 280
tobacco, xiii, 349, 350, 351, 352, 354, 355, 357, 359, 362
toxicity, xiii, 349, 350, 357, 362
toys, 183, 184
traditional views, 231
training, viii, xi, 2, 16, 17, 18, 19, 20, 21, 25, 31, 119, 201, 208, 209, 211, 216, 220, 221, 223, 259, 260
training programs, 16, 20, 21
traits, 71
trajectory, 416, 424
transformation, 24, 84
transmission, 113, 121, 123, 133
transport, 353, 356, 368
trauma, 58, 70, 178, 180, 366
traumatic brain injury (TBI), 19, 53, 70, 71, 73, 78, 147, 148, 160, 161, 164, 165, 167, 169, 171, 173, 174, 195, 196
traumatic experiences, 354
treatment, viii, ix, xiv, 34, 52, 110, 111, 127, 133, 134, 137, 138, 174, 198, 209, 211, 213, 214, 215, 216, 217, 311, 350, 352, 353, 354, 355, 356, 360, 361, 364, 365, 368, 369, 374, 376, 377, 378, 379
trial, ix, xv, 9, 12, 86, 109, 116, 118, 119, 125, 127, 154, 155, 183, 184, 185, 221, 254, 257, 260, 261, 268, 269, 270, 271, 272, 273, 274, 275, 276, 277, 279, 280, 283, 290, 304, 305, 361, 362, 365, 366, 370, 379
tricyclic antidepressant, 354

true/false, 9, 202, 210
tumors, 144, 194, 195, 227
turnover, 354
twins, 161, 168, 182
twist, 358, 371

U

ultrasound, 198
underlying mechanisms, xiii, 302, 310
undernutrition, 190
unification, 297
united, 24, 25, 27, 29, 167, 311
updating, 50, 55, 64, 67, 78, 89, 90, 92, 99, 156, 211, 212, 217, 252, 270, 420
urban, 99
urine, 351, 363

V

valence, xii, 291, 293, 294, 295, 296, 298, 301, 302, 303, 305, 306, 309, 310, 311
validation, 299, 379
variables, x, 176, 181, 186, 210, 213, 214, 229, 231, 234, 235, 236, 241, 261, 375
variations, 35, 38, 84, 86, 270, 281, 296
vasomotor, 433
vector, 282
vein, 227
velocity, 418
verbal fluency, 71, 163, 243, 369
Verbal IQ, 45
vision, 6, 11, 93, 97, 99, 102, 255, 304, 434
visual acuity, 289
visual attention, 6, 198, 298, 417, 436
visual images, 250
visual modality, 303
visual processing, 46, 166
visual stimuli, 10, 18, 270, 435
visual stimulus, 118, 273, 420
visual system, 101, 156
visualization, 63, 282
visuospatial function, 151
vocabulary, 205, 219, 235, 236
vocalizations, 251
vulnerability, 58

W

walking, 89, 91, 240, 245, 257
watches, 178, 179, 183

water, 131, 265, 358
weakness, 14, 23, 57
Wechsler Intelligence Scale, 44, 45, 69, 79, 223
wells, 178, 183
white matter, xiii, 145, 146, 149, 150, 157, 159, 160, 168, 170, 280, 418, 419, 433, 434
windows, 304
withdrawal, 111, 126, 128, 139, 352, 353
word processing, 260
word recognition, 77, 171
workers, 85, 89, 90, 91, 92, 93, 94, 95

X

xenon, 194

Y

yield, 192
young adults, 5, 7, 97, 240, 436